LIBRARY-LRC
TEXAS HEART INSTITUTE

Complications During Percutaneous Interventions for Congenital and Structural Heart Disease

Complications During Percutaneous Interventions for Congenital and Structural Heart Disease

Edited by

Ziyad M Hijazi MD MPH FSCAI FACC
Rush Center for Congenital and Structural Heart Disease
Rush University Medical Center and Rush College of Medicine
Chicago, IL
USA

Ted Feldman MD FSCAI
Cardiac Catheterization Laboratories
Evanston Hospital,
Evanston, IL
USA

John P Cheatham MD FAAP FACC FSCAI
The Heart Center
Nationwide Children's Hospital
Columbus, OH
USA

Horst Sievert MD FSCAI FESC FACC
Cardiovascular Center Frankfurt
Sankt Katharinen
Frankfurt, Germany

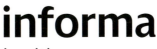

informa
healthcare

© 2009 Informa UK Ltd

First published in the United Kingdom in 2008 by Informa Healthcare, Telephone House, 69-77 Paul Street, London EC2A 4LQ. Informa Healthcare is a trading division of Informa UK Ltd. Registered Office: 37/41 Mortimer Street, London W1T 3JH. Registered in England and Wales number 1072954.

Tel: +44 (0)20 7017 5000
Fax: +44 (0)20 7017 6699
Website: www.informahealthcare.com

All rights reserved. No part of this publication may be reproduced, stored in a retrieval system, or transmitted, in any form or by any means, electronic, mechanical, photocopying, recording, or otherwise, without the prior permission of the publisher or in accordance with the provisions of the Copyright, Designs and Patents Act 1988 or under the terms of any licence permitting limited copying issued by the Copyright Licensing Agency, 90 Tottenham Court Road, London W1P 0LP.

Although every effort has been made to ensure that all owners of copyright material have been acknowledged in this publication, we would be glad to acknowledge in subsequent reprints or editions any omissions brought to our attention.

Although every effort has been made to ensure that drug doses and other information are presented accurately in this publication, the ultimate responsibility rests with the prescribing physician. Neither the publishers nor the authors can be held responsible for errors or for any consequences arising from the use of information contained herein. For detailed prescribing information or instructions on the use of any product or procedure discussed herein, please consult the prescribing information or instructional material issued by the manufacturer.

A CIP record for this book is available from the British Library.

Library of Congress Cataloging-in-Publication Data

Data available on application

ISBN-10: 0 415 45107 8
ISBN-13: 978 0 415 45107 9

Distributed in North and South America by
Taylor & Francis
6000 Broken Sound Parkway, NW, (Suite 300)
Boca Raton, FL 33487, USA
Within Continental USA
Tel: 1 (800) 272 7737; Fax: 1 (800) 374 3401
Outside Continental USA
Tel: (561) 994 0555; Fax: (561) 361 6018
Email: orders@crcpress.com

Book orders in the rest of the world
Paul Abrahams
Tel: +44 (0)20 7017 4036
Email: bookorders@informa.com

Composition by C&M Digitals (P) Ltd., Chennai, India
Printed and bound in India by Replika Press Pvt. Ltd

Contents

SECTION III: STRUCTURAL HEART DISEASE MANAGED BY ADULT AND PEDIATRIC CARDIOLOGISTS

SECTION IV: STRUCTURAL HEART DISEASE MANAGED BY ADULT CARDIOLOGISTS

SECTION V: MISCELLANEOUS INTERVENTIONS

Contributors

Zahid Amin MD FSCAI FAAP
Cardiac Catheterization and Hybrid Suites
Rush University Medical Center
Chicago, IL
USA

Sawson Awad MD
Rush Center for Congenital and
Structural Heart Disease
Rush University Medical center,
Chicago, IL
USA

Amr Bannan MD
Hospital of the University of Pennsylvania
Philadelphia, PA
USA

Yves L Bayard
CardioVascular Center Frankfurt
Sankt Katharinen
Frankfurt
Germany

Lee N Benson MD FRCPC FACC FSCAI
The Hospital for Sick Children
The University of Toronto School of Medicine
Toronto, Ontario
Canada

Peter Block MD
Emory University
Atlanta, GA
USA

Philipp Bonhoeffer
Great Ormond Street Hospital for Children
London, UK

Eric Brochet
Service de Cardiologie
Hôpital Bichat
Paris
France

Gianfranco Butera
Department of Pediatric Cardiology & Adult with
Congenital Heart Defects
IRCCS-Policlinico San Donato
Milan
Italy

Qi-Ling Cao
Rush Center for Congenital and Structural Heart
Disease
Rush University Medical Center
Chicago, IL
USA

Mario Carminati
Department of Pediatric Cardiology & Adult with
Congenital Heart Defects
IRCCS-Policlinico San Donato
Milan
Italy

John P Cheatham MD FAAP FACC FSCAI
The Heart Center
Nationwide Children's Hospital
Columbus, OH
USA

Massimo Chessa
Department of Pediatric Cardiology & Adult with
Congenital Heart Defects
IRCCS-Policlinico San Donato
Milan
Italy

Nicholas J Collins Bmed FRACP
Structural Heart Disease Intervention Program
Division of Cardiology
Peter Munk Cardiac Center
University Health Network – Toronto General
Hospital
Toronto, Ontario
Canada

Matthew A Crystal MD FRCPC
The Hospital for Sick Children
The University of Toronto School of Medicine
Toronto, Ontario
Canada

Karim Diab MD
Pediatric Cardiology
St Joseph Medical Center
Phoenix, AZ
USA

John T Fahey MD
Division of Pediatric Cardiology
Yale University School of Medicine
New Haven, CT
USA

Ted Feldman MD FSCAI
Evanston Hospital
Evanston, IL
USA

Thomas Forbes MD
Detroit Children's Hospital
Detroit, MI
USA

Howard C Herrmann MD
Hospital of the University of Pennsylvania
Philadelphia, PA
USA

Ziyad M Hijazi MD MPH FSCAI FACC
Rush Center for Congenital and Structural Heart
Disease
Rush University Medical Center and Rush College of
Medicine
Chicago, IL
USA

Ralf J Holzer MD MSc
The Heart Center
Nationwide Children's Hospital
Columbus, OH
USA

Eric M Horlick MDCM FRCPC
Structural Heart Disease Intervention Program
Division of Cardiology
Peter Munk Cardiac Center
University Health Network – Toronto General
Hospital
Toronto, Ontario
Canada

Frank F Ing MD
Texas Children's Hospital
Baylor College of Medicine
Houston, TX
USA

Ignacio Inglessis MD
Massachussetts General Hospital
Harvard Medical School
Boston, MA
USA

Bernard Iung
Service de Cardiologie
Hôpital Bichat
Paris
France

Alexander J Javois
Hope Children's Hospital
Oak Lawn, IL
USA

Sachin Khambadkone
Great Ormond Street Hospital for Children
London, UK

Dennis W Kim MD PhD
Sibley Heart Center Cardiology/Children's
Healthcare of Atlanta
Emory University School of Medicine
Atlanta, GA
USA

Rainer Kozlik-Feldmann
Department of Pediatric Cardiology
Klinikum Grosshadern
Ludwig Maximilians University Munich
Germany

Dominique Himbert
Service de Cardiologie
Hôpital Bichat
Paris
France

Daphne T Hsu
Children's Hospital at Montefiore
Bronx, NY
USA

Hani Jneid MD
Harvard Medical School and Massachusetts General
Hospital
Boston, MA
USA

Michael J Landzberg MD
Boston Children's Hospital
Harvard Medical School
Boston, MA
USA

Larry Latson MD
Cleveland Clinic
Cleveland, OH
USA

Trong-Phi Lê
Department of Pediatric Cardiology
Heart Center
University of Hamburg
Germany

Andrew O Maree MSc MD
Harvard Medical School and Massachusetts General
Hospital
Boston, MA
USA

Jean-Bernard Masson MD
St Paul's Hospital
University of British Columbia
Vancouver
Canada

Phillip Moore MD MBA
University of California at San Francisco
San Francisco, CA
USA

Charles Mullins MD
Texas Children's Hospital
Baylor College of Medicine
Houston, TX
USA

David Nykanen MD FRCPC FACC FSCAI
Congenital Heart Institute at APH and MCH
Orlando, FL
USA

Stefan H Ostermayer
CardioVascular Center Frankfurt
Sankt Katharinen
Frankfurt
Germany

Igor F Palacios MD
Harvard Medical School and Massachusetts General
Hospital
Boston, MA
USA

Wes R Pedersen
Minneapolis Heart Institute Foundation at Abbott
Northwestern Hospital
Minneapolis, MN
USA

Jeffrey S Pollak MD
Department of Diagnostic Radiology
Yale University School of Medicine
New Haven, CT
USA

Tim Provias MD
UCLA Medical Center
Office of Graduate Medical Education
Los Angeles, CA
USA

Mark Reisman
Swedish Heart & Vascular Institute
Seattle, WA
USA

David G Reuter MD PhD FAAP
Cardiac Dimensions Inc.
Kirkland, WA
USA

Yoshihito Sakata MD
Ikegami General Hospital
Heart Center
Ikegami
Japan

Dietmar Schranz MD
Universitat Klinikum Giessen
Giessen, Germany

Horst Sievert MD FSCAI FESC FACC
CardioVascular Center Frankfurt
Sankt Katharinen
Frankfurt
Germany

Robert J Sommer MD
Columbia University Medical Center
New York, NY
USA

Karen M Smith MD
University of Florida
College of Medicine
Gainsville, FL
USA

Christian Spies MD
Rush Center for Congenital and Structural Heart
Disease
Rush University Medical Center
Chicago, IL
USA

Jonathan Tobis MD
UCLA Medical Center
Los Angeles, CA
USA

Alec Vahanian
Service de Cardiologie
Hôpital Bichat
Paris
France

Roy P Venzon MD
Rush Center for Congenital and Structural Heart
Disease
Rush University Medical Center
Chicago, IL
USA

Robert N Vincent MD
Sibley Heart Center Cardiology/Children's Healthcare
of Atlanta
Emory University School of Medicine
Atlanta, GA
USA

John G Webb MD
St Paul's Hospital
University of British Columbia
Vancouver
Canada

Robert White MD
Department of Diagnostic Radiology
Yale University School of Medicine
New Haven, CT
USA

Neil Wilson
Children's Hospital Oxford
Oxford
UK

Preface

Over the last decade, interest in interventional therapies for congenital and structural heart disease has increased significantly. About two years ago, Sievert and colleagues published an important textbook on this subject. That book sparked our interest in editing a book that describes in detail all that the chosen experts' knowledge of possible complications associated with advanced interventional therapies for complex congenital and structural heart disease. We hope that it serves you well in those stressful times that lie ahead for all of us.

Each chapter follows a certain format, starting with a very brief discussion of the lesion, followed by what is required (equipment needed) to carry out a successful intervention, tips on how not to get into a problem and, finally, if you get into trouble, how to get out and navigate yourself from this problem.

We have assembled the best of the best in this field and we believe that you'll find the answer to almost every imaginable complication that can be encountered.

No doubt as newer procedures emerge (valvular replacement/repair techniques) in the future, one needs to update the knowledge based on the specific technique or device used.

Acknowledgments

First, I want to dedicate this book to Mr. Alan Burgess, whose insight, wit, kindness, friendship and suggestions through the years have resulted in three books! Alan decided to leave editing and publishing to pursue a higher cause, we miss seeing him and we wish him the very best.

I would like to thank my hybrid suite staff: Lesia, Kathleen, Mary, Shari, Tiana and Tom. Their excellence in the lab is very highly appreciated. Their knowledge and skills is what keeps me sane during the most stressful situations. Also, I want to thank my assistant Ms. Michaeleen (Mike) Wallig for her help during this project! Finally, special thanks to all the contributors in this book, without their hard work there wouldn't be a book!

Ziyad M Hijazi

Special thanks to our patients, who have usually escaped our errors, and have sometimes suffered complications even in the absence of errors.

This textbook is intended to help share what we all have learned from these patients, so better outcomes and fewer complications will result.

Ted Feldman

I would like to acknowledge and thank my mentor and friend, Chuck Mullins, who inspired many of us to choose the field of interventional cardiology and to never accept less than our best effort. I would also like to thank all of the outstanding interventional cardiologists that despite being spread all over the world, remain a "family", with a "common goal and passion".

John P Cheatham

I would like to thank all the members of my cath-lab teams who supported me in good days and in bad days over the last 5 years. Especially during complications this support is extremely valuable because it gives us confidence and strength to manage even very difficult situations.

Horst Sievert

1 Set-up and equipment for a pediatric/congenital interventional cardiac catheterization laboratory

Charles Mullins

The plans for the physical arrangement of the pediatric and congenital interventional catheterization laboratory, and the equipment used in these laboratories, including the rationale for its use and its proper use, are gleaned from the experience of the author[1] during 45 years of practice in both his own and many other catheterization laboratories around the world. This author also has been a principal participant in the design and construction of 14 different catheterization laboratories in the various institutions where he has practiced.

Complications can be reduced significantly when the laboratory has the optimal capital equipment as well as all of the necessary consumable or 'expendable' equipment. In addition to the equipment per se, the actual catheterization *room* must be very large in size and the laboratory must be staffed with qualified personnel who are experts in how to use all of the special equipment.

CAPITAL EQUIPMENT

The capital equipment for the modern pediatric/ congenital interventional cardiac catheterization laboratory comprises the major pieces of 'machinery' in every laboratory. The capital equipment represents a very large initial monetary investment as well as a very large continuing expense. The capital equipment, in general, is very reliable, but at the same time is very complex and requires special and continual maintenance. Service for the continued maintenance must be part of the contractual arrangement in the purchase of the major capital equipment. Because of the rapid developments in the electronics and now in computer and digital technology, most of the capital equipment has a built in obsolescence, with an operational life of 7–10 years. Although the equipment often still is functional after 10 years, the improvements in the technology make upgrading to newer equipment essential for the reliability of its use and the improved quality provided by these updates, and for the safety of the patients and the operating personnel.

The catheterization room

The total space and arrangement within the actual cardiac catheterization room for a pediatric/congenital interventional catheterization laboratory suite in 2008+ must be planned in advance and needs to be very large. In new construction, it is optimal to plan and build the catheterization laboratory/suite before the 'internal' construction of the hospital building is initiated. A minimum of 900 square feet of *free* floor space is recommended for the *actual catheterization room*. This 'free floor space' must be *in addition* to any space required for fixed cabinets, 'racks,' sinks, or counters which might be built into the room. The fixed X-ray equipment occupies the greatest amount of space within the catheterization room. In addition to the floor space occupied by this fixed equipment, a large additional amount of the 'free' floor space also must be available *within the catheterization room* in order to accommodate multiple additional pieces of large but mobile capital equipment, along with the required personnel, all of which are absolutely essential in the modern interventional catheterization laboratory.

In the prospective planning of the initial construction, adequate space should be allocated in the actual catheterization room to accommodate the planned or emergency conversion of an interventional catheterization procedure into an 'open heart' surgical procedure, which can be performed in the same room and on the same table without having to move the patient.

The total area of the catheterization *suite* requires more than quadruple the space of the catheterization room itself in order to allow the space for additional separate rooms, which will accommodate the large electrical equipment (X-ray), a control room, a 'consumables' storage room, administrative support, and often an admitting/holding/recovery area for patients.

Fixed capital equipment

Of the capital equipment, the biplane X-ray imaging equipment, with its compound angulation and monitoring and replay capabilities, is the most essential equipment in a pediatric/congenital interventional catheterization laboratory. In hearts where there often are no 'normal' cardiac structures or locations, it is absolutely essential to have the capability of visualizing corresponding perpendicular views of the heart instantaneously or even simultaneously. The liberal use of the second plane eliminates unnecessary 'blind' probing in a direction 180°

away from the desired direction, which occurs when using only a single plane, and avoids the dangerous pushing of catheters or wires into totally unacceptable locations. Biplane visualization and imaging allows the precise, simultaneous positioning of catheters or devices and of more than one device (e.g. stents) simultaneously into multiple lesions, even when they are in different planes of view. The use of biplane imaging significantly reduces the duration of *every* catheterization procedure and, of equal or greater importance, significantly reduces the radiation to both the patient and the operator.

This fixed X-ray equipment occupies the largest single area of the original 'free' space in the actual catheterization room. The two X-ray tubes, their respective imaging detectors, and the large and complex suspension system for the compound angulation of this X-ray system, all are permanent in their location. In addition to the actual X-ray equipment and its suspension system, an extra long catheterization table is recommended to accommodate the variety of very long pieces of expendable equipment used on the catheterization table during interventional procedures. Adequate space on the actual table helps to avoid contamination of this equipment.

There are three or four major manufacturers of biplane X-ray equipment which are suitable for the congenital catheterization laboratories. These are Siemens (Siemens Medical Systems, Inc, Iselin, NJ), Phillips (Philips Medical Systems, Inc, Shelton, CT), Toshiba (Toshiba America Medical Systems, Inc, Tustin, CA), and General Electric (GE Marquette Medical Systems, Milwaukee, WI) who also stake a claim in this market. All of these systems now have a cesium iodide layer on a flat panel uptake detector, which converts the X-ray energy to photons and then directly to a digital signal which is used for viewing or storage. The flat panel detectors for a usual cardiac catheterization laboratory are either 9 or 12 inches square and are mounted on suspension systems, which allow various degrees of compound angulation. The larger flat panel detectors, which do cover a larger area and are better for imaging the larger patient, are available on all of these systems but, at the same time, the large detectors significantly compromise the potential for the more extreme angulation of the X-ray systems. This makes the 9 inch image detectors more satisfactory for the pediatric interventional laboratory.

Several of the manufacturers (Toshiba, Siemens) are specifically addressing the added requirements of configuring a combined 'hybrid' catheterization/surgical suite. The hybrid suites require a suspension system for the biplane X-ray with more 'mobile' bases for the X-ray tubes and very special tables, which have the special combined requirements for either a catheterization, a surgical procedure, or both procedures in combination.

In order for the operators within the room to be able to continually view the active X-ray images as well as simultaneously view any replayed moving scenes or stored images, multiple, large, high-definition digital monitoring screens are required. These monitors must be in clear view of the catheterization table. The combination of monitors includes separate, large, flat panel digital screens for the active images from both the posterior-anterior (PA) and lateral (Lat) X-ray tubes, as well as separate, equal-sized screens for freeze frame and/or active playback of the images, again from both planes. These monitors are suspended on mobile arms, which are on overhead tracks so that they always can be positioned in close proximity to the catheterization table, and always within a convenient view of the operators. At the same time, the position of the monitors must not interfere with the compound angulation of the X-ray equipment or the overall mobility of the personnel and other equipment within the room. Occasionally, to accomplish this 'universal visibility' duplicate 'banks' of monitoring screens are necessary. In order to visualize the display of the ongoing physiologic data and the images from echocardiograms performed during the procedure, one or two additional large flat panel digital display screens usually are mounted on the same large suspension system for the X-ray screens. All of the display screens also must be duplicated in a separate 'control' room for the personnel working in there.

The generators for the X-ray equipment are located in a completely separate electrical room and never should be in the actual catheterization room. All large pieces of electrical equipment aggressively attract dust and dirt, plus, the modern X-ray generators require a separate room with special 'environmental' cooling. The X-ray generator does need to be close enough to the X-ray table to allow for the high-tension electrical connections, but there is no requirement for any of this equipment to be close to the patient or in the patient's environment. As an added bonus to a separate generator room, when maintenance is required on the equipment, the personnel performing this usually do not have to enter the sterile catheterization room.

In addition to the sophisticated X-ray imaging equipment, the congenital interventional catheterization laboratory requires the monitoring of multiple simultaneous channels of physiologic data electrocardiogram (ECG) multiple pressures, systemic oxygen saturation, core temperature, respirations with a continuous display of this data as well as the capability of accurately recording the same information either intermittently or continuously. The monitoring equipment often comes as a 'package' by the manufacturer of the X-ray systems, although separate monitoring equipment from different manufacturers is available. Each of these have their own particular advantages and disadvantages. The consoles for the monitoring equipment have the capability of displaying and permanently recording 10 to 16 channels of different types of data and, as a consequence, usually are very large. Fortunately, these consoles can and should be positioned remotely in an adjacent 'control' room with only under floor cables running from the consumable monitoring sensors on the catheterization table to the console. The remote display screens for viewing the physiologic data in the catheterization room usually are mounted along with the X-ray display screens.

Other more or less fixed items of capital equipment in the catheterization room are the 'operating field' lights for the catheterization table. These lights must be located for repeated, intermittent, and convenient use. There are many types of surgical 'operating' lights, most of which are mounted on mobile arms and can be angled in multiple directions over the 'field' using these arms. There also are very special lights, which can be recessed in the ceiling and have an electronic, strobe, remote control for the angulation of the light. These lights are particularly helpful in relieving the 'equipment congestion' over and about the table.

A power injector for contrast media is another essential piece of capital equipment, which, however, does not have to be in a single fixed location in the catheterization room, while at the same time, the injector head must be close to the table and available to be attached to a catheter easily and quickly. The injector heads of the power injectors from several different manufacturers can be separated from their consoles or controllers (MedRad, Inc, Indianola, PA; Mallinckrodt, Inc, Hazelwood, MO). The injector head is mounted on an articulated arm, which optimally can be ceiling mounted on a track over the table. This allows the bulky electrical console or controller to be located well away from the table or even in a separate room. This arrangement again helps to alleviate the congestion on the floor around the patient.

Mobile capital equipment

The cardiac catheterization table and X-ray equipment must be arranged to allow free access to the patient by multiple additional pieces of more 'mobile' capital equipment. The most critical piece of this mobile capital equipment, which always must be available in each catheterization room, is a cardiac defibrillator. It is stored in the room on a mobile 'emergency' cart, which also contains the other resuscitation equipment. In order to accommodate the range of patients from very small to very large, the defibrillator in the congenital cardiac laboratory must have a complete range of adjustable voltage outputs and have paddles of at least two sizes. The defibrillator always must be in the catheterization room, and always plugged into the power source with a cord which can extend the console to the side of the patient's chest, with the appropriate paddles attached according to the size of the patient and the contact jelly immediately available adjacent to the paddles.

The resuscitation equipment on the emergency cart includes a child and an adult Ambu™ bag, various sized laryngoscopes, a complete range of sizes of both oral airways and endotracheal tubes, equipment for starting intravenous lines (IVs) and equipment for insertion of a chest tube. All of this equipment should be checked at least daily, before each case begins, and rechecked after any use. Emergency medications usually are kept with the other medications used in the catheterization lab.

Sources of oxygen, compressed air, and vacuum are built into the room construction as fixed, either wall or ceiling outlets. Access to the patient for these gas and vacuum outlets is usually through a console, which is on a ceiling-mounted mobile arm or within a mobile floor console, either of which can be positioned in a convenient location near the head of the catheterization table.

The anesthesia machine, which usually is quite large, along with the anesthesiologist, requires access from the head of the table and in close proximity to the gas and vacuum source. This access usually is from the right side of the *patient*, which positions this equipment to the patient's right of the posterior-anterior (PA) image detector and cranial to the lateral X-ray tube. In this fairly tight area, it must be easy for the anesthesiologist and anesthesia equipment to move toward and away from the patient in order to accommodate angulation of the X-ray equipment and/or operator access to the neck vessels of the patient. This is especially true in the case of the hybrid catheterization/ surgical procedures.

Still more space must be allocated in very close proximity to the catheterization table for one or two separate, 3 × 4–5 foot long equipment 'work' tables. These tables are mobile and almost always positioned immediately behind or adjacent to the operating physicians where they do occupy a relatively large area of space. During procedures, these tables are covered with sterile drapes and accommodate the large array of the often very long, expendable equipment used during an interventional catheterization procedure.

In the interventional catheterization laboratory, transthoracic echo (TTE), transesophageal echo (TEE), intracardiac echo (ICE), and even intravascular ultrasound (IVUS), have become essential adjuncts in many procedures. Each of the consoles for the different echo machines is different for each type of echo; they are all quite large and also must be available easily and immediately, and be capable of being moved expeditiously to positions adjacent to the patient. As a consequence, when in use, each echo machine occupies a significant amount of very specific floor space in the catheterization room.

The TTE machine can be fairly simple and does not have to be the 'latest model'; however, it should be stored actually within the room and, like the defibrillator, be continually attached to a power cord, which will allow the console to reach to the side of the patient's chest. Additionally, the TTE transducer always should be attached to the console and the 'echo jelly' must be kept available immediately adjacent to the transducer. This is mandatory in order to be able to *instantaneously* screen the heart and pericardium by TTE whenever cardiac tamponade is considered even a possibility during a catheterization. If the machine is not *in the room* and not *immediately ready for use*, valuable and possibly life-saving minutes will be lost while locating the machine, moving it to the room, plugging it in, finding and plugging the transducer in, and then finding the jelly.

The exact type of TEE, ICE, and IVUS machines used in the catheterization laboratory varies almost weekly and according to the particular type and generation of echo machines which are available in the hospital, the type of probes used, the institutional/individual's preferences, and the capability for purchase of new or upgraded equipment by the laboratory. The consoles for the TEE, ICE, and IVUS can be stored outside of the catheterization room when not actually being used, but all of these units should be readily accessible to the room, as any delay in retrieving them would result in a delay of the entire lab. When in use, each console must be in close proximity to the catheterization table, but each type of echo requires a different area of access to the patient.

The usual approach to the patient for the standard TTE is from the left side of the patient's thorax, *caudal* to the lateral image detector. The TEE machine approaches from the left side of the patient's head, *cephalad* to the lateral image detector (in order for the TEE probe to be introduced into the mouth), while the ICE and IVUS machines usually approach from either side of the patient's lower trunk (in order for the ICE or IVUS catheters to be introduced into the femoral vessels).

There are several other small and relatively simple echo machines, which usually are not, but maybe should be, considered essential. These machines are very portable, do not take up any space, and can be shared and stored between several catheterization rooms. The Site-Rite 2-D Echo System™ (Dymax Corporation, Pittsburgh, PA) is invaluable for locating relatively superficial vessels. It provides excellent 2-D images of vessels which are within 5–15 millimeters of the skin surface, and it allows a needle to be visualized as it is directed through the subcutaneous tissues to, and into, the vessel. The availability of this simple machine eliminates the blind 'harpoon' stabbing of the carotid vessels in particular, and increases the safety of this approach infinitely.

Many operators also feel that a small portable 'pencil' Doppler™ probe (Parks Medical Electronics, Aloha, OR) or, alternatively, a Doppler™ needle probe (Escalon Vascular Access, New Berlin, WI) should be available to help locate small vessels which are deeper in the tissues and neither visible nor palpable. Both the needle and the pencil probes utilize a Doppler™ signal, which detects blood flow directly in front of the tip of the probe, while neither probe gives an indication of the depth of the signal (vessel) from the tip of the probe. The probes of the needle Doppler™ are disposable and come in three sizes, while the pencil probe can be resterilized and is reusable. In addition to finding elusive vessels during introduction, the pencil Doppler™ probe is invaluable for the evaluation and follow-up of diminished or absent peripheral pulses following prior cannulation of an artery. Both Doppler™ systems attach to their own small console, which can be placed on the table in a sterile wrap and thus reused.

A portable pacing generator is the final piece of mobile capital equipment, which does not take up any fixed space and always must be *available instantaneously* in a congenital cardiac catheterization laboratory. Temporary intracardiac pacing originally was used primarily at times of accidentally induced complete heart block. Like other emergency situations this is very rarely necessary, but, when necessary, the equipment must be available immediately. The pacing generator often was stored on the defibrillator 'cart' along with the pacing catheters and other emergency equipment. The temporary pacing generators now are used electively and far more frequently to purposefully lower the cardiac output by rapid ventricular pacing during

aortic valvotomies, and during the implant of various devices. As a consequence, they now are more readily accessible in every congenital interventional laboratory.

A small but finite amount of additional floor space in the catheterization room is required for a patient warmer, a cardiac output computer, and the equipment for measuring blood oxygen saturation. Patient warmers like the K-Pad™ or Bear-Hugger™ usually are positioned, respectively, under or around the patient with their small consoles at the foot of the table. The Dualtherm™ CO computer (B Braun Medical, Inc, Bethlehem, PA) is relatively mobile, on a small stand, and capable of being moved to a position adjacent to the catheterization table in order for the sterile cables from the cardiac output catheter, which is in the patient, to be attached to the computer.

A readily accessible, rapid, and convenient means of measuring multiple blood oxygen saturation values on very small blood samples is absolutely essential in all pediatric/congenital catheterization laboratories. The apparatus for measuring blood oxygen saturation does not have to be immediately adjacent to the patient but *must be* located *within* the catheterization room in order for the circulating catheterization laboratory personnel to operate the machine efficiently and without significantly interrupting their other duties. Most laboratories now utilize an indirect spectrophotometric oxygen analyzer which operates on a whole blood sample as small as several tenths of a milliliter. Very accurate instruments are available from Waters, Inc (Waters Instruments, Inc, Rochester, MN) and A-Vox™ (A-VOX Systems, Inc, San Antonio, TX). In both machines the sample is placed in a special cuvette and, as certain wavelengths of light pass through the minute sample of the blood in the cuvette, the different saturation of the blood causes a difference in the frequency of the light emitted from the sample. The analyzer calculates the blood oxygen saturation from this directly.

The electrical spectrophotometric equipment for the oxygen determination now is very sophisticated and very accurate, however, the *overall procedure* for obtaining and recording oxygen saturation within most modern catheterization laboratories remains archaic and very prone to human error. In most catheterization laboratories, a blood sample is withdrawn from the patient and the syringe is handed to a nurse or technician who *verbally is provided* with the location of the sample. The sample is injected into the special cuvette and inserted into the densitometer by this nurse. After 10–15 seconds, the densitometer provides a *digital read-out* of the time of the reading and the saturation. This numeric reading is *visualized* by a nurse or technician who *either mentally or manually with pen or pencil* on a 'scrap' paper, *records* the saturation value and the location of the sample. This nurse or technician then 'transmits' these values to a separate recording nurse or technician – who usually is in a completely *separate and often busy control room* – by a verbal 'shout.' The values, *which happened to be heard* by the recording nurse or technician (who also is recording pressure, locations, medications, and other events or numbers from the lab) in turn are *typed manually* into the permanent, timed computer record at the time on the record when the nurse/technician obtains the valve from the room, not at the time when the sample was drawn. This archaic part of the catheterization laboratory system with its many 'human steps' leads to many potential (and real) inaccuracies in the eventual permanent recording of the saturation in the computer record.

As an alternative to this cumbersome system, the digital output of an AVOXimeter™ oxygen analyzer is transmitted electronically and directly to a computer, which, along with the OxyView™ computer program (Scientific Software Solutions, Charlottesville, VA), records and displays the *time*, the *location*, and the *oxygen saturation* of each sample on a separate computer and exactly as they are displayed on the densitometer. The time, location, and oxygen saturation values also are displayed automatically and immediately on a large, separate display screen, which is visible continuously to the operators in the catheterization room. In addition, all of the accurate, timed, values, along with the location of the sample as seen on the display screen, can be printed for a separate, timed, and accurate permanent record.

Several pieces of semi-fixed equipment, which often are considered in the domain of the chemistry laboratory of the main hospital, however, are absolutely essential to the catheterization procedure and, although they do not have to actually be in the catheterization room, they must be within the congenital interventional laboratory *suite*. The first of these is a blood gas analyzer (Radiometer, Copenhagen, Denmark). The analyzer may be in a room adjacent to but separate from the actual catheterization room, but it must be convenient for the *catheterization laboratory staff* to analyze the samples and to have results available immediately. A result from a blood gas sample, which becomes available after even 5 minutes, is past history and is not representative of what is happening from minute to minute during an emergency resuscitation.

The second piece of 'laboratory' equipment which must be present in the catheterization laboratory area is the machine for measuring the activated clotting time of blood, such as the Hemo Tec ACT™ apparatus (Hemo Tec, Inc, Englewood, CO). Particularly with the long duration of many of the interventional procedures and with the multiple exchanges of catheters, wires, sheaths, and devices, essentially all patients undergoing interventional procedures receive heparin anticoagulation. In order to assure the optimal level of anticoagulation, the activated clotting time must be measured periodically throughout the procedure and, like the blood gases, the results must be available expeditiously.

Although, in the past, the 'cabinetry' in the catheterization room has been considered part of the room and not as part of the 'equipment' of the catheterization laboratory, in the modern pediatric/congenital catheterization laboratory all fixed or installed cabinetry, counters, racks, and sinks, including 'scrub areas', should be outside of the actual catheterization room, and the fixed cabinets in the room should be replaced with mobile storage units. Mobile cabinets are available in multiple configurations to accommodate different items. The mobile units in the room are used for all of the very frequently used consumable items, which include the commonly used percutaneous needles, wires, introducers,

and catheters as well as the frequently used medications. The majority of the less frequently used consumable supplies are stored in a separate but, at the same time, adjacent and accessible storage room. Sinks and scrub areas are a source of dirty water, both on the floor and splashed about the room, and also definitely must be outside of the actual catheterization room.

The use of the mobile cabinet units totally eliminates the need for any fixed or permanent storage cabinets or 'catheter racks' mounted within the catheterization room. Any fixed cabinets, counters, racks, or sinks within the catheterization room not only occupy a finite amount of valuable space (3 feet × the length of the cabinetry) which is lost to the room, but they continuously collect dirt and dust, and are impossible to keep adequately cleaned. In addition, when cabinets or racks are installed permanently in the room, the stocking and inventory of supplies in these cabinets must be carried out within the sterile catheterization room. This, of course, requires additional personnel frequently and unnecessarily coming in and out of the sterile catheterization environment. Between procedures, the mobile cabinets are moved out of the catheterization room for stocking and for more frequent and thorough cleaning. Mobile storage cabinets also can be moved about within the catheterization room to accommodate the special configurations of the room for each unique procedure. This is particularly important in the case of a medication cart, which can be moved to a location in close proximity to the site of vascular access at the time of an emergency.

In addition to the space for the multiple varieties of both fixed and mobile capital equipment, the floor space in the actual catheterization room also has to accommodate two, three, *or more* physicians or other specifically trained personnel, who are wearing gowns and sterile gloves, and actually are performing the interventional procedure. Finally, the catheterization room must have adequate space to allow the *efficient and unimpeded movement* of a minimum number of ancillary personnel. In addition to producing a comfortable and more pleasant working environment, this is very important to avoid contamination of the various sterile work areas in the room. The ancillary personnel include at least one person to operate the manifold(s) and/or to maneuver the X-ray table and tube angulation, plus an additional 'circulating' person to operate the oxygen analyzer, retrieve additional expendable equipment, and to move the various pieces of mobile capital equipment into place as needed.

The total environment of the interventional catheterization laboratory is maintained absolutely sterile, similar to an operating theater. In all interventional procedures, multiple catheters, wires, and devices are introduced, withdrawn, and reintroduced repeatedly and frequently into the vascular system and, with many interventional procedures, foreign materials are being implanted permanently in the body. In addition, catheterization procedures often are planned and/or are converted to open chest, combined, or 'hybrid' catheterization/surgical procedures. To accomplish this environment, the catheterization room itself should have a filtered circulating air source and a positive air flow out of the room, and *all personnel who enter* the room are required to wear clean hospital scrub clothes, hats, and masks, with those actually participating in the procedure wearing sterile gowns and gloves.

Potential additional major and fixed capital equipment

When considering building a new catheterization laboratory in the 2008+ era, the concept of the combined or 'hybrid' catheterization surgical room should be considered and carefully investigated. This requires special planning for the choice of a special, combined catheterization/surgical table as well as very special allocations of additional 'space' for the surgeon and his 'team' with their separate equipment. Their equipment includes one or more separate and different portable equipment tables for the extensive array of 'operating' tools, as well as space for the pump oxygenator and its access to the patient via connecting lines in the event that the patient must be placed on cardiopulmonary bypass.

There currently is a growing enthusiasm for very special diagnostic suites, which combine a cardiac catheterization room with complex imaging equipment, which does not involve radiation. These rooms combine either an entire magnetic resonance imaging (MRI) suite or large stereotaxis magnets with an interventional cardiac catheterization suite/room. Because of the bulk and the special additional requirements of this imaging equipment, both of these imaging systems significantly compromise the function of the basic biplane interventional laboratory. A combination suite prohibits the independent use of either the catheterization laboratory or the imaging equipment without tying up the other unit. Additionally, both of these imaging modalities are *extremely* expensive and still at the 'concept' end of practical use in the congenital interventional procedures. Unless funded by a research grant as *an additional catheterization room*, the purchase and installation of either of these imaging modalities does not seem warranted at this time.

CONSUMABLE EQUIPMENT

The proper consumable as well as capital equipment and the expert use of this equipment are paramount in the early recognition, the prevention and, if necessary, the treatment of complications when they occur. All of the consumable equipment used in the modern congenital interventional catheterization laboratory now is available packaged and sterile from the manufacturers and is intended only for one time use. The availability and proper, skilled use of all of this consumable equipment represents the most important 'treatment' of complications; that is, the prevention of their occurrences in the first place.

Consumable equipment required in every procedure

The monitoring of each patient begins with a dependable, continuously visualized ECG, which can be recorded either continuously or intermittently. It is preferable to have an ECG system connected to the patient with at least four disposable leads physically attached to the patient. This allows for the reliable, routine display of ECG tracings from multiple different but simultaneous ECG leads. In the not so unusual event of one, or even two, electrode leads coming loose from the patient under the drapes (from sweat and/or tension on a cable), there still will be at least one usable ECG tracing displayed for uninterrupted monitoring

All congenital interventional procedures require the continuous visualization of accurate intravascular pressures with the capability of permanently recording multiple, simultaneous pressures at any time. The manifolds, which contain the transducers for pressure measurement, multiple three-way stopcocks, and the connecting tubing to the catheters, now are all 'disposable.' They are available from NAMIC USA Corp, Glens Falls, NY, Advanced Medical Designs, Inc, Marietta, GA, and Merit Medical Systems, Salt Lake City, UT, and although all are disposable equipment, the transducers and manifolds which are not exposed to blood often are reused for several cases. The transducers may be positioned on the sterile field or, preferably, are attached to the side or foot of the catheterization table out of the immediate operative field.

Intravascular pressures routinely are visualized through fluid columns from at least one catheter, and often from several catheters, which are being manipulated within all or any area of the heart and blood vessels. All interventional procedures should have an additional indwelling line in a peripheral artery for continuous, uninterrupted pressure monitoring. The continuously displayed intra-arterial pressure tracing is essential, particularly in the more complex procedures, in order to detect very early *trends* in the patient's blood pressure before a major adverse event occurs! This is as opposed to suddenly visualizing a very low blood pressure, which is obtained by an intermittently inflated blood pressure cuff *after* an adverse event has occurred. This arterial monitoring does *not require* a retrograde catheterization with even as small as a 4 or 5 French *catheter*. The peripheral arterial pressure can be monitored equally well and continuously through a secured, but very small, percutaneously introduced, 20 gauge, indwelling plastic arterial cannula.

During every catheterization procedure, each transducer and the lines connecting it to the patient must be checked repeatedly for the accuracy of the pressures. The transducers are balanced when 'opened' to zero atmospheric pressure at the patient's mid chest level. The tubing of the lines from the catheters to the transducers must be flexible, but non-compliant tubing and the catheters, connecting lines, and transducers must all be free of air or other foreign material. Air bubbles anywhere in the system cause either damping or overshoot of the true pressure, while contrast or clot will dampen the pressure.

The transducers, the manifolds, the connecting tubing, and the catheters themselves all require frequent flushing with small amounts of sterile physiologic fluid. Disposable, plastic fluid containers, which are maintained under pressure with an inflatable cuff, provide the most convenient but at the same time a potentially dangerous source of flush fluid. Meticulous attention must be paid when the fluid bags are prepared for use. The flexible bags first and always must be vented to remove all air. The bags are turned upside down, which places the drainage ports at the top. In this inverted position they are squeezed until *emptied completely of the air*, which has risen to the top. The venting and emptying of air always must be performed meticulously before the bags are placed in the pressure cuff and before they are attached to the manifold/tubing/catheter system. If this preparation is not always completed properly, this system creates the potential to force any air left in the system into the patient under high pressure.

The electrical integrity and calibration of the transducers also must be checked at least once during each case. Two transducers easily can be checked against each other with two separate connecting lines and two catheters. The tips of the two separate catheters are positioned in a common location. The pressure from the two catheters in this single, common site is recorded through the two catheters and their connecting lines by the two separate transducers. The pressures visualized (and recorded) from the two catheters through the two accurately calibrated transducers should produce a *single pressure curve* (two overlapping and identical curves) when the transducers are accurately balanced.

Several other parameters are monitored, particularly in the cyanotic, the young, and/or the cachectic patients during any catheterization procedure. These patients routinely have continuous peripheral oximetry and core temperature monitoring. Continuous cutaneous oximetry is readily available using pulse oximetry probes placed on a digit of the patient and connected to an appropriate amplifier in the monitoring system. These probes are interchangeable between various monitoring systems, so also are invaluable for transferring patients to and from the catheterization laboratory. Like the intravascular arterial pressure monitoring, the continuously monitored systemic saturation is displayed on the monitor and will demonstrate early *trends* toward adverse events, often allowing correction before a complication occurs.

Temperature monitoring is equally essential, particularly in the small or cachectic patient. A significant increase or decrease in core temperature is absolutely predictive of an impending problem and allows preventive measures before a major complication occurs. Again, the disposable temperature probe is connected to the appropriate amplifier in the monitor and displayed on the monitor screen. The placement of the actual temperature probes for monitoring temperature is more controversial. The cutaneous probes are more convenient to use but are less reliable, having a propensity to come loose because of body sweat. A transesophageal or rectal probe is more reliable and preferred, but definitely more invasive.

Specific consumable items, their requirements and uses

There is a huge and infinite variety of one time use, case-specific, consumable equipment in the modern congenital cardiac catheterization laboratory. Unfortunately, most of this equipment used in the pediatric congenital catheterization laboratory is used 'off label,' never having been approved by the Food and Drug Administration (FDA) *specifically for children*. At the same time this equipment does have approval for 'human use,' has been used successfully and without complication – often for decade – and now is accepted as the *standard of care in infants and children*. The variety of types and sizes of the consumable equipment is certainly too great for each piece to be described in detail. In order to eliminate or reduce complications, there are some major groups of consumable equipment which must be available in every catheterization laboratory. The specific items which are available often are used because of the individual experience or the preference of the operator, as opposed to any documented superiority of one product over another. Having the proper consumable equipment available, as well as making the correct choice of which piece of equipment to use, often represents the difference between success and failure in a procedure, or the difference between preventing and causing a complication.

Needles

All modern congenital catheterization laboratories utilize percutaneous entry for the introduction of dilators, sheaths, catheters, and other equipment into the vascular system. In order to reduce the local trauma to the vessel, the introduction should be as atraumatic as possible. The entry into the vessel should occur as the needle is being *introduced* into the tissues, with a *single wall puncture* of the vessel, and with as few puncture attempts as possible. There are certain requirements for the needles to facilitate a *precise* and atraumatic percutaneous entry. The needles should have a thin-walled shaft and a very short, non-cutting bevel at the tip. The needle used in each individual patient should be of as small a gauge as possible and yet still able to accommodate the wires being used loosely within its lumen. It is advantageous to have the percutaneous needle as short as possible for the size of the patient and to have a clear hub on the needle; both these attributes facilitate the visualization of even very minute fluid movement within the needle and at the earliest possible instant during puncture into the vessel. There are several manufactures of satisfactory percutaneous introductory needles, which include, but are not limited to, Argon Medical, Inc. (Athens, TX) and Cook, Inc (Bloomington, IN).

There also are several *special* needles to facilitate difficult and/or special intravascular entry. The P.D. Access Doppler™ Needles (Escalon Vascular Access, New Berlin, WI) were discussed previously. The Chiba™ needle (Boston Scientific, Natick, MA) is a 20 cm long, 22 gauge needle, which is utilized for transhepatic vascular entry in the cardiac catheterization laboratory. The needle has a solid, central stilette with a thin-walled, outer plastic cannula. Unlike the ideal single wall percutaneous entry into a vessel, this needle is introduced to its full length with the stilette in place, presumably transecting the vessel along with other tissues during the introduction. The stilette is withdrawn completely and then, as the plastic cannula is withdrawn, the tip of the cannula enters the lumen of the vessel as it is withdrawn back through the vessel. When the cannula tip is free in the lumen of the vessel, blood will return through the cannula. A small amount of contrast can be injected through the cannula to verify which vessel has been entered. The wire is introduced once the proper vessel is identified.

Wires

There are multiple types, sizes, and lengths of wires, which are used for many different purposes in the pediatric and congenital interventional cardiac catheterization laboratory. These can be divided arbitrarily into wires for percutaneous entry into the vascular system and those utilized for special manipulations within the heart and great vessels.

Wires for percutaneous entry

The ideal wire for percutaneous entry has an extremely soft, even floppy, and short distal tip. The wire should be as small a diameter (size) as subsequently can support the introduction of the sheath/dilator, which will be used after the wire has entered the vessel. Wire sizes of 0.015, 0.018, and 0.021 inch diameter are commonly used for percutaneous entry. When the wire size, which also is the outside diameter (OD) of the wire, is significantly smaller than the internal diameter (ID) of the needle, it allows a slight amount of looseness or 'play' within the lumen of the needle. This play, in turn, allows the tip of the wire to deflect away from the precise direction of the needle and deflect into the lumen of the vessel at a sharper angle. Occasionally a very small wire (0.014 or 0.015 inch) will be used to enter very small vessels. Subsequently a very small plastic cannula (Medi-Cut), with a slightly larger lumen than the small wire, is introduced into the vessel over the small wire. The original very small wire is replaced through the cannula with a larger and stiffer wire, which will be used for the introduction of a sheath/ dilator. The overall lengths of the introductory wires are less important. A short introductory wire is more convenient to use, especially in small patients, but a significantly longer wire is safer since it is less likely to accidentally have the entire length of the wire advanced entirely into the vessel through the needle or sheath/dilator.

Wires for special procedures and/or maneuvering into particularly difficult locations

Like the rest of the consumable equipment, there are an infinite variety and numerous sizes of 'spring guide' wires, which are used for many special procedures and maneuvers within the heart and vascular system. Although it is impossible to have every single size, type, and length of wire available in any one laboratory, a representative sample of each type of wire is essential. The different 'guide wires' for manipulations within the vascular system are available from most of the manufacturers of catheters and other intravascular consumables and are manufactured from several different materials, which include stainless steel, nitinol, platinum, and other alloys.

Most of the 'routine' intracardiac wires are stainless steel 'spring guide wires.' These consist of a uniform winding of an extremely fine stainless steel wire around a central, straight, thicker and stiffer, slightly shorter shaft or 'core' wire of stainless steel. The core wire ends up slightly shorter than the windings of wire. There usually is a second, even finer, 'ribbon' safety wire which extends from tip to tip of the wound wire. The 'size' of the guide wire is the outer diameter of the windings of the composite wire and is expressed in thousandths of inches. These wires have a soft tip, which is the short extension of the windings and the safety wire beyond the long, stiffer core wire. The soft tip is of variable length (from 1 to 10 cm) and is connected to the stiffer shaft of the wire through a transition zone, which also can be of variable length, between a very soft tip and the stiff shaft.

Guide wires are particularly useful as an aid to selective maneuvering procedures when the wire is advanced beyond the tip of a catheter and into hard to reach locations – particularly those which arise at an acute angle off the more central vessel. In order to be able to turn the tip of the wire in a different direction from the direction of the catheter, the wire and/or catheter must have a curve at the tip. 'Spring-guide' wires are manufactured with various curves preformed at their tips, or as straight wires, which can be individually curved to suit the operator. In addition to the curve at the tip, in order to be selectively maneuvered the wires must have the capability of being rotated or 'torqued' in a 1:1 ratio over the entire length of the wire. Typical guide wires are available in sizes from 0.014 to 0.045 inch, with various lengths and types of 'soft' tips and varying degrees of stiffness. They are manufactured from a variety of materials, or a combination thereof, and are usually 145 to 165 cm in length.

A few wires are available which are manufactured with a solid shaft of nitinol. This material makes them both somewhat stiffer and 'springier' than the stainless steel spring wires. The nitinol wires have a hydrophilic coating, which makes them very slippery and allows them to 'glide' through both the catheters and vessels more easily. At the same time this combination of properties also makes the nitinol wires much more difficult to hold and maneuver, and it makes them more dangerous to manipulate outside of catheters, where their stiffness and slipperiness make them very capable of *penetrating* into and through tissues – particularly just as the tip of the wire is being extruded out of the tip of a catheter.

In addition to selective maneuvering within the vasculature, stiffer and extra long guide wires are utilized to add extra support within less rigid sheath/dilators, catheters, and various intracardiac therapeutic devices, and for the exchange of various catheters and/or sheath/ dilator sets within the vascular system. Extra long (240–300 cm) wires must be available particularly for the exchange of long catheters and long sheaths in taller patients. Some of these wires must be extra stiff, such as the Amplatz Super Stiff™ wire (Boston Scientific, Natick, MA) in order to support the passage of long and stiff sheath/dilator sets, catheters, devices, or combinations of these through tortuous routes within the heart and great arteries.

An absolutely essential adjunct to complex catheter manipulations is the ability to use wires to deflect or bend the tips of catheters at acute or particularly difficult angles into locations or orifices, which arise even perpendicular to the main vessel. Acute and/or unique curves can be created on the tips of catheters using one or two basic types of 'deflector' wire.

There are special Amplatz™ Active Deflector Wires (Cook, Inc, Bloomington, IN) in which a curve is formed in the distal 1–2 cm of the tip of the wire by a handle incorporated at the proximal end of the wire. The active deflector wire is introduced into the catheter as a straight wire with a relatively soft tip. Once the wire reaches the distal tip of the catheter, a predetermined curve, which is manufactured into the wire, is formed by compression of the 'deflector' handle built onto the proximal end of the wire. Thus, a tight curve is formed actively on the tip of the previously straight wire (and catheter) by squeezing the handle on the wire. As the curve is formed on the distal end of the wire within the tip of the catheter, the tip of the catheter bends to conform to the curve on the wire. The combination can be rotated or advanced together until the tip of the catheter points exactly at the desired orifice. The *catheter then is advanced off* the wire toward the specific new direction, while the wire is fixed in position and the curve is maintained on the wire. The tip of the catheter can be bent or 'deflected' in a direction as acute as 90° off the long axis of the catheter, but the active deflector wire only deflects in a single direction, with no 'lateral' control of the curve. The direction of the acute curve at the tip is only in the direction of any overall *concavity* on the more proximal course of the wire and catheter.

An alternative type of deflector wire utilizes a 'hand formed' fixed curve on any stiff intracardiac wire. This curve is formed by hand bending the proximal or stiff end of a standard spring guide wire, or one end of a special, smooth, stainless steel Mullins™ Deflector Wire (Argon Medical, Inc, Athens, TX) into the desired acute curve while the wire is outside of the catheter. The curves on the stiff wires can be formed or shaped into greater than right angles, or even into 'three-dimensional' curves. When the stiff curve at the end of the wire is advanced within a catheter, the fixed curve bends or deflects the catheter in a direction corresponding to the preformed curve on the wire as the curve passes through the catheter. When the fixed curve on the wire reaches the distal tip of the catheter, the tip of the catheter will be deflected in the direction(s) of the wire curve(s). The catheter then is *advanced off the wire*, which is fixed in place, into difficult angles/locations off the course of the straight catheter.

Using the stiff end of a standard wire or a Mullins™ wire as the 'deflector' has the advantage over the active deflector wire in that the curve formed can be in multiple directions and can actually be three-dimensional. If desired, and in contrast to the active deflector wire, the curve at the tip can be formed so it will point *away* from the overall concavity in the more proximal course of the catheter. At the same time, the stiff, preformed curve on the wire must be advanced through the entire length of the catheter in order to reach the tip of the catheter. This increases the probability of displacing the tip of the catheter from its original position during the introduction of the tightly curved wire. The stiffer the wire and the more acute or complex the curve on the wire, the greater the probability of the catheter being displaced before the curve arrives at the tip of the catheter.

Both deflector wires are used only *within* the tip of the catheters, with the catheter being *advanced off* the curved tip of the wire. Whenever a wire is used for any length of time within a catheter in the circulation, the wire should be introduced through some sort of a wire back-bleed valve with a side port for flushing. The valve is essential to prevent unnecessary bleeding around the wire. The flush port is essential to allow intermittent or even continual flushing of the catheter around the wire in order to prevent thrombus formation on the wire in the catheter. The flush port also allows pressure measurements through the catheter with any type of wire still in place within the catheter.

The pressure wire (Radi Medical Systems, Uppsala, Sweden) is a third type of wire with very special diagnostic capabilities. The pressure wires have a minute transducer incorporated in the tip of a wire from which pressures can be recorded directly from the tip of the wire, which is only 0.014 inch in size. As a consequence, rather than serving only as a support for introducing or maneuvering catheters, these wires are diagnostic instruments in themselves. The pressure wires are extremely useful, if not essential, in the pediatric interventional catheterization laboratory. When only a pressure or a pressure gradient is required from a particular location, the wire alone can be passed into the location or across a very narrow obstruction and pressures obtained without the need for the additional manipulation of a catheter into the area.

Sheath/dilator sets

Introductory sheath/dilator sets   Relatively short sheath/dilator sets are used routinely for the introduction into the subsequent manipulation of catheters and devices within the peripheral vessels, and the exchange of catheters and devices within vessels. These *introductory sheath/dilator sets* are available as matched units of a sheath with a dilator and are available in a wide range of sizes (diameters) from 3 French to 16 (even 24) French, and in sheath lengths from 7 to 15 to 30 cm. The French size (diameter) of a dilator (or of a catheter) refers to the *outer diameter* (OD) of the dilator (or catheter) while the French size of the sheath refers to the *internal diameter* (ID) of the sheath with no indication of its outer diameter. Ideally the difference, or tolerance, between these two diameters should be as close to zero as possible, be absolutely uniform, and yet still allow easy motion of the dilator or catheter within the sheath. The sheath ID can never be any less than the dilator or catheter OD. Like most of the other consumable equipment, these sheath/dilator sets are available from many different manufacturers, each having slightly different, but often very similar, characteristics. The manufacturers of the most commonly used sheath/dilator introducers include Argon Medical, Inc, Athens, TX; Boston Scientific, Natick, MA; Cook, Inc, Bloomington, IN; Cordis Corp, Miami Lakes, FL; Daig Corp, Minnetonka, MN; and Medtronic, Inc, Minneapolis, MN.

The sole purpose of the dilator of the sheath/dilator sets is the smooth introduction of the accompanying sheath into the vessel. The matching dilator of a 'set' usually is 2–3 cm longer than the sheath. The distal tip of the ideal dilator should have a long and *smooth* taper, decreasing from the maximum diameter of the shaft of the dilator down to a tight fit at the tip, both internally and externally, over an introductory wire passing through the distal tip. When this taper is smooth, long enough, and the fit over the wire is very tight, even large sheath/dilator sets (9–11 French) can be introduced over small (0.018 inch) wires with relative ease and minimal trauma to the vessels.

The 'introducer' sheaths are designed to remain indwelling in the peripheral vessel throughout the procedure. The indwelling sheath not only provides a smooth access into the vessel for subsequent catheters and devices, but also provides protection for the intima of the vessel against the constant abrasion caused by the to and fro movements of the catheters within the vessel. When catheters are used through indwelling sheaths, vessel spasm around the catheter is unheard of. The introducer sheath also provides a readily available, atraumatic access to allow the rapid and or repeated exchange of catheters and devices. The introductory sheath should be thin walled, but fairly stiff and kink resistant, and at least the tip of the *sheath* should taper tightly over the matching *dilator*.

Almost all introductory sheaths are manufactured with an attached, combined back-bleed valve and flush port assembly at their proximal end. The back-bleed valve is imperative to prevent excessive blood loss and/or air entry while dilators and catheters are being exchanged. The side port allows clearing of the sheath of air or clots, in addition to allowing flushing into the sheath to keep any catheter within it continuously lubricated and free of clots.

It is advantageous for these back-bleed valve/flush ports to be detachable from the sheath (Argon Medical, Inc, Athens, TX). A sheath which is accurately manufactured with precise tolerances to match with the dilator or catheter of the same size will not bleed around a catheter even when the back-bleed valve is removed completely from the sheath. At the same time, when the valve is loosened from the sheath and 'parked' by withdrawing it back to the hub of the catheter which is being used, it removes the constant resistance or binding, which always occurs with the movement of the catheter against the valve when the valve is fixed on the sheath. Withdrawing the valve onto the catheter eases the catheter movement within the sheath and allows the operator to actually 'feel' the tip of the catheter moving against *tissues* with far more sensitivity as the catheter is maneuvered. In turn, when the valve is not on a sheath, the added sensitivity to the touch on the catheter helps to prevent the catheter from being forced unnecessarily into or through tissues.

Long delivery sheath/dilator sets In addition to the standard 'introductory' sheath/dilator sets there are many longer and *specialized sheaths*, which are used to introduce catheters and intravascular devices to specific locations well within the heart or great vessels. These special sheath/dilator sets are as long as 90 cm and usually larger than the sheaths used primarily for the introduction of catheters into the peripheral vessels. The precise length and size of the special sheath/dilators vary with their proposed use. The original special, long sheath/dilator sets were developed as a component of the Mullins™ *modified* transseptal procedure. The dilators of these sets are matched in length to be 1 cm shorter than the lengths of the two different Brockenbrough™ transseptal needles. The very fine tapers and internal diameters of the tips of the dilators are matched to the outer diameter of the finely tapered portion of the distal tips of the transseptal needles.

Subsequent generations of these long sheath/dilator sets have been developed primarily for the delivery of specific devices to particular locations well within the heart and vascular system. The long sheath/dilator sets are available from many manufacturers, including, but not limited to, AGA Medical Corp (Golden Valley, MN), Cook, Inc (Bloomington, IN), Daig Corp (Minnetonka, MN), and Medtronic, Inc (Minneapolis, MN). These specialized long sheath/dilator sets are available in lengths which are both shorter as well as much longer than the standard transseptal sheath/dilator sets. The current sheaths have special, thicker, and kink resistant walls, better radio-opacity, which is often augmented at the very tip, and, often, special, preformed curves at the distal ends. For the same reasons, but of even more importance than on the short introductory sheaths, all long sheaths must have a back-bleed valve with an attached side flush port.

The tips of the longer dilators are not designed specifically for the 'penetration' of skin or any other structures but rather for the delivery of the sheath/dilator to often very circuitous locations over large diameter and often very stiff, prepositioned wires. As a consequence, the dilators on the long sheath/dilator sets have a tip which is much blunter and tapers to accommodate a wire even as large as 0.038 inch. Sheath/dilator sets which are significantly longer than the transseptal sets are used to deliver many different types and sizes of occlusion devices, for the delivery of balloon-mounted stents and cutting balloons, and are used with all types of foreign body retrieval equipment.

Intermediate length sheath/dilator sets which are longer than the standard introducer sheath/dilator sets but *shorter* than the standard transseptal sets are available for the delivery of the balloon septostomy and blade catheters (usually used in smaller patients) and to introduce and position bioptomes when they are introduced from the jugular veins.

Special long sheaths are available with wire braiding incorporated within their walls to prevent kinking in situations when the sheaths must be positioned through a course involving fairly acute angles. These are available from Arrow International, Inc (Reading, PA), Cook, Inc (Bloomington, IN), and AGA Medical Corp. (Golden Valley, MN). In addition to wire braiding to reinforce sheaths, a large diameter, long sheath can be used coaxially over a slightly smaller diameter long sheath in order to deliver devices through a very tortuous vascular course, which contains multiple sharp bends within the heart or great vessels.

In order to facilitate the withdrawal of deployed intravascular devices, which after being deployed have become larger and/or irregular in configuration, very large diameter, and at the same time very short, sheaths are used prophylactically as 'recovery sheaths.' The extra large, short sheath is placed coaxially over the long sheath and withdrawn to the proximal hub of the long sheath before the latter is introduced into the patient. The large, short sheath is not advanced or introduced into the skin or vessel unless the recovery of a device is required.

The latest development in the long sheath/dilator sets is a sheath with the capability of the sheath itself being deflected as an integral part of the sheath. This allows the tip of the sheath to be deflected and maintained in a relatively specific direction, after which a catheter or device can be delivered out of the sheath in that direction without some additional support of a deflector wire. This capability is particularly useful when directional manipulations are required from within a large chamber into selective side orifices.

There are many different procedures where the long sheath/dilator sets are necessary and, in order to accomplish all of these procedures, a very wide variety of both size and length of the long sheath/dilator sets must be available in every congenital interventional laboratory. With the large variety of long sheath/dilator sets available, the exact set used depends not only upon the specific use intended for the sheath but also upon the operator preference.

Diagnostic cardiac catheters

Of all of the consumable equipment used in the catheterization laboratory, the greatest variety occurs in the types and sizes of the cardiac catheters themselves. There are three *basic types* of catheters used for diagnostic catheterization: the *extruded* catheters, the *balloon floating* catheters and the *woven Dacron*™ catheters. Each of these is also subdivided by the design of the individual catheter into either a *hemodynamic catheter* or an *angiographic catheter*.

The hemodynamic catheters are used to obtain pressures and blood samples for oxygen saturation determination from every necessary area and to deliver guide wires to specific locations within the circulation. Most of the hemodynamic (or pressure) catheters have a single lumen, which extends the entire length of the catheters including straight through the distal tip of the catheter. In addition to the single distal opening, these catheters can have anywhere from two to four additional small holes opening on the sides of the catheter very close to its tip. The lumen extending straight through both ends of the catheter allows the hemodynamic catheters to be advanced over prepositioned wires or vice versa, wires can be advanced through and beyond the catheter into difficult locations.

The angiographic catheters were designed primarily so that they do not move or are not displaced during the injection of a large volume of contrast medium at a high rate of flow, at a high pressure, and over a short period of time. They generally have a closed distal tip with *only* side holes, or as an alternative, a special configuration of the distal tip of the catheter, which produces significant resistance to flow through the very distal area. The special designs of the distal end/tip helps to prevent a 'fire hose' recoil of the catheter during rapid, high pressure injections of contrast. The angiographic catheters can be used to obtain blood samples and certain pressures, but they cannot be wedged into distal capillary locations nor can the closed-ended angiographic catheters be delivered over wires in order to position them in very difficult locations. Hemodynamic catheters can be used to perform angiograms, but only at low pressure with low flow rates of contrast, which almost always results in less than satisfactory angiograms.

Extruded catheters By far and away, the most commonly used of the three basic types of catheter is the extruded catheter. As the name implies, different plastic materials are extruded into a tubing of uniform diameter. When the tubing is cut to a specific length, a proximal hub is added, with possibly some extra holes near the distal end and some special distal shaping; this tubing then becomes a catheter. The extruded tubing and, in turn, the catheters are available in a wide range of materials, diameters, and tubing (wall) thickness. The material or the mixture of materials from which the tubing is extruded includes polyethylene, Teflon™, and mixtures of other plastics. The materials themselves and how the material is extruded impart most of the individual characteristics into these catheters. A few of the extruded catheters even have a fine weave of wire incorporated into the wall of the tubing to improve stiffness, wall strength, and torque of the final catheter. The length of an extruded catheter depends only on how long each segment of tubing is cut to 'a catheter length' and, as a consequence, these catheters are available in an infinite variety of lengths. The extruded catheters are available from many manufacturers, including Argon Medical, Inc, Athens, TX; Arrow International, Inc, Reading, PA; B Braun Medical, Inc, Bethlehem, PA; Boston Scientific, Natick, MA; Cook, Inc, Bloomington, IN; Cordis Corp, Miami Lakes, FL; Edwards Lifesciences, Irvine, CA; and Medtronic AVE, Santa Rosa, CA.

The tubing in the extruded catheters has the characteristic that it can be formed or shaped readily after exposing it to only a moderately high temperature and, after cooling while in the formed shape, the tubing (catheter) fixes quite permanently into any angle or combination of bends. In order to enter almost every conceivable branch or orifice in the vascular system in any size patient, an infinite variety of different configurations and shapes of the distal tips has been designed, and these are available in the extruded catheters. The preformed shape of the extruded catheter does have a 'memory,' even in the warmer temperature of the circulatory system, and, as a consequence, the desired shape persists during even the longest catheterization procedures.

Unfortunately this memory of the extruded materials of these catheters also applies to the shaft of the catheters. This allows for good torque control of the shaft, but tends to result in a catheter shaft which is relatively stiff, with a very poor capability of following or 'flowing' after the tip when the catheter is being manipulated through tortuous vessels. As a consequence of these characteristics, the tip of the appropriately curved catheter can be maneuvered easily from a vessel or chamber into the orifice of the desired side branch, even when the branch arises at a very acute angle. However, advancing or following into that side branch with the straight shaft of the catheter becomes very difficult, if not impossible, with most of the extruded catheter. This is particularly true when the branch does arise at an acute angle off the main vessel. The stiff shaft, along with the curved tip of the catheter, when pushed forward tends to continue in a straight direction, which, in turn, displaces the tip out of the area instead of the catheter 'following' into, through, or around sharp curves.

The appropriately curved tip of an extruded catheter almost always can be pointed accurately toward any conceivable angle or direction and engaged in a particular orifice. Advancing a soft wire from the catheter into the side orifice arising at an acute angle also almost always is possible. However, advancing the catheter over the wire around the angle is similar to advancing the catheter by itself. The relatively stiff, extruded catheter shaft again tends to advance straight and not follow the wire, particularly when the direction of the wire angles acutely or in multiple different planes from the original direction. Instead of following the wire, the advancing, straight shaft of the catheter usually pushes the fixed curve of the catheter along with the wire out of the desired location.

The extruded angiographic catheters have similar handling characteristics to the extruded hemodynamic catheters. The angiographic catheters are available in a range of sizes between 3 and 9 French, and in various lengths. The larger the diameter (of the lumen) and the shorter the length of the angiographic catheter used, the less is the resistance to the flow of the contrast and the faster the contrast can be delivered. The extruded angiographic catheters have either a closed distal end with multiple side holes close to the tip or, more frequently, they have a tight (~1 cm) 360° curve (or 'pig-tail') at the distal end of the catheter, with side holes along or immediately proximal to this curve. The extruded 'pig-tail' catheters are delivered to the location for injection over a relatively stiff, prepositioned wire, while the closed-ended angiographic catheters must be selectively manipulated to the desired area.

Even with their shortcomings, the extruded hemodynamic and angiographic catheters are essential equipment in any congenital interventional laboratory. They are significantly less expensive than the other types of catheters, which allows a wider variety of them to be inventoried in the laboratory, and each laboratory should have a large variety of these precurved extruded catheters for the selective cannulation of difficult intravascular locations. It is advantageous to have a good working relationship with an adult interventional laboratory, as active adult catheterization laboratories usually will have every conceivable variety and shape of the extruded catheters.

The Multi-track™ Catheter (NuMED, Inc, Hopkinton, NY) is a special 'extruded' catheter, which is available as either an angiographic closed-ended or a hemodynamic open-ended catheter. This catheter has a small, very short loop of 'catheter lumen,' which is attached to, but also off-set to one side of the distal tip of the main catheter shaft and lumen. A guide wire passes adjacent to and alongside of the length of the catheter and through this separate loop at the tip, without passing into or through the true lumen of the catheter. This allows either a hemodynamic or an angiographic Multi-track™ catheter to be exchanged over a large guide wire, which already has been positioned in a very difficult location. Pressures can be recorded and samples or angiocardiograms taken through the catheter lumen, all with the wire maintained in the difficult location. The Multi-track™ catheter does require a larger cutaneous introductory sheath with a very competent back-bleed valve in order to accommodate both the support wire, which lies adjacent to the catheter, and the catheter itself within the introductory sheath, and at the same time prevent bleeding from the wire passing adjacent to the catheter through the sheath and valve.

Floating balloon catheters   The second common type of diagnostic catheter used in a congenital cardiac catheterization laboratory is the 'floating' balloon catheter. These also are extruded catheters, which are, however, manufactured of a somewhat softer plastic than the previously discussed, standard extruded catheters. The distinguishing characteristic of these floating catheters is a small, inflatable, spherical Latex™ balloon attached at (around) the distal tip of the catheter.

Theoretically, when the balloon is inflated with a small amount of gas, it acts like a 'sail' and the force of blood flow against the balloon will pull the balloon (and 'soft' catheter with it) along with the flow of the blood. Theoretically, this eliminates the need for complex, selective manipulation of the catheter in order to enter difficult locations. The floating of the balloon works reasonably well when the long axis of the balloon catheter is aligned precisely in the direction of the flow of the blood and the blood flow is vigorous. However, because of the inherent remaining stiffness of the shaft of all of the floating balloon catheters, the forward flow of blood will not pull the balloon catheter in low blood flow situations, or when the flow of blood is in a direction which is at all perpendicular to the long axis of the tip of the catheter. The balloon catheters are useful for following blood flow within channels with unusual turns or even in *channels* which reverse direction from the original course of the catheter, even when the channel makes a 360° turn. For very acute turns, the flow of blood must be somewhat forceful and the long axis of the tip of the catheter (with the balloon) must be maintained in parallel alignment with the direction of blood flow. As a consequence, the floating balloon catheters do not totally replace, but rather must be used in conjunction with, often complex and skilled catheter manipulations.

For inflation/deflation, the balloon on these catheters communicates with a hub on the proximal end of the catheter through a second, separate, very small lumen, which lies adjacent to the main catheter lumen within the wall of the catheter. In the congenital catheterization laboratory, where right to left shunting is very common and/or manipulations commonly are in the systemic circulation, the balloons always should be inflated with filtered carbon dioxide in order to *prevent all possibility* of systemic air embolization with its related catastrophic complications. The floating balloon catheters are available in sizes between 4 and 8 French, from several manufacturers. Like the extruded catheters, the floating balloon guided catheters are available as both hemodynamic and angiographic catheters.

The hemodynamic balloon catheters are also called Swan Catheters™ (Edwards Lifesciences, Irvine, CA) after their original designer. Similar to the extruded hemodynamic catheters, the floating hemodynamic catheters have a catheter lumen which extends through both ends of the catheter with no side holes. The distal end of the lumen exits through the distal tip of the catheter, passing through, but not communicating with, the balloon at the tip. The floating balloon hemodynamic catheters are used primarily to obtain blood samples and sample or monitor pressures after they have been 'floated' to the appropriate location. With the balloon deflated, and because of their softer material, they are very difficult to selectively maneuver, while, with the balloon inflated at the tip, the catheters are less likely to perforate cardiac structures during attempted manipulations. This makes the balloon catheter safer for the inexperienced operator to maneuver. The hemodynamic balloon catheters are particularly useful for measuring

pressures in very precise locations and for obtaining pulmonary capillary 'wedge pressures' from capillary end vessels in the pulmonary bed.

In the Berman™ Balloon Angiographic catheters (Arrow International, Inc, Reading, PA) the main central lumen of the catheter is closed at distal tip of the catheter and the catheter lumen exits through six small side holes, which are located just proximal to the balloon. The inflated balloon is as effective (or ineffective) as the balloon on the hemodynamic catheters for 'pulling' the catheter to the desired location with the flow of blood. The inflated balloon is effective at keeping the tip of the catheter from digging into the myocardium during high pressure injections and, in turn, preventing extravasation of contrast into the tissues. The second small lumen which is required for the balloon does compromise the size of the main lumen of the catheter, which reduces the maximum flow rate of contrast through these catheters.

In some interventional catheterization laboratories the hemodynamic and the angiographic floating balloon catheters are *the* standard diagnostic catheters used by the laboratory. In every laboratory they can be a useful adjunct to the other types of catheter being used, and are essential for some very special maneuvers. As such, a representative sample of both the hemodynamic and the angiographic floating balloon catheters should be available in every laboratory. With the floating balloon catheters, the laboratory also must have a readily available source of filtered carbon dioxide gas and a simple means of providing it in sterile form to the operative field for repeated filling of the balloons while the catheters are on the sterile table.

A special floating balloon catheter is manufactured for the measurement of thermodilution cardiac outputs (B Braun Medical, Inc, Bethlehem, PA). In addition to the balloon and the standard lumen, these catheters have a thermistor imbedded in the distal tip of the catheter. The thermistor is connected to an electrode at the proximal end via a very fine wire imbedded in the wall of the catheter. There also is a third small lumen within the wall for the injection of the 'sensing' fluid. This third lumen originates from a third stopcock at the proximal end of the catheter and then exits through an opening in the side of the catheter, which is approximately 20 cm proximal to the distal tip of the catheter. Because of the accuracy and reproducibility of the thermodilution cardiac outputs obtained by these systems, almost all congenital catheterization laboratories utilize these catheters along with a thermodilution cardiac output computer (Waters Instruments, Inc, Rochester, MN or B Braun Medical, Inc, Bethlehem, PA) to obtain cardiac outputs.

Woven Dacron™ catheters   The third type of catheter, which is the catheter preferred by this author and still is in common use in certain cardiac centers, is the woven Dacron™ catheter (Medtronic, Inc, Minneapolis, MN). The original woven Dacron™ catheters (United States Catheter, USCI, Bard, Glens Falls, NY) were urologic catheters and, initially, they were the only catheters available in any cardiac catheterization laboratory. As the name implies, these catheters are manufactured from a 'woven' Dacron™ fiber. Multiple fine fibers of Dacron™ literally are woven over a mandrel to form a uniform tube of Dacron™. A fine layer of polyurethane is sprayed uniformly over this tube to create a sealed and smooth catheter.

The woven Dacron™ catheter has several advantages. It has excellent (1:1) torque control and the best 'following ability' during intravascular maneuvering of any catheter. Although these catheters appear quite stiff when they are at room temperature, they soften considerably when warmed even moderately to intravascular temperatures. This softening gives them a unique flexibility, which allows the shaft of the catheter to 'follow' or 'snake' through very tortuous courses as the tip is maneuvered through these channels. Once the tip of a Dacron™ catheter has entered an angled side branch, as the catheter is advanced, the following shaft of the catheter easily conforms to the curves in the course through the channel as it follows the tip, even through very circuitous channels. This characteristic makes the woven Dacron™ catheter essential for entering very complex distal locations within the circulation. The softening with heat of the Dacron™ catheters also allows desired curves to be formed selectively at the tip after brief heating in boiling water or steam. The formed curve then can be 'fixed' temporarily by dipping the newly formed curve into a cold sterile solution.

This softness and conformity of the shaft of the Dacron™ catheter is very different from the characteristics of the extruded catheters, which retain their preformed curve configurations and the 'straightness' of the shaft, whether within or outside of the circulation. This difference is why the extruded catheters do not follow or track easily through tortuous courses.

The 'softening' of the woven Dacron™ catheters also is recognized as their major disadvantage. Because of their softening at body temperature, they do not retain preformed curves at the tip for any duration of time once they have been introduced into the circulation. After as little as 10 minutes in the circulation, the shaft becomes too soft to easily maneuver without using extra support wires within the catheter. When, in order to enter a specific location, a special curve is formed on the tip of a Dacron™ catheter, that particular location must be the first priority and be entered immediately after the catheter is introduced into the patient. Because of the softening of the shaft of the Dacron™ catheters, it also is difficult to maintain them in specific locations or to 'wedge' them into distal capillary beds.

The woven Dacron™ catheters, which are used most commonly for the acquisition of hemodynamic data, have an end hole at the distal tip, which is in continuity with the central lumen. The distal tip also may have a special extra taper at the tip and/or up to four additional side holes very close to the distal tip.

Woven Dacron™ angiographic catheters probably are the best of the various types of angiographic catheters.

The woven Dacron™ construction provides the strongest catheter wall while, at the same time, allowing the largest lumen per catheter size. The woven Dacron™ angiographic catheter has a closed distal tip with multiple relatively large side holes near this tip. The closed tip configuration prevents a 'fire hose' type of recoil of the catheter, which occurs when there is a single opening at the tip. The combination of features of the woven Dacron™ angiographic catheter allows contrast injections at the highest pressures and at the maximum flow rate of any angiographic catheter. Unless all of the holes of the catheter are buried in the tissues, the closed-end configurations also prevent extravasation into tissues, which can occur with the excavating capacity of a high-pressure jet of fluid through a single end hole.

The woven angiographic catheters have identical handling characteristics to the woven hemodynamic Dacron™ catheters, and are more difficult to maneuver into more circuitous locations. Because of their softening when in the circulation they must be positioned expeditiously and very precisely, and it is recommended to place a fine support wire (Mullins™) in the catheter lumen to prevent catheter recoil during rapid, high-pressure injections. The angiographic catheters are available in a range of sizes between 3 and 9 French, and in various lengths. The larger the diameter and the shorter the length of the angiographic catheter used, the less is the resistance to the flow of the contrast.

Special diagnostic catheters   Bioptome catheters are an essential tool in any pediatric/congenital catheterization laboratory. Although not a therapeutic procedure, diagnostic biopsies are performed in almost all laboratories where congenital heart patients undergo cardiac catheterization. Unfortunately, biopsies are performed so frequently that they often are considered 'routine' and, as a consequence, treated very casually. Contrarily, the endomyocardial biopsy is potentially one of the more dangerous procedures performed in the cardiac catheterization laboratory. Each sample represents an excision of a small piece of myocardial tissue. The 'excisions' are obtained relatively blindly and repeatedly from more or less 'random' locations in the myocardium.

Bioptomes are available from multiple manufacturers including, among others, Cordis Corp (Miami Lakes, FL), Argon Medical, Inc (Athens, TX), and CERES Medical Systems, LLC (Stafford, TX). They are available in various sizes from 4 to 7 French, and in several lengths. To facilitate delivery to a specific spot in the tissues they are advanced through a long sheath which has been specifically precurved to match the intracardiac location. The distal end of the bioptome also is precurved manually to conform to the location to be biopsied. The long sheath is prepositioned against the myocardium using biplane fluoroscopic and/or echocardiographic guidance. During the repeated introduction and withdrawal of the bioptome, the long sheath has the potential for the introduction of air or clot and the biopsy procedure itself has the potential for perforation of the myocardium or cutting a chordae with each 'bite.'

Transseptal catheterization 'sets' and electrophysiology catheters are several additional 'special diagnostic catheters' which are essential and must be inventoried in a congenital interventional cardiac catheterization laboratory.

Transseptal catheterization procedures are required in an interventional catheterization laboratory. The equipment for performing a standard transseptal procedure actually is a set of matched equipment. Basic to this set is the Brockenbrough™ transseptal needle, which is available in 'adult' and 'pediatric' sizes from Cook, Inc (Bloomington, IN), Daig Corp (Minnetonka, MN), and Medtronic, Inc (Minneapolis, MN). Both the adult and pediatric needles have a 30° curve at the distal end and an 'arrow' on the proximal end of the shaft of the needle, which is fixed and pointing in the direction of the distal curve. The usable length of the adult needle is 72 cm. The shaft of the needle is 18 gauge, with the last distal 1 cm tapering to 20 gauge. The pediatric needle is 62 cm long, with the main shaft of 19 gauge and the last cm tapering to 21 gauge. The 'adult' needle is not only longer, but, because of its larger gauges, is significantly sturdier than the 'pediatric' needle, and in punctures, which are very tough, can be used in the smaller patients.

Originally these transseptal needles were used with a Brockenbrough™ catheter (United States Catheter, Bard, Glens Falls, NY) which essentially was a long dilator, 1 cm shorter than the needle, which had a moderate taper down to the needle at the tip and several side holes near the distal tip. Once the puncture with the needle and the catheter was completed, the needle was removed leaving the Brockenbrough™ catheter in the left heart. The Brockenbrough™ catheters were very stiff and, with the obligatory end hole, they were unsatisfactory for anything except obtaining pressures and blood samples.

The majority of the transseptal procedures performed currently use a Mullins™ transseptal sheath/dilator set from United States Catheter, Bard, (Glens Falls, NY) or Medtronic, Inc (Minneapolis, MN) with the Brockenbrough™ needles. The Mullins™ transseptal sets are an extra long sheath/dilator combination. The dilators in the set are 1 cm shorter than the particular adult or pediatric needle being used and the comparable sheath is 1.5–2 cm shorter than the dilator. These sets are available in sizes from 5 through 8 French. The Mullins™ transseptal set has the advantage that, after the puncture with the needle and the sheath/dilator set, the needle and dilator are removed, leaving the long sheath as access to the desired location for any and all varieties of catheters or devices.

Electrophysiologic studies and the catheter therapy of arrhythmias are essential in the congenital heart catheterization laboratory environment. These studies and therapies require an entirely different spectrum of both capital and consumable equipment. As a consequence, most active congenital *interventional* catheterization laboratories do not have the capability for extensive electrophysiologic studies or therapy in the same laboratory. At the same time, most interventional laboratories do have a close relationship with a laboratory which does perform the electrophysiologic studies and therapy and stocks the necessary equipment.

One final type of diagnostic catheter is the catheter with a microtransducer mounted in its tip, from Millar Instruments, Inc (Houston, TX). These catheters are used primarily in hemodynamic research studies. They have one or more tiny, very accurate transducers or flow probes built into the distal tip of the catheter. The transducers are connected to the monitoring equipment electronically through fine wires running in the wall of the catheters. Since the transducer is in the actual site where the pressure is being recorded, there is no 'contamination' of the pressure curves by the interposed fluid column and extremely accurate pressures can be recorded. These catheters usually have no lumen, they are relatively stiff, and, as a consequence, more difficult to manipulate. They also are very expensive and can no longer be cleaned, resterilized, and reused. These factors, combined with the accuracy of a correctly prepared and calibrated fluid-filled system, make the routine use of the catheter tip transducers not practical.

Therapeutic catheters and devices

Most therapeutic catheters and devices are very specific to the therapeutic procedure and all of these are discussed in far more detail in the subsequent chapters in this book dealing with that particular procedure. Like the other consumable equipment, and no matter how unusual or expensive, the therapeutic catheters/devices for whichever procedure is being attempted must be available and in a range of appropriate sizes according to the size of patient and/or lesion being treated.

The simplest therapeutic catheter which must be available in all congenital interventional laboratories is the pacemaker catheter. These catheters have an electrode at the distal tip connected to a proximal electrical connector by a wire within the catheter. Pacemaker generators were mentioned in the discussion of capital equipment. Pacing catheters compatible with the particular pacemaker generator which is available in the catheterization laboratory must be available in several sizes and varieties of catheter. In the past these catheters were kept with the other emergency equipment in the laboratory, but now with their more frequent and elective use during interventional procedures they are stocked with the other therapeutic catheters.

Pacing catheters are available as extruded, balloon floating, or woven Dacron™ catheters (United States Catheter, Bard, Glens Falls, NY), but not every type need be available. A very small 4 French pacing catheter can be used in either a small or large patient, however the very small catheters are more difficult to manipulate. Each lab probably should have at least several 4 French and several 6 or 7 French extruded or woven Dacron™ pacing catheters. The balloon floating pacing catheter theoretically should be easier to advance into the heart, but in the circumstance of low and/or no cardiac output the floating will not be effective.

Balloon septostomy catheters   The very first intracardiac therapeutic catheter procedure was the Rashkind™ balloon atrial septostomy, which was performed using a Rashkind™ Septostomy Balloon Catheter (United States Catheter, Bard, Glens Falls, NY). There have been some significant changes in the balloon catheter, but the procedure itself is essentially the same and as effective as it was originally. The septostomy balloon catheters now are available from several manufacturers. They all have a small (1–2 cm) spherical balloon mounted securely on the distal end of a small, extruded catheter and all are inflated with a 1:5 dilution of contrast to flush.

Two sizes of septostomy balloon catheters are available from NuMED (NuMED, Inc, Hopkinton, NY). They are both mounted on an extruded catheter and each has a small balloon manufactured from a thermoplastic elastomer. The balloons on the two different NuMED catheters are two different specific sizes; they inflate with a maximum of 1 or 2 cc of fluid respectively, and reach 9.5 and 13.5 mm in diameter respectively. When inflated with these precise volumes, the two balloons are filled, very non-compliant, and are rigid at these maximum diameters. In addition to the balloon lumen, both catheters have a separate through and through catheter lumen, which allows them to be delivered over a wire and/or allows a pressure recording or even a small angiogram through the lumen to aid in positioning. These balloons are optimal in the very small infant and/or when only a small and temporary septostomy hole is necessary.

The Miller-Edwards™ Balloon Septostomy Catheter (Edwards Lifesciences, Irvine, CA) is an extruded catheter with a *single lumen* connected to a Latex™ balloon at the tip. The Latex™ balloon is very compliant and, in order to be truly effective, it must be inflated with 5–6 cc of fluid to make the balloon even somewhat non-compliant. With a 4 or 6 cc volume the balloon reaches approximately 2 cm in diameter, and at that diameter the balloon does lose most of its compliance. Although not advertised, the burst volume of these balloons is 10–12 cc. This balloon is preferred when a larger, more 'permanent' septostomy is desired. The precautions and expiration date on these balloons must be strictly observed, as Latex™ deteriorates fairly rapidly when in light and/or with time. These balloons do not have a separate true lumen and must be manipulated and positioned visually using fluoroscopy and/or echo. They do come with a very fine stainless steel stylet which is useful, not only for deflecting the tip of the catheter, but also for clearing the very tiny lumen should it become clogged and prevent deflation of the balloon.

Blade septostomy catheters   Very early in the experience with balloon septostomy, it became apparent that a balloon septostomy alone was seldom effective in patients older than 1 month to 6 weeks of age. The Park™ Blade Septostomy Catheter (Cook, Inc, Bloomington, IN) was developed to 'initiate' the septostomy procedure in older patients by first incising a small slit in the septum. There are three sizes of blade septostomy catheters – the PBS 100™, PBS 200™, and PBS 300™. The 100 and 200 are both on a 6 French catheter, while the 300 is on an 8 French catheter. The 100 has a cutting blade which is 9.4 mm in length, the 200 a blade length of 15 mm, and the 200 a blade length of 20 mm.

The PBS 300™ is preferred in all except the very smallest patients. The blade of the 300 is not only longer, but the blade and all of the mechanisms of the blade are significantly sturdier, which prevents the blade mechanism from rotating, distorting, and getting jammed. Although most patients have a pre-existing septal opening and do not require a transseptal puncture, the blade catheters are introduced across the atrial septum through a long transseptal sheath. The sheath must be one French size larger than the blade catheter. The potential for air and clot in the long sheath during introduction of the blade catheter potentially is the most dangerous part of the procedure.

Balloon dilation (angioplasty) catheters   The largest group of therapeutic 'devices' is the balloon dilation or 'angioplasty' catheters. As opposed to the more or less spherical and low pressure, septostomy and 'floating' balloons, the angioplasty balloons are cylindrical, relatively non-compliant, and are inflated to a specified 'fixed' diameter at relatively high pressure. Dilation balloons are used to dilate virtually all and/or any stenotic lesion within the vascular system. They also are used for the delivery and the dilation of most of the intravascular stents which are used in stenotic vessels in the congenital population. The lesions, which can be dilated, include cardiac valves, pulmonary and systemic arteries, systemic veins, septa, baffles, and miscellaneous communicating vessels.

The balloons are categorized according to the *expanded diameter* of the balloon, the *length of the balloon*, the *inflation and burst pressure* of the balloon, the *shape* of the balloon, the *length and diameter of the catheter* on which the balloon is mounted, and the *materials* from which the balloons are manufactured. Each of these characteristics imparts the specific and/or special properties to the balloons. In addition to the basic characteristics mentioned, the material of the balloon also influences thickness of the balloon wall and the folding characteristics of the balloons, both of which will influence the ease or difficulty of introducing and/or removing the balloons from the vascular system.

There is no one ideal balloon. Often a balloon will have some ideal characteristics, but, at the same time, some other equally unfavorable or even dangerous characteristic. The particular lesion to be dilated and the potential adverse event which might occur because of an unfavorable characteristic determine which of the good vs bad characteristics of a balloon are most important.

The diameter to which the lesion is to be dilated is the primary determinant of the diameter of the balloon which will be used. Dilation balloons are available in diameters between 2 and 28 mm and reach their diameter when inflated with the advertised amount of fluid at their listed pressure. The pressure of the balloons varies from as low as 2 atmospheres to over 25 atmospheres according to the type and materials of the balloon. The balloons are inflated only to their maximum, advertised inflation pressure, always using a special balloon pressure manometer (or indeflator) in order to control the inflation pressure very precisely.

The 'length' of the balloon refers to the *usable* length of the balloon, which is the length of the parallel surfaces of the inflated balloon and does not include (nor usually mention) the length of the tapered tips ('shoulders'), which connect the balloon to the catheter. The usable length is demarcated by radio-opaque markers positioned on the shaft of the catheter within the balloon. The balloons vary in shape according to the manufacturer's preferences and the materials used to manufacture them. The type of lesion determines the type and shape of balloon used within the availability of balloons in any particular laboratory. For the dilation of most congenital lesions, a balloon with very short shoulders (a 'stubby' balloon) is preferable. In contrast to the ideal stubby balloon, very high pressure balloons often have very long shoulders, which are required because of the materials in the balloon and in order to assure the balloon is not torn from the catheter under the high pressure.

The angioplasty balloon catheter has a central catheter lumen which must accommodate a relatively large guide wire and, in addition, has at least one additional lumen for the inflation and deflation of the balloon. The balloon lumen(s) must be of sufficient diameter to allow rapid inflation/deflation of the balloon with a dilute contrast solution. As a consequence, the catheter shafts for angioplasty balloons are relatively large in diameter. In addition, most balloons are not recessed into the shaft of the balloon catheter and the extra diameter of the deflated and folded or wrapped balloon around the catheter must be considered in determining the size of the sheath used.

The ideal or universal balloon does not exist. The ideal balloon is a stubby balloon, on a small diameter catheter, capable of inflation at moderate pressure, with the capability of rapid inflation/deflation, and with resistance to puncture, rupture, and tearing. The ideal balloon also should have a very smooth, small diameter of the deflated folds of the balloon (profile) around the catheter shaft before *and after* inflation in order that a sheath no more than one French size larger would be necessary to introduce and remove the balloon. Since there is no ideal balloon, the choice of balloon unfortunately depends upon which balloon has the *least potentially dangerous and the fewest undesirable* characteristics for the particular lesion being dilated.

A congenital interventional catheterization laboratory must have a wide variety of multiple sizes and types of angioplasty balloons available in their inventory. Balloons approved for intravascular dilations *in humans* are available in an extremely wide variety of sizes, types, and materials, and from multiple manufacturers including, but not limited to, NuMED, Inc, Hopkinton, NY; B Braun

Medical, Inc, Bethlehem, PA; Boston Scientific, Natick, MA; Cook, Inc, Bloomington, IN; Cordis Corp, Miami Lakes, FL; and Bard Cardiopulmonary, Tewksbury, MA. At the same time, only those available from NuMED and B Braun are FDA approved specifically for pediatric and congenital use.

Specialized angioplasty balloons In addition to the 'standard' angioplasty balloons, there are 'special angioplasty' balloons, each with additional very unique characteristics. These balloons also must be maintained in the inventory of the congenital interventional laboratory along with the 'usual' angioplasty balloons.

The Balloon In Balloon™ (BIB™) catheter (NuMED, Inc, Hopkinton, NY) is the most essential of these. As the name implies, the balloon of the BIB™ catheter actually is one angioplasty balloon within another. The inner balloon is one half the diameter and 1 cm shorter than the outer balloon. Both balloons are attached to separate 'ports' by separate lumens. The BIB™ allows the controlled, sequential – in two separate steps – inflation of a lesion and, in particular, of intravascular stents within lesions. The stepwise inflation allows repositioning within the lesion during inflation and, of more importance, allows expansion of stents without the 'dumbbell' distortion associated with balloon inflation of a large stent with a single large balloon.

The 'cutting' balloon is another very specialized 'angioplasty' balloon (Interventional Technologies, Inc, San Diego, CA), which is desirable in the therapy of small and very resistant vascular stenosis. These balloons range in size from 2 to 8 mm in diameter and have three or four very fine, retractable Atherotome™ blades mounted longitudinally on their wall. When deflated, the blades lie flat against the surface of the balloon and, as the balloons are expanded, the blades open perpendicular to the balloon wall. When opened the blades are capable of making very fine, 0.005 inch deep, longitudinal incisions in the intima of the vessel and, in turn, creating what appears to be a more permanent dilation of the vessel. These balloons require very special handling and manipulation within the circulation. If significant angulation occurs at the site of balloon inflation, the blades can become dislodged from the balloon, making withdrawal very difficult.

Extra high-pressure balloons are still another required type of specialized angioplasty balloon. Although extra high-pressure angioplasty balloons are not required for dilation of most stenoses, they occasionally are essential for the dilation of very resistant vascular lesions. As a consequence, a variety of sizes of these balloons should be available in every congenital interventional laboratory. To accommodate the high pressures, the larger diameter, high-pressure balloons are manufactured either from different materials, as in the Atlas™ balloons (Bard, Covington, GA), or are multilayered materials, as in the Mullins™ balloons (NuMED, Inc, Hopkinton, NY). Their deflated diameters usually are larger and/or significantly more irregular than standard angioplasty balloons of the same size.

As a consequence, these balloons usually require an introductory sheath several French sizes larger than a comparable standard angioplasty balloon, especially for their withdrawal. High-pressure Blue Max™ balloons (Boston Scientific, Natick, MA) also are available, but only in 12 mm or smaller diameters.

The final specialized 'angioplasty' balloon is the sizing balloon. These balloons are not actually used for the dilation of any lesion, but rather for the more precise sizing and 'shaping' of stenotic lesions and intracardiac defects. The sizing balloons are manufactured from similar but thinner plastic materials (NuMED, Inc, Hopkinton, NY) or from Latex™ (AGA Medical Corp, Golden Valley, MN) and are designed to be inflated at very low (zero!) pressures. When inflated appropriately, these balloons conform exactly to the diameter and shape of the vascular lesion without distorting or dilating it at all. When used properly, these balloons are very safe to use and provide invaluable information about the treatment of many stenotic lesions.

Intravascular stents   For the more permanent treatment of vascular stenosis, intravascular stents are an essential and frequently used part of the standard armamentarium of the pediatric and congenital interventional cardiologist. Although considered the standard of care for many pediatric and congenital lesions, all of the available larger intravascular stents used in the United States were designed and FDA approved for adult use and, as a consequence, have been used 'off label' for the pediatric/congenital lesions. Although stents often are implanted in small children, any stent which is implanted should be capable of dilation to the *adult diameter* of the vessel into which it is implanted. Otherwise the stent itself creates a new lesion as the patient outgrows it, and this new lesion will be treatable only by subsequent, complex, and possibly otherwise unnecessary, surgical intervention.

There are two very different types of the larger intravascular stents. These two types are the balloon expandable stents and the self-expanding stents. The balloon expandable stents are those used for the most part in the pediatric/congenital population. The self-expanding stents have been shown to produce excessive neointimal proliferation and rapid restenosis in growing patients and, as a consequence, generally are not recommended in pediatric patients.

The large balloon expandable stents are available from several manufacturers, each with their own special properties and in a variety of lengths and diameters. Regardless of manufacturer, the larger stents which are available in the US are all manufactured from stainless steel. Some stents which are available only outside of the US are manufactured from platinum and other alloys. The major difference between the various balloon expandable stents, regardless of material, is the design of the 'mesh' which makes up the wall of the stent.

The Genesis X-D™ stents (Johnson & Johnson-Cordis Corp, Miami Lakes, FL) and the C-P™ stents (NuMED, Inc, Hopkinton, NY – only available outside of the US and in one recent FDA clinical trial), are 'closed cell' designs, each with side spaces or 'cells' of a maximum, uniform, and predetermined size and shape. This design makes these stents more rigid in both their compressed and expanded configurations, however these closed cell design stents tend to be stronger, with a greater resistance to compression.

The Mega™ and Maxi™ Stents (ev3, Plymouth, MN) are an 'open cell' design with side cells which are larger and have variable, irregular shapes. These characteristics allow more flexibility to the overall stent and allow each individual cell to be dilated considerably larger than the fixed cells. This ability of the individual cells to be dilated allows access through the side of the stent to side or branch vessels which may have been crossed and 'jailed' by the implanted stent. Which exact stent is used for a particular configuration of a lesion often represents a compromise between either the strength or the flexibility of the stent, the availability of the exact type and size of stent, and the individual preference of the operator.

The larger balloon expandable stents are all hand mounted or 'crimped' onto the surface of the delivery balloon and then delivered through a long sheath of a large enough diameter to accommodate the balloon with the stent mounted on it. The optimal balloon for the delivery of a stent is one with short shoulders and one which is exactly or very slightly shorter than the length of the stent. Deviations from these optimal balloon characteristics definitely contribute to the complications during the delivery of the stent. A BIB™, which has an outer balloon the exact length of the stent, has the optimal characteristics and allows undistorted expansion of the larger stents, but requires the use of a significantly larger delivery sheath.

In addition to the standard bare stents described above, there is a definite place for stents which are covered with a very thin layer of an elastic and yet impervious material such as polytetrafluoroethylene (ePTFE™) (WL Gore & Associates, Flagstaff, AZ). A covered stent becomes absolutely essential for an emergency 'bailout' device in the event of rupture of a vessel during any balloon dilation procedure. It also would be preferable to use a covered stent to *prevent* extravasation during dilation or stent implant in vessels suspected of being very weak. 'Covered' stents are available routinely outside of the United States. In the US, covered stents have been hand prepared during emergencies by operators in individual laboratories and, somewhat at the whim of the FDA, have been intermittently available commercially for emergency use. Any catheterization laboratory performing vessel dilations with or without intravascular stent implants should have several sizes of covered stents prepared, sterile, and always available for emergency use. In the case of a ruptured vessel there seldom is time to 'prepare' a covered stent from 'scratch,' even if the various materials are available and sterile.

Occlusion devices   There presently are a number of devices available and approved by the US FDA for the occlusion of a variety of abnormal intravascular openings and communications in pediatric and congenital heart patients. All varieties of the various approved occlusion devices, including a range of each of their different sizes, are required consumable equipment in a valid pediatric and congenital interventional cardiac catheterization laboratory. In a patient who is in the catheterization laboratory for treatment of a lesion, the lack of the proper equipment/device is never a valid excuse for the failure of a procedure.

The oldest and still the most commonly used occlusion devices are the intravascular coils. Like many catheters, etc., the coils are FDA approved for 'human use', but not specifically for congenital or pediatric lesions. The Gianturco™ coil (Cook, Inc, Bloomington, IN) is the most commonly used of the coils. These basically are a short length of spring guide wire, which is formed into a tight 360° or other concentric loop of the wire with short, fine strands of Nylon™ fiber enmeshed in the 'spring' of the wire. The coil wires are either stainless steel or platinum and are available in multiple sizes of coil wire, loop diameters, and multiple lengths of wire, creating a very wide variety of 'coil sizes.'

Coils can be delivered by simply pushing the straightened coil through a small catheter with a guide wire until the coil is extruded, unconstrained, out of the end of the catheter. This is the 'free release' technique, which still is in common use. There also are several techniques and modifications available for controlling the release and allowing retrieval of the coils, which do make their delivery safer. These include specific attach/release mechanisms (Jackson™ Coils [Cook, Europe] and Flipper™ Coils [Cook, Inc, Bloomington, IN]), the use of a small bioptome for gripping the coil until the time of purposeful release, or the use of a small snare for controlling or retrieving the coil after release. The coils are especially useful for the occlusion of small aberrant end vessels, but also are optimal for occluding the small persistent ductus arteriosus.

In addition to the coils, there now is a variety of approved devices designed for the occlusion of specific intracardiac defects, including the patent ductus arteriosus (PDA), atrial septal defect (ASD), the patent foramen ovale (PFO), and the ventricular septal defect (VSD), as well as miscellaneous large vascular communications.

The one device approved in the US by the FDA specifically for the PDA is the Amplatzer™ Patent Ductus Occluder (AGA Medical Corp, Golden Valley, MN). Like all of the Amplatzer™ family of devices, the PDA occlusion devices are a mesh made out of a continuous weave of Nitinol™ wire. The weave is formed into a particular shape, according to the type of device, for a particular lesion. The PDA device is a slightly tapered plug, which is available in increasing lengths between 5 and 8 mm according to the increasing size of the device, and with a small disk-like rim extending 2 mm around the circumference of the larger end of the plug. The Amplatzer™ PDA devices are available in sizes between 5-4 and 16-14, the first number representing the diameter of the *plug* at its largest end and the second number the diameter of the plug at its smaller end. To enhance occlusion, the device contains disks of polyester. The device is connected to a special Amplatzer™ delivery cable with a tiny screw mechanism which connects to a special attachment on the proximal (smaller) end of the plug.

These device are delivered to the ductus through a prepositioned, special long sheath. Once the device is screwed onto to the cable the expanded device is withdrawn into a short sleeve or loader, which compresses the device into a long strand the diameter of the delivery sheath. The elongated device is advanced from the loader into the proximal end of the long, prepositioned, delivery sheath. The device is pushed through the sheath with the cable, out of the sheath, and into the exact position in the ductus, where it expands to occlude the PDA. Once securely in the proper position it is unscrewed from the cable. Similar to all of the Amplatzer™ family of devices, even after it has been deployed but as long as it has not been unscrewed for a purposeful release, the PDA device can be easily withdrawn back into the delivery sheath.

There are several other devices available for the occlusion of the PDA. The Gianturco-Grifka™ Vascular Occlusion Device (GGVOD) (Cook, Inc, Bloomington, IN) is a small Nylon™ sack which is stuffed with a long length of spring guide wire to form an occluding mass. This is only useful in long tubular structures, as it is quite complicated to deliver and difficult to retrieve. As a consequence, the use of the GGVOD has been replaced for the most part by one of the Amplatzer™ devices.

In Europe the PFM Duct Occlud™ device and the newer Nit Occlud™ devices (PFM [Produkte fur die Medizin AG] Cologne, Germany) are available for PDA occlusion. These are tight coils of stiff stainless steel guide wires and Nitinol™ wire, respectively. They are preshaped into cones or double cones of various sizes and are implanted in the ductus with a special delivery system, with which they are retrievable until purposefully released. Both devices depend upon the mass of tightly wound wire to produce the occlusion. These are not yet commercially available in the US.

A variety of occlusion devices has been developed for occlusion of the ASD. There now are two varieties of Amplatzer™ ASD occluders (AGA Medical Corp, Golden Valley, MN) and the Gore, Helix™ Device (WL Gore & Associates, Flagstaff, AZ), all three of which are approved in the US by the FDA. In addition, the STARFlex™ Device (NMT Medical, Inc, Boston, MA) has been used successfully for ASD occlusion in Europe for years and is now in clinical trials in the US for PFO occlusion.

With all of the ASD devices, the ASD must be accurately sized to determine the proper size of device for the occlusion. Undersizing leads to displacement and embolization of the device, while oversizing seems to be the main contributor to erosion through adjacent tissues by the devices. The sizing is performed with transesophageal (TEE) or intracardiac echo (ICE), and is usually confirmed using a sizing balloon inflated at low (no) pressure within the defect. When *used properly*, the sizing balloon provides a more accurate, non-stretched diameter of the defect and, in addition, will demonstrate when the rims of the defect are unusually compliant. Balloon sizing, along with the TEE or ICE, adds an additional step to the implant of ASD devices, but also adds an additional degree of accuracy and, in turn, reduces complications.

Both of the Amplatzer™ devices for the occlusion of the ASD are woven from Nitinol™ wire similar in technique to the construction of the Amplatzer™ PDA device, but the ASD devices are both formed into double opposing disks connected by a central hub. The standard Amplatzer™ ASD device (AGA Medical Corp, Golden Valley, MN) has a large diameter hub between the opposing disks which is 14 mm smaller in diameter than the larger, left atrial disk of the two opposing disks. The diameter of the hub is the size of the standard Amplatzer™ ASD device.

The standard Amplatzer™ ASD device is available in sizes between 4 and 40 mm, in increments of 1–2 mm. The size of the Amplatzer™ ASD device used is usually the same size as the accurately sized (not stretched) diameter of the ASD. The standard Amplatzer™ ASD occluder is the simplest and safest ASD device and is currently the most commonly used device for catheter occlusion of the secundum ASD.

The Amplatzer™ Cribriform ASD Occluder (AGA Medical Corp, Golden Valley, MN) has been approved recently by the FDA for use in the US. It also is a double disk of Nitinol™ mesh construction, but the hub between the two disks is very narrow and relatively flexible. This device was designed for use in the multi fenestrated or 'Swiss cheese' atrial septum. The device is positioned through the most central of the multiple holes, with the idea that the broad expanse of the wide disk extending around the narrow central hub would cover the adjacent holes in the septum. In order to prevent embolization of the device after release, the disks of the Cribriform™ device should be at least twice the diameter of the actual hole through which the device is passed. The size of the Cribriform™ ASD devices is the diameter of the disks. They are available in sizes of 18–40 mm, in increments of approximately 5 mm.

The Helex™ ASD Occluder (WL Gore & Associates, Flagstaff, AZ) is the third ASD device available in the US. As the name implies, it is a spiral (or helix) of Nitinol™ wire, which has a curtain of ePTFE™ (WL Gore & Associates, Flagstaff, AZ) mounted along the length of the wire. The wire is preformed so that, in its 'relaxed state,' it forms loops or circles, each of equal diameter. The maximum diameter of the loops represents the size of the particular Helex™ device. The ePTFE™ curtain is of variable widths and is attached according to the diameters of the loops to make the different sizes (diameters) of devices. The Helex™ ASD device is available in 5 to 35 mm diameters in 5 mm increments.

For delivery, the Helex™ device is first stretched into a 'straight' wire as it is withdrawn into its own delivery catheter. The Helex™ device is delivered to the ASD in this catheter without a long sheath. Once across the ASD the device is slowly pushed out of the catheter, which allows it to reloop. Half of the loops are extruded on the left side of the septum and the other half on the right side of the septum. Once in proper position, it is locked in place and released by a fairly complex system. The Helex™ device does allow a fairly straightforward retrieval of the device until a final 'safety string' is cut after deployment. Since the device has no centering mechanism, a device twice the size of the defect must be used to prevent embolization after release. This significantly limits the maximum size of ASD which can be treated with this device.

The next specific lesion for which there is an FDA approved device in the US is the muscular ventricular septal defect (VSD). The Amplatzer™ muscular VSD occluding device (AGA Medical Corp, Golden Valley, MN) has full FDA approval. Like the other Amplatzer™ devices, the VSD device is a weave of Nitinol™ wire, but with a different configuration from the other devices. The VSD devices also are double opposing disk devices, but with a broad, 7 mm long waist or hub, the diameter of which determines the size of the device. The VSD devices have a 'disk' at each end of the hub. The disks, which will be positioned on the left side of the defect, are 8 mm larger in diameter than the hub. The disks on the end of the hub, which will be on the right side of the defects, are 6 mm larger in diameter than the hub of the device. The Amplatzer™ Muscular VSD Occluders are available in 4–18 mm sizes, varying in 2 mm increments between sizes. The device used is 2–4 mm larger than the accurately measured size of the defect.

The Amplatzer™ muscular VSD occluders usually are delivered from the jugular approach, through a prepositioned long sheath which has been positioned across the defect by a double approach, wire retrieval technique, which produces a through and through wire. The attachment to the cable, the delivery, the release, and/or withdrawal of the device when necessary, are all similar to the other Amplatzer™ occluders.

In addition to the Amplatzer™ Muscular VSD Occluder, the CardioSEAL™ device (NMT Medical, Inc, Boston, MA) has FDA humanitarian use approval for catheter closure of the muscular VSD. This device is a true 'double umbrella' with two alloy wire framed, opposing umbrellas, which fold away from each other at a very small central connecting pin. The opposing umbrellas are covered with a Dacron™ fabric. These devices are available in 17, 23, 28, and 33 mm diameters (sizes). They are delivered similar to the Amplatzer™ VSD device, from the jugular vein through a prepositioned long sheath. A device at least twice the diameter of the muscular VSD is necessary to secure fixation in the defect. Complete closure of the defect often takes from weeks to months after the implant of the CardioSEAL™ device. Once even one disk is deployed, these devices are very difficult to withdraw and/or remove.

In addition to the devices already discussed, which are available for very specific lesions, there are two versions of the Amplatzer™ Vascular Plug (AGA Medical Corp, Golden Valley, MN) now FDA approved for the occlusion of miscellaneous abnormal communications in the vascular system. These occlusion devices are short cylindrical 'plugs,' again manufactured from the woven Nitinol™ material similar to the other Amplatzer™ devices, with similar attach, release, and delivery techniques. All of the plugs are designed to occlude larger and more or less tubular lesions. The standard Amplatzer™ Vascular Plugs are satisfactory for relatively low-flow and/or low-pressure communications, and are available in 4–16 mm diameters. The Amplatzer™ Vascular Plug II (AGA Medical Corp, Golden Valley, MN) has additional 'disks' at each end of the cylindrical plug, which provides greater resistance to flow. The Plug II is available in 3–22 mm diameters.

In the US, there are no devices with full FDA approval for occlusion of the PFO. However, there are four devices used for PFO occlusion in one of several FDA authorized clinical trials in the US, and all of these same devices are in routine use outside of the US.

The first of these is the CardioSEAL™ device. Its design and characteristics have been discussed previously under muscular VSD devices. The CardioSEAL™ device for PFO occlusion is exactly the same device as the muscular VSD device and is available in the same sizes. The second PFO device, the STARFlex™ device (NMT Medical, Inc, Boston, MA) is a slight modification of a CardioSEAL™ device. In addition to the same double umbrellas, it has four micro Nitinol™ spring wires extending from the tip of an arm of one umbrella to the tip of the closest arm of the opposing umbrella. When the umbrellas are open across a defect, these wires create four equally placed 'elastic slings' between the four tips of the opposing umbrellas. The tension on these wires as they pass from umbrella to umbrella through the defect tends to force the umbrellas toward the center of the defect, pulling all four corners of the devices toward the center.

The narrow connector between the two umbrellas of both the CardioSEAL™ and the STARFlex™ devices makes them ideal for closing the very small, potential opening of the 'typical' PFO. These devices are less satisfactory when the remaining septum primum and septum secundum of the defect overlap significantly and create a long tunnel-like opening.

The third device, the Amplatzer™ PFO Occluder, is manufactured from the same materials and with the same general concepts of the other Amplatzer™ devices. The PFO Occluder has a double disk configuration with the two disks attached by a narrow, flexible, and eccentric waist or hub, giving it the appearance of a double umbrella device. The diameter of the right-sided disk determines the size of the Amplatzer™ PFO Occluders, which are available in 18, 25, and 35 mm diameters. With the idea of preventing predominately right to left shunting, the left-sided disks on the 25 and 35 mm devices are only 18 and 25 mm in diameter, respectively. These occluders also are ideal for the short, very small diameter PFO and, because of their greater flexibility, are probably slightly better for the 'tunnel-like' PFO.

The fourth PFO occluder in trials in the US is the CARDIA™ device (Cardia, Inc, Burnsville, MN). These also are opposing double umbrella occluders. Each 'umbrella' has six arms created by three crossing 'bows' of specially woven Nitinol™. The three bows are attached together at their crossing point at the center, creating six arms on each umbrella. The two umbrellas are attached to each other by a very narrow and short (either 3 or 5 mm) connecting post. Each umbrella has a hexagonal sheet of Ivalon™ as the occluding fabric.

The length of a bow of the umbrella determines the size of the device. The CARDIA™ devices are available in 20–35 mm sizes in 5 mm increments. A tiny ball-like pin on the CARDIA™ device attaches to a small bioptome-like delivery cable and the device is delivered to the PFO through a long prepositioned sheath similar to the other PFO devices. The advantages and/or disadvantages of the CARDIA™ device are still to be determined.

In Europe, the Helix™ ASD occluder and the Sideris Reverse Button™ device (Pediatric Cardiology Custom Medical Devices, Athens, Greece) have also been used for occlusion of the PFO. Neither of these seem to have any great advantages over the previously mentioned devices. There is also a bioabsorbable modification (NMT Medical, Inc, Boston, MA) of the CardioSEAL™ device, which is in trial for PFO occlusion. The potential advantage of this type of device is that, after a period of time, there would be little or no remaining foreign material in the body. A favorable outcome of this trial may change the entire concept for the occlusion of the PFO and other intravascular/intracardiac lesions.

Miscellaneous therapeutic items In addition to opening narrowed areas and closing abnormal openings, occasionally totally occluded areas need to be crossed. Initially this was accomplished using the stiff end of a wire protruding out of a catheter or using the standard transseptal equipment. Using either of these types of equipment required the lesion to be more or less in a straight line of approach from the entry site of the catheter or needle, and required a significant amount of mostly uncontrolled force.

As an alternative to the brute force, several different sources of energy were used outside of the US to perforate through totally occluded tissues. The first of these energy sources attempted was Excimer Laser™ (Spectranetics, Colorado Springs, CO) energy delivered through a fiberoptic 'wire.' This proved very effective in perforating through tissues by vaporizing the tissue in front of it. The use of Laser™ was reported in several types of congenital cases; however, the depth or distance of the Laser™ perforation was hard to control and to produce the energy required an expensive and fairly complicated Laser™ generator, which was only available in a very few laboratories. Laser™ never gained much popularity and never was approved for perforations of congenital lesions in the US.

The second source of energy tried was high-energy radiofrequency. When applied to the tip of a wire, this energy did perforate tissues, but only for a short depth.

A source of radiofrequency energy was readily available in the radiofrequency generators used widely in electrophysiology ablations. The ablation generators did require a modification in order to convert the energy into high-impedance, high-voltage (150–180 volts), low-power (3–5 watts) generators which would deliver the energy capable of perforation for a very short (1–2 s) duration. Eventually a dedicated, relatively inexpensive and simple to use generator was developed strictly for perforations.

Radiofrequency perforation using the special Baylis generator (Baylis Medical Co, Inc, Montreal, Canada) was approved by the FDA in 2001 as an alternative technique for the puncture of the atrial septum in the US. Since that time, radiofrequency has been used 'off label' for the perforation of other congenital structures – in particular the atretic pulmonary valve. This use has become the standard of care for the initial treatment of pulmonary valve atresia as well as other discrete obstructive lesions, and requires that every pediatric interventional catheterization laboratory has the necessary generator and the catheters as well as the expertise in their use available for these patients, which inevitably all appear as emergencies. The substitution of the high-energy radiofrequency for the previous brute force does not eliminate the risk of a perforation procedure, but rather introduces a whole new spectrum of potential complications related to the procedure and the equipment.

A final area of equipment, which is becoming more desirable (and maybe essential) for the therapy of particularly the older and postoperative, complex, congenital cardiac patients, is one or more varieties of mechanical thrombolytic equipment. Large in situ thrombi occur, particularly in low-flow situations, in fresh surgical areas, or in or adjacent to implanted devices.

Thrombolytic agents often are not effective in the larger or older clots and require mechanical disruption for removal. In addition to simple 'baskets' for grasping or suction for hopeful withdrawal of the clot, there is a variety of specific devices for mechanically disrupting the clot. These include the Helix Clot Buster™ (ev3, Plymouth, MN), the Thrombex™ device (Edwards Lifesciences, Irvine, CA), the Angiojet™ (Possis Medical, Inc, Minneapolis, MN), the Oasis™ Thrombectomy Device (Boston Scientific, Natick, MA), and the Trerotola™ Percutaneous Thrombectomy Device (Arrow International, Inc, Reading, PA).

None of these devices has an absolutely perfect way of removing the particulate debris which they create. As a consequence, particles can embolize distally, which is often systemically in the congenital patients. In spite of this shortcoming, one or more of these types of devices should be available on short notice to a congenital interventional laboratory.

Emergency equipment

Unfortunately, there always will be times when the emergency treatment of a complication becomes necessary. In spite of all of the proper equipment and the skill and caution used in performing a particular

procedure, complications occur. Like all of the other procedures in the catheterization laboratory, both the proper capital and consumable equipment are necessary for the successful treatment of a complication.

Besides the standard equipment for the congenital interventional catheterization laboratory, there is no additional capital equipment required; but in these circumstances, biplane fluoroscopy is absolutely essential in order to accomplish any retrieval within a reasonable amount of time and with the minimal utilization of radiation. The retrieval of errant intravascular foreign bodies is an especially complex procedure and obligatorily requires 'three-dimensional' visualization for the localization and capture of any foreign body.

Of the consumable equipment necessary for emergencies, pacing catheters have already been discussed for the treatment of arrhythmias, as have 'covered stents' for the emergency treatment of vessels which tear or rupture during dilations. The multitude of different implantable devices which are now in use creates a huge potential for the embolization of 'foreign bodies' into errant positions in the circulation. When these devices are being implanted in the catheterization laboratory, as much capability as possible of safely retrieving and removing these errant devices in the laboratory must be available. This capability does require the availability of some special consumable equipment and, additionally, some 'preplanning.'

Special retrieval equipment The first type of extra equipment which is necessary in the retrieval of most foreign bodies is extra large diameter, long sheaths. Large means 2 to 4 French sizes larger than the original delivery sheath. Even when the errant device is still attached to its delivery system, many of the devices cannot be withdrawn back into the same sized sheath through which they were delivered.

For those devices known to require more frequent withdrawal, and yet known to be difficult to 'recompress' for a withdrawal, a larger diameter, *short* sheath is placed over the delivery sheath prior to its insertion into the patient. The large short sheath is withdrawn to the proximal hub of the long delivery sheath before the long sheath is introduced initially. Then, when an errant device is recaptured but cannot be withdrawn totally into the original long delivery sheath, the larger, short sheath is introduced into the vessel over the long sheath. This allows the partially collapsed device, along with the long sheath, to be withdrawn totally into the short sheath for withdrawal out of the vessel and through the skin.

For errant devices, the first order of business is to replace the original long delivery sheath with a new, larger diameter, long sheath. The new sheath should be as large in diameter as possible, and certainly large enough to accommodate an only partially compressed device. An 'exchange cable' is available for all of the Amplatzer™ device delivery systems. This cable allows replacement of the long delivery sheath with the larger diameter, long sheath *without* releasing the device from the original delivery cable. This makes exchanging for a larger sheath relatively straightforward, without the fear of more distal embolization of the device if it must be released to exchange sheaths.

When devices have become completely free from their delivery system, or must be released in order to introduce a larger sheath, the retrieval becomes significantly more difficult. The distal tip of the large retrieval sheath should be positioned in the same vessel or chamber, and as close to the errant device as possible. It is imperative that the sheath be advanced all of the way *through* any intervening valves or any intervening ventricle. This is in order that once the errant device is retrieved it can be withdrawn *completely* into the retrieval sheath before being withdrawn across a valve or through a ventricle.

Another piece of the standard consumable equipment which is not usually considered a retrieval tool, but at the same time is very useful during foreign body retrieval, is the Amplatz™ Controllable Active Deflector Wire (Cook, Inc, Bloomington, IN). Although the curved tip of the deflector wire is not strong enough to withdraw a foreign body back into a large sheath, the wire can be used to dislodge foreign bodies which are 'plastered' against the wall of a vessel and have no free or exposed ends. The straight deflector wire is advanced or 'drilled' between a foreign body and the vessel/chamber wall. When the deflector is activated, the tip of the wire forms a loop and encircles the foreign body, which allows it to be dislodged or moved to a more favorable position for grasping with a true retrieval device.

The bioptome is another standard consumable catheter and, like the active deflector wire, is not a retrieval tool per se, but a bioptome can also be very useful for grasping and dislodging foreign bodies, particularly those which have no free ends or protrusions into the vessel or chamber.

Specific retrieval tools   There are four very specific types of retrieval tool, all of which should be available in a congenital interventional cardiac catheterization laboratory. In addition to their inherent catheters, all of these retrieval tools are used through a long sheath, which should be large enough to accommodate the retrieved device in its partially collapsed state.

The first available, the most essential, and still the most commonly used of these tools, are the snare retrieval devices. These are basically one or more loops of wire, which extend from the end of catheter. Withdrawing the loops or one strand of a loop into the catheter tightens the loops. The extended wire loop encircles an object. As the loop is pulled into a catheter the loop tightens around the object, grasping it securely. Originally, snares were hand made in each laboratory from an extra long, stainless steel spring guide wire and a long end hole catheter. These snares did not have much memory for the loop and were eventually replaced by a variety of more sophisticated commercial snares. In order for a snare to grasp an object, the loop must be able to encircle at least part of the object.

Of the commercial snares the Amplatz Goose Neck™ snare (Microvena Corp, White Bear Lake, MN) is still probably the most versatile and most commonly used.

These snares are manufactured from Nitinol™ spring wire, giving them a very permanent memory for the loop, which always protrudes perpendicular to the catheter when the snare is extended. The perpendicular orientation of the loop facilitates encircling objects which are aligned along the long axis of the catheter (and vessel). These snares are available in a variety of wire sizes and loop diameters, the latter determining the 'snare' sizes. They are available in sizes between microsnares of 2–7 mm and standard snares of 10–35 mm.

Another snare which is quite similar in its basic design to the original hand made snare, is the Medi-tech™ snare (Medi-tech, Boston Scientific, Natick, MA). This snare has a single elongated hexagonal-shaped 'loop' of memory spring material. The loop extends out of the end of the catheter at a very slight angle off the long axis of the catheter. It is available in 20 and 35 mm wide hexagons. To capture a foreign body, at least a piece of the foreign body must extend approximately perpendicular to the long axis of the vessel/catheter in order to prolapse into the opened loop.

A third and essential snare is the En Snare™ (Medical Device Technologies, Gainesville, FL). This snare is almost a combination of the Goose Neck™ and The Medi-tech™ snare technologies. The loops of this snare also are made from Nitinol™, but each snare has three loops, which extend 45° out from the long axis of the catheter shaft and are aligned ~ 120° to each other. When opened, this creates a sort of 'cup' approaching the foreign body, allowing the capture of objects which are aligned at different angles to the catheter. The size of these snares is also determined by the diameter of the loop. These snares are available in a mini and a standard size, with a range from 2–4 mm to 27–45 mm.

Because of the different angle of the snare loops off the catheters, each of these three types of snare has a different approach for grasping objects and, as a consequence, a slightly different application. With enough time, persistence, and additional radiation any one of the snares probably could be used to retrieve any specific object with a free end. However, for the sake of expediency and patient and operator safety, a representative variety of each type of snare is desirable in the inventory of every interventional laboratory.

In addition to these three more common snare catheters, there are at least three additional snares which are less common or not available in the US and do not add anything to the capabilities of the first three mentioned.

The second major type of retrieval tool is the basket retrieval device. As the name implies, this device resembles a basket being extruded from a catheter. The 'baskets' are formed by four parallel, fine stainless steel wires which are attached together at their tips and at a location 4–8 cm proximal to their tips. The wires are prebent or precurved away from each other in the area between the two spots where they are attached to each other. When within the catheter, the wires are compressed together as parallel strands of wire; however, when the curved areas of the wires are advanced out of the tip of their catheter, they expand away from each other according to their preformed curve to form the 'basket.' The length, diameter, and shape of the basket depend upon the distance between the spots where the wires are attached, and upon the curves which were preformed on the wires. Because of the multiple wires required to form the baskets, these are often fairly large and stiff catheters.

There still are several manufacturers of basket retrieval devices. The Medi-tech™ Retrieval Baskets (Medi-tech, Boston Scientific, Natick, MA) consist of four very fine wires, which form a slightly spiral configuration as they expand out of the catheter. They are available in 15 or 25 mm diameter baskets and are contained within a special 5 French catheter. The Dotter™ Intravascular Retriever (Cook, Inc, Bloomington, IN) also has four wires, which are somewhat thicker than the Medi-tech™ wires and spiral approximately 90° in addition to expanding to 3 cm in diameter. This basket is delivered through an 8 French catheter. This basket is larger and sturdier and, when it can be maneuvered around a foreign body, is usually more capable of compressing the foreign object.

The baskets are used to completely encircle a foreign body and then to compress it for retrieval. The wires of the open basket pass along the side of the foreign body, allowing at least part of the foreign body to 'herniate' between several of the wires of the basket into the 'lumen' of the basket. As the wires (the basket) are retracted into the catheter, the wires compress together, compressing the foreign body between them. The baskets are particularly useful for grasping and compressing large and/or irregular foreign bodies, including intravascular stents.

The next most useful and again absolutely essential specific tool for foreign body retrieval is the Grasper™ Forceps (Medi-tech, Boston Scientific, Natick, MA) or grabber. The forceps portion of this device consists of four parallel, small, stiff, spring wires, which are prebent so that, when extruded from the end of a catheter, they angle approximately 45° away from the catheter tip. Each wire is separated from the adjacent wire by 90° so the four wires extend as an expanding 'square.' The tip of each of these wires has a 0.5 mm long, fixed 90° angle toward the center, which creates an acute 90° hook facing centrally at the end of each of the wires. As the wires are retracted into the tip of the catheter, they, along with their distal 'hooks,' compress together, making a very effective grabbing tool. The catheter for the grabber is only a 5 French so most of the positioning of the grabber must be through the long, large recovery sheath.

This Grasper™ forceps is an absolutely essential component of the armamentarium for the retrieval of foreign bodies. It is uniquely useful for foreign bodies which have no protrusions or ends extending into the lumen. The tip of the grabber, when it is positioned flush against and even perpendicular to an object, can grasp an almost flat surface of that object. This allows objects imbedded in end vessels to be grasped and withdrawn – for example, a 'wad' of coil wedged into a distal pulmonary artery with no 'end' hanging loose. The down side of this device is that the grabbing forceps tend to grab all and anything in the area while grasping

the foreign body. Occasionally a small amount of vascular adventitia will accompany the foreign body out of the body, but this has caused no permanent sequelae.

The final specific retrieval tool which is very useful for the pediatric interventional laboratory is the Vascular Retrieval Forceps™ (Cook, Inc, Bloomington, IN). This device usually is referred to as the 'jaws' device. It is on a 3 French catheter and has a 1 cm long arm, which is recessed in the catheter and is hinged at the center like a seesaw. When opened, the two 5 mm long halves of the arm extend away from the catheter on the opposite sides of the catheter. The proximal end of the arm is attached to a control wire, which opens and closes the 'jaw' when pushed or pulled, respectively. The distal half of the arm opens away from the tip of the catheter. There are two tiny 'teeth' at the tip of this distal arm. These teeth point toward the catheter, which when closed against the catheter forms a 'jaw.' To facilitate maneuvering through vessels, the catheter of the jaws has a 1 cm segment of flexible spring wire attached to the tip just distal to the jaw mechanism.

Like the 'grabber,' this tool can seize a relatively flat surface of a foreign body, even when there are no protruding parts. This allows the foreign body to be dislodged, but usually the jaws are not strong enough to retrieve a foreign body of any size.

PERSONNEL

The most critical element of any congenital interventional catheterization laboratory is the personnel. The physicians performing the procedures must be trained, skilled, and experienced in the entire spectrum of procedures performed in a particular laboratory. A single physician may perform most of these procedures, but only when assisted by very skilled and trained ancillary personnel. All nurses and technicians should be experts with their particular duties and with any specialized procedure which is being performed. If there are physician or ancillary personnel in training, they should be *in addition* to the adequate number of experienced personnel. There should be adequate numbers of ancillary personnel for each particular assignment. Short staffing of a congenital interventional catheterization laboratory represents a very false economy. When there is just one essential person missing during the procedure, the entire procedure (along with all of the physician and other ancillary personnel) must stop and wait *each time* one of the remaining, equally essential, personnel must leave their position to perform the missing person's task. The cost in time of any waiting time is a multiple of the hourly cost of the *total* number of personnel involved plus a domino effect caused by the delay on the function of the catheterization laboratory and any support services.

By the prevention of complications which otherwise would not occur, an ideal complement of personnel, along with the optimal equipment, are the most effective treatment of complications.

REFERENCE

1. Mullins CE. Cardiac Catheterization in Congenital Heart Disease: Pediatric and Adult. Oxford, UK: Blackwell, 2006.

2 How to stock an adult cardiac catheterization laboratory for congenital and structural heart disease

Ignacio Inglessis and Michael J Landzberg

INTRODUCTION

Until recently, cardiac catheterization procedures in patients with adult congenital heart disease (ACHD) have been performed predominantly by pediatric cardiologists in pediatric cardiac catheterization laboratories. However, as the result of improved medical and surgical therapies for children with congenital heart disease, there has been a rapidly growing population of patients reaching adulthood, many of whom have residual complex lesions.[1] Furthermore, the aging ACHD population frequently suffers from comorbidities not commonly seen in childhood, such as obstructive coronary disease, obesity, chronic lung disease, peripheral atherosclerosis, etc., beyond the level of comfort of many pediatric interventional cardiologists and catheterization laboratory staff for the care of these patients. Technologic advances and the better understanding of the mechanisms and long-term results of individual procedures currently allow for the percutaneous treatment of various forms of congenital, valve, and myocardial heart diseases. For example, percutaneous mitral and pulmonary valvuloplasty is now considered standard of care in patients with suitable anatomy and there is an increasing experience in the percutaneous repair of mitral insufficiency, replacement of pulmonary and aortic valves, and alcohol septal ablation for hypertrophic cardiomyopathy. Consequently, there is a growing need for developing the necessary operator, supporting staff, and technician expertise as well as infrastructure in adult cardiac catheterization laboratories for the optimal care of adult patients with complex congenital and structural heart disease.

In this chapter, we discuss the basic organization, infrastructure, and stocking of the cardiac catheterization laboratory required for the performance of adult congenital and structural heart disease procedures.

DEDICATED PERSONNEL

Undoubtedly, expertise in the anatomy and physiology of adult congenital and structural heart anomalies is essential for all personnel taking part in cardiac catheterization procedures, including physicians, nurses, and cardiovascular technicians. For procedures involving complex ACHD patients, close interaction between pediatric and adult cardiologists may be crucial, as their expertise may be complementary, especially if they are not ACHD-subspecialty trained. Although adult interventional cardiologists with expertise in complex ACHD are relatively rare, fortunately, an increasing number of fellowship programs is now offering dedicated training in the field. The performance of percutaneous/surgical hybrid procedures for the treatment of complex congenital and structural cases, i.e. periventricular device closure of apical muscular ventricular septal defects and percutaneous aortic valve replacement, has brought interventional cardiologists, cardiac surgeons, and anesthesiologists working together in the same arena. Cardiac surgery fellowship programs are offering training in interventional techniques (some including ACHD interventions) to their graduates and, ultimately, true 'hybrid operators' will soon be common.

Echocardiography guidance facilitated by experts in congenital and structural heart disease is crucial for many procedures. While the expert interpretation of transesophageal echocardiography (TEE) studies remains in the domain of the echocardiography specialists, interventional cardiologists are increasingly gaining expertise in the interpretation of intracardiac cardiac echocardiography (ICE) images.

Close interaction with peripheral interventional cardiologists and vascular surgeons is also very important, as large introducers are usually required for congenital and structural heart disease procedures in an aging population with increasing peripheral vascular disease in which surgical or endovascular vessel repair is frequently needed. Furthermore, much of the equipment utilized in adult congenital and structural interventions has been developed primarily for the treatment of peripheral vascular disease and undergoes initial testing by the peripheral vascular interventionalist.

Many complex ACHD patients require concomitant diagnosis and treatment of arrhythmias in addition to cardiac catheterization procedures. An example is the performance of left-sided electrophysiology testing and ablation in patients with Fontan circulation via a fenestration prior to its percutaneous device closure. The modern cardiac catheterization suite should allow for this complex interaction to occur smoothly.

Nurses and cardiovascular technicians play a vital role in the cardiac catheterization team. A core group of nurses and technicians should be identified and trained in adult congenital and structural heart disease, as familiarity with the complexity of many procedures improves case flow and safety.

ROOM INFRASTRUCTURE

A spacious room is essential and should allow comfortable placement of ancillary equipment such as an anesthesia station, echocardiography and left ventricular assist device consoles, and even extracorporeal membrane oxygenation (ECMO) equipment, when needed. Space should be available for a large sterile table needed for the assembly of large stents, closure devices, and percutaneous valves.

Setting up of a combined hybrid operating room/ cardiac catheterization laboratory suite imposes great challenges, as the typical catheterization lab frequently lack the prerequisites required to function as operating rooms. A strategy planning multidisciplinary team involving medical staff, nursing managers, perfusion technicians, business administrators, infection control, applications specialists, architects, and engineers needs to work in unison in dealing with the particular challenges of each site.[2] Efficient space utilization is of the utmost importance in hybrid rooms due to the large amount and complexity of equipment required for their functioning, and mobile cabinetry for storage of catheterization and surgical equipment improves space efficiency. Other design requirements include non-paneled ceilings, laminar air flow with greater than 10 air exchanges per hour, temperature and humidity control, overhead surgical lights and wall-mounted connections for electricity, air, and gases required by anesthesia, cardiopulmonary bypass, and ECMO consoles, electrocautery equipment, fiber optic light sources for bronchoscopy procedures, etc.[3] Finally, infection control policies impose mandatory stringent access to the catheterization suite and the use of traditional surgical attire for all hybrid procedures.

ANCILLARY MONITORING SYSTEMS

The hemodynamic monitoring system should allow quality recordings of three pressure transducers simultaneously, which ought to be easy to calibrate and interexchange, and at least three simultaneous electrocardiogram leads, with an option for 12-lead recording when electrophysiology studies are contemplated. Adequacy and fidelity of electrocardiographic monitoring cannot be overemphasized, as some of the most common serious complications occurring in the ACHD or structural heart disease catheterization laboratory may involve breech of adequate coronary arterial flow for a host of supply or demand reasons, and most rapid recognition of such is mandated for optimal safety. Similarly, strategies for optimal sedation strategies, coupled with 'on-line' assessment of CNS function and perfusion abnormalities, should be arranged between anesthesia, nursing, and medical support staffs. Accurate oximeters and a metabolic rate meter to measure (rather than estimate) oxygen consumption are required for the precise measurement of cardiac output by the Fick oxygen principle. The hemodynamics software should allow for the easy calculation of cardiac output, shunts, and vascular resistances.

Overdrive rapid right ventricular pacing decreases ventricular ejection and is required to prevent valve embolization during percutaneous aortic and pulmonary valve implantation. A temporary pacing system that allows for pacing rates greater than 200 per minute is often necessary.

URGENT-USE MEDICATIONS

The adult congenital or structural heart disease patient poses novel physiologies in addition to anatomies for the sole pediatric or adult-trained specialist. Familiarity with and rapid availability of:

- periprocedural assessment for, and utilization of, renal-protective strategies
- intravenous and oral nitrate preparations, intravenous nitroprusside, and calcium antagonists
- intravenous IIb–IIIa inhibitors and thrombolytics for treatment of acute thrombosis
- intravenous prostanoids, acetylcholine, adenosine
- inhaled nitric oxide

are strongly suggested for the ACHD or structural heart disease catheterization laboratory.

IMAGING SYSTEMS

Biplane digital imaging systems are mandatory for congenital and structural interventional cases. The flat panel X-ray detector technology offers improved image quality over the traditional image intensifier and is gaining acceptance. A larger detector size (30 × 40 cm) is now preferred for the anteroposterior (AP) plane to facilitate imaging of larger areas of the circulatory system in adults, however steep angulations are limited. A smaller detector (20 × 20 cm) is usually sufficient for the lateral plane. Flexible architecture using floor or ceiling mounts is becoming important in the design and adequate function of the crowded hybrid catheterization laboratory.

Current X-ray equipment offers automatic selection of the optimal X-ray exposure, significantly reducing the radiation dose, digital subtraction angiography, and road mapping capabilities.

At least four flat panel digital monitors are required, two for live AP and lateral fluoroscopy, one to display a stored image as a 'road map', and one for pressures/EKG display. An additional monitor for the display of ancillary imaging, such as transthoracic echocardiography (TTE), TEE, ICE, or intravascular ultrasound (IVUS) is increasingly required.

ICE and TEE are essential for the performance of device closure of intracardiac defects, percutaneous mitral valve repair and aortic valve replacement, and transseptal placement of the Tandem Heart mechanical assist devices. TTE is required for monitoring percutaneous mitral valvuloplasty and alcohol septal ablation for hypertrophic cardiomyopathy procedures. Catheterization laboratories with a large volume of adult congenital and structural heart cases usually own an ICE console, which also allows for TTE and TEE studies, using the appropriate probes.

Three-dimensional TEE has recently emerged as a promising technique with the potential for improving the geometric analysis of intracardiac defects, optimizing closure procedures. IVUS is an excellent technique for the accurate assessment and tissue characterization of vascular lesions, as well as to evaluate the results of endovascular interventions. IVUS has been extensively used in coronary interventions, with a growing experience in larger vessels utilizing lower frequency catheters with deeper penetration.

Portable ultrasound consoles with Doppler capabilities (Site-Rite 3™, Bard; SonoSite 180™, SonoSite) are useful to localize blood vessels and facilitate accurate needle placement in patients with difficult vascular access, particularly in the venous system. These devices have small handheld probes, which can be brought to the sterile field with the use of sleeves.

BASIC EQUIPMENT

Beyond the basic equipment required for the performance of diagnostic catheterization in patients with coronary, valvular, and peripheral vascular disease, additional stocking is required for the performance of congenital and structural heart disease interventions. A complete description of each individual piece of equipment is beyond the scope of this chapter; however, many devices have similar performance characteristics and individual operators only need to become familiar with a small number of them in each category.

Needles for percutaneous puncture

An 18-gauge 7–8 cm long single-piece and thin-walled needle is commonly used for femoral arterial and

venous access in adult patients. In those patients with femoral arterial or venous occlusive disease, or when internal jugular/subclavian venous or radial/brachial/axillary arterial access is required, a Micropuncture kit is preferred. This kit consists of a 21-gauge needle, a 45-cm 0.018-inch guide wire, and a 4 or 5 French introducer, and is available from several manufacturers (Bard, Abbot, Cook).

Transseptal puncture is performed when direct recording of left atrial hemodynamics is warranted, and in percutaneous mitral valvuloplasty and repair, mitral prosthetic perivalvular leak closure, and device closure of apically located ventricular septal defects. The standard equipment for transseptal puncture in adults includes a 72 cm long Brockenbrough™ needle (USCI-Medtronic) in combination with an 8F Mullins transseptal sheath/dilator set (Cook, Cordis, Arrow, Medtronic), although additional needle and sheath potentials should be trialed and stocked, per needs of staff. The Brockenbrough needle tapers from an 18-gauge shaft to a 20-gauge tip and accepts a 0.025-inch guide wire. In the ideal Mullins sheath/dilator set the dilator should be 2 cm shorter than the needle and the sheath 2 cm shorter than the dilator. The sheath should also have a radio-opaque band at the tip.

Transhepatic venous access is occasionally needed in adult patients with severe iliofemoral venous occlusive disease and requires a 22-gauge 15 cm long Chiba needle (Cook). Direct left ventricular apical puncture is the only possible access to the left ventricle in patients with mechanical prostheses in the aortic and mitral positions, and is indicated when accurate left ventricular hemodynamics and angiography are required and for the evaluation of mitral perivalvular leaks. This procedure can be performed with a single-piece 18-gauge needle followed by placement of a 4 French pigtail over a 0.0035-in guide wire, or a commercially available 22-gauge needle/6 French pigtail assembled set (Cook), primarily used for pleural drainage.

Guide wires

Standard 0.035-in 145-cm long, soft J-tipped wires are the workhorses for arterial and venous vascular access in adults. In patients with vascular obstructive disease, or when navigation over significantly tortuous vessels is required, the 0.035-in Wholey High Torque™ (Mallinckrodt) or the Magic Torque™ (Boston Scientific) wires are safer and more successful. For severely tortuous vessels, hydrophilic coated glidewires (Terumo, Boston Scientific) have excellent tracking capabilities; however, they often offer inadequate support for the delivery of catheters or balloons. The potential for these coated glidewires to subtend atherosclerotic plaque and facilitate dissection is recognized. When stiffer shaft wires are needed for delivery of large catheters, sheaths, or dilation balloons, moderate support (Rosen™,

Mallinckrodt) or heavy support (Amplatzer Extra or Supra Stiff™, Boston Scientific; Lunderquist™, Cook) wires are preferred. Multiple 0.014-in and 0.018-in standard (145–190-cm long) or exchange length (260–300-cm long) wires, primarily developed for coronary and peripheral interventions, are certainly useful to facilitate access and deliver interventional equipment to small vessels.

Although the list of available wires in the market is large, each operator should become familiar with a short list of low (Hi-Torque Floppy II™, Guidant), moderate (Balance Middle Weight™, Guidant), and high (Iron Man™, Hi-Torque Spartacore and Hi-Torque Steelcore™ [0.018-in], Guidant; Platinum-Plus™, Boston Scientific; Stablilizer Plus™, Cordis) support wires, as well as hydrophilic wires (PT Graphix™ and V-18 control™ [0.018-in], Boston Scientific; Whisper™, Guidant). More recently, steerable deflecting tip guide wires (Steer-IT™, Cordis) have been developed to facilitate access to vessels with right or acute angle of origin.

Diagnostic catheters

There are multiple diagnostic catheters available for adult cardiac catheterization, both for angiographic and hemodynamic assessment. Side-hole catheters such as the Pigtail, Multi-track, and Omni Flush are usually sufficient for angiography and pressure recording of cardiac chambers and greater vessels. The Swan–Ganz and other flow-directed balloon-tipped catheters are used mostly for evaluation of right-sided hemodynamics and pulmonary arterial angiography. Several preshaped end-hole catheters are available to facilitate access to side branches or cross stenotic orifices, such as the Judkins, Amplatz, Multipurpose, Internal mammary, Berenstein, Benson, and Cobra catheters. Use of these shaped, highly controlled, torqueable catheters can frequently save the operator substantial time in the intubation of desired vessels.

Sheaths and guide catheters

Long sheaths or guide catheters are used for the delivery of interventional equipment to the desired location and there are important distinctions between them. For a similar French size, long sheaths have a larger lumen diameter compared to guide catheters and allow delivery of larger size equipment. Sheaths are usually more kink resistant than catheters, as they have a thicker braided wall. An advantage of guide catheters over long sheaths is the multiple preshaped curves available, facilitating access to difficult to engage vessels.

Multiple long sheaths are available from Cook, Arrow, and Medtronic, from 5 to 24 French in diameter and 45 to 90 cm in length, all containing a hemostatic valve and flush ports. The Check-Flow Performer™ sheaths (Cook) are the most versatile and widely used, as they are available in multiple sizes, lengths, and preshaped curves (Mullins, Balkin, HausdorfLock, Raabe). A recent modification of the traditional Cook sheath design led to the Flexor Check-Flo™ line, which are more flexible and kink resistant. The Flexor Check-Flow™ sheaths are available with the option of a Tuohy-Borst™ valve to facilitate delivery of large equipment and decrease the risk for stent dislodgement from delivery balloons, occasionally seen with the use of sheaths with traditional hemostatic valves. Metal-braided sheaths (Super Arrow-Flex™, Arrow), available up to 11 and French and 80 cm long, are particularly kink resistant, although sometimes difficult to track around severe tortuousity. A number of tip-deflecting steerable guide catheters designed for use in electrophysiology settings may have particular use in congenital and structural heart disease settings, and familiarity with the available inventory is suggested.

Balloon dilation catheters

Similar to guide wires and catheters, there are numerous (perhaps hundreds) angioplasty balloons available for adult interventional procedures.

Medium diameter dilation balloons (6–12 mm)

Dilatation balloons in this size range include the Ultra Thin Diamond™, SDS™ (both from Boston Scientific), and Opta Pro™ (Cordis) balloons. These balloons are relatively non-compliant, tolerating 10 to 15 atm of pressure. The new Blue Max™ (Boston Scientific) and Conquest™ (Bard) balloons are highly non-compliant, tolerating pressures up to 25 atm, making them ideal for dilation of rigid vascular structures. The Conquest™ balloon has very long shoulders and should be used with caution when dilating tortuous or angulated vascular segments.

Large diameter dilation balloons (> 12 mm)

These balloons are typically used for the dilation of and stent delivery to large vascular structures, such as for the treatment of coarctation of the aorta and stenotic conduits, and for balloon valvuloplasty.

The most commonly used large balloons include the Tyshak X™, Z-MED X™, and Z-MED II X™ (NuMED); XXL™ (Boston Scientific), and Maxi LD™(Cordis). The NuMED balloons are also available in medium diameter sizes, making them a versatile line facilitating stocking and inventory. The Tyshak X™ is a thin-walled balloon with the lowest profile and is ideal for patients with significant vascular disease; however, the trade off is a very low maximum burst pressure and poor trackability in the larger sizes. The Z-MED X™ and Z-MED II X™ balloons have thicker walls, tolerating higher pressures, and are the most frequently used balloons for valvuloplasty in adult patients who can tolerate sheaths in the 12 to 14F range.

The Atlas™ (Bard) balloon is made of the same, very non-compliant material as the Conquest™ balloon, tolerating up to 16 atm of pressure for the 20 mm balloon; however, they also have very long shoulders that limit their use in curved structures.

Specialty balloons

The Balloon in Balloon (BIB)™ (NuMED) includes by an inner balloon which is half the diameter and 1 cm shorter than the outer balloon and has a separate inflation port. The unique sequential inflation property of this balloon renders it ideal for the deployment of stents.

The Cutting balloons™ (Boston Scientific) have small and sharp blades along the longitudinal axis of a non-compliant balloon, emerging to the surface upon inflation. The blades are intended to incise the intima and media of highly resistant stenosis, improving the final lumen and facilitating stent deployment. The Inoue balloon™ (Toray) is the preferred technique for percutaneous mitral valvuloplasty in the adult and it has been increasingly used for percutaneous antegrade aortic valvuloplasty as well.

Endovascular stents

Currently, there are no stents specifically manufactured for the endovascular treatment of adult congenital and structural lesions. Therefore, the adoption of stents developed for the treatment of atherosclerotic lesions or biliary tree obstructions is mandatory.

Large vessel stents (> 12 mm)

The Genesis XD™ (Cordis) is the mostly commonly used stent for the treatment of congenital lesions up to 18 mm in diameter. Its 'closed cell' design with round ends provides flexibility and minimal edge injury to the vessel. As is the case for all large stents available in the United States, the Genesis XD™ stent has to be hand mounted to the delivery balloon.

The Palmaz™ P308 (Cordis) was the only balloon-expandable stent available for many years and was used extensively in congenital heart disease. However, its use has fallen out of favor as it is relatively rigid, difficult to deliver through tortuous segments, and its sharp edges increase the risk for vessel damage upon deployment.

Other large-vessel balloon-expandable stents available include the Mega LD™ and Maxi LD™ (ev3) and the Cheetham-Platinum C-P™ (NuMED); the latter is not available in the United States except in clinical trials.

Medium size vessel stent (6–12 mm)

The Medium and Large Genesis™ (Cordis), Express™ Biliary (Boston Scientific), ParaMount™ (ev3), Palmaz Blue™ (Cordis), and Formula 418™ (Cook) stents are available for medium sized vessels. All these stents are premounted on delivery balloons, improving safety of delivery.

Closure devices

The Amplatzer ASD, PFO, PDA, VSD, and Vascular plug™ (AGA), CardioSEAL, STARFlex, and BioSTAR™ (NMT Medical), Helex™ (Gore), and Premere™ (St Jude) closure devices are available or undergoing testing in the US and abroad. The merits of each device are discussed in different chapters.

Vascular closure devices for appropriate arteriotomies and larger venotomies, as discussed elsewhere in this text, are used more frequently in adult patients. It remains unclear whether such devices add to the overall safety profile in the general population of catheterization suites, but their use may be appropriate in particular laboratories.

Retrieval devices

The snare retrieval devices are the most widely used systems for the extraction of foreign bodies due to their simplicity and versatility. Commercially available systems include the Amplatz™ Goose-Neck snare (Microvena), Medi-tech™ snare (Boston Scientific), and En Snare™ (Medical Device Technologies). The latter is constructed with three separate interlaced loops, increasing the ability to retrieve large foreign bodies.

Basket retrieval devices, such as the Medi-Tech™ basket (Boston Scientific) and Dotter™ Intravascular retriever (Cook) are specially constructed for the extraction of large foreign objects and require very large sheaths for use.

MECHANICAL ASSIST DEVICES

Mechanical assist devices have been used extensively for supporting patients with acute myocardial infarction and cardiogenic shock secondary to severe left ventricular dysfunction, severe mitral insufficiency, or ventricular septal rupture, as well as for patients with refractory ventricular arrhythmias or undergoing high-risk percutaneous coronary interventions.

The intra-aortic balloon pump (IABP) remains the most commonly used support device due to its simplicity, ease of insertion, and long track record. Nevertheless, IABP support requires active left ventricular ejection and a normally functioning aortic valve, and can only increase the cardiac output by 10–15%. More recently, innovative left ventricular assist devices have been developed that depend much less on active myocardial ejection for increasing cardiac output, including the Impella Recover® (Abiomed) and the Tandem Heart PTVA™ (CardiacAssist) devices. The Impella device is a microaxial blood pump placed through the aortic valve, aspirating blood from the left ventricle and expelling it into the ascending aorta. The Impella LP 2.5 model is inserted percutaneously via the femoral artery through a 13F sheath, providing flow up to 2.5 l/min, and can be used for up to 5 days. The Impella LP 5.0 model is inserted via cutdown in the femoral artery, providing up to 5.0 l/min of flow, and can be used for up to 10 days. The Tandem Heart percutaneous venous assist (PTVA) device is an extracorporeal blood pump that drains blood from the left atrium via a transseptally placed 21 F sheath, actively pumping blood back into the body via a percutaneously placed 15 or 17F femoral sheath. Obviously, peripheral vascular disease is a major limitation for the use of either device. Both of these technologies are now being modified for right ventricular assistance.

There is growing experience on the use of the newer generation left ventricular assist device in adult congenital or structural heart percutaneous procedures. The most extensive experience so far is on the use of the Tandem Heart assist device in performing high-risk percutaneous aortic valvuloplasty or percutaneous valve replacement.

CONCLUSIONS

The rapidly growing field of adult congenital and structural heart disease interventional procedures imposes great organizational challenges to the traditional adult cardiac catheterization laboratory. A well designed and coordinated effort led by a core group of personnel with expertise in the field, involving significant changes in the catheterization suite infrastructure and stocking of numerous accessory equipment and material, is required for success.

REFERENCES

1. Warnes CA, Liberthson R, Danielson GJ et al. Task Force 1: the changing profile of congenital heart disease in adult life. J Am Coll Cardiol 2001; 37: 117–15.
2. Hirsch R. The hybrid cardiac catheterization laboratory for congenital heart disease: from conception to completion. Cathet Cardiovasc Int 2007; 71: 418–28.
3. The American Institute of Architects. Guidelines for the Design and Construction of Hospitals and Health Care Facilities (Section 7.10.H1-H11). Washington, DC: The American Institute of Architects, 2001; 49–50.

3 How to build a hybrid congenital heart disease program

John P Cheatham

BACKGROUND

The advances in surgical therapy for congenital heart disease (CHD) have mirrored the progress in transcatheter techniques and materials, especially in the past two decades. Yet the disciplines of cardiothoracic surgery and interventional cardiology have taken decidedly different paths for success. In the world of acquired heart disease, adult cardiologists and surgeons frequently have been at odds, or competitive, in their quest to treat coronary artery disease. However, a 'team approach' has always been required to build a successful program dedicated to CHD. It takes a cooperative spirit between multiple specialists, such as cardiologists, surgeons, anesthesiologists, intensivists, nurses, and technicians, to treat infants, children, and adults with complex CHD. None-the-less, surgical management strategies have differed from transcatheter options – similar to our adult colleagues.

Sometimes, the challenges and obstacles confronting the CHD surgeon in the operative theater mirror the barriers facing the CHD interventional cardiologist for success in the cardiac catheterization laboratory. As time has passed, it has become more obvious to both specialists that, if they combine their talents, they may in fact eliminate some of these obstacles and improve outcomes. So, we have coined the term *Hybrid Therapy* to signify this new spirit of collaboration. According to *Webster's, Revised Unabridged Dictionary*, 1996, the definition of Hybrid \Hy"brid\, n. [L. hybrida, hibrida, (Biol.)] is the offspring of the union of two distinct species; an animal or plant produced from the mixture of two species. Some would argue that the cardiothoracic surgeon and the interventional cardiologist are definitely two different species – different training, different manners, different expectations, and definitely different salaries! However, those differences continue to disappear as the disciplines come closer and closer together and new management strategies emerge.

So, exactly what *is* a Hybrid approach? First, it starts with a collaborative effort between the cardiothoracic surgeon and interventional cardiologist. It continues with careful planning of a management strategy involving the other services within The Heart Center – namely, the other cardiologists, anesthesiologists, intensive care team, nurses, perfusionists, and even outside services such as neonatology and radiology. This type of approach encourages the sharing of ideas, expertise, equipment, and techniques. It allows one to think 'outside the box' and to develop novel treatment strategies. We have coined the term *Two Perspectives. Single Focus.* to represent the spirit of the Hybrid approach.

The goals of Hybrid therapy are many: (1) to reduce both morbidity and mortality, (2) to reduce the cumulative impact of multiple interventions often required to treat those with complex CHD, (3) to improve the quality of life, (4) to deliver more efficient and cost-effective care, and (5) to encourage *teamwork*. However, there are a few requirements for initiating a successful Hybrid program. First and foremost, there can be *no competition* between the surgeon and interventionalist, economically or professionally! There must be mutual respect for each other and the talents and limitations that each possess. It is important that no individual's opinion is weighted more than the other – it is a *partnership*. All members of The Heart Center team must also be supportive of this new concept, for someone must refer the patients for treatment, someone must care for them while recovering in the CICU (cardiac intensive care unit) and ward, and someone must closely follow the patients in the outpatient clinic to assess the outcome.

A NEW VENUE

As the level of collaboration between the surgeon and interventionalist increased, the need for a specially designed therapeutic suite that allows both disciplines to 'feel at home' became evident. In the past, the surgeon would be called to the 'cath lab' when there was trouble. This necessitated an emergent intervention without the conventional operative equipment, such as overhead surgical light, instruments, headlight, electrocautery, and a place for the perfusionists and cardiopulmonary bypass circuit. Conversely, when the interventionalist was called to the 'OR' it meant that a possible misdiagnosis was made. This required that a portable X-ray angiographic unit be available and wheeled into the room; someone then had to be found to run it; there were no catheters or devices, no monitors, and a surgical table that had metal railings with metal surgical instruments spread throughout the field to ensure that no X-ray image could be obtained easily. So, the idea of a *Hybrid Suite* was born.

It is fundamental that a decision is made as to whether this Hybrid Suite will be a primary venue for cardiac catheterization or surgery, because the design, space, personnel, equipment, and cost will be different. Typically, the staff involved in a Hybrid CHD case will obviously be the interventionalist and surgeon; cardiac anesthesiologist; echocardiographer; nurse practitioners, physicians assistants, and fellows as first assistants; ancillary staff such as scrub nurses (surgical and interventional), cath lab and radiology technicians; perfusionists; and sometimes the electrophysiologist – making quite a large number of people in a single suite, all trying to do their jobs! One must not forget that each of these specialists requires equipment to be present to allow them to be successful. So, in planning a Hybrid Suite, there are two major considerations: *adequate space* and *information management and transport*. Currently, it is possible to install the needed integrated systems in an existing catheterization or surgical suite. However, incorporating a systematic approach in all stages of planning and construction is optimal for maximum functionality.

In a perfect world, a minimum of 900 square feet would be allowed for the procedure space in a Hybrid Cardiac Catheterization Suite (Figure 3.1) and 800 square feet in a Cardiac Hybrid Operative Suite (Figure 3.2), allowing for the difference of installing a biplane versus a single plane X-ray imaging system, respectively. One must also account for a large control room with optimal viewing, a cold computer room, an induction room for anesthesia, and a supply room. Floor space reserved for surgical and catheterization trays and tables, anesthesia and echocardiography machines, along with the cardiopulmonary bypass circuit must be available. All of these machines and equipment are located on the floor, but one should plan all other equipment and monitors to be ceiling mounted in order to optimize working space. This includes equipment booms and strategically placed flat panel video monitors to ensure that at least two monitors are in view to any operator or staff, regardless of the location within the Suite. An information management system is essential to control the staggering amounts of information generated in the healthcare environment and Hybrid Suite, and to make these data available at any time and at any place during the procedure. Consider the images from angiography, echocardiography (transthoracic, transesophageal, intracardiac, intravascular, epicardial), computer assisted tomography, magnetic resonance imaging, as well as strategically placed video and endoscopic cameras and then one can get an idea of the importance of careful planning – and the financial resources required! The next area for Hybrid development is a procedural table that is suitable for both the surgeon and the interventionalist, possessing the movement, size, shape, and fluoroscopic integration into the X-ray imaging equipment. Several manufacturers are currently working on this project.

Having said all of this, one interventional colleague perhaps summarized what is *really* most important to start a Hybrid program for CHD. Evan M Zahn MD,

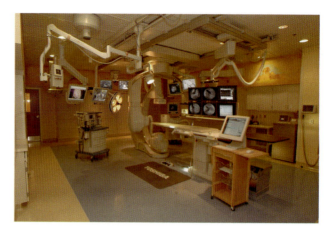

Figure 3.1 This picture is one of two Hybrid Cardiac Catheterization Suites that opened at Nationwide Children's Hospital in June 2004. Note the strategic location of the equipment and video monitor booms, surgical equipment, and the necessary space to allow all team members to easily perform their duties – even in a biplane configuration.

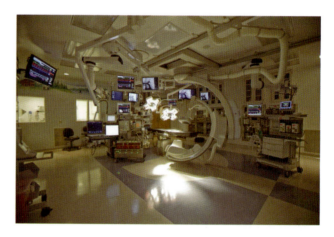

Figure 3.2 In comparison to Figure 3.5, the Cardiac Hybrid Operative Suite has a single plane X-ray imaging system incorporated into the Suite design, with equipment and video monitor booms easily manipulated around the 'fluoro friendly' surgical table and cardiopulmonary bypass circuit. This Hybrid Suite opened in November 2007.

Director of Pediatric Cardiology at Miami Children's Hospital stated:

For the better part of the past decade I have been getting questions regarding the details of our 'hybrid suite.' The reality is that we have never had one (although we too are currently in the planning stages to build one) … My point is that with the right approach, right personnel, surgeons who really want the procedure to work, and some creativity you can reproducibly perform all of the hybrid procedures I know of (and invent the ones you don't) with excellent results and outcomes … While there is little doubt that these newly designed hybrid rooms will offer some clear advantages in terms of versatility and procedural ease, I firmly believe that they are

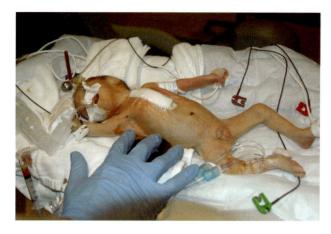

Figure 3.3 Size is not a contraindication to Hybrid therapy, as demonstrated by this 1.1 kg neonate who successfully underwent PA bands and PDA stent for palliation of complex CHD.

NOT a prerequisite to performing these types of procedures and that people should not feel that because they don't have large patches of real estate … that they can't begin a hybrid program … In my opinion the most important determinants of success with regard to hybrid procedures are not the room size, or even room design, but rather the ability to truly create a new operating philosophy among your entire team, a new way of thinking about treating patients and a team desire to innovate.

Stated more succinctly and perhaps in more *surgeon talk*, my surgical partner, Mark Galantowicz MD, Chief of Cardiothoracic Surgery and C-Director of The Heat Center at Nationwide Children's Hospital, stated 'A Hybrid approach is merely the right attitude and a sense of collaboration.'

HYBRID PROCEDURES AND EDUCATION

So the question should beg, exactly who qualifies for a Hybrid procedure for CHD? As our experience has evolved over the past 8 years, we believe that *anyone*, regardless of size or complexity of disease, who would benefit from a procedure that combines the talents of multiple interdisciplinary teams, qualifies (Figure 3.3). Over a 5-year period at Nationwide Children's Hospital, July 2002 to June 2007, 140 Hybrid cardiac procedures were performed in patients with complex CHD, ranging in age from 2 days to 62 years (median 14 days), weighing from 1.1 kg to 120 kg (median 3.5 kg), and where 75% were < 2 years and 10 kg. The patients were divided into seven groups according to the type of procedure:

  group I: extreme premature neonates and/or vascular access difficulties [9] (Figure 3.4a–f)
  group II: intraoperative stents [12] (Figure 3.5a–d)

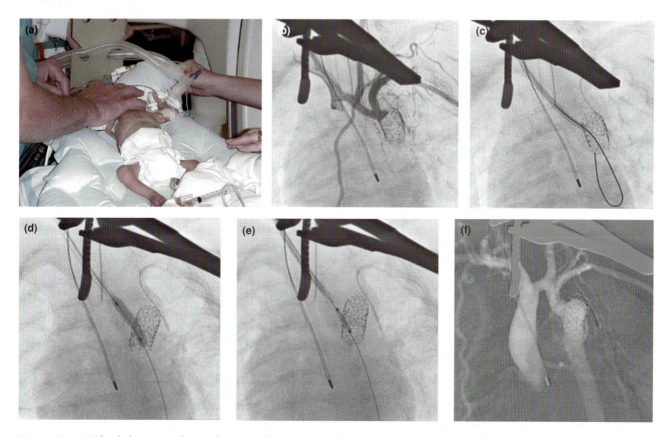

Figure 3.4 Hybrid therapy utilizing the surgical team to perform right carotid artery cutdown (a) in a 1.1 kg neonate with recurrent and complete aortic arch obstruction associated with complex CHD (b). After wire perforation (c), balloon angioplasty was performed (d), followed by stent implantation (e). The final angiogram nicely demonstrates restored antegrade aortic flow (f).

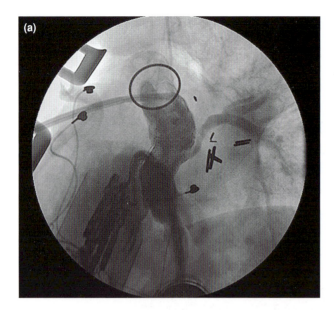

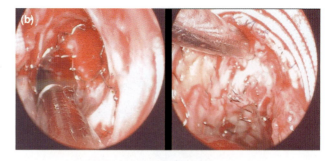

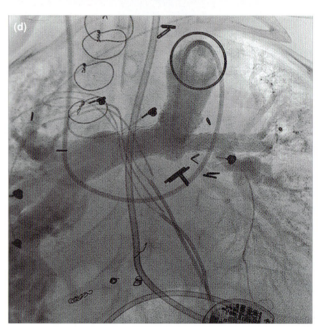

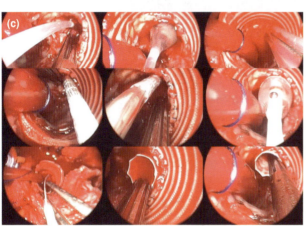

Figure 3.5 Intraoperative stenting can sometimes save the surgeon a great deal of time and effort when performing complete intracardiac repair in a patient with multiple previous surgeries. An RV–PA conduit angiogram demonstrates the complex PA anatomy and severe LPA in-stent stenosis and hypoplasia in this 4-year-old (a). Intraoperative endoscopic imaging demonstrates the previously implanted LPA stent and severe in-stent stenosis (b). In the following series of endoscopic images a guide wire is inserted, followed by cutting balloon angioplasty and then a covered balloon expandable stent (c). The final angiogram nicely demonstrates re-established flow to the LPA with excellent filling of the distal vessels (d).

group III: perventricular muscular VSD closure [6] (Figure 3.6 a-c)

group IV: young adults requiring combined interventional and electrophysiology/pacemaker interventions [33]

group V: unusual and/or uncommon Hybrid procedures [4] (Figure 3.7a–e)

group VI: intraoperative diagnostic angiography [12] (Figure 3.8)

group VII: pulmonary artery bands with PDA stent [64] (Figure 3.9a–f).

Before the two Hybrid Cardiac Catheterization Suites opened in June 2004, procedures were performed in the traditional cath lab [4], cardiothoracic operating room [40], and serially in both locations [16]. Since the specially designed Suites were opened, Hybrid procedures have mostly been performed in this venue [80]. So, as Dr Zahn so eloquently pointed out in an earlier quote, it is not necessary to have these specially designed Suites to begin a Hybrid program – it is just nicer and perhaps easier for everyone to perform their assigned duties.

The new Cardiac Hybrid Operative Suite at Nationwide Children's Hospital opened in November 2007, giving three specially designed venues to perform Hybrid procedures, along with a newly designed second Cardiac Operative Suite without a permanent X-ray imaging system. As expected, the number of Hybrid procedures steadily increased during 2007. Forty-six procedures were performed during August–December 2007, with 26 interventions in the two Hybrid Cardiac Catheterization Suites and 20 performed in the Cardiac Hybrid Operative Suite and second Operative Suite.

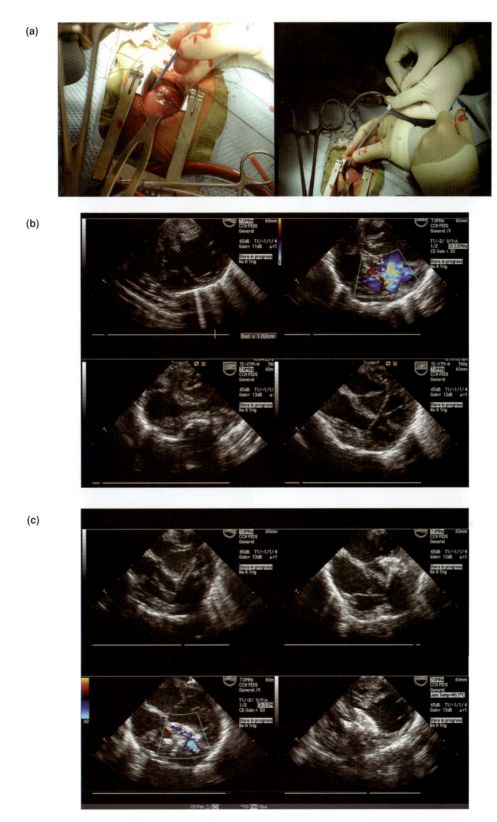

Figure 3.6   A small median sternotomy off cardiopulmonary bypass is performed to allow perventricular closure of a muscular VSD. It is important that the surgeon and interventionalist work closely in a relatively confined space, as evident in this small infant (a). An equally important component to the success of this Hybrid procedure is a skilled echocardiographer. The transesophageal echo nicely demonstrates the defect as well as visualization of the proper angle for needle entry and placing the wire from the RV into the LV (b). After the sheath is carefully inserted, the LV disc, middle waist and RV disc of the Amplatzer device are deployed (c). After device release, the defect is completely closed … all without the need for cardiopulmonary bypass.

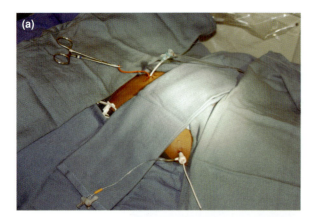

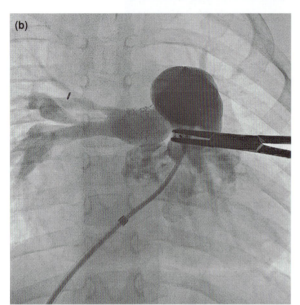

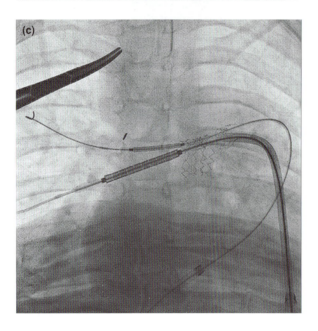

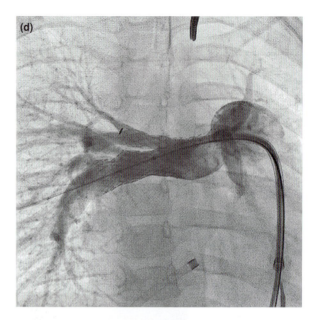

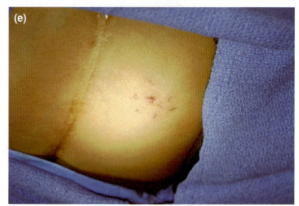

Figure 3.7 By thinking 'outside the box', sometimes impossible challenges are overcome. A 3-year-old with very complex CHD and without conventional vascular access presented with recurrent multiple sites of PA stenoses. After transhepatic access was performed and angiography demonstrated the anatomic position of the RV-PA conduit, percutaneous transthoracic needle entry by the surgeon was performed, which allowed a sheath to be placed (a, b). Two stents were delivered simultaneously (c), with the final angiogram demonstrating significant improvement (d). The suture mediated Perclose device was used to close the hole in the conduit made by the large sheath and prevented bleeding from the chest site (e).

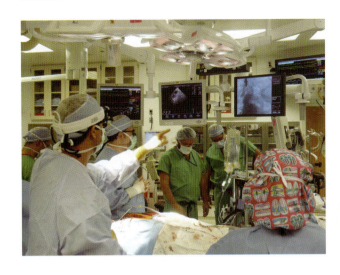

Figure 3.8 Completion angiograms are now more routinely performed in our new Cardiac Hybrid Operative Suite after complex CHD surgery where echocardiography cannot provide adequate imaging.

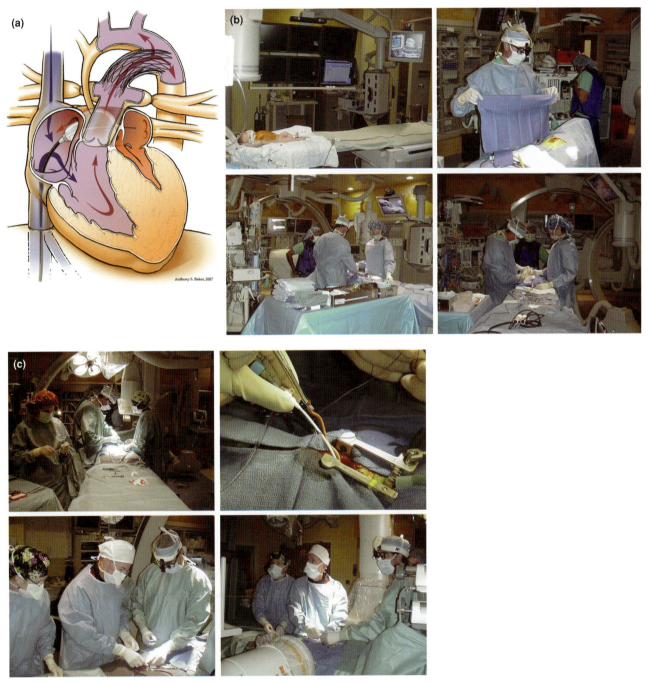

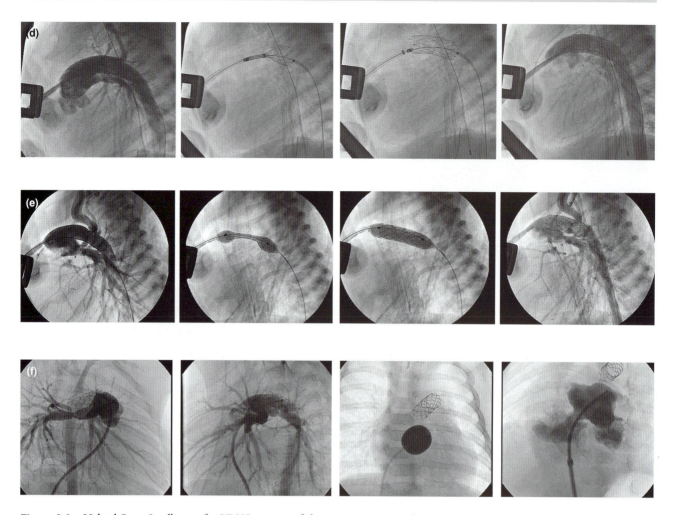

Figure 3.9   Hybrid Stage I palliation for HLHS consists of three components as depicted by this cartoon: PA bands, PDA stent, and creation of an adequate ASD (a). After a median sternotomy off cardiopulmonary bypass, the surgeon places Gore-Tex bands around the LPA and RPA (b). Next, the interventional team moves into place and, after a sheath has been placed in the proximal MPA, the angiographic unit is moved into a lateral position (c). One can use either a self expandable (d) or a balloon expandable stent (e) to effectively maintain patency of the PDA. Balloon atrial septostomy is performed prior to discharge, while the PA bands and PDA stent are also assessed (f).

Currently, it is our policy to perform *completion angiograms* after single ventricle repair, complex two ventricle repair, and those surgeries where the aorta and pulmonary arteries require reconstruction and cannot be imaged by transesophageal echocardiography. We also now routinely perform endoscopic-assisted intraoperative pulmonary artery stenting during complete CHD repair (10 already), rather than spending the extra time on cardiopulmonary bypass for surgical dissection and patch augmentation (Figure 3.10). All of the Hybrid Suites are interconnected via digital audio and video cables through a video router located in each of the three Hybrid Suites and the new Cardiac Operative Suite, which in turn are connected to the Cardiac Teleconference Center which serves as the 'mother ship' for communication. This allows a seamless transfer of information and procedures both within as well as outside The Heart Center at Nationwide Children's Hospital.

In order to improve the collaboration necessary between cardiothoracic surgeons and interventional cardiologists to initiate and sustain a Hybrid Cardiac Program, the International Symposium for the Hybrid Approach to Congenital Heart Disease (ISHAC) was started in 2006 and continues on a yearly basis. During this 3-day conference, an internationally recognized faculty who pioneered new Hybrid therapies presents lectures, moderates interactive discussions, and performs live case presentations demonstrating Hybrid procedures during the 2–day symposium (Figure 3.11 a and b). Also included in this 3-day event is a unique 1-day skills workshop where the faculty teach selected participants Hybrid procedures in a modern cardiovascular research facility (Figure 3.12a-c). In this way, those attending the conference can return to their institutions at home and initiate a Hybrid Program for CHD after actually performing the procedures as a Hybrid team at ISHAC. Hybrid cardiac procedures for complex CHD are now being performed throughout the world and will allow new management strategies to develop for those that dare think *outside the box*![1–21]

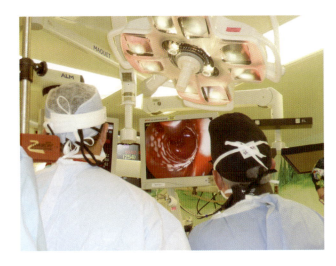

Figure 3.10 In the new Cardiac Hybrid Operative Suite, intraoperative stenting is more routinely performed and is quite easy using endoscopic-assisted delivery and completion angiography.

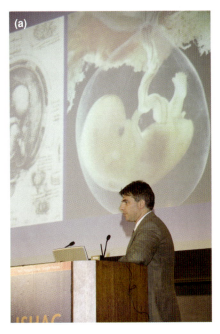

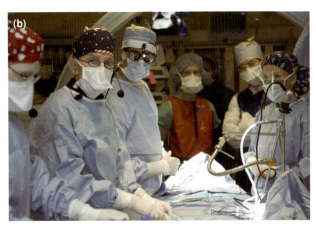

Figure 3.11 In order to facilitate the necessary collaborative spirit required for a successful Hybrid program, the International Symposium on the Hybrid Approach to Congenital Heart Disease (ISHAC) was initiated in 2006. During the two day Symposium, an international faculty who pioneered Hybrid procedures presents lectures, moderates interactive discussions, and performs live case demonstrations of new Hybrid therapies a and b.

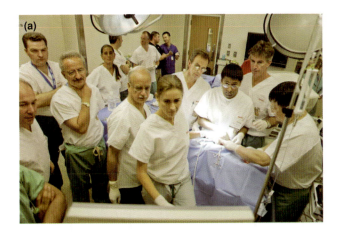

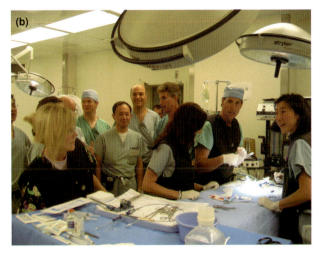

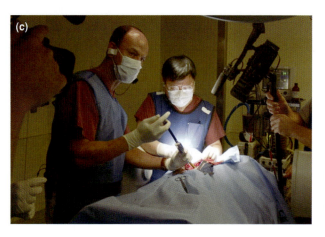

Figure 3.12 A unique aspect of ISHAC is a one day special Skills Workshop where attendees participate in actual Hybrid procedures taught by the faculty in a modern Cardiovascular Research Laboratory (a-c).

REFERENCES

1. Bacha EA, Hijazi ZM, Cao QL et al. Hybrid pediatric cardiac surgery. Pediatr Cardiol 2005; 26(4): 315–22.
2. Hill SL, Galantowicz M, Cheatham JP. Emerging strategies in the treatment of HLHS: combined transcatheter & surgical techniques. Pediatr Cardiol Today 2003; 1(3): 1–5.
3. Akinturk H, Michel-Behnke I, Valeske K et al. Hybrid transcatheter-surgical palliation: basis for univentricular or biventricular repair: the Giessen experience. Pediatr Cardiol 2007; 28(2): 79–87.
4. Galantowicz M, Cheatham JP. Lessons learned from the development of a new Hybrid strategy for the management of hypoplastic left heart syndrome. J Pediatr Cardiol 2005; 26: 190–9.
5. Pigula FA, Vida V, Del Nido P et al. Contemporary results and current strategies in the management of hypoplastic left heart syndrome. Semin Thorac Cardiovasc Surg 2007; 19(3): 238–44.
6. Bacha EA, Daves S, Hardin J et al. Single-ventricle palliation for high-risk neonates: the emergence of an alternative hybrid stage I strategy. J Thorac Cardiovasc Surg 2006; 131(1): 163–71.
7. Caldaron CA, Benson L, Holtby H et al. Initial experience with hybrid palliation for neonates with single-ventricle physiology. Ann Thorac Surg 2007; 84(4): 1294–300.
8. Akinturk H, Michel-Behnke I, Valeske K et al. Stenting of the arterial duct and banding of the pulmonary arteries: basis for combined Norwood stage I and II repair in hypoplastic left heart. Circulation 2002; 105: 1099–103.
9. Galantowicz M, Cheatham JP. Fontan completion without surgery. Pediatr Cardiac Surg Ann Semin Thorac Cardiovasc Surg 2004; 7: 48–55.
10. Diab KA, Cao QL, Mora BN, Hijazi ZM. Device closure of muscular ventricular septal defects in infants less than one year of age using the Amplatzer devices: feasibility and outcome. Cathet Cardiovasc Interven 2007; 70(1): 90–7.
11. Bacha EA, Cao QL, Starr JP et al. Perventricular device closure of muscular ventricular septal defects on the beating heart: technique and results. J Thorac Cardiovasc Surg 2003; 126(6): 1718–23.
12. Murzi B, Bonanomi GL, Giusti S et al. Surgical closure of muscular ventricular septal defects using double umbrella devices (intraoperative VSD device closure). Eur J Cardiothorac Surg 1997; 12(3): 450–5.
13. Amin Z, Danford DA, Lof J et al. Intraoperative device closure of perimembranous ventricular septal defects without cardiopulmonary bypass: preliminary results with the perventricular technique. J Thorac Cardiovasc Surg 2004; 127(1): 234–41.
14. Zeng XJ, Sun SQ, Chen XF et al. Device closure of permembranous ventricular septal defects with a minimally invasive technique. Ann Thorac Surg 2008; 85(1): 192–4.
15. Bacha EA, Cao QL, Galantowicz ME et al. Multicenter experience with perventricular device closure of muscular ventricular septal defects. Pediatr Cardiol 2005; 26: 169–75.
16. Zahn EM, Dobrolet NC, Nykanen DG et al. Interventional catheterization performed in the early postoperative period after congenital heart surgery in children. J Am Coll Cardiol 2004; 43(7): 1264–9.
17. Nykanen DG, Zahn EM. Transcatheter techniques in the management of perioperative vascular obstruction. Cathet Cardiovasc Interven 2005; 66(4): 573–9.
18. Ungerleider RM, Johnston TA, O'Loughlin MP et al. Intraoperative stents to rehabilitate severely stenotic pulmonary vessels. Ann Thorac Surg 2001; 71(2): 476–81.
19. Cheatham JP. Columbus' latest discovery – CCH becomes home to nation's first hybrid cardiac catheterization suites. RT Image 2006; 12: 28–9.
20. Cheatham JP. Columbus Children's Hospital collaborates to build catheterization lab of the future. Cath Lab Digest 2006; 14: 32.
21. Cheatham JP. Where cardiac cath lab meets the OR. HealthImag IT 2006; 4: 31.

4 Complications of vascular access

Neil Wilson

Vascular access to the central circulation is possible via many different routes, each of which carries advantages and disadvantages and potential complications.

Sites of vascular access:

Venous

In order of frequency of use:

femoral vein (right or left, occasionally simultaneously)
internal jugular vein (most often right)
subclavian vein
umbilical vein (predominantly used for balloon atrial septostomy)
umbilical artery
hepatic vein
direct transthoracic cardiac puncture

Arterial

femoral artery
brachial artery
axillary artery
carotid artery
umbilical artery
direct cardiac puncture.

INTRODUCTION

Vascular access is frequently via multiple points of access, particularly for interventional techniques. It almost always involves the use of one or more sheaths. This may mean two venous sheaths from the same access point, such as two sheaths in the femoral vein, or from separate access, such as one sheath in the femoral vein and another in the internal jugular vein.

Venous access is the commonest employed for cardiac catheterization of patients with congenital heart disease, whether that be for a purely diagnostic study for physiologic measurements and angiography or for an interventional procedure. It must be remembered that the very nature of the congenital abnormality may facilitate access to the left side of the circulation by the coexistence of lesions which allow communication between the venous and arterial sides of the circulation.

For example, it is relatively easy to access the left atrium, left ventricle, and aorta through a patent foramen ovale, an atrial septal defect, or a ventricular septal defect when the catheter is initiated from the femoral vein. In more complex forms of congenital heart disease, there may be free communication at the atrial and ventricular level before and after surgical palliation. For example, in a patient who has undergone a Norwood type I style of operation for hypoplastic left heart syndrome, the 'neo-aorta' arises from the right ventricle, and thus can be freely accessed from the femoral vein. Likewise, in such a patient the atrial septum has usually been excised and this gives free access to the left atrium and pulmonary veins from the femoral vein.

The catheter operator should obviously choose the routes of access according to the nature of the procedure, taking into consideration the anticipated maximum size of sheath likely to be used, and the structures which may be involved in the catheter course. As an example, aortic balloon valvuloplasty in the neonate may be performed exclusively from the femoral vein by using a catheter course of right atrium > left atrium > left ventricle > aorta. Some very sick babies may tolerate this approach poorly due to disturbance of myocardial kinetics from the 'splinting' effect of the catheter, or induced mitral regurgitation consequent on catheter position. An alternative would be to perform the valvuloplasty via the femoral, axillary, or carotid artery. Vascular approaches will obviously be discussed fully in the sections addressing specific interventional procedures. Complications may be related to route of access, but they are also related to method and ease of access – such as the Seldinger technique or cut down vessel exposure. The size of sheath/catheter and the length of time it is in situ clearly influence the possibility of local complication. The coexisting use of heparin during the procedure may be mandatory in certain circumstances, such as an interventional closure of an atrial or ventricular septal defect, but may increase the chance of hematoma at the access point. Arterial thrombosis requiring treatment has been reported as complicating almost 4% of cardiac catheter procedures,[1] transient pulse loss not requiring treatment is probably somewhat commoner.

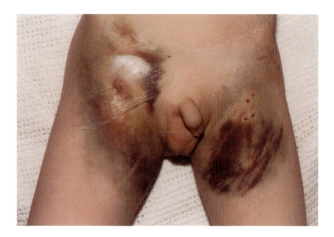

Figure 4.1 Extensive bilateral inguinal hematoma following bilateral arterial and venous access for revascularization of an occluded Blalock Taussig shunt. Heparin had been given during the procedure and hemostasis was felt to be adequate before the patient returned to the ward. The patient became restless some hours afterwards, upon which the hematomas were evident.

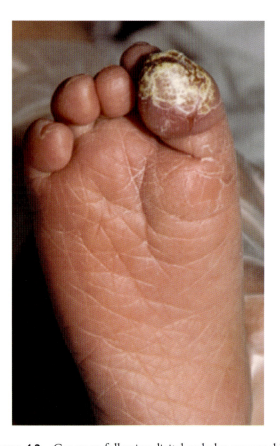

Figure 4.2 Gangrene following digital embolus presumably from an arterial puncture site evident 6 weeks after cardiac catheterization. This patient had well documented femoral, posterior tibial, and dorsalis pedis pulses on discharge after an uncomplicated diagnostic procedure.

Venous thrombosis is probably underdiagnosed as the clinical consequences are less important because rapid development of venous collaterals restores venous return quickly.

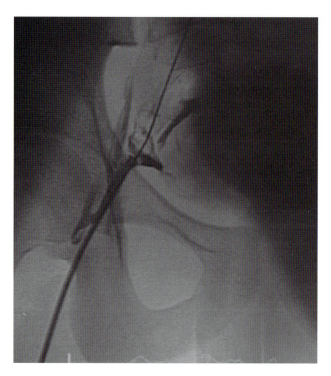

Figure 4.3 Right iliac vein extravasation in a patient who had had multiple venous cardiac catheter procedures from the right femoral vein. It is likely that injudicious forceful dilator manipulation had perforated the vein. Assuming an appropriate initial Seldinger wire position, resistance to sheath advancement should be assessed by passing a short, peripheral venous access cannula over the wire through which an exploratory angiogram is performed.

TYPES OF COMPLICATIONS FROM VENOUS AND ARTERIAL ACCESS POINTS

Local

- Hematoma (Figure 4.1)
- Vessel insufficiency, spasm, and thrombus leading to occlusion (Figure 4.2)
- Extravasation of blood due to vessel perforation may be venous or arterial and retroperitoneal in the pelvis or abdomen (Figures 4.3 and 4.4)
- Arteriovenous fistula
- More serious bleeding leading to compromise of cardiac output
- Puncture of structures related to the site of access, e.g. pneumothorax following internal jugular vein or hepatic venous puncture (Figure 4.5)
- Infection: cellulitis at the site of access is rare. In the context of femoral access in babies and children who are incontinent of urine and feces it is very surprising that this is the case.

Hemobilia may occur as a consequence of communications with the bile ducts and the hepatic veins

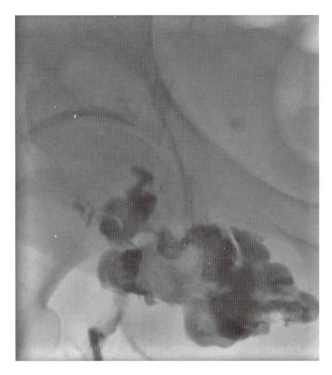

Figure 4.4 Extensive extravasation after perforation of the femoral–external iliac artery junction with a Seldinger wire. Note the calcification in the external iliac artery proximal to extravasation, which is a risk factor for this complication.

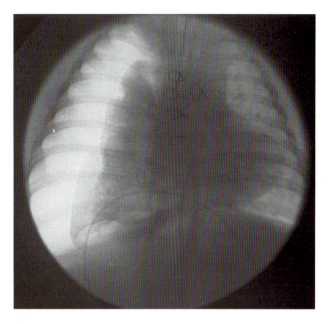

Figure 4.5 Right pneumothorax following transhepatic access for pulmonary artery stent implantation in a bilateral pulmonary artery stenosis postarterial switch procedure.

after transhepatic access. Such communications are usually very small, can often be demonstrated on ultrasound in adults, and are relatively common. They rarely cause symptoms. Tiny intrahepatic arteriovenous fistulae are also a relatively frequent and benign complication of transhepatic access.

Direct cardiac puncture is seldom employed to access the circulation, and when it is it is usually performed through the anterior chest wall in patients who have undergone surgery for complex heart disease in whom access to the left atrium in particular is impossible indirectly.[2,3] The target of access here is relatively large and described using biplane fluoroscopy guidance. Because of the adhesion of scar tissue to the back of the sternum, the risks of bleeding into the pericardium once the sheaths and catheters are removed are reduced. Nevertheless, there are potentially significant complications. Hemothorax requiring drainage and pneumothorax are both reported in these series.

Necrotizing enterocolitis is a rare but well recognized complication of cardiac catheterization in neonates.[4,5] A direct cause–effect relationship with route of access per se is not established, but the effect of vascular sheaths inducing relative stasis in the splanchnic venous and arterial vessels could be implicated in its etiology. These are further reasons therefore to minimize cardiac catheter procedures in the neonatal group.

Minimizing complications

It is commonly understood that vascular access complications are less likely in the hands of experienced catheter operators. In practical terms, the vast majority of hospitals offering cardiac catheter facilities are training establishments of one sort or another. Thus, despite close one to one teaching and proctoring of junior staff, the time taken and number of attempts at achieving access are often suboptimal. Complications of cardiac catheterization are commoner in the hands of trainees.[6]

By definition, some patients undergoing cardiac catheterization will have clinical conditions such as low cardiac output, severe edema, or pulse loss due to the existing lesion such as coarctation of the aorta. The standard palpation landmarks guiding percutaneous puncture in these patients are likely to be distorted or absent. These, patients in the first instance, perhaps should have access attempts by the most senior member of the team. On occasion it may be appropriate in such patients to access by elective cut down, rather than use this approach after multiple, time-consuming percutaneous attempts. The rationale for this is that repeated unsuccessful puncture in a compromised patient may lead to extensive subcutaneous inguinal hematoma, which subsequently renders access by cut down difficult and hazardous.

The advent of small footprint, high-frequency, ultrasound transducers with small, portable screens has facilitated ultrasound-guided vascular access. This technique has slowly crept into the technique of achieving vascular access for cardiac catheterization. It is now commonly used for access via the hepatic veins,[7]

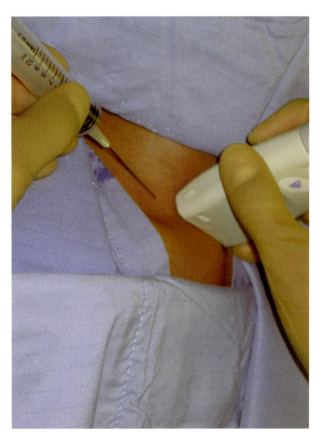

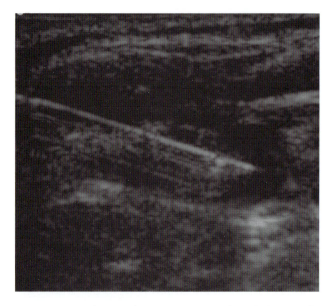

Figure 4.7 The jugular vein is imaged and the needle advanced into its lumen under direct vision.

Figure 4.6 Use of high-frequency ultrasound to guide internal jugular vein puncture. This technique is being increasingly used to facilitate access – typically with transhepatic but also with femoral arterial and venous access.

internal jugular vein, and less frequently the femoral vessels. This technique of ultrasound-guided vascular access has a learning curve and so currently is not in routine use for a standard cardiac catheter procedure in children or adults. Selective use for accessing less frequently used vessels, and use in those patients with compromised landmarks for reason are clearly logical. It is likely to reduce the number of puncture attempts and the risk of vessel disruption (Figures 4.6 and 4.7).

The size of the patient is intimately related to the risk of vascular complication with, significantly, a higher incidence of arterial thrombosis reported in babies weighing less than 5 kg.[8]

It is possible that during the vessel puncture/ Seldinger wire insertion and exchange for sheath the iliac vessels may be dissected by injudicious technique. This complication is more likely when the patient has had numerous previous cardiac catheter procedures, where there have been repeated attempts at access, and when there is tortuosity and or calcification of these vessels (Figures 4.3 and 4.4). Meticulous attention to screening the wire position as it is advanced and the use of a short, narrow gauge (18–22 French) cannula over the wire as an interim maneuver will help to minimize these complications. In the event of a severe bleed from vessel perforation, which may be retroperitoneal, it is important to remove the offending wire or sheath and

reverse the effects of heparin with protamine if relevant. More serious blood loss requires support of blood volume with appropriate blood products. Surgical exploration to stop the bleeding is rarely necessary, but if hemostasis is not achieved quickly, this should be considered.

The size of access sheath is intimately important in the role of thrombus/spasm and subsequent arterial insufficiency. Whilst 'smaller the better' may be intuitive, one has to acknowledge that narrower gauge catheters such as 3 and 4 French try to be kink resistant by having more plastic in their construction. This reduces the lumen caliber down to 0.021 or 0.025 inch, thus angiography quality is compromised because of the relatively poor flow rates physically possible. For the same reason of compromised caliber of the lumen these catheters are more prone to thrombotic occlusion during use. On the other hand, catheters of 5 French and above generally have a 0.035 or 0.038 inch luminal caliber, making them superior for angiography. Modern plastic polymers are such that 5 or 6 French gauge catheters are easily torquable and, with the adjuvant use of hydrophilic steerable wires, they are widely used. It is rare to have to use larger gauge catheters than 5 or 6 French for diagnostic purposes. Most operators would tend to use 4 and 5 French catheters in children on the arterial and venous sides, respectively. Vascular access sheaths and catheters of 3 French gauge are available, but tend to be preserved for use in very small (less than 2.5 kg) patients. In the setting of intervention it is almost always necessary to upsize the sheath for the interventional procedure. In this context, the operator is likely to start with a narrow gauge sheath on the arterial side, achieve the diagnostic information ready for intervention, and then upsize the sheath to the appropriate size depending on the technology being used. On the venous side, say for atrial septal defect closure, the 'working' size sheath is most often positioned at the beginning of the procedure, venous complications on the whole being less likely and troublesome.

Hematoma of the access site of one sort or another is virtually impossible to eliminate. Almost all patients by definition will have at least a small bruise at the access site after cardiac catheterization. It is important that this is understood as part of the consent process. Large hematomas may arise when large caliber sheaths have been used, when anticoagulation has been given, and also when a patient has been restless in the recovery phase and thus standard palpation pressure on the access wound has not been effective (Figure 4.1). Hematoma is therefore best prevented by meticulous attention to the technique of pressure on the wound after sheath removal. This takes time and patience which, in the context of constraints on catheter lab throughput, may not always be appropriately practiced.

Vascular hemostasis devices vary from mechanical pressure 'clamps' to numerous forms of vascular seal technology. Some employ extravascular or intravascular collagen plugs, and some have suture-based technology. These do have some role to play in achieving femoral artery and vein hemostasis but these are restricted to larger and older, cooperative patients. **They must not be used as an alternative to keen nursing observation.** Patients sedated for cardiac catheterization can become disorientated in the recovery period, and attempts to change position in bed for reasons of comfort or otherwise can dislodge and displace the clamp type devices, with the undesirable result of bleeding and hematoma formation. In the case of transhepatic access, some operators advocate closing the 'track' left in the hepatic parenchyma as the sheath is removed, using Gelfoam[9] or embolization coils to avoid intraperitoneal bleeding. This practice appears safe, but in the context of patients who will require multiple access via this route, there is a potential problem of obstructing the future routes of access with the coils.

Another potential hazard, particularly in children, is the misguided concept of a 'pressure dressing' on the femoral access wound. Without the use of a rigid plaster of Paris hip spica it is, of course, impossible to both immobilize the groin area and apply pressure to it. As soon as the hip is flexed, any 'pressure' in this area is completely lost. Conversely, a heavily sedated child may have an overdressed wound which compresses the femoral artery inappropriately, and whilst this may reduce the immediate possibility of hematoma formation, it would of course increase the possibility of causing an intra-arterial thrombus and thus induce ischemia to the leg. Overdressing of the inguinal region with wads of lint type dressing furthermore may obscure the access wound. In this circumstance there may be bleeding under the dressing which is not recognized by the patient's attendant until extensive hematoma and or blood loss is evident (Figure 4.1). It is my recommendation that, following

manual compression of the wound to acceptable dryness, a small, loose dressing is applied which facilitates easy observation.

It is common practice to give heparin as an anticoagulant during cardiac catheterization when accessing from the arterial side, and when an interventional procedure involves device implantation. As most procedures are relatively short, a standard dose of 100 u/kg is sufficient for adequate anticoagulation. Some operators will monitor activated clotting time (ACT) and give further aliquots of heparin, depending on the desired level of anticoagulation, which for most catheter procedures is to keep the ACT around 220–250 seconds. Heparin reversal with protamine is not commonly employed in the catheter laboratory, but this may be advocated at the end of the procedure if there is unacceptable persistent bleeding at the site of vascular access.

CONCLUSIONS

Tips and tricks to minimize access site hematoma and reduce the possibility of postprocedure arterial insufficiency:

- Plan the routes of access before getting to the table.
- Critically assess the need to keep the procedure as short as possible.
- Employ an experienced operator.
- Narrow gauge needle and flexible Seldinger wire.
- Use high-frequency ultrasound as a guide for access when landmarks are constrained.
- Use smallest gauge sheaths and catheters wherever possible. When upsizing a sheath use gradual dilation.
- Use heparin as anticoagulant; monitor ACT accordingly.
- Consider reversing the effect of heparin, depending on the procedure.
- Be vigilant and assiduous when applying pressure to the wound.
- Do not obscure the wound with overzealous dressing and maintain meticulous observation.
- The concept of 'pressure dressing' in a child is flawed.
- There is no substitute for experience, technical excellence, anticipation, and vigilant observation.

When arterial insufficiency is of concern, compare with the 'normal' contralateral limb where possible. Signs to note are:

- Loss or weakness of the distal pulse. Assess the pulse distal to the access site. Palpation at the groin, for example, will be painful and obscured by hematoma. Use of an ultrasound 'Doppler' probe may be helpful in identifying distal pulsatile flow, but does not necessarily provide complete reassurance that perfusion is sufficient.

- Pale color, taking into consideration that a limb that has had simultaneous venous access may appear dusky and blue rather than white.
- Cool temperature on palpation. In the appropriate context an electronic temperature probe may be useful for monitoring the progress of improving or worsening perfusion.
- Pain in the limb (other than at the site of puncture access) is a late sign and usually indicates severe ischemia.
- Be vigilant and assiduous when applying pressure to the wound.

Management of arterial insufficiency

If the leg is warm and an appropriate color an expectant policy may be worthwhile in the anticipation that there is mild arterial spasm and flow stasis, which will improve spontaneously. For more established signs of insufficiency the options are for anticoagulation with heparin or thrombolysis with thrombolytic drugs such as streptokinase, urokinase, or modern agents such as tissue plasminogen activator. Surgical thrombectomy or more extensive revascularization is very rarely employed in the modern era of anticoagulation and thrombolysis, but if there is a tissue viability question there should be no delay in referral for exploration.

Management of venous insufficiency

Thanks to the relatively rapid development of venous collaterals when there is local venous thrombosis in the groin, this is a relatively benign complication. In the days of infant cardiac catheterization via cut down on the femoral vein it was common practice to ligate the femoral vein at the end of the procedure.[10] Discoloration and resulting edema of the leg may be dramatic and disconcerting, and often incur comments from the attendant observers. In practice, resolution of this venous congestion is effected in a matter of hours with the natural mobilization of the limb which occurs as the patient recovers. Coexisting arterial insufficiency may hinder progress, so this of course should be treated concurrently if present. Elevation of the leg may expedite recovery in heavily sedated or anesthetized patients. More invasive attempts to expedite recovery of pure venous congestion such as anticoagulation are likely to have a deleterious effect on outcome and result in bleeding and hematoma formation.

It is understandable that a recurring theme in this text of complications as a consequence of cardiac catheterization procedures is 'prevention is better than cure.' Practice and experience with discipline are obvious bywords, but have to be practiced in the context of training and educating junior interventionists and the nursing and ancillary staff we rely upon to observe our patients in the recovery period postcatheterization. The approach to vascular access should start well before the patient reaches the lab by taking into consideration the size and general condition of the patient, the lesion being treated, the merits of each access site being considered, and the potential complications that might be met. Many patients with complex disease will be returning to the catheter lab for repeated intervention, so the necessity for optimizing vessel patency for the future speaks for itself. We must be true to ourselves and to the operators who may be succeeding us in the management of the patient.

The importance of professional application and integrity, which should be employed at all times, can be found in the the the words of the pianist Vladimir Horowitz (1903–89):

If I don't play the piano for one day I feel it myself …
on the second day the critics will notice it …
and on the third day the audience will hear it …

REFERENCES

1. Vitiello R, McCrindle B, Nykanen D, Freedom R, Benson L. Complications associated with paediatric cardiac catheterisation. J Am Coll Cardiol 1998; 32: 1433–40.
2. Maher KO, Murdison KA, Norwood WI, Murphy JD. Transthoracic access for cardiac catheterization. Cathet Cardiovasc Interven 2004; 63: 72–7.
3. Nehgme RA, Carboni MP, Care J, Murphy JD. Transthoracic percutaneous access for electroanatomic mapping and catheter ablation of atrial tachycardia in patients with lateral tunnel Fontan. Heart Rhythm 2006; 3: 37–43.
4. Dickinson DF, Galloway RW, Wilkinson JL, Arnold R. Necrotising enterocolitis after neonatal cardiac catheterization. Arch Dis Child 1982; 57: 431–3.
5. Sweet DG, Craig B, Halliday HL, Mulholland C. Gastrointestinal complications following neonatal cardiac catheterization. J Perinat Med 1998; 26: 196–200.
6. Agnoletti G, Bonnet C, Boudjemline Y et al. Complications of paediatric interventional catheterisation: an analysis of risk factors. Cardiol Young 2005; 15: 402–8.
7. McLeod KA, Houston AB, Richens T, Wilson N. Transhepatic approach for cardiac catheterization in children: initial experience. Heart 1999; 82: 694–6.
8. Rhodes J, Asnes J, Blaufox A, Sommer R. Impact of low body weight on frequency of paediatric cardiac catheterisation complications. Am J Cardiol 2000; 86: 127–8.
9. Johnson JL, Fellows KE, Murphy JD. Transhepatic central venous access for cardiac catheterization and radiologic intervention. Cathet Cardiovasc Diagn 1995; 35: 168–71.
10. Porter CJ, Gillette PC, Mullins CE, McNamara DG. Cardiac catheterisation in the neonate. A comparison of three techniques. J Pediatr 1978; 93: 97–101.

5   Balloon atrial septostomy and stenting of the atrial septum

Sawsan Awad and Ziyad M Hijazi

INTRODUCTION

The presence of unrestrictive atrial septal defect is crucial for the survival of patients with certain forms of congenital cardiac defects. The interatrial shunting may be important to augment cardiac output in right-sided obstructive lesions, to relieve elevated Fontan and pulmonary pressures in Fontan failure, to relieve pulmonary hypertension in left-sided obstructive lesions, to decompress the right ventricle in postoperative right ventricular failure, and to improve mixing in transposition of the great arteries and similar physiology.

There are multiple techniques to create or enlarge an atrial communication. However, such techniques would be suitable to support oxygen mixing and augment the cardiac output for only a short period of time. We believe that stenting the atrial septum would provide a reliable, longer lasting interatrial communication.

In this chapter we discuss the different techniques used to create and or enlarge an atrial communication and we will cover the potential complications and how to manage them.

PERSONNEL REQUIREMENTS, FACILITIES AND EQUIPMENT

Performing interventional cardiac catheterization in children requires high skills and training. Only trained pediatric/congenital cardiologists with expertise in interventional therapy should perform such complex procedures. The catheterization laboratory should be equipped preferably with biplane fluoroscopy imaging. However, the procedure can be done using single plane fluoroscopy imaging, but the operator would need to rotate the plane in multiple views to assure safety of the procedure. Interventional procedures should not be performed in an institution where there is no surgical back-up and ECMO support capabilities.[1] All types of wires, catheters, balloons (including high-pressure and cutting balloons), retrieval catheters/snares, and devices should be readily available in the catheterization laboratory. A failed procedure or a complication that may lead to untoward events due to lack of proper equipment is inexcusable.

INDICATIONS FOR CREATING/ DILATING INTERATRIAL COMMUNICATIONS

1. Transposition of the great arteries with restrictive/intact atrial communication.
2. Total anomalous pulmonary venous connection with restrictive atrial septal defect (ASD) if needed before surgery.
3. Tricuspid atresia with restrictive ASD.
4. Hypoplastic left heart syndrome.
5. Pulmonary atresia/intact ventricular septum.
6. Pulmonary hypertension, to alleviate the pressure on the right side of the heart. Control of the defect size is crucial to avoid devastating hypoxemia.
7. Failing Fontan circulation. Creation of an interatrial communication helps decrease systemic venous hypertension, improve systemic perfusion, and perhaps improve patients with protein-losing enteropathy.
8. Left atrial decompression during ECMO support.

TECHNIQUES USED TO DILATE PRE-EXISTING BUT RESTRICTIVE INTERATRIAL COMMUNICATIONS

Balloon atrial spetostomy

Balloon atrial septostomy was first described in 1966 by Rashkind and Miller as palliation for patients with transposition of the great arteries to improve saturation.[2] The procedure is basically performed in the catheterization laboratory under fluoroscopic guidance. Some operators perform the procedure at the bedside under transthoracic echocardiography guidance.

Technique

1. Venous (umbilical/femoral) access is obtained with the appropriate size sheath.
2. A balloon septostomy catheter (the Miller catheter [Edwards-Baxter Healthcare Corporation, Santa Ana, CA]; the Rashkind balloon catheter [USCI-CR Bard, Inc, Billerica, MA]; the Fogarty (Paul) balloon catheter [Edwards-Baxter Healthcare], or the Z-5 septostomy catheter [NuMED, Inc, Hopkinton, NY]) is then advanced through the sheath up to the right atrium and through the atrial communication to the left atrium.
3. Appropriate positioning of the balloon at the atrial septum to avoid any potential complication is of crucial importance. The operator should avoid common abnormal positions of the balloon such as:

   - left atrial appendage or the right atrial appendage in patients with juxtaposed right atrial appendage
   - the left pulmonary veins
   - through the left atrioventricular (AV) valve to the left ventricle.

4. The balloon is then inflated in the left atrium. To ensure proper positioning, transthoracic echocardiography can be used. The catheter is then pulled into the right atrium using a rapid and forceful jerk.
5. The forceful jerk/pull motion should be stopped at the right atrium inferior vena cava junction. The catheter should be pushed back to the mid right atrium then deflated as rapidly as possible.
6. The deflated catheter is advanced to the left atrium and the procedure is repeated until adequate atrial communication is achieved and no resistance is felt during passage of the inflated balloon across the defect.
7. At the end of the procedure the balloon is deflated and pulled outside the body.

Complications and management

1. Balloon rupture, and embolization of the balloon fragments. Retrieval can be attempted; however, if the operator is unable to retrieve all fragments, surgery is indicated.
2. Failure of balloon deflation. On rare occasions, the balloon fails to deflate and remains inflated despite negative suction. The operator should attempt to pass a guide wire in the balloon lumen to clear any obstruction. If this does not work, the balloon lumen should be connected to an injector and 3–5 cc of contrast injected under pressure (as for an angiogram) using 300 psi. This will result in balloon rupture and then the operator should be able to remove the balloon catheter outside the body. If this does not work, one may attempt to pass a wire from the contralateral femoral vein using a long sheath, then try to puncture the balloon using the stiff end of a guide wire. Extreme care should be exercised and the procedure should be done under biplane fluoroscopy.
3. Misjudgment of the position of the catheter tip due to absence of the end hole. This can be avoided using echocardiography to guide the procedure.
4. Rupture of the atrial appendage immediately after balloon inflation is the most serious complication, especially in patients having left juxtaposition of the right atrial appendage.

To avoid the occurrence of the last two complications, the use of biplane fluoroscopy together with transthoracic echocardiography will continuously help the operator to adjust the catheter position. Further, we believe that using the newly developed end hole septostomy catheter (Z-5) will give additional confirmation of the catheter tip.

5. Vascular injury due to the large introducing sheath required for the conventional balloons (at least 6–8 French).
6. Transient rhythm disturbances are frequent.[3] The availability of anti-arrhythmic medications in the laboratory is essential. On rare occasions, if the neonate is unstable, DC cardioversion may be required.
7. Failure to create an adequate communication: due to inadequate balloon size, poor technique, or, in older patients, due to thick atrial septum.
8. Other general complications encountered in the catheterization laboratory.

Low-profile balloon atrial septostomy

This new balloon was initially studied by Hijazi *et al.* in 1994[4] in an animal model. It was then used successfully in patients with various cardiac conditions requiring septostomy.[5] This catheter requires a 5 or 6 French introducer sheath and it has special advantages, including the presence of an end hole that allows the operator to pass the balloon catheter over a wire (0.018 inch for the Z-5 and 0.014 inch for the smaller version), the ability to measure pressure or inject contrast through this end hole to confirm catheter position, and the smaller size balloon required to create a large defect. This is of particular importance in both neonates and premature neonates with a small left atrium. The operator can cross the atrial septum to the left atrium using any end hole catheter.

Once the catheter is in the left atrium and the position is confirmed by echocardiography or pressure recording, or by contrast injection, this catheter is exchanged over an appropriate size guide wire. Then the Z-5 or Z-4 catheter is advanced over this wire to the left atrium. Septostomy is performed over the wire in the usual fashion. Once the balloon crosses to the right atrium inferior vena cava junction, the balloon is pushed back to the mid right atrium and deflated. The balloon can be advanced back to the left atrium over the wire. The presence of the wire facilitates the procedure.

Complications encountered using this balloon include a torn-off catheter tip, as reported by Akagi et al.[6] To manage this complication, the operator can attempt percutaneous retrieval and, if this not possible, surgical removal is indicated.

Static balloon atrial dilation

Static balloon atrial dilation was first described in the laboratory animal by Mitchell et al.,[7] and then in humans by Shrivastava et al.[8] This method is very effective in creating adequate atrial communication in situations where the atrial septum is rather thick (age > 6 weeks); it may also be used to follow/supplement blade atrial septostomy.

Technique

1. Venous access is obtained from the femoral vein and a guide wire is advanced to the left atrium.
2. The balloon size is selected to be the largest that may be advanced through the sheath.
3. The selected balloon is advanced over the guide wire and positioned so that it 'straddles' the atrial septum.
4. The balloon is then fully inflated with diluted contrast (20–25%) until the indentation (waisting) caused by the atrial septum is eliminated.
5. Right and left atrial pressures are obtained before and after the procedure.

Complications

1. Inadequate atrial communication that requires the use of blade atrial septostomy or a cutting balloon.
2. General complications encountered in interventional cardiac catheterization procedures.

Cutting balloon atrial septostomy

This method was first used experimentally on piglets in 1996 by Coe et al.[9] The technique proved to be effective in creating adequate size atrial communication. Later, this technique was used in cases of intact atrial septum[10,11] to create atrial communication after septal puncture or radiofrequency perforation. This technique is useful in small infants with a very small left atrium that cannot accommodate the blade catheter.

Technique

1. Femoral venous access is obtained.
2. A catheter is advanced to the left atrium through the atrial communication.
3. A guide wire is then advanced to the left atrium. The primary catheter is then removed, leaving the guide wire in the left atrium.
4. A cutting balloon catheter of the correct size is then delivered over the wire and across the atrial septum.
5. The balloon is inflated to no more than 8 atm (usually a waist is visible that gives way, indicating successful dilation), then the balloon is deflated completely. The balloon is then pulled inside the sheath and removed out of the body.
6. To further enlarge the defect, static balloon dilation using a high-pressure balloon is usually performed after angioplasty with the cutting balloon.
7. Continuous fluoroscopic monitoring is maintained throughout the procedure. Echocardiography can also be used to confirm the correct balloon position.

Complications

Laceration of the left atrial free wall is possible, as reported by Coe et al. in an animal study.[9] To prevent such a complication from happening, the correct balloon position is confirmed by fluoroscopy and or echocardiography.

Blade atrial septostomy

Blade atrial septostomy was first described by Park et al.[12] This procedure is indicated in older patients (6–8 weeks), where the presence of an adequate atrial septal communication is crucial for patient survival. In such patients the atrial septum is usually thick, and conventional balloon atrial septostomy alone is inadequate. The blades (Cook, Inc, Bloomington, IN) are available in three sizes: 9.4, 13.4, and 20 mm. Currently, this procedure is very rarely performed.

Techniques[13]

1. Femoral access is usually obtained using a 7 French sheath.
2. A selective left atrial angiogram is recommended to evaluate the size of the left atrium and the location of the atrial communication.
3. The catheter system is inspected and then introduced into the left atrium. Because the side arm is

in the same plane as the curve of the catheter tip, passage of the catheter into the left atrium can be facilitated by maintaining the side arm in a posterior and leftward orientation.

4. The location of the catheter in the left atrium is confirmed using fluoroscopy and echocardiography.

5. The locking device is loosened from the control wire and pulled backward until the gap between the gasket and the locking device is 12 mm; the holder is then tightened.

6. The blade is extended by advancing the blade control wire holder gently toward the catheter tip under fluoroscopic control. If resistance is met or the blade cannot be fully extended, it should be suspected that the catheter tip is positioned in the left atrial appendage or in a pulmonary vein. In this situation, the control wire holder is withdrawn to fold the blade back into the catheter. Then the entire catheter system is slightly withdrawn and the same maneuver repeated.

7. Once the blade has been extended, the gasket and the locking device are held together. The catheter is then slightly rotated counterclockwise until the blade is facing somewhat anteriorly.

8. The entire catheter system is slowly withdrawn to the right atrium using both hands to maintain the same catheter orientation. Resistance of the interatrial septum is usually encountered in the middle or lower portion of the cardiac silhouette. Gentle but firm force is maintained to withdraw the catheter from the left atrium to the right atrium, until a sudden decrease in resistance is felt. Continued resistance may be felt despite withdrawal of the catheter to the level of the diaphragm or even lower, especially if the left atrium is large or if the interatrial septum is quite stiff. Under no circumstances should rapid withdrawal be attempted as required for balloon atrial septostomy.

9. Once the blade septostomy catheter has been withdrawn across the interatrial septum, the catheter is advanced to the mid right atrial position and the blade is folded back into the catheter lumen by withdrawing the locking device and blade control wire holder.

10. The procedure may be repeated if little resistance was encountered during the initial withdrawal. The angulation of the blade should be changed slightly on subsequent withdrawals to ensure adequate incision of the atrial septum. When the interatrial septum is unusually thick and the atrial communication is very small (less than 4 mm in diameter or in a transseptal approach) the first withdrawal of the catheter is done with only a partially extended blade. This is followed by withdrawal with a fully extended blade. This stepwise manner facilitates initial withdrawal of the blade across the interatrial septum and causes less stress on the delicate blade assembly.

Complications and management

1. Laceration of the left atrial wall is possible, especially in patients with hypoplastic left heart syndrome who often have a small left atrium. Left atrial angiography prior to the procedure is essential to identify the left atrial size and locate the position of the atrial communication.

2. Perforation of the right ventricular outflow tract by the catheter tip. Continuous monitoring of the position of the catheter tip using biplane fluoroscopy is mandated during such a procedure. The introduction of the long percutaneous sheath facilitates rapid introduction of the blade catheter into the left atrium, thus eliminating prolonged and potentially traumatic maneuvering of the blade catheter and minimizing the incidence of major complications.

3. Failure to retract the blade into the catheter. This complication is rather rare. The catheter and wire of the blade should be maneuvered carefully in different directions until the blade folds – if it does not, then surgical exploration and removal of the blade are indicated.

4. Other general complications encountered in any catheterization procedure could happen.

Stenting of the atrial septum

Creation and/or dilatation of an already existing atrial communication may take place using one or more of the previously described methods. However, usually this is not long-lasting palliation. Therefore, if the communication is needed for a long time, stenting of the defect may be the preferred option.

Technique[14]

1. Venous access is obtained (via the femoral vein, or by transhepatic puncture).

2. Diagnostic right and left heart catheterization according to the need for further evaluation of the underlying congenital heart disease is performed.

3. Access to the left atrium is gained, either through the patent foramen ovale or ASD, or using a standard transseptal puncture technique (as discussed elsewhere).

4. A guide wire is positioned in the left upper pulmonary vein. A long sheath is then advanced over the wire and the dilator is removed, ensuring that

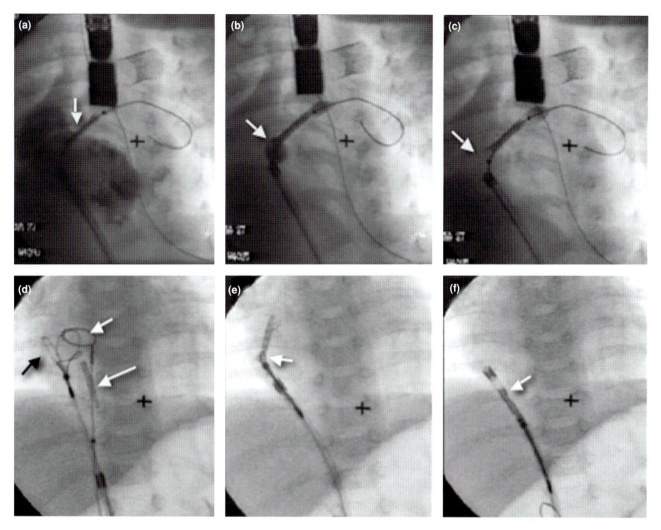

Figure 5.1   Cine fluoroscopic images in a neonate with hypoplastic left heart syndrome who underwent hybrid intervention stage 1 (stent of the ductus and banding of the branch pulmonary arteries) and is now undergoing stent implantation for a restrictive atrial septum. This procedure resulted in balloon rupture prior to stent deployment. (A) Angiogram in the right atrium via the side arm of a delivery sheath to show the position of the atrial septum, with the stent (arrow) straddling the septum prior to balloon inflation. (B) Cine image during balloon inflation (arrow) when the balloon ruptured. (C) Cine image showing that the proximal part of the stent is flared (arrow). (D) The stent migrated off the wire and is now in the right atrium (thin long arrow), Note, there are two snares in the right atrium: the gooseneck snare (thin white arrow) and the Ensnare (black arrow). (E) The Ensnare capturing the proximal part of the stent with coaxial alignment with the long sheath (arrow). (F) The stent was brought inside the long sheath.

the sheath tip is in the left atrium. This can be confirmed by angiography using the side arm of the sheath. Careful deaeration of the sheath is mandatory to avoid air embolism.

5. To achieve a restrictive atrial communication outside the body a 5.0 Prolene ligature is placed around the central strut of the stent; the diameter of the ligature should be no more than 5–6 mm. The stent is crimped on a large balloon (10–14 mm). The balloon/stent assembly is introduced inside the sheath as usual. Proper positioning of the stent across the atrial septum is confirmed by fluoroscopy. The balloon is inflated; this will create waisting in the stent corresponding to the diameter of the ligature, and the ends of the stent dilate to the same size of the balloon. The balloon is deflated and removed carefully.

6. To achieve a non-restrictive atrial communication, the stent is directly mounted on a 10–14 mm angioplasty balloon catheter.

7. The implant catheter is advanced through the sheath and across the atrial septum.

8. Half of the stent is exposed by pulling back the sheath, and the balloon is inflated in the left atrium, expanding the distal half of the stent.

9. The entire system is firmly pulled back against the atrial septum, and the right atrial portion of the stent is unsheathed and expanded. This will ensure that the stent has slight waisting to prevent the stent from slipping off the septum.

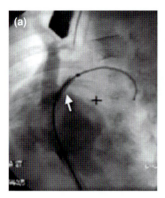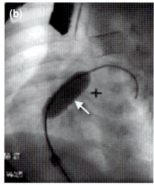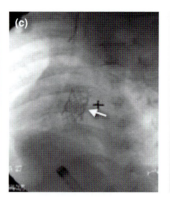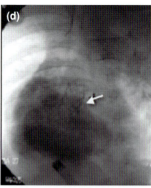

Figure 5.2   Cine fluoroscopic images during successful stent deployment in the patient shown in Figure 5.1. (A) Angiogram via side arm of the sheath demonstrating a good position to deploy the stent (arrow). (B) Balloon inflation of the stent (arrow). (C) Cine image after the balloon has been removed, demonstrating good stent position (arrow). (D) Final angiogram showing good stent position across the septum (arrow).

Complications and management[14,15]

1. Thrombus formation on the stent is possible, especially on the right atrial side of the stent, with the consequent potential for embolic phenomena and other clinical sequelae. This complication is of great concern in patients with Fontan physiology and sluggish flow across the Fontan circuit. Use of generous anticoagulation to keep the ACT above 250 seconds is recommended. Desaturation is also another potential complication due to significant right-to-left shunt. Therefore, appropriate sizing of the defect is important.

2. Stent erosion through the free wall of the right atrium could happen, particularly if long stents are used. The use of shorter stents (the shortest possible stent to provide stability and avoid migration) is important to avoid this complication.

3. Stent migration is of great concern since the only mechanism to keep the stent in place is by flaring both ends of the stent using the above techniques. Migrated stents may be retrieved over the balloon used for their deployment. The assembly must be carefully maneuvered until the stent is in the inferior vena cava. Further dilation with a larger balloon will firmly appose the stent struts against the vessel wall. If this is not possible, surgical exploration and removal are indicated. Placing patients on long-term antiplatelet and or anticoagulation regimen is of crucial importance. Serial echocardiographic follow-up to look for clot formation and stent patency is recommended. On occasion, if the balloon ruptures prior to stent inflation, the stent can be retrieved using snaring techniques. The stent can be captured using the Ensnare (MD Technologies) (Figures 5.1 and 5.2). A larger sheath is of course needed to bring the snared stent inside the sheath and then outside the body.

4. Atrial stents perform well in the short term but poorly in the long term (8–12 weeks).

The stents are prone to stenosis with restriction and/or loss of the atrial communication in the long term. In our experience, atrial stents are reliable for a period of not more than 3 months. Therefore, close monitoring by echocardiogram and/or angiography if needed is advised.

SUMMARY

There are different techniques to create and maintain an interatrial communication when needed. Each one of these techniques has its own complications. Some of them are major, some are minor and easily avoidable. Having a fully stocked catheterization laboratory and high expertise in performing these procedures is mandatory to avoid and/or manage such complications.

REFERENCES

1. Allen HD, Beekman RH 3rd, Garson A Jr et al. Pediatric therapeutic cardiac catheterization: a statement for healthcare professionals from the Council on Cardiovascular Disease in the Young, American Heart Association. Circulation 1998; 97: 609–25.
2. Rashkind WJ, Miller W. Creation of an atrial septal defect without thoracotomy: a palliative approach to complete transposition of the great arteries. JAMA 1966; 196: 991–2.
3. Parsons CG, Astley R, Burrows FG, Singh SP. Transposition of great arteries: a study of 65 infants followed for 1 to 4 years after balloon septostomy. Br Heart J 1971; 33: 725–31.
4. Hijazi ZM, Geggel RL, Aronovitz MJ et al. A new low profile balloon atrial septostomy catheter: initial animal and clinical experience. J Invas Cardiol 1994; 6: 209–12.
5. Hijazi ZM, Abu Ata I, Kuhn MA et al. Balloon atrial septostomy using a new low-profile balloon catheter: initial clinical results. Cathet Cardiovasc Diagn 1997; 40: 187–90.
6. Akagi T, Tananari Y, Maeno YV et al. Torn-off balloon tip of Z-5 atrial septostomy catheter. Cathet Cardiovasc Interven 2001; 52: 500–3.
7. Mitchell SE, Kan JS, Anderson JH, White RI Jr, Swindle MM. Atrial septostomy: stationary angioplasty balloon technique. Pediatr Res 1986; 20: 173a.

8. Shrivastava S, Radhakrishnan S, Dev V, Singh LS, Rajani M. Balloon dilatation of atrial septum in complete transposition of great artery: a new technique. Ind Heart J 1987; 39: 298–300.

9. Coe JY, Chen RP, Timinsky J, Robertson MA, Dyck J. A novel method to create atrial septal defect using a cutting balloon in piglets. Am J Cardiol 1996; 78: 1323–6.

10. Schneider MBE, Zartner PA, Magee AG. Transseptal approach in children after patch occlusion of atrial septal defect: first experience with the cutting balloon. Cathet Cardiovasc Interven 1999; 48: 378–81.

11. Hill SL, Mizelle KM, Vellucci SM, Feltes TF, Cheatham JP. Radiofrequency perforation and cutting balloon septoplasty of intact atrial septum in a newborn with hypoplastic left heart syndrome using transesophageal ICE probe guidance. Cathet Cardiovasc Interven 2005; 64: 214–17.

12. Park SC, Zuberbuhler JR, Neches WH, Lennox CC, Zoltun RA. A new atrial septostomy technique. Cathet Cardiovasc Diagn 1975; 1: 195–201.

13. Veldtman GR, Norgard G, Wahlander H et al. Creation and enlargement of atrial defects in congenital heart disease. Pediatr Cardiol 2005; 26: 162–8.

14. Danon S, Levi DS, Alejos JC, Moore JW. Reliable atrial septostomy by stenting of the atrial septum. Cathet Cardiovasc Interven 2005; 66: 408–13.

15. Bacha EA, Hijazi ZM. Hybrid procedures in pediatric cardiac surgery. Semin Thorac Cardiovasc Surg Pediatr Card Surg Annu 2005; 78–85.

6 Transseptal puncture in congenital heart disease

David Nykanen

INTRODUCTION

Transcatheter perforation of the atrial septum was first described in 1959,[1] and subsequently gained popularity as an alternative to transbronchial or transthoracic access to the left atrium for diagnostic catheterization.[2–6] Improved ability to estimate left atrial pressure by pulmonary arterial wedge pressure and hemodynamic assessment by non-invasive echocardiographic Doppler interrogation resulted in a decline in the popularity of the technique. In recent years there has been renewed interest in transseptal puncture of the atrial septum for more accurate hemodynamic assessment and access to the left atrium and ventricle for interventional procedures such as radiofrequency ablation of accessory pathways and arrhythmia control, as well as therapeutic interventional procedures for congenital and structural heart disease. Stenotic aortic valves with significant calcification or vegetations may represent an embolic risk, and the severity of stenosis may preclude accurate retrograde assessment of pressure difference by pullback.[7,8] In general, the direct measurement of the atrial pressure is more accurate than wedge pressures for the assessment of mitral valve physiology. Simultaneous measurement of left atrial and left ventricular or left ventricular and aortic pressures will always yield more precise characterization of mitral and aortic valve hemodynamics, respectively. In addition to providing access to the left atrium, transseptal puncture with creation of an atrial defect has been further utilized as a therapeutic strategy for patients with end stage pulmonary hypertension,[9–11] patients on mechanical cardiopulmonary support requiring left atrial decompression,[9–12] as an adjunct to closure of the long tunnel at times associated with the foramen ovale in cryptogenic stroke,[13] and for patients who, by the nature of their congenital heart defect, require an obligatory atrial shunt or mixing for survival[14–16] (for example: hypoplastic left heart syndrome, tricuspid stenosis, pulmonary atresia with intact ventricular septum). There has been recent interest in primary intervention on the atrial septum for severe forms of congenital heart disease in utero.[14,17] Mechanical perforation of conduits and other surgically created intra-atrial patches has also

been well described.[18] A broad list of the indications for transseptal puncture or intervention of the atrial septum is presented in Table 6.1.

Contraindications include obstruction of the inferior vena cava or a tumor obstructing access to the right atrium, right atrial thrombus or myxoma that may result in embolization, bleeding diathesis or systemic anticoagulation, congenital variations in cardiac anatomy with unusual orientation of the atrial septum, and severe scoliosis that results in unusual septal position. While these may represent relative contraindications, careful consideration prior to proceeding is warranted.

EQUIPMENT AND TECHNIQUES

Mechanical perforation

Venous access is preferred from the right femoral vein, preferably with a horizontal subcutaneous approach to the vein rather than an acute entry. The procedure can be accomplished from the left femoral venous approach, however this is not ideal and can be more uncomfortable to the sedated patient. In general, biplane imaging is utilized although there is accumulating experience with single plane techniques, especially if other imaging modalities such as intracardiac echocardiography are used. If the septal anatomy is complex then intracardiac or transesophageal echocardiography can be of critical benefit. Long transseptal needles may take the form of the 17 gauge Ross needle or a Brockenbrough needle which is 18 gauge but tapers to 21 gauge. The former is used with a Brockenbrough catheter while the latter is typically used in a long Mullins sheath. It is important to ensure that the needle length and sheath length are appropriately matched so that the needle, when fully inserted, protrudes from the dilator only a small amount (a few millimeters). The long needle typically has a flange shaped like an arrow. The needle should be inspected prior to proceeding to ensure that the arrow is oriented to indicate the direction of the curve of the distal end of the needle. A wire is positioned from the

Table 6.1   Indications for transseptal puncture.

Diagnostic

Direct measurement of left atrial pressure

Hemodynamic assessment of aortic valve or mitral valve disease

   Simultaneous measurements for gradient assessment and valve area measurement

   Aortic valves at risk for systemic emboli (severe calcification, vegetations, and excrescences)

Mechanical valve assessment

Pulmonary vein angiography

   Pulmonary vein

   Pulmonary artery via venous wedge injection

Therapeutic

Antegrade mitral or aortic valve valvuloplasty

Transcatheter mitral valve repair (leaflets/annulus) or aortic valve implant

Access for pulmonary vein intervention

Access for left-sided electrophysiologic ablation

   Left free wall, posterior septal, septal bypass tracts

   Atrial fibrillation

Atrial septostomy for improved mixing (e.g. TGA, DORV with subpulmonary VSD)

Atrial septostomy for obligatory shunting (e.g. HLHS, TA, PAT/IVS)

Atrial fenestration creation in Fontan circulation

Atrial septostomy for end stage pulmonary hypertension

Antegrade access to ascending aorta for angiographic and hemodynamic assessment in aortic coarctation intervention

DORV, double outlet right ventricle; HLHS, hypoplastic left heart syndrome; PAT/IVS, pulmonary atresia, intact ventricular septum; TA, tricuspid atresia; TGA, transposition of the great arteries; VSD, ventricular septal defect.

femoral vein to the superior vena cava at the level of the insertion of the innominate vein. This allows the long sheath and dilator to be advanced to the same level over the wire. Care must be taken never to advance the sheath and dilator unless over a wire, to avoid perforation of the heart or great vessels.

Once the sheath and dilator are in position the long needle is gently inserted into the dilator taking care to smoothly advance it, allowing for free passive rotation, to the tip of the dilator. The needle must remain inside the dilator. Some operators will mark the position of the aorta with a pigtail catheter introduced retrograde from the femoral artery to the right coronary cusp of the aortic valve in an effort to avoid inadvertent aortic perforation. At this point operators differ in technique. Some will attach pressure tubing to the needle hub to continuously monitor atrial pressure during the procedure, while others will attach a syringe filled with contrast to stain the septum at the time of puncture. The tip of the needle is rotated to point leftward and slightly posterior, usually by clockwise rotation. There is a tactile component to this procedure and the needle direction has been noted to vary[19] even in anatomically normal hearts. The entire system is withdrawn inferiorly with three typical tactile and visual 'bumps.' The first bump occurs when withdrawing through the junction of the superior vena cava and the right atrium. The second occurs as the needle descends past the aorta, and this can be subtle. The third and most crucial to recognize occurs

as the needle passes over the limbus of the fossa ovalis. After the last 'bump' the system is advanced slightly as a unit to engage the septum. This last maneuver may open the probe patent foramen ovale, hence perforation is not required to enter the left atrium. Note that, even in the anatomically normal heart, the position of the septum may be altered by left atrial enlargement (more horizontal), aortic dilation (more vertical), and right atrial enlargement (more remote). As discussed in the next section, there may be a need to perforate the atrial septum in a more superior or inferior location depending on the procedure contemplated.

Once the septum is engaged at the level of the fossa ovalis the pressure tracing, if monitored, will dampen. The needle is then advanced to its position beyond the end of the dilator. In many instances the needle will advance to the left atrium and an atrial trace will be identified hemodynamically. If the contrast staining technique is utilized, a small amount of contrast is introduced through the needle to stain the location of the intra-atrial septum. If the contrast fills the left atrium naturally, perforation has been successfully achieved. If the septum is too thick, or if it is particularly fibrous, the entire system must be carefully advanced as a unit to perforate the septum. Care must be taken not to advance beyond the position of the left mainstem bronchus if one is to avoid inadvertent perforation (Figure 6.1a). If the pericardium or the aorta is entered at this stage then one can simply remove the

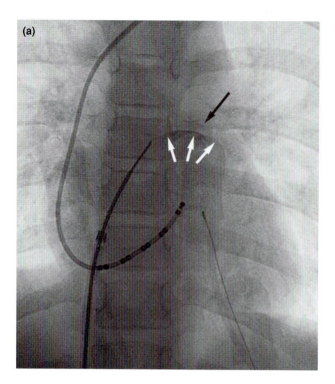

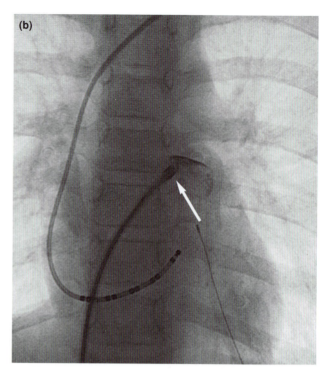

Figure 6.1 Mechanical transseptal atrial puncture. (a) Frontal angiographic view of transseptal needle injection into the left atrium. Note the relation of the superior aspect of the left atrium (white arrows) to the left mainstem bronchus (black arrow). (b) The sheath has been advanced over the needle to facilitate catheter access to the left atrium.

needle and start from the beginning, taking care to ensure that no hemodynamic instability occurs. Recall that at this stage the puncture is only undertaken with a 21 gauge needle tip. If the sheath and dilator are advanced to an inappropriate location then one must assume that a sizable perforation exists and the system should not be withdrawn without having the ability to emergently surgically intervene.

Once the puncture has been confirmed to be successful then the entire sheath and dilator are advanced over the needle to the left atrium (Figure 6.1b). Some have advocated placing a 0.014 inch wire through the needle and into a left pulmonary vein or curled in the atrium to ensure that the system does not puncture the heart during sheath advancement.[20] In this setting a stained intra-atrial septum can be useful in ensuring that the septum does not advance over the sheath and dilator during this maneuver. This is particularly troublesome in the thick or fibrotic septum. Once the sheath is confirmed to be in the left atrium the dilator can be withdrawn, taking care not to introduce air into the system. This can be accomplished with a continuous flush or by underwater seal. The system must be aspirated and flushed to ensure there is no air or clot in the sheath. Meticulous attention to sheath detail should be employed to avoid major embolic complications. At this point the patient can safely receive systemic administration of heparin and catheters can be introduced to the left atrium through the long sheath.

Radiofrequency-assisted transseptal techniques

There can be many challenges associated with mechanical perforation of the atrial septum. These include inadvertent perforation of the atrial wall with pericardial effusion or perforation of the aorta superiorly, causing an aorta-atrial fistula. The small neonate with a hypoplastic atrium, the patient with a sclerotic septum, and the patient with a redundant aneurysmal atrial septum can pose significant challenges to the mechanical techniques described above. More recently, there has been accumulating experience with radiofrequency-assisted perforation of cardiac and vascular tissue. A discussion of the biophysics of radiofrequency perforation is beyond the scope of this chapter, however systems have been developed which limit the damage to surrounding tissue, which is unlike the objective desired with radiofrequency ablation of tissue. It is important to understand the difference between perforation and ablation (Table 6.2). Histologically these lesions result in a discrete injury to tissue wherein the initial thermal coagulation necrosis with adherent microthrombi is limited to a few cell layers and replaced by local inflammation and fibrosis[21] (Figure 6.2). Perforation by radiofrequency is achieved by a combination of rapid cellular heating, resulting in vaporization, cellular electroporation, and the dielectric effect, all of which are evidenced by the sudden appearance of microcavitations or bubbles with successful perforation (Figure 6.3).

Table 6.2 A comparison of radiofrequency-assisted perforation and ablation.

	Radiofrequency perforation	Radiofrequency ablation
Objective	Discrete local perforation	Large non-penetrating lesion
Conditions	Low power (5–10 watts), short (< 2 seconds), high voltage (150–180 volts)	High power (35–50 watts), long (60–90 seconds), low voltage (30–50 volts)
Impedance	High (2000–4000 ohms)	Low (150–300 ohms)
Active catheter tip	Small (short and thin – 1.3 French)	Large (long and thick – 7–8 French)

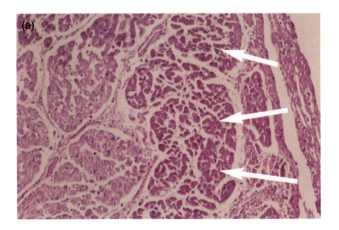

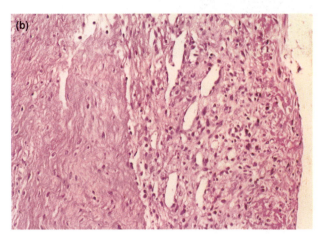

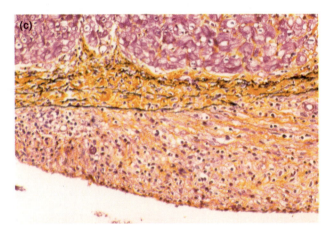

Figure 6.2 Histology of radiofrequency-assisted perforation. (a) Hematoxylin and eosin stain of initial perforation of porcine atrial tissue is marked by thermal coagulation necrosis with denaturation of myocardial protein (white arrows) that is only a few cell layers thick. (b) Hematoxylin and eosin stain demonstrates early healing with local lymphocytic inflammation. (c) MOVAT pentachrome stain demonstrates completed fibrosis.

Currently a system exists that utilizes a 0.024 inch flexible wire (Baylis Medical Company) which can act as an exchange wire (Figure 6.4). Typically, the wire and a coaxial catheter are advanced into a catheter that is opposed to the atrial septum. The wire is advanced through the catheter to the septum and 5–10 watts of energy are applied while advancing the wire across the atrial septum. There is minimal tactile feedback to the procedure, hence attention must be paid to the fluoroscopic or echocardiographic image to ensure that the perforation does not continue through the left atrial wall. The coaxial catheter is advanced into the left atrium and then the guiding catheter is advanced. At this point any wire can be exchanged for the system through the guiding catheter. While this technique can prove useful in the small neonate,[14,16] in larger patients the system proves to be too flexible for routine use. As a result a specific radiofrequency system

has been developed for the patient with more normal septal anatomy,[22,23] The transseptal perforation is achieved utilizing a perforating catheter (Toronto transseptal system, Baylis Medical Company, Mississauga, Canada) that is flexible but thicker than the previous wire. It has an internal lumen to measure pressures and deliver contrast, and the distal end is curved to avoid anterior dissection of the perforating catheter. The perforating catheter is preloaded into a sheath that has been specifically designed for septal perforation (TorFlex Transseptal Guiding Sheath, Baylis Medical Company, Mississauga, Canada). This sheath is shaped like a Brockenbrough needle, is braided for torque, and has a foreshortened dilator tip. The sheath is opposed to the atrial septum and 5–10 watts of energy are applied for 2 seconds. The sheath is connected to the pressure monitoring system continuously, hence the left atrial position is confirmed. If doubt exists then contrast can

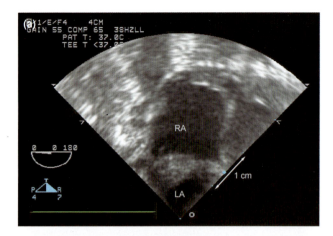

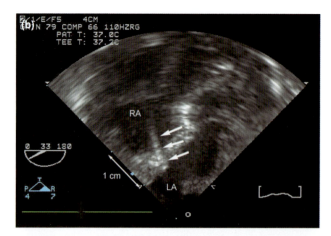

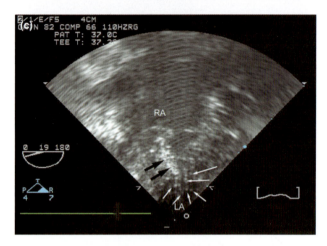

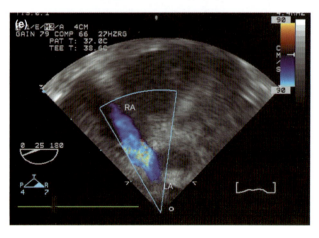

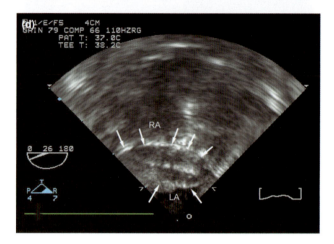

Figure 6.3 Transesophageal images of radiofrequency perforation of the atrial septum. (a) Transesophageal image of a newborn with hypoplastic left heart syndrome and a thick intact atrial septum. Mechanical perforation in this setting is difficult, hence a radiofrequency strategy is employed. (b) The radiofrequency wire (white arrows) is advanced through the atrial septum with application of energy. (c) Perforation is signaled by the sudden appearance of microcavitations or bubbles (white arrows) in the left atrium (LA). The perforating catheter is indicated by the black arrow. (d) To enlarge the created septostomy, static balloon dilation (arrows) is performed. (e) Postseptostomy color flow indicates flow from LA to right atrium (RA).

be injected to the left atrium to confirm. The entire sheath and dilator can then be advanced to the left atrium and the procedure continues. It is important to note that perforation can result in a more permanent tract as the histology demonstrates healing by inflammation and fibrosis of a thermal injury, however small. Knowing where the perforation is located on the septum can be of considerable importance, hence the importance of imaging. The lack of mechanical force required to achieve perforation in radiofrequency systems can contribute a margin of both precision and safety.

COMPLICATIONS

There are few little published data on the complications of radiofrequency-assisted perforation of the atrial septum, likely in view of the relatively novel nature of the technique and limited broad experience. Mechanical perforation of the atrial septum has endured the test of time and, fortunately, the majority of procedures are free of major complications. Several case series have resulted in a major complication rate that is less than 2% and is generally related to puncture to the pericardial space. Tamponade seems to be fortunately rare (<1%).[8,24,25]

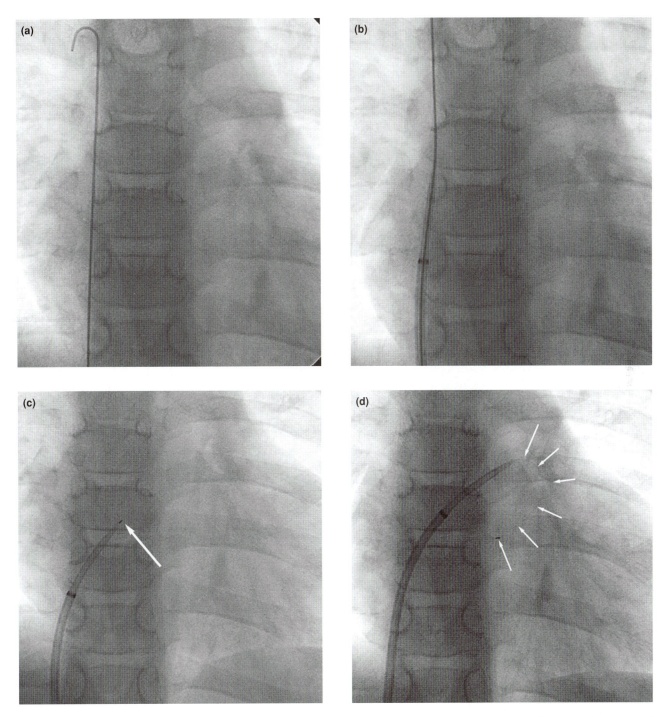

Figure 6.4 Angiographic appearance of radiofrequency-assisted transseptal perforation. The technique of transseptal perforation of the atrial septum is similar to mechanical perforation. (a) A wire is introduced from the femoral vein to the superior vena cava. (b) The sheath and dilator are advanced over the wire. (c) The wire is removed and the sheath withdrawn as described in the text to engage the fossa ovalis with the dilator. The tip of the radiofrequency wire is applied to the septum (white arrow) and energy is applied while gently advancing. (d) The sheath and dilator are advanced over the perforating wire curled in the left atrium to avoid perforation of the left atrial wall (white arrows). The dilator and wire are then removed and the sheath de-aired, thus providing access to the left atrium.

Other complications include perforation of the right atrium or the inferior or superior vena cava, systemic embolization of clot or air to the coronary, cerebral, splanchnic, renal, and femoral vessels, bleeding, vasovagal responses, aortic perforation, inability to engage the atrial system, and tamponade resulting in death.[8,25–29]

Complications are being addressed by new technology such as the radiofrequency-assisted systems described above, and by improvements in imaging. A biplane fluoroscopic system for the difficult patient is traditionally recommended, however there is accumulating evidence for single plane safety and efficacy.[24] Complementary

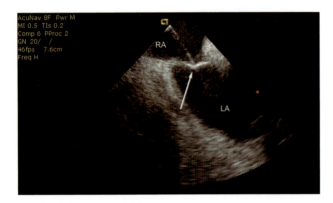

Figure 6.5 Intracardiac echocardiography. This intracardiac echocardiographic image demonstrates the location of a needle or wire on the atrial septum to precisely determine the location of the transseptal puncture. Note as well the clear image of the left atrium. The wire or needle can be easily tracked as it advances into the left atrium, providing precision and safety.

imaging modalities utilizing real-time three-dimensional echocardiographic imaging,[30] transesophageal echocardiography,[31,32] computerized tomography of the fossa ovalis,[32] and intracardiac echocardiography[33,34] have all been employed to further increase safety. The latter technique, now widely employed in electrophysiology offers the advantage of projecting where the system will be heading after the septum is punctured, so that the position of the puncture is of best advantage to the anticipated application (Figure 6.5).

SUMMARY

Transseptal access to the left atrium is an important tool to the invasive cardiologist. Mechanical perforation has endured the test of time, but newer techniques utilizing radiofrequency-assisted systems may offer an advantage, especially in the setting of the very thick septum or the small atrium in congenital heart disease. Consideration should be given to complementary imaging modalities, especially transesophageal and intracardiac echocardiography, depending on the patient and procedure.

REFERENCES

1. Cope C. Technique for transseptal catheterization of the left atrium; preliminary report. J Thorac Surg 1959; 37: 482–6.
2. Brockenbrough EC, Braunwald E, Ross J Jr. Transseptal left heart catheterization. A review of 450 studies and description of an improved technic. Circulation 1962; 25: 15–21.
3. Duff DF, Mullins CE. Transseptal left heart catheterization in infants and children. Cathet Cardiovasc Diagn 1978; 4: 213–23.
4. Mullins CE. Transseptal left heart catheterization: experience with a new technique in 520 pediatric and adult patients. Pediatr Cardiol 1983; 4: 239–45.
5. Ross J Jr, Braunwald E, Morrow AG. Transseptal left heart catheterization: a new diagnostic method. Prog Cardiovasc Dis 1960; 2: 315–18.
6. Roveti GC, Ross RS, Bahnson HT. Transseptal left heart catheterization in the pediatric age group. J Pediatr 1962; 61: 855–8.
7. Carabello BA, Barry WH, Grossman W. Changes in arterial pressure during left heart pullback in patients with aortic stenosis: a sign of severe aortic stenosis. Am J Cardiol 1979; 44: 424–7.
8. Schoonmaker FW, Vijay NK, Jantz RD. Left atrial and ventricular transseptal catheterization review: losing skills? Cathet Cardiovasc Diagn 1987; 13: 233–8.
9. Galie N, Seeger W, Naeije R et al. Comparative analysis of clinical trials and evidence-based treatment algorithm in pulmonary arterial hypertension. J Am Coll Cardiol 2004; 43: 81–8S.
10. Law MA, Grifka RG, Mullins CE et al. Atrial septostomy improves survival in select patients with pulmonary hypertension. Am Heart J 2007; 153: 779–84.
11. Rothman A, Sklansky MS, Lucas VW et al. Atrial septostomy as a bridge to lung transplantation in patients with severe pulmonary hypertension. Am J Cardiol 1999; 84: 682–6.
12. Seib PM, Faulkner SC, Erickson CC et al. Blade and balloon atrial septostomy for left heart decompression in patients with severe ventricular dysfunction on extracorporeal membrane oxygenation. Cathet Cardiovasc Interven 1999; 46: 179–86.
13. McMahon CJ, El Said HG, Mullins CE. Use of the transseptal puncture in transcatheter closure of long tunnel-type patent foramen ovale. Heart 2002; 88: E3.
14. Cheatham JP. Intervention in the critically ill neonate and infant with hypoplastic left heart syndrome and intact atrial septum. J Interven Cardiol 2001; 14: 357–66.
15. Javois AJ, Van Bergen AH, Cuneo BF et al. Novel approach to the newborn with hypoplastic left heart syndrome and intact atrial septum. Cathet Cardiovasc Interven 2005; 66: 268–72.
16. Justino H, Benson LN, Nykanen DG. Transcatheter creation of an atrial septal defect using radiofrequency perforation. Cathet Cardiovasc Interven 2001; 54: 83–7.
17. Vlahos AP, Lock JE, McElhinney DB et al. Hypoplastic left heart syndrome with intact or highly restrictive atrial septum: outcome after neonatal transcatheter atrial septostomy. Circulation 2004; 109: 2326–30.
18. El Said HG, Ing FF, Grifka RG et al. 18-year experience with transseptal procedures through baffles, conduits, and other intra-atrial patches. Cathet Cardiovasc Interven 2000; 50: 434–9.
19. Gonzalez MD, Otomo K, Shah N et al. Transseptal left heart catheterization for cardiac ablation procedures. J Interven Card Electrophysiol 2001; 5: 89–95.
20. Hildick-Smith D, McCready J, de Giovanni J. Transseptal puncture: use of an angioplasty guidewire for enhanced safety. Cathet Cardiovasc Interven 2007; 69: 519–21.
21. Veldtman GR, Hartley A, Visram N et al. Radiofrequency applications in congenital heart disease. Expert Rev Cardiovasc Ther 2004; 2: 117–26.
22. Sakata Y, Feldman T. Transcatheter creation of atrial septal perforation using a radiofrequency transseptal system: novel approach as an alternative to transseptal needle puncture. Cathet Cardiovasc Interven 2005; 64: 327–32.
23. Sherman W, Lee P, Hartley A et al. Transatrial septal catheterization using a new radiofrequency probe. Cathet Cardiovasc Interven 2005; 66: 14–17.
24. Croft CH, Lipscomb K. Modified technique of transseptal left heart catheterization. J Am Coll Cardiol 1985; 5: 904–10.
25. Roelke M, Smith AJ, Palacios IF. The technique and safety of transseptal left heart catheterization: the Massachusetts General Hospital experience with 1,279 procedures. Cathet Cardiovasc Diagn 1994; 32: 332–9.
26. Adrouny ZA, Sutherland DW, Griswold HE et al. Complications with transseptal left heart catheterization. Am Heart J 1963; 65: 327–33.

27. Ali Khan MA, Mullins CE, Bash SE et al. Transseptal left heart catheterisation in infants, children, and young adults. Cathet Cardiovasc Diagn 1989; 17: 198–201.

28. Lindeneg O, Hansen AT. Complications in transseptal left heart catheterization. Acta Med Scand 1966; 180: 395–9.

29. Nixon PG, Ikram H. Left heart catheterization with special reference to the transseptal method. Br Heart J 1966; 28: 835–41.

30. Baker GH, Shirali GS, Bandisode V. Transseptal left heart catheterization for a patient with a prosthetic mitral valve using live three-dimensional transesophageal echocardiography. Pediatr Cardiol 2007; [ePub Ahead of print]

31. Tucker KJ, Curtis AB, Murphy J et al. Transesophageal echocardiographic guidance of transseptal left heart catheterization during radiofrequency ablation of left-sided accessory pathways in humans. Pacing Clin Electrophysiol 1996; 19: 272–81.

32. Van Der Velde ME, Perry SB. Transesophageal echocardiography during interventional catheterization in congenital heart disease. Echocardiography 1997; 14: 513–28.

33. Daoud EG, Kalbfleisch SJ, Hummel JD. Intracardiac echocardiography to guide transseptal left heart catheterization for radiofrequency catheter ablation. J Cardiovasc Electrophysiol 1999; 10: 358–63.

34. Ren JF, Marchlinski FE, Callans DJ, Herrmann HC. Clinical use of AcuNav diagnostic ultrasound catheter imaging during left heart radiofrequency ablation and transcatheter closure procedures. J Am Soc Echocardiogr 2002; 15: 1301–8.

7 Pulmonary valvuloplasty

Ralf J Holzer

TECHNIQUE

Balloon pulmonary valvuloplasty was first introduced as an interventional procedure by Kan and colleagues in 1982,[1] and is now accepted as the standard therapeutic procedure for valvar pulmonary stenosis.[2–4] The procedure can be successfully performed at any age, ranging from a newborn infant with critical pulmonary valve stenosis to the adult population.[5] With its excellent results and low rate of procedure-related adverse events, peak instantaneous systolic echo gradients of as little as 35 mmHg, when combined with evidence of right ventricular hypertrophy, should be considered an indication for balloon pulmonary valvuloplasty.[6]

Even though the procedure is frequently performed using general endotracheal anesthesia, this is not always necessary and in most patients the procedure can be performed safely using a combination of deep sedation and local anesthesia. Vascular access is obtained in at least a single femoral vein, with an additional monitoring cannula being placed in the femoral artery. Additional femoral venous access is required when the double-balloon technique is employed, and may also be helpful to facilitate periprocedural right ventricular pressure monitoring and angiography as well as emergent drug administration. Standard right heart catheterization is performed preferably using a floating balloon-tipped end hole catheter. In most patients, the pulmonary valve can be readily crossed without inducing hemodynamic instability. However, if the pulmonary valve cannot be crossed easily, or in patients with very severe pulmonary valve stenosis and/or very high right ventricular pressures, right ventricular angiography is performed before further attempts are made at crossing the pulmonary valve, using straight lateral projection as well as a degree of cranial angulation on the frontal tubes. It is important to appropriately measure the hinge points of the pulmonary valve using an accurate calibration technique. The appropriate balloon size is determined at about 120–140% of the pulmonary valve annulus.[4] In general, low inflation pressures of less than 6 atmospheres are usually sufficient to perform balloon pulmonary valvuloplasty for congenital pulmonary valve stenosis with typical valve morphology. The use of a low profile balloon with favorable deflation characteristic, such as the Tyshak II balloon (NuMED, Hopkinton, NY), is usually recommended as the initial balloon type. However, in larger patients and especially when a single-balloon technique is employed, the rated burst pressure in these balloons can be very low and then the use of a higher pressure balloon, such as ZMed II (NuMED, Hopkinton, NY) may be required. The same applies in the presence of a very thickened, dysplastic pulmonary valve.

After the appropriate balloon size has been determined and the balloon has been prepped meticulously, the pulmonary valve is crossed and the catheter placed in a distal branch pulmonary artery. When the catheter does not readily cross the pulmonary valve, an exchange length wire with a very soft tip, such as the 0.035 inch Magic wire (Boston Scientific, Natick, MA) can be used to carefully probe the pulmonary valve, and this can be further facilitated through small incremental hand injections of contrast underneath the pulmonary valve. However, this is rarely required beyond infancy. In smaller patients the 0.018 inch Hi-Torque Flex-T guide wire (Mallinckrodt, Hazelwood, MO) may be used for the purpose of crossing the valve. Once a distal catheter position has been obtained with a larger end hole catheter, the soft-tipped floppy wire is removed and exchanged for an exchange-length extra stiff wire, preferably with a short floppy tip, which is curved only gently prior to positioning into the branch pulmonary arteries. The balloon is then advanced carefully over the wire and through the tricuspid valve and right ventricle across the pulmonary valve. On rare occasions when the balloon does not cross the pulmonary valve with ease, predilatation with a lower profile smaller diameter balloon may be required. A roadmap obtained from the initial right ventricular angiogram should be readily available during inflation of the balloon to show the relationship of the pulmonary valve to fixed bony structures, usually part of the sternum. An inflation device that facilitates pressure monitoring is utilized for balloon inflation, preferably controlled with a single hand, while the other hand controls the position of the balloon and maintains it centered across the valve during inflation, avoiding 'see-saw' motions across the valve annulus. If the balloon cannot be stabilized across the valve and milks either proximally or distally, the inflation is aborted and the balloon repositioned. One should expect the waist to disappear completely during the balloon inflation, and a repeated inflation should not demonstrate a significant residual waist, unless the pulmonary valve is severely dysplastic, in which case an optimal result frequently cannot be achieved. Once a satisfactory balloon inflation has been performed, the balloon is deflated and removed carefully over the wire. If a second femoral venous line has been in place for monitoring purposes, simultaneous main pulmonary artery (MPA) and right ventricular pressure recordings can be obtained. If only a single femoral venous sheath has been placed, a multitrack catheter (NuMED, Hopkinton, NY) can be used to obtain a pressure gradient across the pulmonary valve and, if satisfactory, catheter and wire are removed and a final angiography is performed within the right ventricle.

The single-balloon technique requires some modification in neonates and small infants (Figure 7.1). Right ventricular angiography has to be evaluated carefully, to exclude the presence of any right ventricle dependent coronary circulation. If in doubt, an aortic root injection may be helpful, and in some patients even selective coronary angiography may be required to better delineate the coronary circulation. Frequently a balloon-tipped wedge catheter may not easily advance into the right ventricular outflow tract or across the pulmonary valve. Therefore a 5 French 2.5 curve Judkins right coronary catheter may be required to allow torquing of the catheter underneath the pulmonary valve, where careful hand injections of contrast are very important to visualize the frequently very small pulmonary valve opening. The valve can then be crossed by advancing a soft-tipped wire, such as the 0.018 inch Hi-Torque Flex-T guide wire (Mallinckrodt, Hazelwood, MO), across the pulmonary valve. In patients with critical pulmonary valve stenosis this wire may be manipulated through a persistent arterial duct into the descending aorta. In other patients where a position within a distal branch pulmonary artery has been obtained, the fairly long transition of the Hi-Torque Flex-T wire may not be sufficiently stiff to advance the balloon across the pulmonary valve and the wire may therefore need to be exchanged for the stiffer 0.018 inch V18 wire (Boston Scientific, Natick, MA), which provides better pushability and control when advancing the balloon across the pulmonary valve. In most patients the Tyshak II balloon is the best choice for initial valvuloplasty, and the use of the Tyshak Mini balloon (NuMED, Hopkinton, NY) is usually not recommended due to its slow deflation characteristics. However, in patients with a persistent arterial duct, or when the standard Tyshak II balloon does not readily cross the valve, the

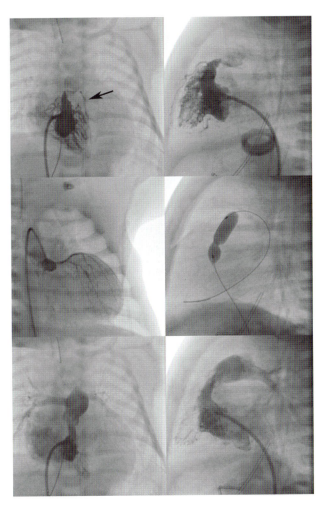

Figure 7.1   Balloon pulmonary valvuloplasty in a 5-day-old infant with critical pulmonary valve stenosis. The initial right ventricular angiogram (top two images) demonstrates a tripartite right ventricle with an extremely muscle-bound apical trabecular component and an extremely small pulmonary valve opening. Of note is a fistula from the right ventricle to the left circumflex coronary artery (arrowhead). The pulmonary valve plate is poorly developed and cone shaped. The annulus is measured at about 4 mm, using a combination of right ventricular (RV) angiography and aortogram (delineating the PDA and pulmonary valve). Selective left coronary angiography demonstrates a non-stenotic left coronary system (middle left image). Balloon valvuloplasty is performed using a 6 mm * 2 cm Tyshak II balloon (middle right image), completely abolishing the transvalvar gradient and reducing the RV/systemic pressure ratio from 200% to 65%. Final RV angiography demonstrates significantly improved antigrade flow across the pulmonary valve (bottom images).

use of the Tyshak Mini balloon may offer advantages through its lower profile.

The double-balloon technique is very similar to the single-balloon technique (Figure 7.2). However, the appropriate size of the combined diameter of the two balloons is about 170% of the pulmonary valve annulus.[6,7] The pulmonary valve is crossed in the same fashion as for the single-balloon technique, but an

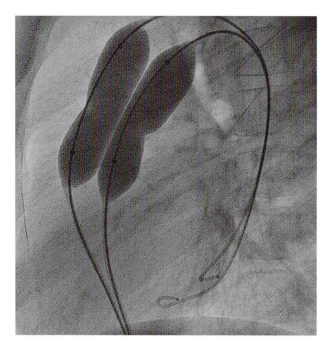

Figure 7.2 Balloon pulmonary valvuloplasty in a 5-year-old boy with valvar and supravalvar pulmonary stenosis, using the double-balloon technique to facilitate the use of higher inflation pressures.

additional stiff wire is placed in a distal pulmonary artery branch. During balloon inflation, additional personnel are usually required to handle one of the inflation devices, while the operator handles the other inflation device with one hand, and uses the other hand to maintain position of both balloons across the pulmonary valve annulus.

HOW NOT TO GET INTO TROUBLE

If performed accurately, balloon pulmonary valvuloplasty is an extremely safe procedure with virtually zero mortality and minimal morbidity. The double-balloon technique is not required in all patients but has several distinct advantages. Not only does it limit the sheath size that is required to accommodate the individual balloon catheters, thereby resulting in a lower risk of femoral venous injury and thrombosis, but it also offers the advantage of not completely obstructing the valve annulus during inflation, thereby allowing still a small amount of antegrade blood flow across the pulmonary valve, with less temporary strain on the right ventricle and lower chances of significant vagal response. This technique should therefore be considered especially in adult-size patients with a large pulmonary valve annulus, or in patients with very high right ventricular pressures who may be more likely to decompensate during balloon inflation.

Taking extra time to place an arterial monitoring cannula does increase the safety of the procedure, and any patient who is hemodynamically unstable or who has

very high right ventricular pressures may benefit from an additional femoral venous line that can solely be used for right ventricular pressure monitoring and angiography, as well as drug administration throughout the procedure. The patients most likely expected to show more significant hemodynamic instability, especially during balloon inflation, are infants just beyond the immediate neonatal period who have high right ventricular pressures, but without the presence of a patent foramen ovale (PFO) or atrial septal defect (ASD) to decompress the right ventricle, and no persistent ductus arteriosus (PDA) to maintain pulmonary blood flow during balloon expansion. In these patients it is of the utmost importance to have all equipment that is required (or potentially required) ready and prepared before crossing the pulmonary valve to facilitate immediate valvuloplasty. These patients may not tolerate a catheter or sometimes even a wire across the valve, and therefore advancement of the balloon may have to be performed quickly to decompress the right ventricle before encountering significant hemodynamic instability.

When positioning a wire in distal pulmonary arteries, wires with a short floppy J-tip are preferred, and care has to be taken not to push the wire too far within a small distal pulmonary arterial branch, as this can lead to small vascular injuries that may be associated with bleeding via the endotracheal tube, especially in small patients. Advancing the balloon catheter across the tricuspid valve has to be performed with great caution, and any resistance encountered should be considered a warning sign of the wire possibly having passed through tricuspid valve chordae, rather than the central lumen of the valve. Forcing the balloon catheter in this situation across the tricuspid valve may lead to injury or disruption of chordal attachments, with the patient then potentially requiring surgical tricuspid valve repair or replacement in the future. The best method to minimize the chance of traversing the chordal apparatus is to use a floating balloon-tipped end hole catheter with the balloon fully inflated when crossing the tricuspid valve, rather than just a torque-controlled catheter. Similarly, the sharp extra stiff wire may potentially damage tricuspid valve tissue, and it is therefore helpful to leave the standard catheter in place over the wire in a distal pulmonary arterial position, until the operator is ready to advance the balloon catheter.

By being meticulous about the chosen balloon size, one can usually avoid any complications related to the balloon expansion itself, especially valve and valve annulus disruption. Use of the appropriate calibration techniques helps to prevent overestimation or, more importantly, underestimation of the pulmonary valve annulus. In addition, it is important to emphasize the need to measure the pulmonary valve annulus at the hinge point. If the initial angiographic projection is suboptimal to obtain good biplane imaging of the valve annulus, the projections should be modified, using more or less cranial angulation on the frontal

Table 7.1 Complications of balloon pulmonary valvuloplasty reported in four series.

Study	Patients	Total reported adverse events	Mortality	Avulsion or annular tear or perforation	Tricuspid valve injury	Venous injury	Arrhythmia orconduction anomaly
Stanger et al. 1990[3]	n = 822 mainly peds	37/822 (4.5%)	2/822 (0.2%)	3/822 (0.4%)	2/822 (0.2%)	7/822 (0.9%)	8/822 (1%)
Gildein et al. 1996[10]	n = 18 all critical PS	7/18 (38.9%)	1/18 (5.5%)	3/18 (16.7%)	0	0	2/18 (11.1%)
Chen et al. 1996[9]	n = 53 adults	0	0	0	0	0	0
Fawzy et al. 2007[8]	n = 90 mainly adults	1/90 (1.1%)	0	0	0	0	0

Peds, pediatric patient; PS, pulmonary valve stenosis.

tubes, until accurate measurements can be obtained. Preparing the balloon with too much contrast (more than 20–30%) does prolong the time it takes for the balloon to deflate, thereby prolonging the time the right ventricle is exposed to significant obstruction of antegrade flow across the pulmonary valve. Being diligent when prepping and purging the balloon and only using the maximum recommended inflation pressure is also important to prevent inadvertent balloon rupture during inflation. The operator should aim to avoid rapid see-saw movements of the balloon across the pulmonary valve as this may damage the annulus itself.

The procedure is not completed with successful balloon valvuloplasty alone until the balloon catheter has been completely removed. The deflated balloon catheter often has very sharp wings which, if removed against resistance, can easily damage chordal attachments of the tricuspid valve or the valve itself. If any resistance is encountered the balloon is carefully inflated, deflated, and rotated to allow it to pass easily through the valve. While one should try to use the smallest sheath size possible, in general the operator should choose a hemostatic sheath size that is at least 1 French larger than the shaft size of the dilation catheter. This is much less traumatic then having to remove a deflated balloon with its sharp wings directly through the femoral vein, because of an inability to capture it back into an undersized hemostatic sheath.

In small infants and neonates, and patients with critical pulmonary valve stenosis, it is extremely important to use only soft-tipped wires when crossing the pulmonary valve and to confirm the appropriate position by selective hand injections of contrast through the catheter before crossing the valve itself with a larger catheter. The right ventricular outflow tract (RVOT) is extremely thin and vulnerable in these patients and sharp wires, such as for example angled glide wires, may just cross directly through the RVOT and into the pericardial space.

COMPLICATIONS

Table 7.1 lists the most common complications reported in several larger series of balloon pulmonary valvuloplasty.[2,6,8–10] Not surprisingly, complications are more common in infants and neonates with critical pulmonary valve stenosis.[10] However, in general, complications of balloon pulmonary valvuloplasty are rare, and can be almost completely eliminated through the use of the appropriate technique and choice of the correct equipment. Complications include those associated with any cardiac catheterization procedures that have been discussed in preceding chapters. Complications specific to balloon pulmonary valvuloplasty include, at the most severe end of the spectrum, valve and valve annulus disruption. Tricuspid valve injury through the wire and/or balloon have been described,[11] as has injury of pulmonary arterial branches as a result of wire manipulation or wire movement. Balloon rupture, especially circumferential, is rare if care is taken not to exceed the rated burst pressure. Hemodynamic instability and/or cardiac arrest can occur during balloon inflation, as discussed above. Additional complications include femoral venous injury, rhythm and conduction anomalies, as well as the creation of pulmonary insufficiency. The latter is rarely clinically significant, and in the presence of otherwise normal heart and lungs, the regurgitant fraction is usually small.

HOW TO MANAGE COMPLICATIONS

When performing balloon pulmonary valvuloplasty, the best way to 'manage' most of the complications is to avoid getting into trouble in the first place. At the most severe end of the spectrum of complications, if annulus disruption does occur in a patient without previous cardiac surgery, this complication is usually fatal. Blood needs to be readily available and a large pericardial drain is placed. If the patient can be stabilized emergent surgery is necessary, but unfortunately, in the presence of a larger tear, resuscitation attempts are usually futile. In patients with previous cardiac surgery, a tear may not necessarily comprise an acute emergency, and instead present as a false aneurysm seen on postvalvuloplasty right ventricular angiography. Frequently these patients do not present with any hemodynamic instability and, depending on the nature of the tear and the associated cardiac and extracardiac anatomy, surgical repair may or may not be required at the same admission. In most patients follow-up including a CT-scan is recommended the day following the procedure and after 2–4 weeks to monitor the false aneurysm for any potential increase in size, with cardiac surgery then being performed electively when suitable to the patient and family.

Injury to the pulmonary arterial branches can be caused by the stiff guide wire. This usually presents with blood being noted on suctioning of the endotracheal tube. An angiography should be performed, using for example a multitrack catheter (NuMED, Hopkinton, NY), excluding any obvious loss of vascular integrity of a pulmonary arterial branch. In most circumstances, bleeding is due to the end of the wire causing a minor injury to a distal small pulmonary arterial branch. In this scenario, suctioning of the endotracheal tube should not be performed too aggressively and the bleeding usually stops spontaneously without any additional intervention. Administration of blood products is usually not required.

If hemodynamic instability with bradycardia and a drop in blood pressure is encountered during balloon inflation, the best course of action is to deflate the balloon quickly and remove it from the right ventricle into an inferior vena cava (IVC) position. Atropine should be readily available and occasionally a small dose of epinephrine or brief cardiac massage may be required. However, while this loss of cardiac output appears dramatic at the time, in general the vast majority of patients regain a normal heart rate and blood pressure very quickly, especially if valvuloplasty was performed successfully prior to balloon removal.

On occasion, the placement of a stiff guide wire in distal pulmonary arteries may be poorly tolerated, especially in infants, through stenting open the tricuspid valve. If the wire or wire loop causes hemodynamic instability, heart block, or arrhythmias, relieving the tension on the wire and/or the wire loop is usually sufficient to restore hemodynamic stability. In some patients, however, hemodynamic stability may only be fully restored after successful balloon valvuloplasty when the wire is being removed from the right ventricle. Injury to the tricuspid valve can usually not be ameliorated within the catheterization laboratory once it has occurred, and therefore prevention of its occurrence in the first place through careful catheter, wire, and balloon manipulation is the only effective 'treatment' of this complication.

At the severe end of the spectrum, a patient may require surgical tricuspid valve repair or even replacement after a catheter- or balloon-induced injury to the valve or the valve apparatus. The same applies to femoral venous injury, and therefore the use of low-profile balloons is very important in reducing the trauma to the femoral venous vasculature.

Balloon rupture is a very rare complication when the necessary care is taken not to exceed the rated burst pressure during balloon inflation, but calcified pulmonary valves in older patients or protruding sharp edges from stents that have previously been placed in proximal branch pulmonary arteries may induce such a rupture. On most occasions, balloons rupture longitudinally and can be safely removed. Very rarely, a circumferential rupture is encountered and removal of the balloon may disintegrate the distal balloon portion from the catheter shaft. If this is recognized after balloon removal and inspection of the balloon catheter, a large sheath is advanced over the wire to a position where the balloon fragment is likely to be expected. It is important to keep the wire in position as the wire will remain through the balloon fragment, thereby allowing a more controlled retrieval and preventing the fragment from embolizing further distally. The balloon fragments are noticeable as filling defects on angiography. At this point a gooseneck snare (ev3, Plymouth, MN) or the Ensnare (MD Technologies, FL) can be advanced, with part of the snare loops being fed over the wire and then advanced through the sheath. This should enable the balloon fragment to be caught and retrieved into the long sheath. Alternatively, a snare can be advanced next to the wire, snaring the distal end of the wire and recapturing it as a U-loop back into the sheath, with the balloon fragment being trapped in the mid portion of this wire. Finally, if all else fails, a snare can be positioned just distal to the balloon fragment. The wire is then removed very slowly and gradually, and the balloon fragment is grabbed immediately after the wire has been pulled back.

REFERENCES

1. Kan JS, White RI Jr, Mitchell SE, Gardner TJ. Percutaneous balloon valvuloplasty: a new method for treating congenital pulmonary-valve stenosis. N Engl J Med 1982; 307(9): 540–2.
2. Stanger P, Cassidy SC, Girod DA et al. Balloon pulmonary valvuloplasty: results of the Valvuloplasty and Angioplasty of Congenital Anomalies Registry. Am J Cardiol 1990; 65(11): 775–83.
3. Rao PS, Galal O, Patnana M, Buck SH, Wilson AD. Results of three to 10 year follow up of balloon dilatation of the pulmonary valve. Heart 1998; 80(6): 591–5.
4. McCrindle BW. Independent predictors of long-term results after balloon pulmonary valvuloplasty. Valvuloplasty and Angioplasty of Congenital Anomalies (VACA) Registry Investigators. Circulation 1994; 89(4): 1751–9.
5. Jarrar M, Betbout F, Farhat MB et al. Long-term invasive and noninvasive results of percutaneous balloon pulmonary valvuloplasty in children, adolescents, and adults. Am Heart J 1999; 138(5 Pt 1): 950–4.

6. Mullins CE. Pulmonary valve balloon dilation. In: Mullins CE, ed. Cardiac Catheterization in Congenital Heart Disease. Malden: Blackwell, 2006: 430–40.

7. Mullins CE, Nihill MR, Vick GW et al. Double balloon technique for dilation of valvular or vessel stenosis in congenital and acquired heart disease. J Am Coll Cardiol 1987; 10(1): 107–14.

8. Fawzy ME, Hassan W, Fadel BM et al. Long-term results (up to 17 years) of pulmonary balloon valvuloplasty in adults and its effects on concomitant severe infundibular stenosis and tricuspid regurgitation. Am Heart J 2007; 153(3): 433–8.

9. Chen CR, Cheng TO, Huang T et al. Percutaneous balloon valvuloplasty for pulmonic stenosis in adolescents and adults [see comment]. N Engl J Med 1996; 335(1): 21–5.

10. Gildein HP, Kleinert S, Goh TH, Wilkinson JL. Treatment of critical pulmonary valve stenosis by balloon dilatation in the neonate. Am Heart J 1996; 131(5): 1007–11.

11. Berger RM, Cromme-Dijkhuis AH, Witsenburg M, Hess J. Tricuspid valve regurgitation as a complication of pulmonary balloon valvuloplasty or transcatheter closure of patent ductus arteriosus in children < or = 4 years of age. Am J Cardiol 1993; 72(12): 976–7.

8 Radiofrequency perforation of the pulmonary valve in patients with pulmonary atresia and intact ventricular septum

Ralf J Holzer and John P Cheatham

TECHNIQUE

Even though patients with the diagnosis of pulmonary atresia with intact ventricular septum (PA/IVS) and a single-ventricle pathway usually have a very poor long-term outcome, the outlook for those patients with a biventricular or a 'one-and-a-half ventricle' circulation is much better. Achieving antegrade pulmonary flow through perforation of the atretic pulmonary valve plate is an important treatment modality, not only to decompress the right ventricle (RV), but more importantly to serve as an incentive to facilitate further growth of an initially hypoplastic right ventricle.[1] A variety of sharp instruments as well as laser-guided techniques have been used to perforate the atretic pulmonary valve. However, these techniques are often poorly controlled and associated with a risk of creating inadvertent injury to surrounding structures, often with disastrous results. As a result, the use of radio frequency (RF) energy was introduced into therapeutic cardiac catheterization in the early 1990s as an alternative to laser-guided perforation of the pulmonary valve plate.[2] Not all patients with PA/IVS are suitable candidates to be taken to the cardiac catheterization laboratory. A thorough echocardiographic assessment is required prior to the procedure and minimal requirements in most cases include the presence of a tripartite RV as well as a membranous atretic pulmonary valve with a well formed infundibulum.[3]

All procedures are performed under general endotracheal anesthesia using a dedicated pediatric cardiac anesthetist. Vascular access is obtained via right femoral venous cannulation as well as placing a femoral arterial pressure monitoring line. Baseline hemodynamic evaluation should include right ventricular and systemic arterial pressures. Right ventricular as well as left ventricular angiographies are obtained using the same projection with 20° cranial angulation of the frontal tubes and standard lateral projection. This not only facilitates measurement of the pulmonary valve plate diameter and exclusion of RV-dependent coronary circulation (Figure 8.1), but also facilitates a better understanding of the exact relationship between the blind ending

right ventricular infundibulum and main pulmonary artery which is fed via the PDA. The equipment most frequently used to achieve perforation of the atretic pulmonary valve with RF energy is the Nykanen RF perforation wire with its coaxial catheter and the Baylis radiofrequency puncture generator (all: Baylis Medical Corporation, Montreal, Quebec, Canada). Even in smaller patients, for better torquability a 5 French Judkins 2.5 right coronary catheter is placed below the pulmonary valve within the right ventricular outflow tract. A Touhy Borst adapter is used to allow passage of the RF wire while being able to simultaneously inject contrast to confirm appropriate positioning of the catheter tip. Once the RF wire and coaxial catheter are loaded, and accurate positioning is confirmed, RF energy is applied while gently pushing the RF wire toward the valve membrane. The initial RV and left ventricle (LV) angiography should serve as orientating roadmaps and one should pay diligent attention that the RF wire is advancing towards the main pulmonary artery (MPA). A power setting of 5 W/s is usually sufficient to perforate the pulmonary valve plate. RF energy is discontinued once the wire has advanced through the valve plate, which is frequently notable with the wire suddenly advancing a few millimeters. Before advancing the coaxial catheter, it is necessary to confirm that the RF wire has in fact entered the main pulmonary artery, using a small injection of contrast through the Touhy Borst adapter. The coaxial catheter is then advanced over the RF wire into the main pulmonary artery and the RF wire is exchanged for a 0.014 or 0.018 inch coronary wire (depending on the balloon), which can be directed either to a position in a distal branch pulmonary artery or preferably through the persistent ductus arteriosus (PDA) into the descending aorta. The chosen balloon size should be about 120–130% of the pulmonary valve plate annulus, and preferably a low-profile balloon valvuloplasty catheter is used, such as the Mini-Tyshak (NuMED, Hopkinton, NY) (Figure 8.2). If the balloon does not easily cross the valve plate, predilation can be performed using an even lower profile

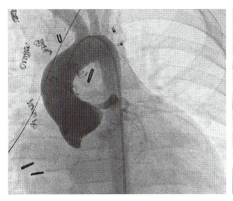

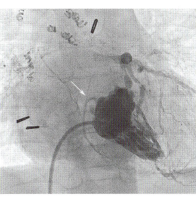

Figure 8.1 Male infant with PA/IVS and RV-dependent coronary circulation. The aortogram (left) demonstrates a single left coronary artery giving rise to a circumflex and anterior descending branch. There was no evidence of any right coronary artery. RV angiogram (right) demonstrates a small hypoplastic right ventricular cavity and multiple coronary fistulas. The left circumflex system appears to have multiple stenoses and a small right coronary branch (arrow) is supplied by the RV cavity without any communication with the ascending aorta.

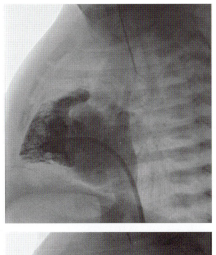

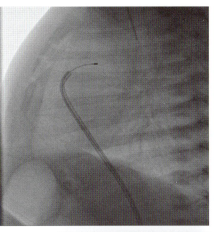

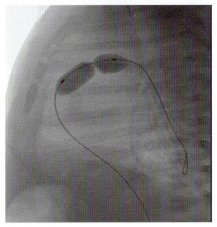

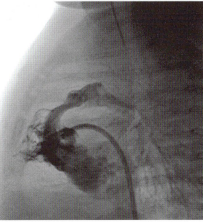

Figure 8.2 RF perforation of the pulmonary valve in a neonate with pulmonary atresia with intact ventricular septum. Top left: RV angiogram delineating the RVOT. Top right: RF wire across the pulmonary valve plate. Bottom left: Balloon valvuloplasty with a wire positioned in the distal right pulmonary artery. Bottom right: RV angiogram demonstrating the newly created continuity between the right ventricle and main pulmonary artery.

2.5–3 mm coronary balloon. If the wire has been passed through the PDA into the descending aorta, rather than any of the pulmonary arterial branches, then the wire can either be fixed through manual compression above the femoral artery, or through snaring the wire within the descending aorta.[4] After at least two inflations have been performed that document abolition of the waist of the balloon catheter, a final hemodynamic evaluation is performed that includes assessment of the transvalvar gradient, as well as the RV–systemic pressure ratio. A final RV angiography should document the lack of any aneurysm formation or extravasation, as well as improved antegrade flow

across the pulmonary valve. Patients are usually continued on prostaglandin for at least 5–7 days before attempting to wean, to allow the RV to dilate and grow through the improved antegrade flow. If a patient cannot be weaned off prostaglandin, further palliation will be required, either in the form of a surgical shunt or through transcatheter stenting of the arterial duct.

HOW NOT TO GET INTO TROUBLE

Many of the comments made when discussing balloon pulmonary valvuloplasty in Chapter 7 also apply to the management of patients with PA/IVS. Being diligent in the diagnostic and angiographic evaluation is essential to avoid many of the more serious complications seen in this group of patients. Patients with RV-dependent coronary circulation are clearly a contraindication for this procedure, and, if in doubt, one may have to repeat RV angiographies in various projections as well as perform selective coronary angiography. An attempt to perform RF perforation in the presence of a muscle-bound right ventricular outflow tract (RVOT) without a clear path to the pulmonary valve plate is a futile undertaking, and clearly associated with an increased risk of creating a false tract and perforation.

In patients with PA/IVS the right ventricular cavity is usually very small and at times it may be difficult to advance the JR catheter underneath the pulmonary valve plate. A tip deflector or the stiff preshaped end of a standard wire may aid in advancing the catheter carefully into the right ventricle. While a 4 French JR catheter is softer than a 5 French one, its use is clearly counterproductive in these patients. The lack of sufficient torque makes it very difficult to advance the catheter underneath the pulmonary valve, and the operator will frequently find himself changing to the 5 French variety after multiple unsuccessful attempts that may have caused unnecessary arrhythmias as well as always being associated with a small risk of creating damage to the very thin myocardium of the RVOT if not used cautiously. The 5 French catheter can be torqued more easily, but while torque is necessary to advance the catheter to the RVOT, one has to be constantly aware of the very thin nature of the RVOT myocardium in these patients. If the catheter does not advance easily when rotating it clockwise towards the RVOT, it may be necessary to withdraw the catheter tip as it may be buried in blind-ending right ventricular myocardium.

When the catheter tip is positioned within the RVOT, a hand injection of contrast should outline the smooth pulmonary valve plate, and it is important to distinguish this from a more muscle-bound RVOT. Several hand injections may be necessary to achieve an appropriate position. For this purpose, the initial RV and LV angiography are extremely important, not only in allowing accurate sizing of the pulmonary valve plate, but more importantly by showing the relationship of the RVOT and valve plate to the blind-ending MPA stump. If this relationship is not well defined using an LV angiogram, the arterial monitoring cannula can be exchanged for a 3 French short hemostatic sheath and a simultaneous hand injection of contrast performed at the mouth of the PDA during RV angiography.

When advancing the RF wire, care has to be taken that the wire follows a course that is in alignment with the main pulmonary artery. Quite frequently, especially when the catheter tip is not aligned with the central portion of the valve plate, the wire may follow a course that is too superior and anterior to the course of the genuine MPA. In this context, it is very easy to miss a wire extravasation and therefore the accurate position has to be confirmed through injection of contrast through the Touhy Borst adapter before attempting to advance the coaxial catheter over the RF wire. One should be particularly suspicious about the possibility of creating a false tract if high power settings are required on the RF generator, despite the angiographic and echocardiographic appearance suggesting a thin pulmonary valve plate.

While it is important to achieve a wire position in the distal pulmonary arteries, or preferably across the PDA, this should not be attempted with the Nykanen RF wire, as it can easily cause perforation of the main pulmonary artery.[1] Once the RF wire has crossed the valve plate it should only be advanced a few millimeters, just about enough to allow the coaxial catheter to track into the MPA without losing wire position. Under no circumstances should the RF wire be pushed against any resistance after successful RF perforation of the valve. If, for any reason, wire position is lost, then a small hand injection frequently shows the newly created perforation within the valve plate, and a coronary wire can often be advanced directly through the created perforation back into the MPA. This is similar to the technique employed when using the Osypka RF system (Cordis Webster, Inc, or Dr Osypka GmbH), which has the clear disadvantage of not having a coaxial catheter to track into the MPA.

Hemodynamic instability, as well as rhythm and conduction anomalies, are usually the result of either a perforation with pericardial tamponade, or tension of the guide wire within the right ventricular cavity and/or right atrium. This may be aggravated if the balloon catheter does not cross the valve plate easily and pushing too forcefully in this scenario may not only induce temporary bradycardia, heartblock, or atrial arrhythmias, but may also be associated with a sudden loss of wire position. To reduce the risk of hemodynamic instability or loss of wire position when attempting to advance the ballon catheter across the valve the operator may need to consider using a smaller coronary balloon to predilate the valve plate, or to snare the wire in the descending aorta to achieve a more stable wire position.

COMPLICATIONS

Complications that are seen after standard balloon pulmonary valvuloplasty apply also to patients with PA/IVS who undergo RF perforation of the pulmonary valve plate. Most series that have reported on the

Table 8.1 Procedural complications after RF perforation of the pulmonary valve plate in patients with PA/IVS, reported in three larger series between 2000 and 2003. pts: patients.

Study	Patients	Total pts with complications	Procedural death	Perforation	Arrhythmia heart block	Other
Alwi et al. 2000[12]	21	6	1	3	2	1
Humpl et al. 2002[10]	30	—	1	6	7	2
Agnoletti et al. 2003[11]	33	6	2	3	3	—

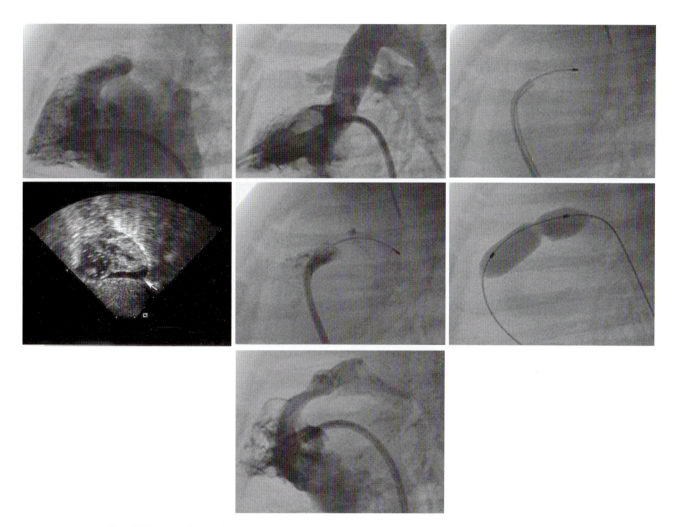

Figure 8.3 Two-day old female infant with PA/IVS. From top to bottom: RV angiogram with a small right ventricular cavity and a blind-ending RVOT. The second angiogram was obtained inside the left ventricle (in same projection as RV angiogram), demonstrating the main pulmonary artery being supplied via a PDA. The third image demonstrates the RF wire slightly too anterior in relation to the main pulmonary artery. Injection of contrast through the JR catheter did not help to better define the wire position (not shown), but the patient gradually became hypotensive and echocardiography (fourth image) demonstrated a pericardial effusion. The wire was withdrawn and, after stabilizing the patient (including pericardiocentesis), a repeat attempt at RF perforation demonstrated an improved wire position (more inferior), which was confirmed angiographically (fifth image). The sixth image demonstrates balloon valvuloplasty, followed by a final RV angiogram documenting appropriate antegrade flow across the pulmonary valve.

results of transcatheter management of patients with PA/IVS are small and include fewer then five patients.[5–9] Table 8.1 lists the complications reported in three larger studies with more than 20 patients.[10–12] The overall incidence of procedure-related complications ranges from 18 to 28%, with procedural deaths in the cardiac catheterization laboratory (or within a few hours of the procedure) being reported in 4–6%. The most common reported complications include atrial arrhythmias and conduction anomalies, as well as cardiac, infundibular, or MPA perforation (with or without pericardial effusion/tamponade) (Figure 8.3). Other rare complications include MPA aneurysm, damage to the tricuspid valve apparatus with tricuspid regurgitation, as well as decompressing an RV with an RV-dependent coronary circulation.

HOW TO MANAGE COMPLICATIONS

Complications related to valvuloplasty itself are managed in a similar way to those encountered in patients with critical pulmonary valve stenosis (and have been discussed in Chapter 7, pulmonary valvuloplasty). When complications do occur as a result of RF perforation, they are usually more profound, and associated with significant hemodynamic instability. It is therefore of the utmost importance to limit the occurrence of these complications through the use of a very careful and diligent technique, to avoid having to deal with a major adverse event.

If perforation does occur, it is important is to recognize this before advancing any catheter over the RF wire. Diagnostic clues are the wire not following the course into the MPA, or the wire tracking along the cardiac silhouette within the pericardial space. At this point, the perforation can be confirmed by injecting a small amount of contrast through the JR catheter. Unless contrast is clearly seen entering the main pulmonary artery without any staining, the wire position should be regarded as doubtful and no further attempts be made to track any catheter over the wire. The cardiac surgical colleagues need to be aware of the procedure and any potential complication. At this point the wire is carefully pulled back and the patient observed for any hemodynamic instability or any sign of pericardial effusion/tamponade. For this purpose, the cardiac catheterization laboratory should have echocardiography readily available and set up to evaluate the patient for the presence of a pericardial effusion, if any hemodynamic instability is encountered. If the patient remains hemodynamically stable without any evidence of pericardial effusion, fresh attempts can be made to perforate the pulmonary valve plate. If a patient develops a significant pericardial effusion, pericardiocentesis needs to be performed rapidly and blood products need to be readily available. In most cases the bleeding stops spontaneously, but surgical back-up is important if hemodynamic stability cannot be achieved. The risk of inducing rhythm and conduction anomalies can usually be reduced by avoiding significant tension and looping of the guide wire. If the anomaly persists despite releasing the wire tension, the appropriate medical and/or electrical therapy needs to be initiated.

Decompressing an RV with an RV-dependent coronary circulation is an extremely rare event, and should ideally be avoided by carefully evaluating RV angiography as well as possible using selective coronary angiography. However, if it does occur the presentation is usually quite dramatic, with ST/T-wave changes and hypotension following balloon deflation. The only way to achieve any degree of stability in this situation is to try to occlude the RVOT at least temporarily, until further surgical intervention can be performed. The standard Tyshak II or Tyshak Mini Balloon catheters (NuMED, Hopkinton, NY) are usually too long to keep inflated across the RVOT, as they would either potentially obstruct part of the PDA flow, or some of the RV cavity. A suitable alternative could be the 1 ml NuMED Septostomy Balloon Catheter (NuMED, Hopkinton, NY), which could be advanced quickly over the wire that is already in place and positioned in such a way that it just occludes the RVOT. The inflation will have to be maintained until surgical intervention can be performed.

REFERENCES

1. Holzer RJ, Hardin J, Hill SL, Chisolm J, Cheatham JP. Radiofrequency energy – a multi-facetted tool for the congenital interventionist. Congen Cardiol Today 2006; 4: 1–8.
2. Redington AN, Cullen S, Rigby ML. Laser or radiofrequency pulmonary valvotomy in neonates with pulmonary atresia and intact ventricular septum – description of a new method avoiding arterial catheterization. Cardiol Young 1992; 2: 387–90.
3. Cheatham JP. To perforate or not to perforate – that's the question … or is it? just ask Richard! Cathet Cardiovasc Diagn 1997; 42: 403–4.
4. Latson L, Cheatham J, Froemming S, Kugler J. Transductal guidewire 'rail' for balloon valvuloplasty in neonates with isolated critical pulmonary valve stenosis or atresia. Am J Cardiol 1994; 73(9): 713–14.
5. Benson LN, Nykanen D, Collison A. Radiofrequency perforation in the treatment of congenital heart disease. Cathet Cardiovasc Interven 2002; 56(1): 72–82.
6. Gournay V, Piechaud JF, Delogu A, Sidi D, Kachaner J. Balloon valvotomy for critical stenosis or atresia of pulmonary valve in newborns. J Am Coll Cardiol 1995; 26(7): 1725–31.
7. Walsh KP, Abdulhamed JM, Tometzki JP. Importance of right ventricular outflow tract angiography in distinguishing critical pulmonary stenosis from pulmonary atresia. Heart 1997; 77(5): 456–60.
8. Wang JK, Wu MH, Chang CI, Chen YS, Lue HC. Outcomes of transcatheter valvotomy in patients with pulmonary atresia and intact ventricular septum. Am J Cardiol 1999; 84(9): 1055–60.
9. Justo RN, Nykanen DG, Williams WG, Freedom RM, Benson LN. Transcatheter perforation of the right ventricular outflow tract as initial therapy for pulmonary valve atresia and intact ventricular septum in the newborn [see comment]. Cathet Cardiovasc Diagn 1997; 40(4): 408–13.
10. Humpl T, Soderberg B, McCrindle BW et al. Percutaneous balloon valvotomy in pulmonary atresia with intact ventricular septum: impact on patient care. Circulation 2003; 108(7): 826–32.
11. Agnoletti G, Piechaud JF, Bonhoeffer P et al. Perforation of the atretic pulmonary valve. Long-term follow-up. J Am Coll Cardiol 2003; 41: 1399–403.
12. Alwi M, Geetha K, Bilkis AA et al. Pulmonary atresia with intact ventricular septum percutaneous radiofrequency-assisted valvotomy and balloon dilation versus surgical valvotomy and Blalock Taussig shunt. J Am Coll Cardiol 2000; 35: 468–76.

9 Complications of percutaneous pulmonary valve replacement

Sachin Khambadkone and Philipp Bonhoeffer

INTRODUCTION

Percutaneous pulmonary valve replacement was introduced in 2000 by Bonhoeffer et al.[1] to treat stenosis and regurgitation in a prosthetic conduit in the right ventricular outflow tract (RVOT).[2] Since then, over 300 such procedures have been performed successfully worldwide. Balloon dilatation and bare metal stenting have been successfully used to relieve conduit obstruction at the expense of causing free pulmonary regurgitation. Percutaneous pulmonary valve replacement with a Melody percutaneous pulmonary valve (Medtronic, Inc) effectively relieves stenosis without causing severe regurgitation and is very effective in treating regurgitant conduits.

In this chapter, we will outline our experience with percutaneous pulmonary valve replacement, particularly emphasizing the complications of the procedure seen during the evolution of this new technique, right from its inception and first-in-human application.

INDICATIONS

Percutaneous pulmonary valve replacement is applicable in patients with repaired congenital heart disease with residual or recurrent lesions causing RVOT dysfunction. Patients with tetralogy of Fallot with pulmonary stenosis or pulmonary atresia, double outlet right ventricle with pulmonary stenosis, truncus arteriosus, transposition of great arteries with ventricular septal defect and pulmonary stenosis, and the Ross operation with a homograft in the pulmonary position, amongst others, usually require valved conduits in the pulmonary position. These conduits usually degenerate over time with calcification, fibrosis, and degeneration of valve leaflets leading to stenosis, regurgitation, or both.

Indications of treatment for RVOT conduit dysfunction are:

- RV systolic pressure > 2/3 of systemic pressure in symptomatic patients
- RV systolic pressure > 3/4 of systemic pressure in asymptomatic patients

- Moderate to severe pulmonary regurgitation (PR) with symptoms or
  - moderate to severe RV dilatation
  - moderate to severe RV dysfunction
  - impaired exercise capacity (<65% of predicted)

Patients suitable for using the Melody percutaneous pulmonary valve:

1. Presence of valved-conduit in the right ventricular outflow tract.
2. Diameter of the conduit between 16 to 22 mm either at implantation or as measured prior to the procedure.
3. RVOT not distensible to more than 22 mm, that may preclude secure anchoring of the device.
4. Coronary artery origin or course not closely related to RVOT preventing any coronary compression after implantation of the device.
5. Venous access available through the femoral or jugular approach.

Pregnancy, active infection, and absence of venous access through the femoral and jugular veins are absolute contraindications. Weight less than 20 kg is a relative contraindication.

INVESTIGATIONS

- Complete history including the surgical history and availability of the detailed surgical notes at the time of repair
- ECG
- Chest X-ray to look for calcification of the conduit
- Echocardiography with attention to tricuspid regurgitation to assess RV systolic pressure, and RVOT Doppler and color flow maps to quantify the gradient and assess severity of regurgitation, respectively
- Magnetic resonance imaging is very helpful in assessing the morphology of the RVOT, and quantifying

RV volumes, systolic function, and regurgitation by determining regurgitant volume and fraction
- Cardiopulmonary exercise testing to assess functional status

The procedure should be performed ideally in a cardiac catheterization suite with the availability of biplane fluoroscopy. All procedures are performed under general anesthesia. A fully stocked catheterization suite equipped with materials used for pediatric and adult patients with congenital heart disease is absolutely essential for this procedure.

EQUIPMENT

- Introducer sheaths (5 or 6 French for artery, 7 or 8 French for vein)
- Pigtail catheter, a curved-tip or balloon-tipped catheter for right heart catheterization
- Stiff guide wire (e.g. 0.035 inch, exchange length 260 cm, Ultrastiff Cook)
- Multitrack catheter for right heart hemodynamics and angiography
- High-pressure balloons (Mullins 14 to 22 mm × 3.5 to 4 cm)
- Indeflators for high-pressure inflation
- Stents (CP stent or Max LD eV3, 26 or 36 mm length)
- Long sheaths for stent delivery (Mullins, appropriate for stent–balloon assembly)
- Dilators (14 and 22 French)
- Melody valve
- Ensemble delivery system of appropriate size (18, 20, or 22 mm, determined by the size of the outer balloon of the BIB catheter in the system)

STEPS IN PERCUTANEOUS PULMONARY VALVE REPLACEMENT

1. Access

    (a) femoral or internal jugular vein
    (b) femoral artery.

2. Heparinization as standard.
3. Assess hemodynamics

    (a) systemic pressure (aorta, left ventricle)
    (b) right ventricular pressure, pulmonary artery pressure
    (c) rule out additional lesions.

4. Angiography

    (a) aortogram to assess coronary artery arrangement (pigtail catheter)

    (b) RVOT angiogram to delineate morphology and assess stenosis and regurgitation (Multitrack angiographic catheter over an Ultrastiff Cook 0.035 inch wire).

5. If conduit is severely stenosed, predilatation and bare-metal stenting may be necessary to facilitate delivery of the valve to the site of implantation. A Mullins sheath (10–12 French) is guided over a stiff wire into the RVOT, the dilator is removed, and a stent crimped on a balloon is delivered and deployed by standard techniques. The balloon used to deploy the stent is at least 2 mm smaller than the delivery system for the Melody valve.
6. The Melody valve is washed in 3 saline baths for 5 minutes each, to clear the glutaraldehyde preservative.
7. The Ensemble delivery system is flushed and the balloons are de-aired and prepared with diluted contrast.
8. The venous access is dilated sequentially to 22 French (using 14 and 22 French dilators).
9. The valve is crimped on to the balloon catheter of the delivery system carefully to orientate it in the direction of flow. This is always checked by at least one other member of the staff other than the operators. The correct orientation is clearly indicated by the label on the device and also color-coded sutures at the ends of the valved-stent (blue to blue on the dilator of the delivery system, and white to white).
10. The outer sheath on the delivery system covers the valved stent and prevents it from moving over the balloon catheter until it is delivered to the site of implantation.
11. The valve is uncovered at the optimum site of implantation. Check angiography can be performed through the side arm of the outer sheath of the delivery system.
12. Sequential dilatation of the inner and outer balloons deploys the valved stent.
13. The delivery system is carefully pulled out, without losing guide wire position.
14. Repeat hemodynamic assessment and angiography is then carried out with the Multitrack catheter.
15. Further dilatation with a high-pressure Mullins balloon (up to 10–12 atm) may be necessary if significant residual gradient is detected.

COMPLICATIONS AND MANAGEMENT

Local

1. Access may be difficult due to previous catheterization and surgery. Ultrasound-guided access may help.

2. As large sheaths are used, hemostasis may need due attention. External occlusion devices may be used; nevertheless, a good assistant providing manual compression of the access site always provides excellent hemostasis and reduces the risk of hematoma and bruising.

Minor complications

Complications related to various generic steps include those associated with the use of stiff guide wires, the insertion of long sheaths, high-pressure balloon dilatation, stent implantation, and implantation of devices.

Some early complications were related to design of the delivery system (there were two cases of dislodgment of the dilator tip of the delivery system requiring retrieval with a snare). These were resolved with improved design, and no further cases have been seen.

The use of stiff guide wires could result in injury to the pulmonary artery during manipulation of the delivery system guide wire assembly to deliver the device to the implantation site. The guide wire should be preshaped into a curve, to allow good tracking of the large sheaths around the curvature of the right heart structures. During manipulation of the delivery system, care should be taken to avoid pushing the tip of the stiff wire against the vessel wall. If the guide wire position is lost during manipulation, the large sheath or delivery sheath should be taken out and a curved tip catheter (Judkins right coronary catheter) should be used over the wire to position its tip securely into the distal pulmonary artery branches.

Injury to the tricuspid valve could result in severe tricuspid regurgitation due to chordal rupture or leaflet injury. Due care should be taken to cross the tricuspid valve during initial right heart catheterization to avoid the subvalvar tension apparatus. If there is significant resistance to a large sheath as it crosses the tricuspid valve, while positioning it into an RVOT, it is always useful to remove the sheath and guide wire and recross the tricuspid valve rather than force the sheath and increase the risk of trauma.

Major complications

These events could have important clinical implications, either in the form of hemodynamic instability or required emergent or elective surgery.

Procedural complications

Stent dislodgement and instability

An unstable valved stent needs to be stabilized on the guide wire to prevent hemodynamic compromise.

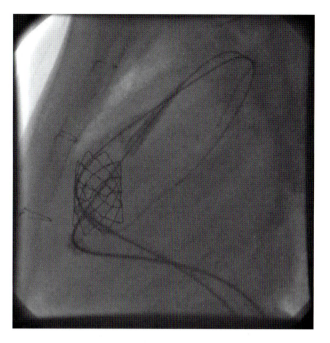

Figure 9.1   Dislodgement or embolization of the device, stabilized in the guide wire, needing surgical exploration.

Surgery is the only way to remove an expanded valved stent that has embolized (Figure 9.1). This occurred in two patients in our early experience, requiring surgical explantation of the stent with insertion of homograft. Both patients had outflow tract characteristics which prevented safe anchoring of the device. One patient had a homograft too large (24 mm) for the current device, and the other had a non-circumferential homograft patch used to augment the right ventricular outflow tract. There was no hemodynamic instability related to these events and the surgery was uneventful with a successful outcome. This experience contributed to the learning curve of case selection and there have been no further cases of device instability. If there is a doubt about the RVOT dimension, use of a sizing balloon (PTS sizing balloon, NuMed, Inc) inflated in the RVOT may improve the assessment of RVOT characteristics to determine the site of implantation.

Homograft rupture

Balloon dilatation of the calcified homograft can lead to homograft dissection or rupture. The bleeding may be limited by the fibrous and scar tissue around the homograft, or may lead to hemodynamic compromise from bleeding into the mediastinum or pleural space. Fluoroscopic evidence of fracture of the calcification is more commonly seen without hemodynamically significant consequences. Homograft rupture caused hemothorax in four patients, and was treated acutely with autotransfusion. Surgical exploration was required in two patients to control bleeding; however, in one the valve remained competent and was not explanted.

Rupture of homograft is not predictable. Oversizing of the balloon homograft ratio should be avoided;

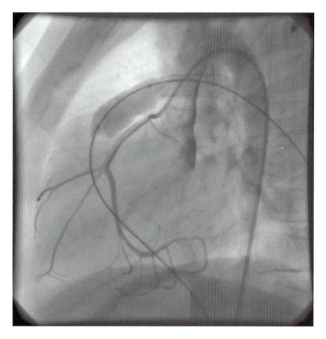

Figure 9.2 Compression of the left coronary artery after valve replacement with no flow seen on aortography.

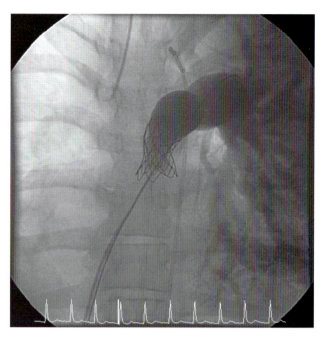

Figure 9.3 Complete occlusion of the right pulmonary artery by the valved stent needing explantation.

nevertheless, for severely calcified and stenosed homograft conduits, the risk of dissection and rupture remains, when high-pressure balloon dilatation is carried out. Careful hemodynamic monitoring of arterial pressure to detect hypotension, screening of lung fields to detect hemothorax, and angiography to detect extravasation of the contrast are means of early detection of this complication. Early treatment with pleurocentesis and autotransfusion can stabilize the hemodynamics. Persistent hemorrhage and hemodynamic compromise require surgical exploration and explantation of the device.

Coronary compression

Unusual anatomy leading to compression of the left coronary artery by the implanted stent valve resulted in ischemic left ventricular dysfunction requiring cardiopulmonary resuscitation in one patient. During cardiac massage, the stent became compressed and moved away from the posteriorly located left coronary artery with re-establishment of flow and recovery of left ventricular function. Emergency surgery was then undertaken to explant the valve and insert a homograft.

It is important to assess the coronary anatomy to diagnose anomalous coronary origin or course around the RVOT that may be compromised by an increase in the RVOT dimension. A thorough knowledge of morphologic diagnosis, a review of surgical notes of the conduit implantation, and confirmation of coronary anatomy by MRI and aortography or selective coronary angiography[3] before the final decision of valve implantation should help to prevent this complication (Figure 9.2).

Occlusion of the pulmonary artery

The Melody valve is, in essence, a covered stent, and implantation close to the pulmonary artery bifurcation would lead to occlusion of the pulmonary artery. This complication was seen only in one patient in our experience, and was potentially avoidable (Figure 9.3). Meticulous imaging of the relationship of the pulmonary artery bifurcation to the site of implantation, if necessary by measuring distances in MRI, CT angiography, or during conventional biplane angiography in different projections, should identify the risk of this consequence.

Balloon rupture

This complication should be anticipated for any procedure involving balloon dilatation. Guide wire position should be maintained until the balloon catheter is removed and examined diligently to ensure complete removal of the ruptured balloon segments. In circumferential tears and embolization of the distal tip of the balloon catheter, a snare inserted through additional venous access can be used to remove the remnants. There has been no procedural mortality related to percutaneous pulmonary valve replacement in the entire clinical experience, right from the first-in-human implant.

Device-related complications

The most common consequence of this group of complications was residual obstruction or restenosis. The

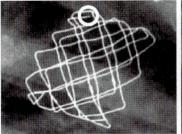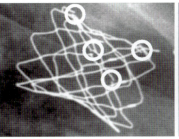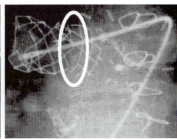

Figure 9.4 Stent fracture on X-ray surveillance with three grades: I with single fracture, II with multiple fractures without loss of stent integrity, and III loss of stent integrity and stent embolization.

'hammock effect' resulted from the walls of the bovine venous valve 'hanging in' along the length of the stent. The first design had the vein sutured only at its ends to the stent, leaving the wall unsupported. The current generation device, which is sutured along its length, has solved this problem.

Stent fracture is an unavoidable complication of any device placed within the circulatory system that is exposed to cyclic compressive stress. Implantation into a native RVOT, absence of calcification in the RVOT, and presence of recoil of the valved stent during deployment or postdilatation were the risk factors identified for stent fracture. One consequence is restenosis; however, when there are multiple fractures, there is a risk of loss of integrity and stent embolization (Figure 9.4). Regular surveillance with chest X-rays in the PA and lateral projections at regular intervals (3, 6, and 12 months, and annually after that) helps in anticipatory management. If echocardiography detects an increasing gradient across the valve, re-intervention should be planned electively before loss of integrity of the valve stent.[4]

Endocarditis

Infection of the implanted valve may occur after bacteremia, and prophylaxis during elective procedures should be a rule. Infection of the valve is treated with intravenous antibiotics, and indications for explantation would be failure of medical therapy. The hemodynamic consequence of endocarditis, usually pulmonary regurgitation, has not been significant enough to warrant surgery.

Residual stenosis

A conduit with severe external constraints (e.g. sternal compression) may not be expandable to its nominal dimension or be suitable for percutaneous pulmonary valve replacement. Predilation with a high-pressure balloon allows one to judge the compliance of the conduit and the ability to dilate it to a particular dimension. A rare complication of intravascular hemolysis from a severe residual stenosis in a retrosternal small stenosed conduit was seen early in our experience. Surgical explantation was performed, with replacement with a larger conduit.

Mortality

There were three deaths in the entire world experience of 324 patients until August 2007. In two patients, who presented in cardiogenic shock and multiorgan failure, percutaneous pulmonary valve replacement was performed as a palliative strategy. The first had a history of five previous operations, deteriorated 6 weeks after a technically successful procedure, and died from a chest infection. The second presented with multiorgan failure and with severe fluid overload. Despite successful percutaneous pulmonary valve replacement and dilatation of severe re-coarctation, the patient died of pulmonary edema 24 hours after the procedure. One patient with repaired pulmonary atresia and pulmonary hypertension experienced sudden cardiac death at 35 months after a successful procedure. The patient had stent fractures with no hemodynamic consequences and a peak velocity of 2.8 m/s across the device at the last follow-up (11 months before death). The death was presumed to be due to arrhythmia.

SUMMARY

Complications of a novel technique are related to every aspect of the device development, patient selection, and procedural experience over a learning curve. An analytic approach to complications helps in understanding, modifying, and anticipating them, with the intention of avoiding them completely or intervening early for the unavoidable events. Modification of the device and delivery system, better selection of patients, rigorous follow-up to detect clinically insignificant events, and initiating further research into redefining the indications have all helped to limit major clinical adverse events.

REFERENCES

1. Bonhoeffer P, Boudjemline Y, Saliba Z et al. Percutaneous replacement of pulmonary valve in a right-ventricle to pulmonary-artery prosthetic conduit with valve dysfunction. Lancet 2000; 356(9239): 1403–5.

2. Khambadkone S, Coats L, Taylor A et al. Percutaneous pulmonary valve implantation in humans: results in 59 consecutive patients. Circulation 2005; 112(8): 1189–97.

3. Sridharan S, Coats L, Khambadkone S, Taylor AM, Bonhoeffer P. Images in cardiovascular medicine. Transcatheter right ventricular outflow tract intervention: the risk to the coronary circulation. Circulation 2006; 113(25): e934–5.

4. Nordmeyer J, Khambadkone S, Coats L, et al. Risk stratification, systematic classification, and anticipatory management strategies for stent fracture after percutaneous pulmonary valve implantation Circulation 2007; 115(11): 1392–97.

10 Aortic valvuloplasty complications

Alexander J Javois

Concerns for major complications related to balloon aortic valvuloplasty have been documented ever since Lababidi first reported its application in humans in 1983.[1] Not surprisingly, with expanded knowledge and enhanced technology, major complications have diminished. However, the improved and miniaturized equipment has motivated pediatric interventionalists to attempt smaller patients, bringing additional concerns not initially realized. Complications of aortic balloon valvuloplasty can be broadly categorized as vascular, valvular, myocardial, and embolic. The incidence of all complications is greater in the neonate. Mortality from all causes is < 2% in older children, but is 5% in non-duct-dependent and as high as 38% in ductal-dependent neonates.[2,3]

VASCULAR COMPLICATIONS

Vascular complications include pulse loss, vessel aneurysm, dissection, rupture, aortic perforation, and aortic arch intimal tears. Death from acute iliac artery tear in a neonate has been reported.[3] The smaller the child, the higher the likelihood of vascular complications. In the initial report of the Valvuloplasty and Angioplasty of Congenital Anomalies (VACA) Registry in 1990, in which 204 procedures were reported, there was a 12% incidence of femoral thrombosis or damage, which was successfully treated in 80% of cases.[4] In the 1996 follow-up VACA Registry report of 630 procedures, transection of the femoral or iliac artery was seen in 2.1% of patients.[2] The incidence of pulse loss has been reported to be as high as 7%;[5] the need for surgical intervention is less than 1%. Pulse loss may also be asymptomatic and permanent. Egito reported in 1997 a series of 33 neonates of which 20 had the retrograde femoral approach.[6] All 20 (100%!) had pulse loss and were treated with thrombolytic therapy. The pulse returned in 35%. At mid term follow-up (on average 4.3 ± 1.8 years), 9/20 (45%) still had absent femoral pulse but no obvious leg discrepancy. Extremity growth retardation has been reported, but its exact incidence is unknown.[7]

With technologic advances resulting in smaller profile balloons, catheters, and sheaths, femoral artery complications in neonates have become less frequent (the original reports of iliofemoral arterial complications were in neonates and children in whom 8 and 9 French balloon catheters were used *without* a sheath).[8] In 2006, Zain *et al.* reported a neonatal series in which 4/12 (33%) had femoral artery thrombosis.[9] All were successfully treated with thrombolytic therapy. The incidence of vascular complications is much lower in older children; Echigo reported in 2001 a multi-institutional series from Japan of 77 patients for whom the mean age of intervention was 8.3 ± 5.5 years. Only one case (1.3%) had femoral artery thrombosis.[10]

For neonates, carotid and umbilical artery access may reduce the risk of vascular complications. A right carotid approach was first advocated by Fischer *et al.* in 1990.[11] This approach may be associated with residual carotid stenosis. The neonatal right carotid approach in 95 cases from a multi-institutional review in 2000 reported follow-up on 64 patients. A technically feasible approach in 97% carotid dissection occurred in one patient. Follow-up evaluation revealed an 8% incidence of ultrasound-proven narrowing of the carotid artery and 2% had total occlusion; there were no neurologic sequelae.[3] Successful long-term outcome with carotid artery ligation with extracorporeal membrane oxygenation has further minimized the concern for residual mild carotid obstruction in the neonatal valvuloplasty population. The transumbilical approach has been widely accepted since Beekman reported a series in 1991.[12] Rarely, umbilical artery rupture has been reported.[13] Alternatively, a subscapular artery approach has been reported but not widely used.[14]

Rare vascular complications include transverse aortic arch trauma. In Egito's neonatal series of 33 patients, 2 patients were incidentally found to have transverse aortic arch flaps on echocardiogram. Both cases were felt to be related to the use of a 0.018 inch torque wire with a stiff mandril along with a balloon with larger internal diameter lumen (a wire lumen mismatch). It was recommended by the authors that the guide wire should be preshaped for the aortic arch and that the wire diameter should be matched to the balloon catheter lumen.[6] The 1996 VACA registry reported a 0.2% incidence of aortic perforation.[2] Also rare is aortic aneurysm. In a multi-institutional series from Japan of 77 children with non-critical aortic stenosis, only one case (1.3%) of aortic aneurysm was seen.[10] A single case of aortic dissection involving the ostia of the left coronary artery in a neonate has been reported; ischemic changes were noted immediately after balloon valvuloplasty, with subsequent demise 20 days later.[15]

Prevention and treatment

Use of the smallest available balloon and sheath profile will minimize the risk of arterial damage. Currently, the lowest profile balloons are the Tyshak Mini balloons (NuMed, Hopkinton, New York). They range in diameter from 4 to 8 mm × 2 cm length introduced through a 3 French sheath and 9 to 10 mm × 2 or 4 cm length through a 4 French sheath. Rated burst pressures are correspondingly lower (3.5–6.0 atm), but are typically not an issue for the native valve tissue of the neonate. Experience with these balloons has been excellent.[16]

Avoiding femoral artery damage from a single large balloon can be accomplished by using the double-balloon technique; both femoral arteries can be used to further minimize trauma to a single artery.

Heparinization during the procedure reduces the likelihood of arterial thrombosis; reinitiation of heparin shortly after the procedure for diminished or absent pulses has been recommended even early in the valvuloplasty experience.[17] Mullins has advocated heparinization with high activated clotting time (275–350 seconds) for left heart interventions.[18] I have found an initial bolus of 150 units/kg and a 35 unit/kg/hour drip typically maintains an ACT between 250 and 300 seconds. Only partial reversal of heparin with protamine is performed at the end of the case to achieve ACT < 200 seconds. Obviously, if aortic perforation occurs, reversal is necessary.

A pulseless leg is initially treated with heparin. A weight-based heparin protocol should be utilized. Thrombolytic therapy is considered if ischemic changes in the leg are noted (pale, painful, cold). Recombinant tissue plasminogen activator (r-TPA) is most commonly used in children at 0.5 mg/kg/hour systemic intravenous therapy; it is given in addition to the heparin therapy. The response to thrombolytic therapy should be monitored by prothrombin time (PT) International normalized ratio (INR), APTT, and fibrinogen level 4 hours following the onset of the infusion and every 6–8 hours thereafter. If a patient has received thrombolytic therapy for more than 6 hours, consider treating with heparin alone for 24 hours before reinstituting thrombolytic therapy. There may be ongoing thrombolysis even in the absence of continued administration of the thrombolytic agent. Bleeding may occur in 30–50% of patients; usually this is oozing from a wound or puncture site and should be treated with local pressure and supportive care. If severe bleeding occurs, stop the infusion of the thrombolytic agent and heparin. Consider administration of factor VIIa (discuss with Hematology). Administer cryoprecipitate (usual dose of 1 unit/5 kg) to increase the fibrinogen concentration. Fresh frozen plasma may also be indicated in the presence of severe bleeding if factor VIIa is not administered.[19–22]

A useful resource for extensive experience in pediatric thrombolytic therapy is available 24 hours a day, 7 days a week, from the Division of Pediatric Hematology-Oncology at McMaster University Children's Hospital (Hamilton, Ontario) by telephone: 1-800-NO-CLOTS.

If an aortic perforation is suspected, confirmation should be made without removing the offending guide wire or catheter. When perforation is confirmed by angiography or echocardiography, it may be elected to remove the perforating device in the operating room with the pediatric cardiovascular surgeons in attendance. Bleeding may be self-limiting; if not, it may require emergency surgery. If perforation is detected after the guide wire or catheter has been removed, pericardiocentesis or thoracocentesis may be urgently needed. Significant blood losses are replaced with previously cross-matched blood. Rapidly aspirated blood from the pericardial or thoracic space can be returned immediately to the patient intravenously. Heparin should be reversed in such situations. Other rare vascular complications (exact incidence unknown) include femoral artery aneurysms and pseudoaneurysms.[5]

VALVULAR COMPLICATIONS

Aortic balloon valvuloplasty has been described as a 'blind' technique; the exact location and extent of the leaflet tear is unknown and unpredictable.[23] Suboptimal gradient reduction has been associated with a balloon:annulus ratio of < 0.9 in the 1996 VACA registry.[2] Such a result can be addressed with further balloon valvuloplasty. A complication that may not be simply treated is severe aortic insufficiency (AI). Many series support the notion that a balloon:annulus ratio ≤ 1.0 reduces the risk of aortic regurgitation.[12,17,24] However, the risk for AI is not simply just related to balloon size. In the largest retrospective evaluation, the VACA registry of 1996, larger valve size, oversized balloons, and the presence of more than trivial pre-existing aortic regurgitation were found to be significant independent predictors for the development of aortic regurgitation complications.[2] Overall, the incidence of severe aortic insufficiency was 1.6%. Valve annulus size was associated with risk for increasing AI grade by ≥ 2 grades, or the development of severe AI when the annulus was < 8 mm and ≥ 16 mm. The VACA study group theorized that this may be due to degenerative changes in larger valves and dys-plastic changes in smaller valves. Preexisting AI of mild or more had greater risk for developing severe AI. A balloon:annulus ratio > 1 was also associated with increased risk for severe AI. Interestingly, previous surgical valvotomy and the double-balloon tech-nique were not independent risk factors for aortic regurgitation.

Not only acute, but progressive aortic insufficiency may be considered a complication of balloon valvulo-plasty. Some data support the notion that such aortic insufficiency is, however inevitable, not related to the balloon:annulus ratio but perhaps related to progressive valve deterioration. Shaddy *et al.* noted the develop-ment of aortic valve prolapse in 7/32 (22%) with no cor-relation to the balloon:annulus ratio.[25] As a matter of fact, no patient with increased insufficiency had a bal-loon:annulus ratio > 1. Echigo reported a multi-institu-tional series from Japan of 77 patients; the average age of intervention was 8.3 ± 5.5 years and there were 7 cases (9%) with moderate or severe regurgitation with balloon size 90–100% of the annulus.[10] In another large series of 70 patients, of whom 21 were neonates, free-dom from moderate or severe regurgitation was initially lower in the neonates (75% vs 90% in older children), but after 2 years the difference was not significant (50% vs 61%).[26] In this series, small balloons (the mean bal-loon:annulus ratio was 0.9, with a range of 0.67–1.0) did not seem to protect against the late development of sig-nificant aortic insufficiency. Across all age groups, in a series of 113 patients undergoing balloon valvuloplasty between 1985 and 2002, moderate or severe aortic insufficiency eventually developed in 15%.[27]

Many studies have noted this high incidence of the development of progressive insufficiency after bal-loon valvuloplasty. In a retrospective review of 148 children, Moore *et al.* noted that, on average follow-up of 45 months, significant progression of regurgita-tion was seen; 38% had greater than or equal to moderate grade insufficiency as compared to 13% immediately after dilation and 3% prior to dilation.[5] The degree of pre-existing insufficiency was also an important risk for progressive late insufficiency; less than 8% of patients with trivial or no regurgitation before balloon dilation developed severe insuffi-ciency after ballooning. Another independent risk factor for the development of significant regurgita-tion was the presence of a thick valve (all leaflets ≥ 2 mm). Age also played a role; children aged 1–5 years were more likely to have aortic regurgitation greater than or equal to moderate after balloon dilation. Interestingly, in contrast to the VACA registry, Moore's data suggested prior surgical valvotomy *was* a risk factor for developing regurgitation greater than or equal to moderate after balloon dilation, but the balloon:annulus ratio *did not* influence the severity of regurgitation or the increase in regurgitation in response to balloon dilation.

Severe acute valve damage may require immediate surgery to treat severe left heart volume overload. Aortic valve avulsion had a 0.2% incidence in the 1996 VACA registry.[2] Aortic valve perforation was seen in 0.5% of cases in the same series. In the series reported by Moore, traumatic damage to the mitral valve occurred in 1/148 (0.7%), requiring surgery within one month of balloon dilation for repair of a tear in the anterior leaflet during an anterograde approach.[5] However, Peuster has demonstrated that the antero-grade approach can be done safely. In 17 consecutive neonates with critical aortic stenosis (AS), the antero-grade approach from either the femoral or the umbili-cal vein was performed with no damage to the mitral valve.[28] Mitral valve damage can occur with a retro-grade approach also. Brierley *et al.* reported two such cases in a 2-day-old and an 11-month-old.[29]

Some consider restenosis and the need for re-intervention to be a complication of aortic balloon valvuloplasty. Others do not see this as a complication, but, rather, an inevitability, referring to aortic balloon valvuloplasty as a 'palliative' procedure.[3,10,30] Unfortunately, there is a high incidence of repeat interventions after balloon dila-tion.[5] Some sort of intervention for either repeat steno-sis or regurgitation was required in 25% of patients at 4 years and 50% of patients at 8 years after balloon dila-tion. Overall, 30% of patients required surgical inter-vention 8 years after balloon dilation. Egito *et al.* showed neonatal reintervention rates were higher at 40% during a mean follow-up of 4.3 years compared to 25% in non-neonates, as mentioned above.[6]

Prevention and treatment

Prevention of aortic insufficiency has focused on the balloon:annulus ratio since the 1980s. Most series have concluded that the balloon should be 80–100% of the annulus, or 1mm smaller than the annulus.[2,10,31] A conservative balloon approach would be to start at 90% of the annulus and increase its size by 1 mm if the gradient has not been adequately reduced and there is no significant increase in insufficiency.[32]

Single-balloon migration resulting in valve damage or even avulsion may be prevented with the double-balloon approach; some forward flow around the balloons may minimize the expelling force on the balloons. However, in the 1996 VACA registry data, the single-balloon tech-nique did not influence gradient reduction or procedural risk compared to the double-balloon technique after con-trolling for the balloon:annulus ratio.[2] Rapid right ventric-ular pacing at 220 to 240 beats per minute is another method of decreasing cardiac output to help stabilize bal-loon position during inflation. The appropriate rate can be determined by test pacing and noting not only a drop in aortic pressure but a flattening or narrowing of the aortic pulse pressure. The risk of ventricular pacing is of inducing sustained ventricular arrhythmias from an already strained

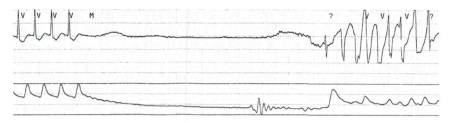

Figure 10.1 Adenosine administration resulted in asystole. The escape rhythm, however, was not a sinus rhythm but polymorphic ventricular tachycardia requiring cardioversion. Response to adenosine is unpredictable.

left ventricle (LV); a charged defibrillator adjacent to the patient is a necessity.[33] Adenosine has been advocated to temporarily stop cardiac output.[34] However, the response and duration may be unpredictable, especially in a hypertrophied and strained LV; note the unexpected ventricular arrhythmia seen in my lab in Figure 10.1.

Balloon migration is difficult to quantify as a risk factor for the development of aortic insufficiency. The natural tendency is for the balloon to be ejected from the LV, but this outward movement is counteracted by the inward force provided by the interventionist. Such in-and-out balloon movement may be the cause of excessive valve trauma and result in severe insufficiency. Balloon migration may be multifactorial. A floppy guide wire, a large balloon with a long inflation/deflation time, and an overly viscous balloon inflation medium, also resulting in slower inflation and deflation, are all more likely to allow excessive balloon movement. To avoid migration, the use of a long balloon (even 6–8 cm in older children) that reaches the cardiac apex allows the inward force on the catheter to stabilize and minimize ejection of the balloon. A safe wire tip position in the ventricular apex coursing anterior to the mitral valve in the lateral view is critical if long balloons are used to prevent mitral apparatus damage. Minimizing the inflation/deflation time is also important; the more dilute the contrast, the faster the balloon can be inflated and deflated.

With an anterograde approach, the risk for mitral valve damage may be minimized with an inflated, balloon-tipped, end hole catheter which is passed through the mitral valve and deflected up toward the aortic valve. Soft-tipped guide wire probing in the left ventricular outflow tract for the aortic orifice minimizes the chance of the guide wire engaging mitral chordae. The risk of mitral damage from a retrograde approach can be minimized by avoiding a posterior position of the guide wire; the apical position is best.[29] Aortic valve perforation may also be minimized by the anterograde approach, since the catheter and guide wire will tend to follow the outward stream.[28] Some studies have even purported that the anterograde approach may be associated with a lower incidence of aortic insufficiency.[27,35]

MYOCARDIAL COMPLICATIONS

Guide wire perforation of the LV occurred in 1.1% of 630 patients in the 1996 VACA registry.[2] This complication is more likely to happen in neonates. A recent report indicated an incidence of LV perforation in neonates as high as 17%.[9] Accordingly, neonatal procedural mortality has been much greater than older children. Overall mortality has been reported at 1.9%, but, in the original 1990 VACA report, neonatal mortality was 13%, then 9.6% in the 1996 report.[2,4] In recent smaller series, neonatal mortality has still ranged between 12% and 34%.[6,10] Mortality is not always related to perforation and tamponade but, rather, to issues of myocardial 'reserve' or the ability to tolerate a transient severe rise in LV pressure, wall strain, and cessation of myocardial perfusion. Thus, asystole was seen in 12% of neonates in a series reported by Peuster et al.[28] A rare anatomic finding that may contribute to cardiac arrest immediately postballoon is the so-called 'hooded coronary'; in such an entity, the coronary ostia is deep within the coronary sinus and becomes occluded by a freed up or flail aortic leaflet.[36]

Pressure or trauma from the balloon on the myocardium and conduction tissue can lead to left anterior hemiblock or even a complete left bundle branch block (LBBB). This condition is almost always transient and requires no treatment. Transient LBBB has been seen as often as in 13% of cases.[5]

I experienced a previously unreported myocardial complication related to aortic balloon valvuloplasty in a 10-year-old status post (s/p) two previous surgical valvuloplasties. He suffered a traumatic ventricular septal defect (VSD) from balloon valvuloplasty. A 90 Torr gradient and aortic annulus of 18–20 mm were identified in the catheterization lab. The valve was crossed with ease with a floppy-tipped Cook Bentson wire (Cook, Inc, Bloomington, IN), over which a pigtail catheter was placed. Ultimately, a Cook Amplatz Superstiff 0.035 inch guide wire with a 1 cm floppy tip was preshaped to create a curve to fit in the LV apex. A single inflation with a 16 mm × 6 cm Meditech XXL balloon (Boston Scientific, Natick, MA) was performed. Figures 10.2a and 10.3a show the balloon and guide wire positioning at peak inflation. The gradient dropped to 40 Torr but immediate postvalvuloplasty angiography revealed a small left to right shunt through a small VSD, but what appeared to be a larger linear laceration of the septum (Figures 10.2b, 10.3b, and 10.4). Approximately 20 hours later, the patient developed sudden severe chest pain, dyspnea, and desaturation; the VSD had suddenly enlarged along the length of the 'laceration.' He was intubated; pink frothy secretions of acute pulmonary edema were aspirated. He underwent emergency aortic valve

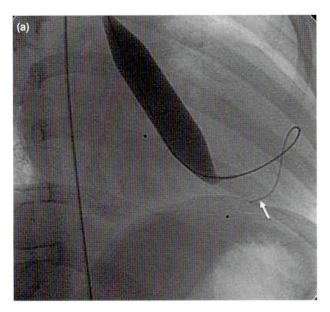
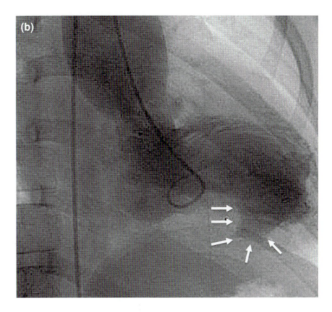

Figure 10.2 Right anterior oblique (RAO) views during and postvalvuloplasty. (a) Balloon and wire position at end inflation. (b) Postballoon angiogram with left to right shunt through a small VSD. Arrows indicate wire tip position and the edges of the septal laceration.

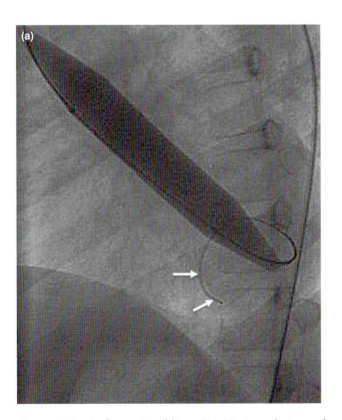
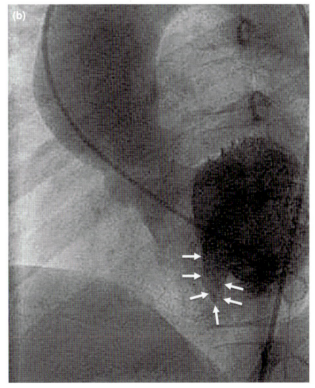

Figure 10.3 Left anterior oblique (LAO) views during and postvalvuloplasty. (a) Balloon and wire position at end inflation. (b) Postballoon angiogram with left to right shunt through a small VSD. Arrows indicate wire tip position and the edges of the septal laceration.

replacement and VSD closure. Evaluation for failure to extubate revealed residual VSD that was closed with an Amplatzer Muscular Occluder by a hybrid approach. Severe diastolic dysfunction resulted in the need for orthotopic cardiac transplantation, which has resulted in good long-term survival.

Presumably, the shape and position of the Amplatzer Super Stiff guide wire in a hypercontractile ventricle resulted in a 'sawing' effect on the ventricular septum (hence the appearance of a linear laceration on the LV side of the septum). The acute finding of a small VSD within the septal laceration immediately

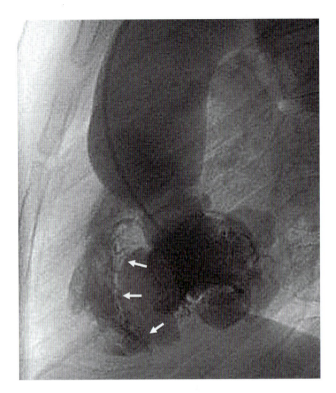

Figure 10.4 Straight lateral view. LV angiogram in this view best portrays the extent of the septal laceration; the arrows indicate the smooth edge of the laceration on the left side of the septum.

after balloon removal speaks for traumatic origin rather than infarction.

Prevention and treatment

Myocardial trauma in most cases is directly related to the stiffness of the guide wire being placed across the aortic valve. Treatment of perforation is drainage of symptomatic effusion. To prevent perforation, crossing the aortic valve should be done with a floppy, soft-tipped wire. The Cook Bentson wire is a 0.035 inch wire with a very long straight soft tip. Even smaller caliber 0.014 inch coronary guide wires can be used. It is not uncommon for the wire to 'bounce off' the valve and enter a coronary artery. Using a soft-tipped wire as small as possible will avoid not only coronary trauma/spasm but also perforation of the aortic valve. The soft-tipped wire can then be curled in the LV apex for passage of an angiographic catheter. Crossing the valve with a stiffer wire increases the likelihood of inducing ventricular arrhythmias and perforating the LV. It is not uncommon for the guide wire to enter the LV posteriorly and pass through the mitral apparatus. In such cases, the guide wire may be redirected anteriorly with an angle-tipped catheter.

In severe AS, particularly with myocardial dysfunction, total occlusion of LV output may result in LV failure or life-threatening arrhythmias. Use of the double-balloon approach, especially in older children, permits some forward flow, allowing not only partial decompression of the LV during inflation but also some systemic and coronary perfusion.

The case of the traumatic VSD emphasizes that great caution is needed with placement and positioning of a stiff wire; a stiff guide wire had been used in an attempt to minimize the degree of large diameter balloon migration during inflation. The complication may have been prevented by creating a tighter 'J' at the apex of the LV. Too wide a 'J' or loop within the LV with a stiff guide wire may have resulted in the hypertrophied and hypercontractile LV, with cavitary obliteration during systole, squeezing down on the wire and 'slicing' the myocardium. Making the 'J' at the end of the wire as tight as possible will reduce the chance for myocardial trauma. This case demonstrated that a chronically pressure overloaded, hypertrophied LV can be a poor candidate for emergency open heart surgery. Acute heart failure from a large VSD likely worsened existing diastolic dysfunction of the severely hypertrophied ventricle. Overall, this case highlights that the best treatment is prevention.

EMBOLIC COMPLICATIONS

Thrombus formation is a risk of long-standing left heart catheters and guide wires. Stroke was seen in 0.2% of the 630 balloon aortic valvuloplasty procedures in the VACA registry report from 1996.[2] Stroke was reported early in the aortic balloon valvuloplasty experience with heparinization of 50 units/kg, prompting a recommendation to increase heparinization to 100 units/kg.[37] Acute myocardial infarction was seen in a neonate with critical AS; the infant died 3 days postballoon procedure.[38] Other end organ infarctions have not been commonly reported.

Prevention and treatment

Systemic air embolism, always a possibility during left heart catheterization, is fortunately rare and avoided by meticulous attention to technique. Backbleeding and placement of sheaths and catheters under a water seal are ways of minimizing the risk of introducing air into the system. Prepping the balloon with carbon dioxide reduces the risk of air embolism from balloon rupture; this is accomplished by leaving the sheath or factory covering on the balloon and gently forcing CO_2 in and out of the balloon. Likewise, very dilute contrast can additionally be forced in and out of the factory covered balloon to de-air it. Operating the balloons under the rated burst pressure is another necessity in the aortic position to prevent air embolism.

Heparin administration immediately after vascular access is obtained will reduce the likelihood of thrombus formation on catheters and guide wires that may chronically reside across the aortic valve. Use of a heparin drip after bolus administration also reduces the likelihood of the ACT dropping during an unexpectedly long procedure. I utilize a 150 unit/kg bolus followed by a 35 unit/kg/hour drip. ACTs are checked 10 minutes after the bolus and then every 20 minutes; the ACTs are typically in the range of 250–300 seconds. Additional precautions include keeping unused catheters out of the LV or ascending aorta as well as removing balloon catheters from the LV immediately after use.

SPECIAL SUMMARY STATEMENTS FOR THE NEONATE

Risk for poor outcome of balloon valvuloplasty in a multicentered study of 95 neonates with critical AS included ductal dependency, mitral stenosis, an LV which did not form a cardiac apex, and aortic valve diameter less than 6 mm.[3] Neonatal mortality ranged from 9.6% to 34%; this is significantly greater than for older children. This higher mortality is both technical in etiology (perforation, valve avulsion) and myocardial reserve in etiology (asystole with balloon inflation).[2,10,28] The highest risk patient is the neonate with LV dysfunction; crossing the aortic valve has been associated with ventricular fibrillation. Under such circumstances, the valve should be quickly dilated (the balloon catheter should be already de-aired and attached to the indeflator prior to crossing the valve). It is believed that an unobstructed ventricle is more likely to be successfully defibrillated than a severely obstructed one.[39]

Umbilical artery retrograde catheterization may avoid femoral artery complications but may be a higher risk for sepsis, especially in the older infant; Egito reported death related to umbilical artery sepsis after balloon valvuloplasty.[6] Overall, in Egito's series there was a 9% incidence of procedure-related deaths, including wire perforation of the LV causing tamponade and wire perforation of the cusp with sudden severe regurgitation upon dilation. Anterograde dilation of the valve is not necessarily associated with a higher risk of mitral valve damage if care is taken to course through the mitral valve and out toward the aortic valve with an inflated balloon-tipped catheter.[29] To prevent complications of femoral artery damage and minimize the risk of mitral damage from an anterograde approach, some authors have declared the umbilical approach to be the preferred technique.[40] Overall, neonatal cases need to be followed closely over time as repeat intervention, either transcatheter or surgical, is common. Specifically, freedom from reintervention after 3 years was found to be significantly lower in neonates (35%) compared to older children (80%) in Balmer's series of 70 consecutive children.[26]

REFERENCES

1. Lababidi Z. Aortic balloon valvuloplasty. Am Heart J 1983; 106: 751–2.
2. McCrindle BW. VACA registry investigators: independent predictors of immediate results of percutaneous balloon aortic valvotomy in childhood. Am J Cardiol 1996; 77: 286–93.
3. Robinson BV, Brzezinska-Rajszys G, Weber HS et al. Balloon aortic valvotomy through a carotid cutdown in infants with severe aortic stenosis: results of the multicentric registry. Cardiol Young 2000; 10(3): 225–32.
4. Rocchini AP, Beekman RH, Ben Shachar G et al. Balloon aortic valvuloplasty: results of the Valvuloplasty and Angioplasty of Congenital Anomalies Registry. Am J Cardiol 1990; 65: 784–9.
5. Moore P, Egito E, Mowrey H, Perry SB, Lock J. Midterm results of balloon dilation of congenital aortic stenosis: predictors of success. J Am Coll Cardiol 1996; 27: 1257–63.
6. Egito ES, Moore P, O'Sullivan J et al. Transvascular balloon dilation for neonatal critical aortic stenosis: early and midterm results. J Am Coll Cardiol 1997; 29: 442–7.
7. Peuster M, Freihorst J, Hausdorf G. Images in cardiology: defective limb growth after retrograde balloon valvuloplasty. Heart 2000; 84(1): 63.
8. Burrows PE, Benson LN, Williams WG et al. Iliofemoral arterial complications of balloon angioplasty for systemic obstructions in infants and children. Circulation 1990; 82: 1697–704.
9. Zain Z, Zadinello M, Menahem S, Brizard C. Neonatal isolated critical aortic valve stenosis: balloon valvuloplasty or surgical valvotomy. Heart Lung Circ 2006; 15: 18–23.
10. Echigo S. Balloon valvuloplasty for congenital heart disease: immediate and long-term results of multi-institutional study. Pediatr Int 2001; 43: 542–7.
11. Fischer DR, Ettedgui JA, Park SC, Siewers RD, del Nido PJ. Carotid artery approach for balloon dilation of aortic valve stenosis in the neonate: a preliminary report. J Am Coll Cardiol 1990; 15: 1633–6.
12. Beekman RH, Rocchini AP, Anden A. Balloon valvuloplasty for critical aortic stenosis in the newborn: influence of a new catheter technology. J Am Coll Cardiol 1991; 17: 1172–6.
13. Sasidharan P. Umbilical arterial rupture: a major complication of catheterization. Indiana Med 1985; 78(1): 34–5.
14. Alekyan BG, Petrosyar YS, Coulson JD, Danikov YY, Verokwurov AV. Right subscapular artery catheterization for balloon valvuloplasty of critical aortic stenosis in infants. Am J Cardiol 1995; 76: 1049–52.
15. Carminati M, Giusti S, Spadoni I et al. Balloon aortic valvuloplasty in the first year of life. J Interven Cardiol 1995; 8: 759–66.
16. Kim DW, Raviele AA, Vincent RN. Use of a three French system for balloon aortic valvuloplasty in infants. Cathet Cardiovasc Interven 2005; 66(2): 254–7.
17. Kasten-Sportes CH, Piechaud J, Sidi, D, Kachaner J. Percutaneous balloon valvuloplasty in neonates with critical aortic stenosis. J Am Coll Cardiol 1989; 13: 1101–5.
18. Mullins CE. Cardiac Catheterization in Congenital Heart Disease: Pediatric and Adult. Malden: Blackwell Publishing, 2006: 261.
19. Ino T, Benson LN, Freedom RM et al. Thrombolytic therapy for femoral artery thrombosis after pediatric cardiac catheterization. Am Heart J 1988; 115: 633–9.
20. Leaker MT, Massicotte MP, Brooker LA, Andrew M. Thrombolytic therapy in pediatric patients: a comprehensive review of the literature. Thromb Haemostas 1996; 75(2): 132–4.
21. Manco-Johnson M, Kemahli AS, Massicotte MP et al. Recommendations for t-PA thrombolytic in children. Thromb Haemostas 2002; 88: 157–8.
22. Monagle P, Chan A, Massicotte P, Chalmers E, Michelson AD. Antithrombotic therapy in children. Chest 2004; 126: 645S–87S.
23. Solymar L, Sudow G, Berggren H, Eriksson B. Balloon dilation of stenotic aortic valve in children: an intraoperative study. J Thorac Cardiovasc Surg 1992; 104(6): 1709–13.

24. O'Connor BK, Beekman RH, Rocchini AP, Rosenthal A. Intermediate-term effectiveness of balloon valvuloplasty for congenital aortic stenosis: a prospective follow-up study. Circulation 1991; 84(2): 732–8.

25. Shaddy RE, Boucek MM, Sturtevant JE, Ruttenberg HD, Orsmond GS. Gradient reduction, aortic valve regurgitation and prolapse after balloon aortic valvuloplasty in 32 consecutive patients with congenital aortic stenosis. J Am Coll Cardiol 1990; 16: 451–6.

26. Balmer C, Beghetti M, Fasnacht M, Friedli B, Arbenz U. Balloon aortic valvoplasty in paediatric patients: progressive aortic regurgitation is common. Heart 2004; 90: 77–81.

27. McElhinney DB, Lock JE, Keane JF, Moran AM, Colan SD. Left heart growth, function, and reintervention after balloon aortic valvuloplasty for neonatal aortic stenosis. Circulation 2005; 111(4): 451–8.

28. Peuster M, Fink C, Schoof S, Von Schnakenburg C, Hausdorf F. Anterograde balloon valvuloplasty for the treatment of neonatal critical valvar aortic stenosis. Cathet Cardiovasc Interven 2002; 56: 516–20.

29. Brierley JJ, Reddy TD, Rigby ML, Thanopoulous V, Redington AN. Traumatic damage to the mitral valve during percutaneous balloon valvotomy for critical aortic stenosis. Heart 1998; 79: 200–2.

30. Borghi A, Agnoletti G, Poggiani C. Surgical cutdown of the right carotid artery for aortic balloon valvuloplasty in infancy: midterm follow-up. Pediatr Cardiol 2001; 22: 194–7.

31. Zeevi B, Keane JF, Castaneda AR, Perry SB, Lock JE. Neonatal critical valvar aortic stenosis: a comparison of surgical and balloon dilation therapy. Circulation 1988; 80(4): 831–9.

32. Reich O, Tax P, Marek J et al. Long term results of percutaneous balloon valvoplasty of congenital aortic stenosis: independent predictors of outcome. Heart 2004; 90(1): 70–6.

33. Daehnert I, Rotzsch C, Wiener M, Schneider P. Rapid right ventricular pacing is an alternative to adenosine in catheter interventional procedures for congenital heart disease. Heart 2004; 90: 1047–50.

34. De Giovanni JV, Edgar RA, Cranston A. Adenosine induced transient cardiac standstill in catheter interventional procedures for congenital heart disease. Heart 1998; 80(4): 330–3.

35. Magee AG, Nykanen D, McCrindle BW et al. Balloon dilation of severe aortic stenosis in the neonate: comparison of anterograde and retrograde catheter approaches. J Am Coll Cardiol 1997; 30(4): 1061–6.

36. Mullins CE. Cardiac Catheterization in Congenital Heart Disease: Pediatric and Adult. Malden: Blackwell Publishing, 2006: 490.

37. Treacy EP, Duncan WJ, Tyrrell MJ, Lowry NJ. Neurological complications of balloon angioplasty in children. Pediatr Cardiol 1991; 12: 98–101.

38. Saiki K, Kato H, Suzuki K et al. Balloon valvuloplasty for congenital aortic valve stenosis in an infant and children. Acta Paediatr Jpn 1992; 34(4): 433–40.

39. Torres AJ, Hellenbrand W. Aortic valve stenosis in neonates. In: Sievert H, Qureshi SA, Wilson N, Hijazi ZM, eds. Percutaneous Interventions for Congenital Heart Disease. Informa Healthcare, Oxon, 2007: 166.

40. Reich O. Aortic valve, congenital stenosis. In: Sievert H, Qureshi SA, Wilson N, Hijazi ZM, eds. Percutaneous Interventions for Congenital Heart Disease. Informa Healthcare, Oxon, 2007: 157.

11 Complications of stenting the right ventricular outflow tract

Matthew A Crystal and Lee N Benson

INTRODUCTION

Right ventricle to pulmonary artery conduits are used to palliate a variety of congenital heart lesions[1] and have significantly improved care for the child with complex congenital heart disease. While these conduits have allowed effective palliation for many years, there is an increasing incidence of conduit dysfunction, either stenosis or insufficiency, that ultimately limits conduit effectiveness. As a palliative intervention, conduit stenting can extend conduit lifespan.[2,3] For the purposes of this chapter we will focus on complications associated with bare metal stent implantation to conduits in the setting of stenosis. Additionally, stenting of the native cardiac outflow tract as a palliative technique in newborns is under investigation and comments about the observed complications with that approach will be discussed as well. Complications of stent-valve implantation will be discussed in another section.

BACKGROUND

Balloon dilation of extracardiac conduits was initially performed in attempts to decrease right ventricular outflow tract obstruction, and increase the longevity of the implant. Such angioplasty, however, proved to be an ineffective therapy, associated with a high incidence of complications (bleeding, exteriorization of wires, myocardial staining, and balloon rupture). Isolated balloon dilation results in clinical benefit in only one-third of patients, with the mechanism of failure typically due to conduit elasticity and recoil, or a fixed non-dilatable lesion. In addition, such obstructed conduits may cause balloon rupture and, if heavily calcified, are at risk of cracking or rupturing.[4–7] Almagor and colleagues reported the first successful bare metal stent implantation in an animal model of an obstructed right ventricle to pulmonary artery conduit in 1990.[8] Since that time, numerous clinical studies have demonstrated that bare metal stent implantation can successfully relieve stenosis and prolong conduit lifespan.[9–15]

A number of stents are available for application in extracardiac conduits. Ideally, a stent should be biocompatible (to avoid neointimal proliferation and be resistant to thrombosis), have a low profile for use with a small delivery system, be flexible, have good radial strength, and be durable. The most commonly used and reported stents in conduits are balloon-expandable closed cell designs. Self-expanding implants may be an option, but generally have lower radial strength[16] and are constrained when the conduit is calcified in association with a sclerotic valve. Balloon-expandable stents, on the other hand, reliably expand to rated balloon diameters (although they suffer from recoil due to collapsing radial forces, and the effects of a non-compliant lesion) and can undergo subsequent expansion/re-expansion to finite diameters. Disadvantages include their relative stiffness, potential sharp edges (possibly rupturing the balloon), and large delivery systems,[17] a factor which limits their application in very small children or infants.[18] For the purposes of this chapter, only balloon-expandable stents (which are primarily used in this setting) will be discussed. Balloon-expandable stents can be an open-cell or a closed-cell design. The open-cell design has increased flexibility, lower radial strength, and less scaffolding for the conduit wall compared to the closed-cell design, which offers better radial strength, increased stiffness, but significant foreshortening.

There are a number of studies reporting the safety and effectiveness of stent implantation to an obstructed right ventricular outflow conduit.[9–11,19] Sugiyama et al.[13] and Powell et al.[11] noted that such interventions may extend the lifetime of the conduit by 3 to 4 years before surgical replacement is required. Often times, this was due to the child outgrowing the conduit effective outflow area, rather than in-stent stenosis. In this regard, at the time of surgical replacement of a stented conduit, there are no reports of complications or technical difficulties related to the stent.

Complications of conduit stent implantation can be viewed as having both an early and a late phase hazard. Early events include malposition and embolization, vessel perforation, and side branch obstruction, in addition to technical problems with stent delivery.

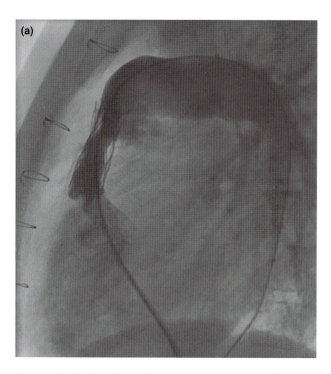
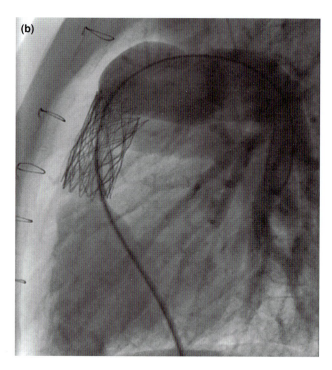

Figure 11.1 (A) Lateral projection of a previously stented conduit which has become compressed in its anteroposterior dimension. (B) After a second stent is implanted, there is improvement in the cross-sectional area and reduction in the right ventricle to pulmonary artery gradient.

Peng and colleagues[14] reported stent fracture in 43% of children undergoing follow-up catheterization and a 30% overall incidence (56 out of 126). Fractures were felt to be associated with stent compression in a substernal location. While there were no acute hemodynamic consequences, it can be associated with a recurrent stenosis. Late phase events include stent compression and fracture, migrations, and in-stent stenosis.

INDICATIONS FOR CONDUIT STENT IMPLANTATION

Right ventricular outflow tract stent implantation can be considered for obstructed conduits (pulmonary or aortic homografts, or bioprosthetic valves – e.g. Hancock™, Carpentier-Edwards™, Simbion™). Additionally, a previously stented conduit with compression in the anteroposterior dimension due to sternal and/or cardiac structures can have some improvement in the cross-sectional outflow area (from an ellipse to a circle) with implantation of a second stent[13] (Figure 11.1).

Consideration for a catheter-based intervention is the same as that for surgical conduit replacement. General guidelines include a right ventricular systolic pressure greater than or equal to three-quarters of the systemic pressure in an asymptomatic child, or two-thirds the systemic pressure in a symptomatic child (e.g. exercise intolerance, fatigue, dyspnea). Assessment of the child's age and size relative to the

original conduit impacts decision-making (i.e. is the conduit stenotic or has the child simply outgrown the implant?). If the child has outgrown the conduit, the benefits of stent implantation are marginal. Ultimately, catheter-based interventions are intended to postpone conduit replacement during times of somatic growth. The complete avoidance of surgical conduit management is neither plausible nor achievable in the growing child.

TECHNIQUES INVOLVED IN MANAGEMENT

Generally, under general anesthesia, a complete right heart catheterization study is performed. Hemodynamics are obtained in the right ventricle and the pulmonary arteries with angiography in the right ventricle, the conduit, and the branch vessels as required. Technically, right ventricle angiography and conduit angiography are obtained with a 90° left lateral projection and an anterior projection with 10° to 15° cranial angulation, as necessary.[7] Stents of lengths appropriate for the conduit can be implanted based on the diameter and length of the obstruction and the original conduit size. A length sufficient to span the stenotic area with a single stent is ideal, although multiple tandem stents may be needed. With a heavily calcified conduit, risk of rupture increases and a covered stent should be considered. Short segment stenoses are best palliated with a single stent, whereas long segment stenoses may be better served by multiple overlapping stents.

Stents are mounted on balloon catheters and delivered by way of a long guide sheath placed in the right ventricular outflow tract. The sheath is positioned with the distal end of the sheath beyond the area of stenosis. A 0.035 inch stiff interventional exchange wire should be placed into the distal pulmonary artery (the left pulmonary artery is preferred due to the trajectory of the outflow tract) to aid in the stabilization and positioning of the sheath and balloon across the target lesion. Stents are crimped manually onto an appropriately sized balloon and introduced over the wire. The sheath is then retracted and the balloon dilated with a 30:70 contrast to saline mixture. Sheath sizes range from 7 French to 11 French, depending on the size and type of the balloon and stent being introduced. We recommend that all patients receive preintervention heparinization and antibiotic prophylaxis during the procedure.

In order to avoid the problem of traversing the potential tight curves of the right ventricular outflow tract, the sheath and balloon stent can be inserted as a single unit over the exchange wire (so-called front loading). This technique avoids potential angles that can dislodge the stent from the balloon during advancement in the sheath.[9] Alternatively, a non-kinkable sheath (Flexor™, Cook, Bloomington, IN) can be used, or a tapering tip placed on the balloon can help traverse the outflow tract (Brite Tip™ Interventional Sheath, Johnson & Johnson, Cordis Endovascular).

Balloon dilation of the conduit prior to stent implantation is not mandatory, although it is recommended. Predilation testing is indicated in heavily calcified conduits to assess for expandability. In this setting, serial dilations may be required to expand the conduit to a diameter that will have a hemodynamic impact, followed by stenting to maintain or enhance the diameter achieved. It is also important to consider coronary angiography before implantation to ensure the stented conduit will avoid coronary arterial compression.

HOW TO AVOID TROUBLE: SKILLS AND EQUIPMENT REQUIRED

- Angioplasty balloons (regular and high-pressure types):
  - Tyshak II (NuMED, Inc, Hopkinton, NY)
  - Atlas or Conquest High Pressure Balloons (Bard Peripheral Vascular, Inc)
  - Mullins High Pressure Balloons (NuMED, Inc, Hopkinton, NY)
- Balloon-expandable stents:
  - Palmaz (Johnson and Johnson, Cordis Endovascular)
  - Genesis (Johnson and Johnson, Cordis Endovascular)
  - MaxiLD (eV3, Intrastent)
  - Cheatham-Platinum (CP) 8 Zig stent (Numed, Inc, Hopkinton, NY)
  - Cheatham-Platinum Covered stent: (Numed, Inc, Hopkinton, NY)
- Retrieval snare:
  - Ensnare (InterV, Medical Device Technologies)
  - Amplatz Gooseneck Snare (eV3, Vasocare Co Ltd)

When choosing an appropriate stent for a given patient it is important to account for stent shortening, strength, flexibility, rigidity, and a smooth surface. A comparison of the radial strengths between different stents has been obtained both in vivo and in vitro. Closed-cell designs in general are stronger (increased radial strength) compared to open-cell designs. By the nature of the anatomy of the right ventricular outflow tract and the potential risk for conduit compression, closed-cell designs are favored. The Genesis™ stent has demonstrated radial strengths in vitro that are equal to or better than its Palmaz counterpart, and twice that of the Intrastent LD stent,[20] but in vivo results favor the Palmaz™ over the Genesis™ stent.[14] The CP stent demonstrates good radial strength, albeit less than the Palmaz™ stent.[17] Their use, however, especially the covered stent variation with a PTFE membrane, is very helpful as a bail-out option in the setting of conduit fracture to avoid a hemothorax and hemodynamic compromise.[21] We recommend the use of the Palmaz™ stent for right ventricle to pulmonary artery conduits, with the CP covered stent available as a safety implant. A novel use for the covered stent can also be in the setting of initial stent implantation in preparation for a concurrent percutaneous pulmonary valve implant at the same procedure.

POSSIBLE COMPLICATIONS AND TECHNICAL DIFFICULTIES

Complications experienced with right ventricular outflow tract conduit stenting can be divided into early and late events. Early complications are related to technical issues such as sheath placement, stent–balloon delivery, balloon–stent deployment, or hemodynamic responses to balloon inflation. During inflation within the conduit the stent–balloon complex may move (generally forward) during inflation or the stent may migrate off the balloon, if inflation is not uniform. A hardened, calcified conduit may cause balloon rupture and result in an incompletely expanded stent or rupture of the conduit, causing acute hemothorax and tamponade. Rarely, the stent position can jail a branch pulmonary artery, compromising the flow. Importantly, coronary artery compression during implantation can result in significant hemodynamic compromise. This possibility should be considered if the conduit was inserted to address an anomalous coronary vessel.

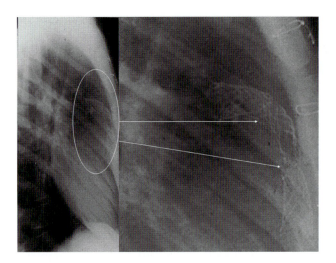

Figure 11.2 Left panel shows a lateral chest roentgenogram several years after conduit stent implantation. Note multi-level fractures, magnified in the right panel.

Late obstruction after implantation is often due to patient growth, particularly if implantation was performed at a young age. However, obstruction may occur secondary to stent fracture, which can develop as result of compression of an anteriorly positioned conduit wedged between the sternum anteriorly and the ventricular mass posteriorly. In a review from Boston Children's Hospital, more then 90% of such fractures were located immediately behind the sternum and were compressed between the chest wall and the heart, with longitudinal or compound fractures occurring in the majority,[11] with fragment embolization to the right ventricle and or pulmonary artery occurring in a quarter of the children (Figure 11.2). Such embolization occurred in the absence of symptoms or had hemodynamic consequences and did not contribute to mortality.

In this regard, stent selection may impact the incidence of stent fracture, with the Genesis™ stent (Johnson and Johnson, Cordis Endovascular) appearing to be at higher risk of fracture than the Palmaz™ XL stent (Johnson and Johnson, Cordis Endovascular). This is due to the slightly lower radial strength with the Genesis implant. Encouragingly, stent fracture was not associated with a shorter freedom from conduit surgery compared to intact stented conduits.[20] The original Cheatham platinum stent (NuMed, Inc) used in the percutaneous pulmonary valve implant was also plagued by fracture, with 21% (26/123) of patients so implanted presenting between 0 and 843 days. Fracture-free survival was 85% at 1 year and 69% at 3 years. The majority (two-thirds) had no deterioration in stent integrity and only one patient experienced separation of the fragments or embolization. With improvements in stent construction (gold brazing/soldering for the joints) the incidence of fracture has been reduced, but not eliminated. Recent studies suggest that implants that experience recoil (that is a reduction in diameter after balloon deflation), regardless of

position, are also at risk of fracture. In this setting, recoil is a surrogate for increased radial wall forces on the implant, perhaps affected by cyclic changes in the stent diameter due to cardiac motion. Other indicators of increased fracture risk are a non-calcified conduit and its repetitive compression by the sternum during the cardiac cycle. Recent reports, however, have not found significance in a substernal location, but this may be related to highly calcified conduits with increased resistance to compression.[22] Additionally, a heavily calcified conduit may be more likely to have a residual gradient after the implantation, compared with a conduit that is more compliant and non-calcified. A high pre- or post-stent right ventricular outflow tract gradient and stent compression or asymmetry after implantation appeared not to be associated with stent fracture.[22]

Pulmonary insufficiency accompanies a successful implant, but frequently is in the setting of pre-existent moderate to severe regurgitation. Long-term so-called 'free' pulmonary insufficiency warrants close observation, although it appears to be clinically well tolerated in the short term. After bare metal stenting, Sugiyama and colleagues demonstrated stable right ventricle (RV) dimensions throughout their follow-up period (median 2.3 years after the procedure, range 4 months to 10 years).[13] It should be underscored that pulmonary insufficiency may be aggravated by distal pulmonary artery obstruction, highlighting the importance of assessing the branch vessels and the need for distal angioplasty (or stenting) prior to conduit stent implantation. From the 15-year experience in the Boston series, there were no deaths, strokes, myocardial infarctions, cardiac perforations, or conduit damage after stent implantation that required urgent surgical intervention.[14]

HOW TO MANAGE COMPLICATIONS

Early complications

The likelihood of stent migration can be diminished by establishing a stable position of the long delivery sheath and the use of a 'stiff' exchange wire (Amplatz, Cook, Boston Scientific). Additionally, use of a short balloon (i.e. one that does not protrude significantly beyond the stent) and the appropriate length stent will prevent the stent from 'milking' off the catheter during inflation. Some operators suggest the use of a balloon-in-balloon catheter (BIB™, Numed, Inc) allowing a partial expansion and repositioning before full expansion as required. Stent migration on the balloon during inflation is inevitably due to non-symmetric inflation of the balloon. This is often due to excessive crimping of the stent on to the balloon shaft (often unavoidable), and forces expansion to begin on the proximal end of the balloon, thus 'milking' the stent forward. This can be avoided by using the BIB™

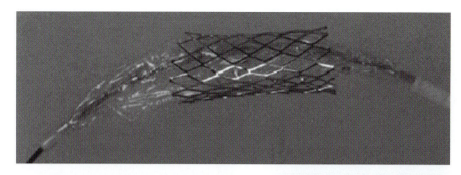

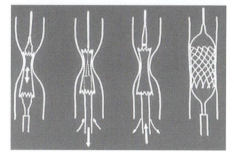 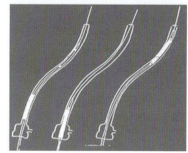

Figure 11.3 Upper panel shows a photograph in vitro of a Palmaz™ XL stent, which has milked backward on the balloon during inflation. The lower left drawing illustrates a technique for removing a balloon that has ruptured before full inflation, using the long sheath as countertraction while removing the failed balloon. The right panel illustrates a further technique to reposition a stent that has come off the balloon while still on the delivery sheath.

balloon as noted above, or by only partial retraction of the sheath over the balloon before inflation. With inflation, the contrast will track to the tip of the balloon, expanding that first, and then, with further sheath retraction, the balloon can be fully expanded. Note also that access from the left femoral vein will result in an inferior-medial direction of the balloon–stent complex as it traverses the long sheath. With a long stent, care must be taken to avoid displacement of the stent onto the balloon shaft, which occurs usually at the junction of the internal iliac to the inferior caval vein. Finally, predilation of the stenotic area has been found to improve the safety of implantation by assessing the unpredictable compliance of the conduit, avoiding implantation to a non-distensible tube, and it helps to identify the locations of additional stenotic areas.[14]

In the event of stent migration, a sequential strategy can be employed to assess and correct the situation. First, stop inflation and determine whether the stent is 'milking' forward or backward onto the catheter shaft. If the former, attempt to withdraw the balloon–stent complex, reposition the balloon in the conduit to the target lesion, and re-expand the balloon in place (Figure 11.3). Ultimately, it matters little if the stent is deployed a little closer to the pulmonary arteries or in the right ventricular outflow tract, as it will not be obstructive and a second stent can be placed to address the remainder of the lesion. If the stent retracts onto the balloon shaft instead of moving forward, try to reposition the stent on the balloon, either alone or with the support of the long sheath, and then try deployment in the conduit again. Remember, so long as the wire is through the stent, it is possible to capture it and position it into a distal branch pulmonary artery or the inferior caval vein.[23]

Crossing the orifice of a branch pulmonary artery with a more distal deployment can be addressed by flaring the distal end of the stent into the branch pulmonary artery. Flaring increases the size of the individual stent cells and can avoid obstruction to flow, although this is rare. Obstruction to a branch pulmonary artery more often occurs due to deformation of the vessel orifice by the stent, thereby 'jailing' the branch. With open-cell stents, the cells can be individually dilated, or, if significant obstruction occurs, an additional stent can be placed in to the vessel to relieve the branch obstruction. At the time of conduit change, the stent can be either removed or cut through as necessary.

Some degree of residual stenosis is common due to the increased right ventricular stroke volume; the conduit is of a marginal diameter or concurrent distal pulmonary artery pathology. By using a high-pressure balloon (Atlas™, Mullins™, Conquest™), even significantly calcified conduits can achieve an adequate diameter. Finally, additional stents may offer greater support by increasing radial forces as noted above.

Balloon rupture without full expansion can be managed in a number of ways, including balloon exchange and dilation with a new balloon if the stent is stable in the conduit, or, if unsuccessful, withdrawal and implantation into the inferior caval vein. More often, if rupture occurs during inflation and the stent is in the proper position, a rapid inflation (using dilute contrast) may allow balloon expansion.[24] One report has suggested attaching the balloon to an angiographic pressure injector and using 30 cc of saline at 5 cc/s (400 psi) to rapidly expand the balloon[25] (Figure 11.4). If that is unsuccessful, one can try 10 cc/s at 600 psi, and for large balloons use 40 cc at 10 cc/s (600 psi). In one series, balloon rupture occurred in 30% of implants ($n = 74$), with 3 children requiring a venous cutdown for stent removal. The remainder of the children had the balloon removed through either the original introducer sheath or a second sheath placed for the purpose of snaring and removing the balloon.[14]

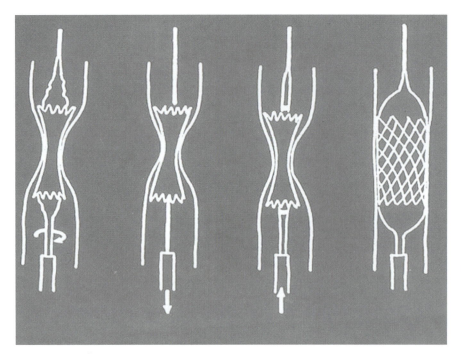

Figure 11.4 If a balloon ruptures before full inflation, this figure illustrates another technique for removing the balloon, by rotating the balloon shaft and withdrawing it into the long sheath.

The potential for coronary arterial obstruction must be appreciated, anticipated, and avoided. If the anatomic risk is present (coronary arterial course in close proximity to the conduit), selective coronary angiography or an aortic root injection should be performed to define the path of the coronary artery in relation to the conduit. This should be performed with test balloon inflation in the presence of continuous electrocardiographic monitoring for evidence of ischemic changes (Figure 11.5). There is little that can be done if coronary compression occurs after implantation, other than urgent surgical intervention. One author has described an instance where chest compressions successfully compressed the conduit stent, relieving the coronary obstruction, but, certainly, this cannot be a technique to rely upon, only avoidance.

A tear in the conduit is uncommon, with 3% of children noted to have extravasation of contrast after dilation and/or stent implantation (Figure 11.6) without accompanying evidence for hemothorax or hemopericardium.[14] However, with the application of high-pressure balloons and covered valve stents, this is probably underrecognized. Evidence of a conduit fracture with contrast extravasation can be addressed with a covered stent if the hemodynamic situation allows. Under circumstances of hemodynamic instability, urgent surgical intervention is warranted.

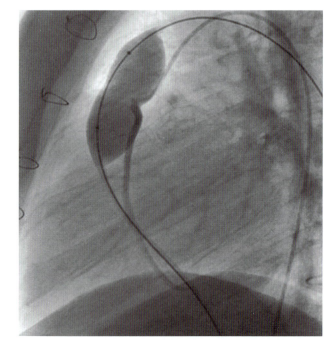

Figure 11.5 A lateral projection angiogram during balloon inflation in a stenotic right ventricle to pulmonary artery conduit, during selective coronary angiography. Note the inflated balloon compresses the coronary. Significant coronary ischemia would occur if this conduit were stented open.

Late complications

Recurrent stenosis should be viewed in the perspective of the natural history of conduits, as opposed to a treatment failure, and is often due to the growth of the child. Data for redilation suggested a significant number of children achieve an additional 1 or 2 years before conduit replacement is indicated.[13] In this regard, if recurrent stenosis is felt to be related to the intrinsic conduit geometry, a repeat catheter intervention is appropriate, with attempted balloon dilation or a second stent-in-stent implantation (Figure 11.7).

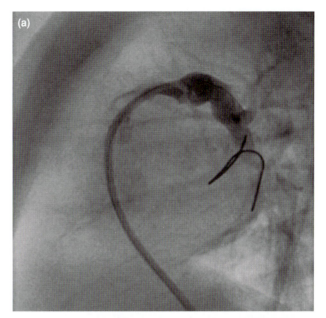

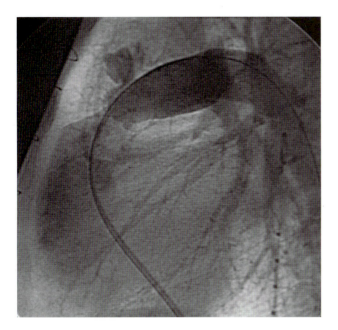

Figure 11.6   A heavily calcified conduit which was balloon dilated in preparation for stent implantation. Note the anterior extravasation of contrast. The child had a covered stent positioned to control the conduit disruption.

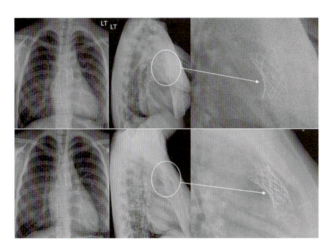

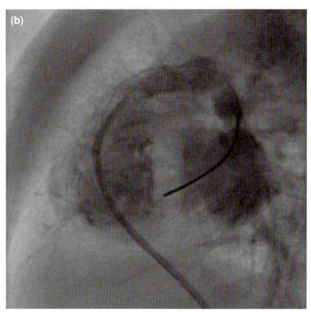

Figure 11.7   Chest roentgenograms immediately after conduit stenting (upper panel) and 6 months later (lower panel). With time, the very anterior stent (immediately under the sternum) has become compressed. This occurred despite restenting (lower panel).

Caution is required during re-intervention, with special attention to the potential for balloon rupture within the first stent, or with the successive implantation of a new stent. Studies have demonstrated successful alleviation of obstruction in approximately 50% of children undergoing a second intervention with a reduction in right ventricular pressure. Attempts beyond a second catheter intervention have been universally unsuccessful, dictating surgical intervention to be the better option.[9]

Finally, in long-term follow-up, surveillance for stent fracture is imperative. Many children will have asymptomatic stent fracture with maintenance of stent

Figure 11.8   (A) Lateral projection of an angiogram taken in a symptomatic (cyanotic) neonate with Fallot's tetralogy denoting severe infundibular stenosis. Because of the child's weight and age surgery was deferred, and a stent placed in the outflow tract with excellent anatomic and clinical effect (B).

integrity, but recurrent obstruction. Routine chest radiography may define such lesions, but fluoroscopy appears to be the best imaging modality.[11,14] The development of a new outflow tract gradient should prompt such investigations.

NATIVE RIGHT VENTRICULAR OUTFLOW TRACT STENT IMPLANTATION

Infants with Fallot's tetralogy presenting with significant hypercyanotic episodes or baseline cyanosis and considered high risk (prematurity, cerebral hemorrhage or injury, growth restriction) for surgical intervention (modified Blalock–Taussig shunt or early primary repair) present an interesting dilemma. We have demonstrated the feasibility of implantation of coronary stents within the right ventricular outflow tract, spanning the entirety of the infundibular mass through the pulmonary valve and into the proximal main pulmonary artery[26] (Figure 11.8). Under these circumstances, the children can be stabilized and grow prior to an elective surgical repair, with the stent removed at the time of surgery. The only observed complication, other than improper stent placement, has been stenosis with subsequent reduction of arterial saturations due to either stent compression or persistence of infundibular tissue outside the margins of the stent. Depending on the age and size of the child, the potential interventions include surgical repair, balloon dilation of the initial stent, or implantation of an additional stent to span the entirety of the infundibulum. Results of this approach are limited by patient numbers and short duration of follow-up, but initial results are promising and will have an important role in management of the small child with tetralogy of Fallot.[27]

SUMMARY

Extending the lifespan of right ventricle to pulmonary artery conduits and limiting cyanosis in newborns with tetralogy of Fallot can be achieved with a strategy of stent implantation to the right ventricular outflow tract. Coordinated efforts between the interventional cardiologist and the cardiac surgeon to optimize the timing of surgical repair or palliation will reduce the number of operations required and the frequency with which they take place. Complications occur in the early and late phases and monitoring the effects of stenting the outflow tract requires vigilance. Persistent obstruction, recurrent stenosis, stent fracture, and conduit disruption can be limited by appropriate stent selection and the precautions described in this chapter. Continued progress in stent technology and deployment strategies will expand current indications for implantation.

REFERENCES

1. Razzouk AJ, Williams WG, Cleveland DC et al. Surgical connection from ventricle to pulmonary artery. Comparison of four types of valved implants. Circulation 1992; 86(Suppl II): 154–8.
2. Salim MA, DiSessa TG, Alpert BS et al. The fate of homograft conduits in children with congenital heart disease: an angiographic study. Ann Thorac Surg 1995; 59: 67–73.
3. Stark J, Bull C, Stajevic M et al. Fate of subpulmonary homograft conduits: determinants of late homograft failure. J Thorac Cardiovasc Surg 1998; 115: 506–16.
4. Sreeram N, Hutter P, Silove E. Sustained high pressure double balloon angioplasty of calcified conduits. Heart 1999; 81: 162–5.
5. Sanatani S, Potts JE, Human DG et al. Balloon angioplasty of right ventricular outflow tract conduits. Pediatr Cardiol 2001; 22: 228–32.
6. Zeevi B, Keane JF, Perry SB, Lock JE. Balloon dilation of postoperative right ventricular outflow obstructions. J Am Coll Cardiol 1989; 14: 401–8.
7. Aggarwal S, Garekar S, Forbes TJ, Turner DR. Is stent placement effective for palliation of right ventricle to pulmonary artery conduit stenosis? J Am Coll Cardiol 2007; 49: 480–4.
8. Almagor Y, Prevosti LG, Bartorelli AL et al. Balloon expandable stent implantation in stenotic right heart valved conduits. J Am Coll Cardiol 1990; 16: 1310–14.
9. Ovaert C, Caldarone CA, McCrindle BW et al. Endovascular stent implantation for the management of postoperative right ventricular outflow tract obstruction: clinical efficacy. J Thorac Cardiovasc Surg 1999; 118: 886–93.
10. Hosking MC, Benson LN, Nakanishi T et al. Intravascular stent prosthesis for right ventricular outflow obstruction. J Am Coll Cardiol 1992; 20: 373–80.
11. Powell AJ, Lock JE, Keane JF, Perry SB. Prolongation of RV-PA conduit life span by percutaneous stent implantation. Intermediate-term results. Circulation 1995; 92: 3282–8.
12. Pedra CA, Justino H, Nykanen D et al. Percutaneous stent implantation to stenotic bioprosthetic valves in the pulmonary position. J Thorac Cardiovasc Surg 2002; 124: 82–7.
13. Sugiyama H, Williams WG, Benson LN. Implantation of endovascular stents for the obstructive right ventricular outflow tract. Heart 2005; 91: 1058–63.
14. Peng LF, McElhinney DB, Nugent AW et al. Endovascular stenting of obstructed right ventricle-to-pulmonary artery conduits: a 15-year experience. Circulation 2006; 113: 2598–605.
15. O'Laughlin MP, Slack MC, Grifka RG et al. Implantation and intermediate-term follow-up of stents in congenital heart disease. Circulation 1993; 88: 605–14.
16. Frias PA, Meranze SG, Graham Jr TP, Doyle TP. Relief of right ventricular to pulmonary artery conduit stenosis using a self-expanding stent. Cathet Cardiovasc Interven 1999; 47: 52–4.
17. Ing F. Stents: what's available to the pediatric interventional cardiologist? Cathet Cardiovasc Interven 2002; 57: 374–86.
18. Zeidenweber CM, Kim DW, Vincent RN. Right ventricular outflow tract and pulmonary artery stents in children under 18 months of age. Cathet Cardiovasc Interven 2007; 69: 23–7.
19. Saliba Z, Bonhoeffer P, Aggoun Y et al. Treatment of obstruction of prosthetic conduits by percutaneous implantation of stents. Archives des Maladies do Coevr et des Vaisseaux 1999; 92: 591–6.
20. Forbes TJ, Amin Z Rodriguez-Cruz E, Benson LN et al. The Genesis stent: a new low-profile stent for use in infants, children and adults with congenital heart disease. Cathet Cardiovasc Interven 2003; 59: 406–14.
21. Cheatham JP. Stents and Amplatzers: what's an interventionalist to do? Cathet Cardiovasc Interven 1999; 47: 39–40.
22. Nordmeyer J, Khambadkone S, Coats L et al. Risk stratification, systematic classification, and anticipatory management strategies for stent fracture after percutaneous pulmonary valve implantation. Circulation 2007; 115: 1392–7.
23. Hoyer MH, Bailey SR, Neill JA, Palmaz JC. Transcatheter retrieval of an embolized palmaz stent from the right ventricle of a child. Cathet Cardiovasc Diagn 1996; 39: 277–80.
24. Order BM, Muller-Hulsbeck S. Management of unexpected balloon rupture during deployment of balloon-expandable stents. J Endovasc Ther 2002; 9: 622–4.
25. Keelan ET, Nunez BD, Berger PB, Holmes Jr DR, Garratt KN. Management of balloon rupture during rigid stent deployment. Cathet Cardiovasc Diagn 1995; 35: 211–15.
26. Laudito A, Bandisode VM, Lucas JF et al. Right ventricular outflow tract stent as a bridge to surgery in a premature infant with tetralogy of Fallot. Ann Thorac Surg 2006; 81: 744–6.
27. Dohlen G, Chaturvedi R, Benson LN et al. Stenting of the right ventricular outflow tract in the symptomatic infant with tetralogy of Fallot. Heart 2008 [Epub ahead of print.]

12 Stenting branch pulmonary arteries

Frank F Ing

BACKGROUND

Stent-implantation to treat a branch pulmonary stenosis in congenital heart disease is well established.[1–9] While its safety and efficacy is well reported in the literature, the procedure can be quite challenging technically and fraught with anatomic limitations, adverse events and complications. Anatomic limitations of this procedure may include small patient size and lack of vascular access due to obstructed femoral veins secondary to prolonged central line placement and/or repeated access previously. Furthermore, anatomy of the pulmonary artery stenosis may be quite varied and complex, and difficult to navigate, especially in the presence of a dilated right atrium and right ventricle. Associated regurgitant tricuspid and/or pulmonary valves also add to the difficulty of maintaining adequate wire control during the stenting procedure. Complex anatomy may include stenosis adjacent to side branches, especially the lobar and segmental branches.[10–11] Noncompliant, long segmental stenosis may pose a particular challenge, even if access is adequate.

ADVERSE EVENTS AND COMPLICATIONS

Adverse events and complications of stenting branch pulmonary arteries are similar to those of other stenting procedures, but because access to the pulmonary vessels has to pass through the right heart and its two valves, once an adverse event or complication develops, it is more difficult to address compared to stenting in other vessels. Hence, it would be best to avoid these mishaps in the first place. Attention to the smallest details is required in all aspects of the stent procedure in order to have excellent results consistently. When a problem arises, the operator must know how to make corrections in order to avoid a potential emergency operation, or even death. The purpose of this chapter is to review anatomic limitations of pulmonary artery stenting, discuss those areas of the procedure where there is the most potential for adverse events which may lead to a complication, as well as to review the techniques of correction and management of the complications.

The majority of adverse events and complications are related to the techniques of stent implantation, including stent slippage on the balloon during placement, balloon rupture during a stent implant, and stent malposition or embolization. Anatomic-based complications include jailing of side branches, aneurysm formation, and vascular dissection or disruption. Other complications include pulmonary thromboembolic events, air embolism and pulmonary edema. Late complications include restenosis, occlusion of jailed side branches and, rarely, stent fracture.

ANATOMIC LIMITATIONS: SMALL PATIENT SIZE

Branch pulmonary artery stenosis (BPS) is most commonly found after surgical correction of tetralogy of Fallot and pulmonary atresia with ventricular septal defect (VSD), and less commonly, but not rare after repair of truncus arteriosus, d-transposition of the great arteries and after various stages of single ventricle repair. Congenital BPS is commonly found in Alagille and Williams syndrome. With the current surgical trend of early repair, it is not uncommon to encounter significant BPS in infants and small children postoperatively. When these patients present with right heart volume and/or pressure overload and varying degrees of right heart failure, an intervention is required to improve their hemodynamics. Often angioplasty alone is inadequate or there is early restenosis requiring a stent procedure.

Early reports recommended the use of an 11 French delivery system to implant large size stents (dilatable to 18 mm diameter) into the proximal pulmonary arteries.[1–3] However, with lower profile balloons and stents, and improved techniques learned over the last decade, delivery systems as small as 7 French size can now be used to implant large size stents into infants as small as 4–5 kg.[12–15]

Access to pulmonary arteries through the tricuspid and pulmonary valves in these small chambers can be difficult, and is associated with hemodynamic instability. The relatively stiff wire and delivery system props

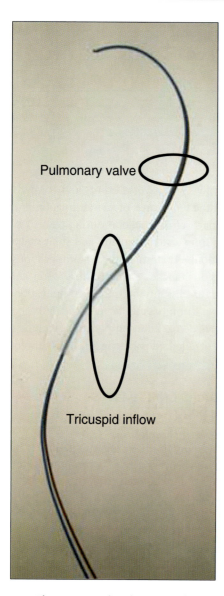

Figure 12.1 Shaping an 'S-bend' on a guidewire to match the natural curves across the tricuspid and pulmonary valves in a small child minimizes the risk of propping open the valves and resultant regurgitation.

open the tricuspid and pulmonary valves, resulting in valve regurgitation. It is important to properly estimate the shape of the intracardiac route and shape the wires appropriately to minimize the valve regurgitation. This is accomplished by bending an 'S'- shape in the wire itself to follow the natural curves across the tricuspid and pulmonary valve (Figure 12.1). This may require several attempts at bending the wire until it matches the natural intracardiac course. Adequate volume loading and even inotropic support may be required in the very small patients. The use of newer, lower profile, and more flexible stents such as the Genesis (Cordis Corp, Miami Lakes, FL), and Doublestrut and Mega-LD (eV3, Plymouth, MN) stents has made it easier to cross the right ventricular outflow tract, but it can still be quite difficult in the smallest and sickest of patients. While

there are published data showing successful use of the premounted medium size stents (dilatable to 12 mm diameter) in the small age range, a major disadvantage is that, while the medium size stents can be implanted successfully into the branch pulmonary arteries, they cannot be dilated beyond 12 mm and will require surgical removal when the patient grows to adolescent size.[14,18,19] It should be noted that premounted 'large' genesis stents, in spite of the 'large' label, are not truly large size stents and can only be dilated to 12 mm diameter with significant shortening of the length. The only true large size Genesis stent is the Genesis XD, which is not available pre-mounted to date.[13]

The technique of intraoperative stent implantation has been reported.[20–25] This technique can avoid all the problems of the small femoral vessels and tight curves around the right heart. However, it is still an operation and should be reserved only for the smallest and sickest of patients, the early postoperative period, or when there is associated surgery required, such as homograft replacement or Glenn or Fontan completion. Another technique to facilitate placement of a large stent in small children (5–10 kg) involves cutting a dilator tip and mounting it on a balloon, and front loading the stent on this balloon.[12,15–17] Once a wire position is achieved the sheath, "dilator-tipped" balloon, and stent unit are advanced to the site of stenosis. The sheath is withdrawn to expose the balloon and stent and, without additional exchanges, the stent can be implanted quite rapidly, even in the presence of hemodynamic instability in a small child. In one series from the Children's Hospital of San Diego, the front-loaded balloon tip dilator technique successfully implanted 70 large size stents in 50 patients.[17] In this group the mean age and weight were 1.1 years and 8.5 kg, respectively. The weight range was 3.3 to 12.0 kg. The minimum diameter increased from 3.1 to 6.8 mm. The pressure gradient decreased from 34.0 to 11.4 mmHg. Right ventricle to femoral artery pressure ratio decreased from 72% to 52%. All cases were stented successfully, thereby avoiding the need for surgery. With the recent arrival of the more flexible and lower profile Genesis XD stent, 6–10 mm diameter balloons can be mounted and advanced through 7 French sheaths without the balloon-dilator tip and front-loading technique. However, preliminary data show that, using the same technique, a Genesis stent can be delivered through a 5 French delivery system.

INTRAOPERATIVE STENT IMPLANTATION

The advantage of this technique is that the size of the delivery system is not an issue. Furthermore, the stent

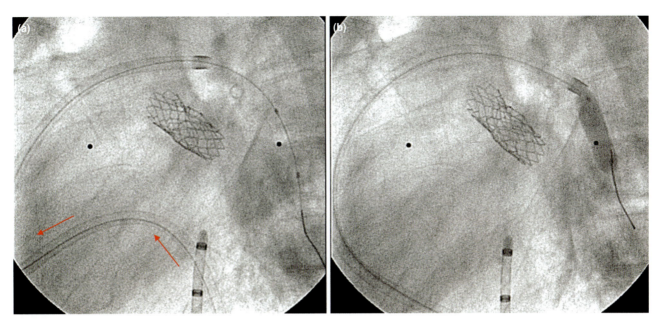

Figure 12.2 (A) Advancing a large delivery sheath into the pulmonary artery over a guidewire results in buckling of the sheath (red arrows) in the dilated right atrium and ventricle. (B) A balloon is advanced into the left pulmonary artery and inflated to 'anchor' the wire, facilitating advancement of the sheath into the left pulmonary artery.

can be modified to fit the anatomy of the small size patients. Delivery through an open technique on bypass or through a sheath placed in the main pulmonary artery without bypass can be performed easily.[20] Associated procedures such as homograft, Glenn and Fontan completion can be performed at the same time. This technique is also particularly useful in the early postoperative days where there is a high risk of rupture of suture lines during stent implantation.[22,25] However, one of the major disadvantages is the need for a portable fluoroscopic unit, which has less resolution and limited angiography compared to a catheterization laboratory suite. The arrival of the new hybrid surgical suites or catheterization laboratories should eliminate this disadvantage.[26] Nevertheless, intraoperative stenting is still an operation that requires cooperation with a cardiovascular surgeon. During the intraoperative procedure, the operating table may be reversed to allow proper placement of the base of the portable C-arm under the table. This maneuver has to be done before the start of the case if intraoperative stenting is considered.

LACK OF VASCULAR ACCESS AND DIFFICULT VASCULAR ANATOMY

Due to the repeated use of femoral veins for cardiac catheterization and surgery, and/or prolonged central line placement during infancy, it is not uncommon to find stenotic or occluded femoral and iliac veins in these patients at the onset of the procedure. While a single femoral venous access is sufficient for the stent procedure, it is preferable to have bilateral access from the onset. There are reports in the literature indicating successful recanalization of stenotic and occluded

femoral vessels, using a combination of angioplasty and stent implantation in order to regain access to the right heart and pulmonary arteries.[27–29] Specific techniques on recanalization are beyond the scope of this chapter. Alternative vascular access including transhepatic access and internal jugular and subclavian vein access have been reported.[30–32]

Not uncommonly, branch pulmonary artery stenosis in congenital heart disease is often associated with pulmonary and/or tricuspid valve regurgitation. The resulting dilatation of the right atrium and/or right ventricle may cause difficulty in accessing and maintaining stable distal wire and sheath position. It is the compromise of optimal wire and sheath position that often results in an adverse event, which leads to a complication. Advancing stiff wires and large sheaths across a dilated right heart can be difficult secondary to upward bending of the wire at the dome of the enlarged right atrium, or downward bending at the apex of the dilated right ventricle. Even when a good distal wire position is achieved, these bends can 'pull' the wire out of position when any forward force is applied on the delivery system during manipulations or exchanges. One technique to facilitate stable placement of a large sheath and stiff wire is the initial use of a smaller gauge exchange guide wire passed to the distal pulmonary arteries, followed by advancement of a smaller balloon to the distal vessel. With the balloon inflated in the small vessel to act as an anchor and to provide countertraction, a larger sheath can be advanced over the smaller guide wire across the right heart into the distal branch pulmonary arteries (Figure 12.2). Once the sheath is in a stable position, the smaller gauge wire is exchanged for a stiffer exchange guide wire that has been

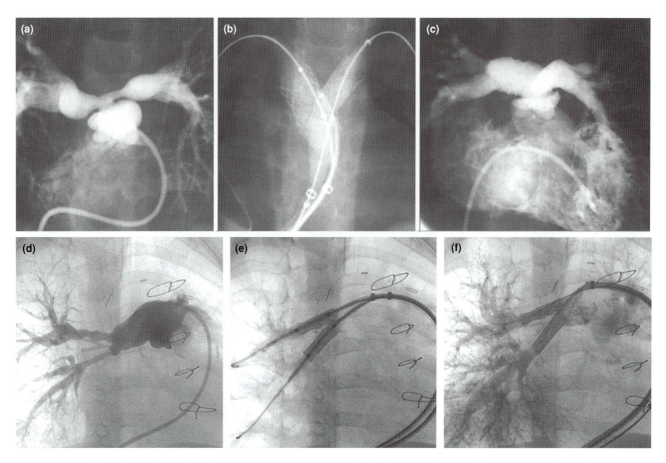

Figure 12.3 (A) Bilateral branch pulmonary artery stenoses with closely related ostia following arterial switch operation. (B) Bilateral simultaneous implantation of stents into the proximal right and left pulmonary arteries. (C) Post stent angiogram showing wide patency of both pulmonary arteries. (D) Right upper and lower lobar branch stenoses in unifocalized aortopulmonary collaterals. (E) Simultaneous implantation of 2 stents in the RUL and RLL. (F) Post stent angiogram showing improved flow to RUL and RLL.

preshaped. Hemodynamic instability can result during this part of the procedure which may require additional volume loading and/or inotropic support. Stable positioning of a large sheath and stiff wire with stable hemodynamics should permit delivery of the stent and balloon.

Long segment stenoses that are non-compliant may be encountered, especially in the unifocalized aortopulmonary collaterals of PA/VSD or in congenital BPS. Predilation in these cases is recommended to test the stability of the balloon prior to stent implantation. Vascular non-compliance can result in the balloon milking backwards during inflation. Similarly, stent and balloon slippage can occur during inflation if the vessel is non-compliant. If predilation demonstrates stable balloon dilation, then stent implantation is performed. If the balloon shifts out of position due to non-compliance, either a smaller, high-pressure balloon or a cutting balloon is used to dilate the segmental stenosis large enough to permit a stable implantation of the stent itself.[34–37] The balloon diameter selected for predilation should be smaller than the final diameter of the stent and balloon selected.[38]

Stenosis can be found anywhere along the course of the pulmonary arterial tree, from the branch pulmonary artery orifices in the main pulmonary artery to the bifurcation of the segmental or subsegmental branches distally. It can be diffusely located in the lobar branches, at the segmental and subsegmental levels. Stenting is usually reserved for the right and left branch pulmonary arteries, and occasionally in the lobar branches. When stenosis is found near the branch PA orifice, special attention is needed to evaluate the contralateral branch. In the case of close proximity of the ostia of the two branch pulmonary arteries, stent implantation of one branch might jail the contralateral orifice. Similarly, when stenosis is located at the bifurcation of the lobar branches, stenting of one lobar branch may jail another lobar branch. A technique of simultaneous implantation of two crossing stents has been reported to prevent jailing of either branch and to permit future access to both branches.[39] The same technique can be used in stenting both the right and left branch pulmonary arteries as well as two lobar branches (Figure 12.3).

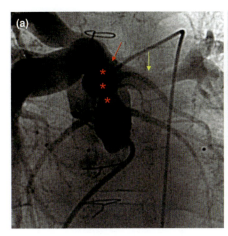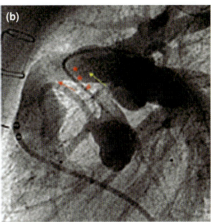

Figure 12.4 Evaluating the adjacent anatomy of a stenotic left pulmonary artery (LPA) and RVOT in a hypoplastic left heart syndrome patient. AP (A) and lateral (B) projections of simultaneous injections of contrast into RVOT and native aorta (A): LPA stenosis (yellow arrow) behind dilated neo-aorta. A second stenosis is at the MPA (red arrow). Note course of adjacent native ascending aorta and left coronary artery (red asterisks). A stent implanted in the LPA and RVOT might risk compressing the native aorta or coronary flow. In this case, a stent was not implanted and patient was referred for surgical correction.

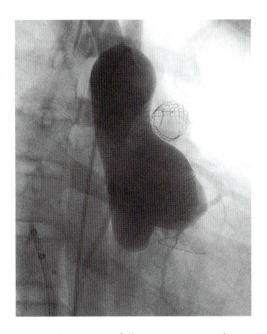

Figure 12.5 Aortogram following stent implantation to treat LPA stenosis in a patient with d-TGA after arterial switch operation. Stent compresses the adjacent ascending aorta.

coronary artery course before implantation in order to avoid compression of the coronary artery that might happen to course in the vicinity of the stented vessel. Occasionally, simultaneous injection of a selective coronary artery while a balloon is inflated in the stenosis is used for careful evaluation of the coronary course (Figure 12.4). Coronary artery compression by a stent is a complication more commonly associated with stenting of an RV to PA conduit. When BPS is found in d-TGA following a Lecompte maneuver, it is usually due to inadequate mobilization and/or overstretching of the branch pulmonary arteries.[40] In this scenario, the aorta sits just behind the bifurcation of the branch pulmonary arteries and stenting of the proximal branches may result in compression of the adjacent posteriorly positioned ascending aorta (Figure 12.5). Stent compression of or erosion into adjacent structures has been reported.[41–44] Simultaneous injection of the aorta with the balloon inflated within the stenotic pulmonary arteries might be useful to evaluate the degree of compression in this region.

STENT MALPOSITION AND BALLOON RUPTURE

Stent malposition and balloon rupture are the two most common adverse events of a pulmonary artery stent procedure.[3,4,6,45–47] Failure to properly manage these events when they do occur can easily result in a complication. First, it is important for the operator to be fully familiar with all the minute details of stent implantation and where these adverse events might occur during the procedure in order to avoid them in the first place. Inevitably, these events will occur and expertise is needed to manage them to avoid a true complication. Specifically, it is important to know how and where to reposition a stent and how to maintain stent position for balloon exchanges.

Obviously, this technique is more challenging because it requires multiple operators and the handling of two sheaths and two stents. Implantation with balloon inflation and deflation must be performed simultaneously in order to prevent balloon rupture by the contralateral stent edge; this will be discussed later.

Occasionally, BPS is associated with an adjacent dilated ascending aorta. This is commonly seen with the left pulmonary artery positioned behind a dilated aorta of a truncus arteriosus or of the neoaorta following a Norwood or a Damus–Kaye–Stansel operation. In this scenario, it would be important to evaluate the

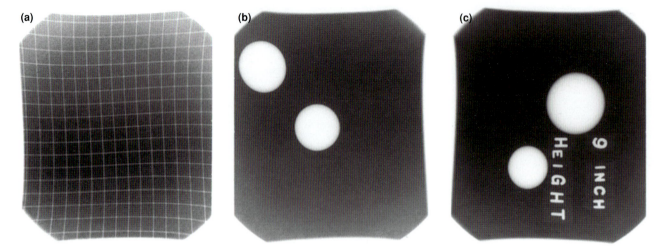

Figure 12.6 Examples of peripheral distortion or magnification which may render measurements inaccurate: (A) A grid placed over an image intensifier (II) shows the slight curves of the straight lines at the periphery of the II. (B) Two balls of equal size with one placed at the center of the II and the other at the periphery showing peripheral distortion of the ball placed at the edge of the II. (C) The same 2 balls placed in the 9 inches apart in height. The ball closer to the II is magnified.

FOUR PHASES OF STENT IMPLANTATION

There are four general phases of the pulmonary artery stent procedure. They are: (1) accurate measurement of the anatomy and appropriate selection of the stent and balloon, (2) stent delivery to the stenotic segment, (3) balloon inflation to implant the stent, and (4) balloon removal out of the stent. Knowledge of the fine details of each phase of the stent procedure will help the operator to pay special attention at certain critical moments of the procedure to minimize the risk of an adverse event which might lead to a complication. The following discussion highlights those critical points of the stent procedure where stent malposition or balloon rupture might occur, and how they can be avoided or managed.

Accurate measurement and selection of stent and balloon

All catheterization laboratory imaging systems have built-in image errors that can render a measurement inaccurate. These include magnification, quantum mottle, image blur, motion blur, quantum blur, and peripheral distortion (Figure 12.6).[6,48] Newer flat panel systems have improved but not eliminated these built-in errors. It is important to position the anatomy of interest at the center of the image intensifier to minimize the peripheral distortion. Angiograms should be taken at no less than 30 frames per second to minimize motion blur and increase the chance of finding the optimal frame for measurement.

It is important to use large reference markers for accurate measurement. While adult cardiologists use the diameters of catheters as measurement references for coronary artery interventions, these dimensions are simply too small for the larger sizes of the pulmonary arteries. The diameter of the stenosis, and the adjacent normal vessel segment, as well as the length of stenosis, should be measured accurately. Pertinent adjacent anatomy such as side branches of the pulmonary arterial tree and the nearby aorta and coronary course should also be evaluated prior to the stent procedure.

It is important to select the frame that shows the widest diameter of the pulsating vessel rather than to select a frame that has the most contrast in the segment of interest. Vessel diameters in the systolic and diastolic phases can range widely. If the widest diameter is not selected, the balloon used for stent implantation might be undersized, resulting in a 'loose' stent which can migrate or embolize. Furthermore, optimal angulation of the image intensifier is needed to properly profile the stenotic segment and side branches. Occasionally, multiple injections at multiple angulations are required for proper measurements. This is particularly important when the stenosis is located at the orifice of the right and left branch pulmonary artery which might be superimposed by a dilated main pulmonary artery (Figure 12.7).

The stent selected should be one whose maximal diameter is the same as that of the adult size pulmonary artery. Generally, for the right and left main branch, a large size stent such as the Genesis XD stent or the Mega-LD stent (maximal diameter 18 mm)

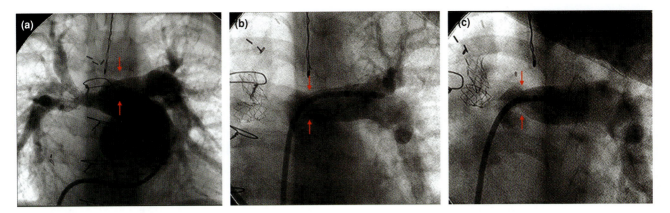

Figure 12.7 (A) Straight AP projection does not reveal LPA stenosis due to superimposition of dilated MPA. (B) Angulation of 20° LAO and 20° cranial suggests LPA stenosis (red arrow). (C) Additional angulation of 30° LAO and 30° cranial reveals clearly profile of LPA stenosis at orifice (red arrow).

should be selected. For lobar branches, a medium size stent (maximal diameter 12 mm) is acceptable. These include all of the premounted Genesis stents. In cases where the patient will require additional surgery in the future (such as homograft replacement), it may be acceptable to use a smaller stent where it can be removed at the time of the next surgery. While it may be easier to implant a smaller premounted stent, keep in mind that, as the child grows to adult size, the smaller stent will become the site of restenosis and will eventually require additional surgery for removal. Some might even consider this an anticipated long-term 'complication.' Balloon size should be selected to be equal or slightly larger than the adjacent normal pulmonary segment. There are limited stent lengths, but the ideal selected stent length should be long enough to cover the stenosis, maintain radial traction against the normal segment, and not cross a side branch.

Stent delivery to the stenotic pulmonary segment

During insertion of the stent and balloon unit into the delivery sheath, the valve of the sheath might 'catch' the stent, resulting in backward shifting of the stent along the balloon. One method to avoid this is to cut a short sheath of equal French size and use it as an introducer to prevent the stent from contacting the sheath valve during its insertion. During advancement of the stent/balloon unit along the length of the sheath, the stent can also milk back over the balloon, especially at the region of tight curves where the internal circular lumen takes on an oval shape. This is particulary true when the sheath selected has a diameter barely large enough to accommodate the stent/balloon unit. Ideally, the selected sheath size

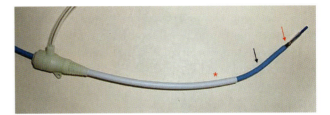

Figure 12.8 A technique to prevent backward shifting of stent on balloon during delivery through sheath: Frontload stent/balloon unit (red arrow) onto a long sheath (black arrow) and introduce it as one unit through a shorter, but larger Fr size sheath (red asterisk) placed at the groin. Stent/balloon unit is protected inside the long sheath as entire unit is advanced into target vessel.

should be 2 French sizes larger than the sheath size needed to pass the selected balloon on which the stent is mounted. However, in order to minimize the delivery system, sometimes the sheath selected is only 1 French size larger and proximal stent slippage on the balloon can occur during its delivery. It is important to avoid using a short delivery sheath, which cannot provide countertraction or prevent proximal shifting of a stent during implantation. A long sheath is imperative for optimal results and for bail-out situations. With the introduction of the newer, more flexible Genesis and EV3 open-cell stents, the incidence of stent slippage on the balloon during delivery has decreased. Another technique to prevent backward shifting of the stent on the balloon during advancement is to front load the stent/balloon unit onto the long sheath and introduce it as one unit though a shorter, but larger French size sheath placed at the groin (Figure 12.8). Using this technique, the stent/balloon unit is protected inside the tip of the long sheath as it is delivered to the stenotic region. But one disadvantage is the need for a larger size, short sheath placed at the groin.

A final moment of potential stent shift on the balloon is during the actual stent positioning within the stenosis, where the stent edge might catch the stenotic segment during its final positioning. To avoid this, the stent should be centered over the stenosis while still inside the tip of the delivery sheath. The sheath is withdrawn to expose the stent/balloon unit to the pulmonary vessel. A small hand injection of contrast through the side port of the sheath should be made to assess stent position on the stenosis. If the stent has to be repositioned more distally, pushing the balloon shaft is acceptable, but if the stent has to be repositioned more proximally, pushing the wire allows finer control than simply pulling on the balloon shaft.

To minimize the risk of stent slippage on the balloon during delivery, the stent should be crimped securely onto the balloon using an umbilical tape (Figure 12.9a). This technique allows even circumferential compression rather than bidirectional force between two fingers. A very small amount of fluid is then injected into the balloon to create a very slight bulge proximal to the mounted stent. This is because fluid enters the balloon from an exit hole located in the proximal end. By tightly squeezing this proximal 'bulge' of the balloon, the fluid is now forced into the distal part of the balloon, forming a 'bulge,' at the distal end. This technique not only results in a firmer grip of the stent on the balloon, but also the 'fluid channel' formed inside the balloon allows for the balloon to secure the stent (with the 'bulges' on both ends of the stent) and for even expansion during inflation (Figure 12.9b).

During stent delivery, even if the stent shifts backward on the balloon, the stent can still be positioned properly. This is accomplished by first centering the stent on the stenosis, then withdrawing the delivery sheath and carefully readvancing the sheath tip to come into contact with the proximal stent edge. By using the sheath tip to maintain stent position at the stenotic segment, the balloon is slowly pulled back to recenter the stent onto the balloon (Figure 12.10a). Small movements should be used to avoid pulling the balloon too far back. The radiopaque markers on the balloon are important landmarks for centering the stent. Occasionally, the stent slips forward on the balloon. In this case, a snare or bioptome can be used to pull the stent back and recenter onto the balloon (Figure 12.10b).

Balloon inflation to implant the stent

If the stent is not well centered on the balloon, the stent can shift either proximally or distally during inflation. This will result in partial and uneven dilation of the stent. Typically, either the proximal or the distal

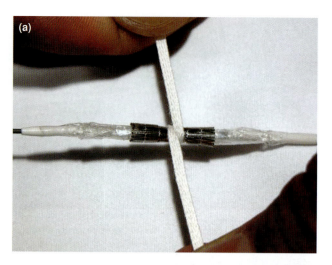

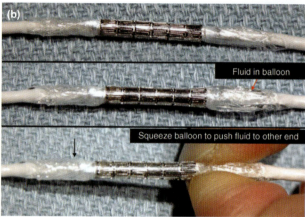

Figure 12.9 (A) Use of umbilical tape to crimp stent onto balloon. This technique allows even 'circumferential' pressure on stent. (B) Inject a small amount of fluid into balloon to form slight 'bulge' in proximal balloon (red arrow). Then squeeze proximal bulge to force fluid into distal balloon to form a distal 'bulge' (black arrow). A fluid channel is formed within the balloon to allow for even expansion of the balloon and stent. This technique decreases the risk of stent slipping off the balloon during inflation.

edge is dilated more than the opposite end, resulting in a cone shape. In this case, the balloon will have to be deflated and recentered for repeat dilation to fully expand the stent. If the balloon shifts forward, the large sheath can be used to stabilize the stent while the balloon is pulled back into the partially inflated stent for recentering. However, if the balloon shifts backwards, advancing the balloon might result in distal migration of the stent. In this case, there is no way of stabilizing the stent while the balloon is advanced further for recentering. If the stent does migrate distally along the guide wire, the stent usually stops at a bifurcation point or when the distal vessel narrows down to a size smaller than the stent. The deflated balloon could still be recentered at the more distal location. With slight balloon inflation, the stent can be recaptured and then pulled back to the site of stenosis. Even if optimal

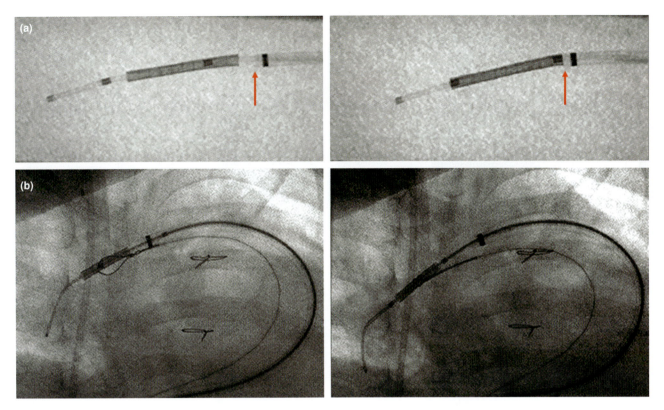

Figure 12.10 (A) Example of stent shifting back on balloon during advancement of stent/balloon unit inside sheath. Once stent is across stenosis, withdraw sheath to expose stent. Then advance tip of sheath (red arrow) to proximal edge of stent to 'hold' stent position while gently withdrawing balloon to recenter stent on balloon. (B) Example of stent shifting forward on balloon during stent/balloon positioning on stenosis. Use snare to capture and pull stent back to recenter on balloon.

repositioning is not possible, at least the stent can be implanted in a pulmonary artery segment where it does not jail a side branch. It is important to maintain good wire position during this maneuver. As a general principal, if there is potential for error, it is better to have the stent migrate distally rather than proximally.

For long segment stenosis, predilation with a balloon alone to test for balloon stability during inflation is highly recommended. Occasionally, resistant long segment stenoses may require use of a cutting balloon to 'score' the stenosis to permit more stable stent positioning. However, currently the largest available cutting balloon is only 8 mm in diameter. During balloon inflation, unless there is hemodynamic instability, one should inflate slowly at the beginning to make sure that both ends of the balloon inflate evenly to avoid shifting of the stent. Also, if the entire balloon/stent unit shifts, one can make adjustments to stabilize its position or to reposition the stent/balloon unit before further inflation. Once the stent is fully inflated, it cannot be repositioned.

Balloon rupture

During balloon dilation and stent implantation, balloon rupture can also occur. This is a common adverse event and, if managed incorrectly, will almost certainly result in stent malposition and embolization. A study from Children's Hospital of San Diego showed that, balloon rupture during stent implantation occurred in 22.4% (28/125 cases).[46] The overwhelming majority of these ruptures were found to be pinholes, located in the vicinity of the edges of the stent. However, circumferential ruptures can occur in calcified regions such as in the RV–PA homografts. Even when the stent implant is in the branch pulmonary artery, the most proximal part of the balloon may come in contact with these calcifications, which can risk balloon rupture. Overinflation with pressures higher than the balloon can handle often result in longitudinal ruptures. When implanting stents, an inflator with a pressure gauge should be used. It is also recommended to capture the images of the balloon inflation itself so that it can be reviewed if balloon rupture or some other adverse event takes place. By observing the pattern of contrast exiting the balloon, one may be able to differentiate a pinhole rupture from a circumferential or longitudinal rupture. Pinhole ruptures result in contrast extravasating faintly into the vessel and the balloon profile remains intact (Figure 12.11a). Sometimes the pinhole rupture is only evident when blood is noted in the inflator syringe during deflation. When circumferential or longitudinal ruptures occur, the

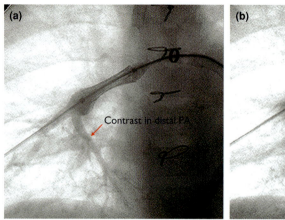

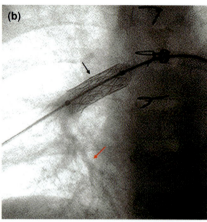

Figure 12.11 (A) A partially expanded stent in the RPA. Contrast is seen in the distal vessel (red arrow) but balloon profile appears intact. This is consistent with a pinhole rupture of the dilation balloon. (B) A 3 cc syringe is used to rapidly inflate balloon with higher PSI forcing more fluid into the balloon than what escapes out of the pinhole. This technique will permit further expansion of the stent (black arrow) in spite of the pinhole rupture and avoids having to exchange balloons in a partially expanded and 'loose' stent.

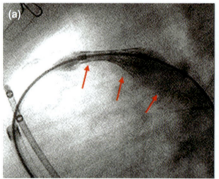

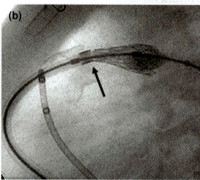

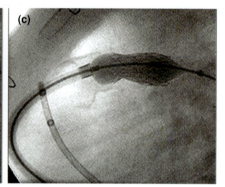

Figure 12.12 (A) Partially expanded RPA stent due to proximal pinhole rupture. In spite of using a 3 cc syringe with rapid inflation technique, the stent did not adequately expand. Contrast can be seen escaping from proximal balloon (red arrows). (B) Long sheath advanced over proximal balloon to cover pinhole (black arrow), (C) Another attempt at rapid inflation with small syringe results in further expansion of stent. Adequate inflation of proximal balloon 'pushes' sheath back. This technique avoided risks of exchanging balloons in presence of a partially expanded 'loose' stent.

dilation balloon appears to 'pop,' followed immediately by the appearance of a large amount of contrast in the vessel.

If a pinhole rupture is noted, one can attempt to further dilate the stent by exchanging the inflator for a smaller syringe (1 cc or 3 cc). By using a smaller syringe, one can achieve higher inflation pressure. The goal is to inject more fluid into the balloon than what escapes through the pinhole, thereby increasing the diameter of the balloon and further expanding the stent (Figure 12.11b). This can be repeated several times until the stent is fully inflated. Some have advocated attaching the balloon to a power injector for a high-power inflation. However, if the balloon is inflated with a pressure higher than its burst pressure, the balloon can rupture further. If the pinhole rupture is located in the proximal aspect of the balloon, the delivery sheath can be advanced over the proximal pinhole rupture to prevent

unfolding of the balloon (Figure 12.12). This would prevent or at least minimize fluid escaping from the pinhole and force more fluid into the balloon, thereby further expanding the balloon and stent. The 'sheath over pinhole' technique cannot be used if the pinhole rupture is located distally. The older Palmaz stents had sharp edges, which increased the risk of balloon rupture during implantation. The newer Genesis and Maxi-LD stents have rounded edges which decrease, but not eliminate, this risk (Figure 12.13). Therefore, crimping of the stent on the balloon should be done with care to avoid excessive pressure of the stent edge on the balloon. Also, balloons with short shoulders should be used. If the stent is to be dilated to larger diameters (greater than 14 mm), a Balloon-in-Balloon (BIB) balloon (Numed Inc., Hopkinton, NY) can also help to minimize the risk of pinhole ruptures. This balloon is designed with a smaller balloon inside a larger balloon. Sequential inflation,

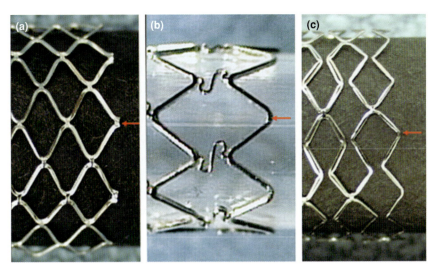

Figure 12.13   Close-ups of stent edges (red arrows): (A) Palmaz, (B) Genesis-XD, (C) Doublestrut/Mega-LD.

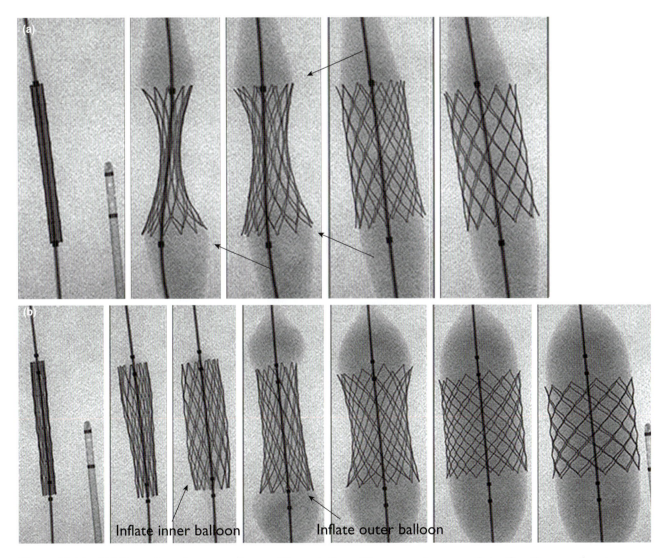

Inflate inner balloon   Inflate outer balloon

Figure 12.14   (A) Expansion of a stent using an 18 mm balloon. The stent edges expand significantly more than its center, creating an acute angle in which the stent edge can puncture the balloon (black arrows). (B) Expansion of a stent using a 24 mm BIB balloon. Inner balloon initially expands the stent evenly to 12 mm (black arrow), then outer balloon expands further to 24 mm diameter. The stent edge is better aligned with the balloon (yellow arrow) which minimizes the risk of balloon rupture.

starting with the smaller inner balloon followed by inflation of the larger outer balloon, allows the stent to be evenly expanded to a smaller diameter (half of the final diameter) before full expansion to the larger intended diameter (Figure 12.14). This technique creates a less sharp angle between the stent edge and the balloon. The use of higher-pressure balloons with tougher balloon material (Kevlar) such as the Atlas balloon (Bard Peripheral Vascular Inc., Tempe, AZ) may also decrease the risk of rupture.

One scenario with high risk of balloon rupture is when there is bilateral branch PS that requires a stent in each proximal branch. The proximal edge of an implanted stent can puncture the contralateral balloon during inflation and stent implantation. To avoid balloon rupture by the opposing stent edge, a balloon should be inflated in the first implanted stent on one branch before the balloon and stent is inflated in the contralateral branch.

For longitudinal tears, the balloon must be replaced with a new balloon without stent malposition. Use of the long sheath to prevent backward shifting of the stent is imperative during balloon removal. After removal of the torn balloon, a new smaller balloon should be inserted into the stent. The insertion maneuver could risk distal migration of the stent. A bioptome or snare from a second venous sheath may be required to 'hold' the stent in place during the exchange process. Sometimes this is unavoidable and the stent might shift distally until the vessel becomes too small, or until a bifurcation point 'catches' the stent. Once the smaller balloon is centered on the balloon, a slight inflation will 'capture' the stent and the entire stent/balloon unit can be brought back for implantation.

While longitudinal ruptures will require replacement with a new balloon, circumferential ruptures have an added risk of separation of the distal tip of the ruptured balloon, which may require additional retrieval after removal of the torn balloon. Snares over the guide wires may be required to pull out the distal segments (Figure 12.15). Occasionally, the torn balloon is entrapped within the stent, which might result in stent malposition during retrieval. This particular type of balloon rupture carries the highest risk for stent embolization. Sometimes it is impossible to separate the balloon fragment from the stent and a surgical intervention may be required. Again, much care should be given to using the long sheath to stabilize proximal shifting of a stent during removal of a torn balloon. When calcium is noted in the area of stenosis, predilation should be performed to test for rupture prior to stent implantation. In this scenario, should the balloon rupture circumferentially, at least there is no entrapped or embolized stent to worry

about. It is recommended to predilate with high-pressure balloons whose balloon material can withstand the sharpness of the calcifications.

Various retrieval devices including bioptomes, grabbers, baskets, and snares should be readily available in the catheterization laboratory during stent implantation. One particularly useful technique is to create a makeshift snare of the desired diameter and angle by inserting both ends of an 0.018 or 0.025 inch exchange guide wire through an end hole catheter to form a loop. This 'loop snare' forms a 180° angle to the endhole catheter. The snare can be bent to form various degrees of angulation for retrieval purposes.

Ballooon removal out of the stent

After successful stent implantation, the balloon must be carefully removed out of the stent. This part of the procedure carries the risk of proximal stent migration. Once inflated, the balloon may not rewrap tightly upon deflation. During balloon withdrawal, the 'wings' of the deflated balloon can catch on the stent and pull it out of position. To avoid this, the long sheath should be advanced back into the stent to capture the deflated balloon before it is pulled out of the stent. The safest way to reinsert the delivery sheath into the stent is to first inflate the balloon within the stent. Then deflate the balloon slowly while advancing the sheath over the balloon. This technique will keep the sheath centered inside the stent to avoid contact with the stent edge or the inside wall (Figure 12.16).[49] Several inflations and deflations while advancing the sheath might be required to completely advance the sheath into the stent to recapture the balloon. Once the balloon is recaptured inside the sheath, the balloon can then be withdrawn out of the body without risk of stent malposition. At this point, if needed, a larger balloon can be passed to the stent inside the sheath for further dilation. Alternatively, the sheath can then be withdrawn out of the stent.

MANAGING STENT MALPOSITIONS

Most stent malpositions are due to technical errors. When this adverse event occurs, it is imperative to maintain good wire position. As long as the stent remains secured along the course of the wire, several techniques have been developed to manage the malpositioned stent to avoid a full blown complication. The general algorithm is as follows: if a balloon is still inside the stent, the balloon should be recentered and inflated to recapture the stent in an attempt to place it back in the stenotic segment. If

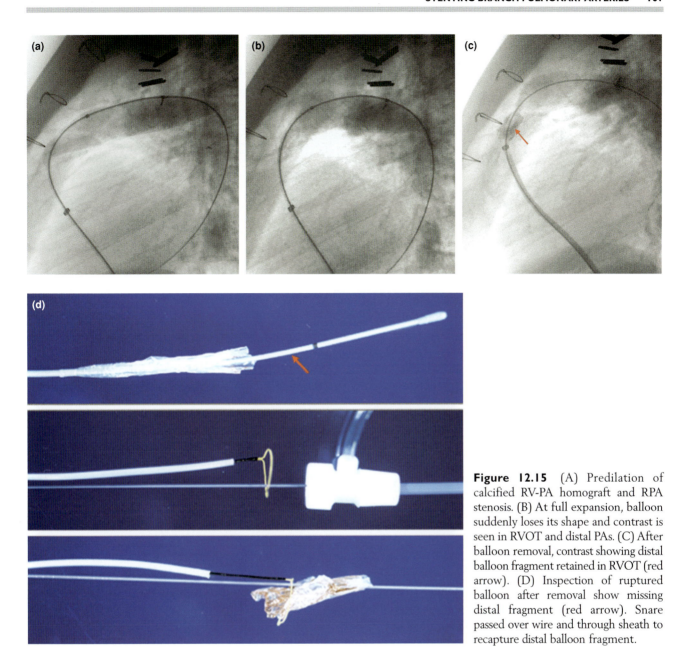

Figure 12.15 (A) Predilation of calcified RV-PA homograft and RPA stenosis. (B) At full expansion, balloon suddenly loses its shape and contrast is seen in RVOT and distal PAs. (C) After balloon removal, contrast showing distal balloon fragment retained in RVOT (red arrow). (D) Inspection of ruptured balloon after removal show missing distal fragment (red arrow). Snare passed over wire and through sheath to recapture distal balloon fragment.

that is not possible, then placing the recaptured stent into a safe but non-therapeutic position should be the next option. This might be in the more distal segment of the branch pulmonary artery, the contralateral pulmonary artery, or even back down to the IVC. The latter option carries some risk because the stent has to traverse the pulmonary and tricuspid valves.[47] The stent should never be pulled back through a valve without being held by an inflated balloon, or if the stent edges are protruding off the balloon. If the stent edges get caught on the tricuspid valve apparatus, not only is there a high risk of damage but the stent can prop open the valve, creating insufficiency and/or ventricular arrhythmias, resulting in the need for an emergency operation. Finally, if the stent cannot be implanted in a safe

position, then it will have to be removed either by transcatheter techniques or by surgery. Distal migration of the stent is usually not a major problem with jailing of a side branch being the major adverse event. Although pulmonary infarction has been reported with an embolized stent, it is exceedingly rare.[50] However, proximal migration into the main pulmonary artery or right ventricle can result in a major complication requiring emergency surgery. One may attempt to inflate a balloon inside the embolized stent and reposition it back into the stenotic branch, but if the stent is already expanded, even partially, it usually cannot be placed back across the stenosis. Fortunately, when unilateral branch stenosis occurs, the contralateral branch tends to be larger and can accommodate the expanded stent.

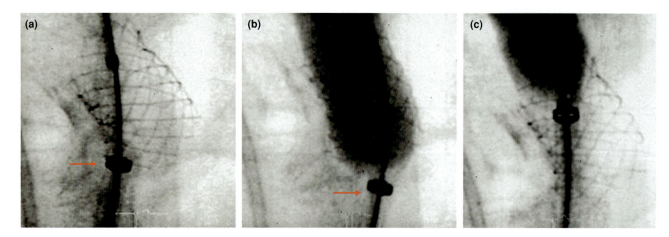

Figure 12.16   (A) To remove a balloon out of a freshly implanted stent and avoid dislodging stent with its deflated 'wings' it is best to advance the sheath back into the stent and then withdraw the balloon into the sheath. But the sheath itself can come into contact with stent and dislodge it (red arrow). (B) First inflate balloon to center the sheath (red arrow), then (C) slowly deflate balloon as sheath is advanced into stent and over balloon.

The technique of transferring an embolized stent in the MPA to the contralateral branch pulmonary artery for safe implantation is as follows: With the loose stent still held by the original guidewire an end hole catheter is passed through the stent and into the contralateral PA, then exchanged for a second long stiff guide wire. Once the second wire in the contralateral branch is secured, the original wire can be withdrawn. The delivery sheath can push the stent along the new wire into the contralateral vessel, or a new balloon can be advanced over the new wire to recapture the stent and then deliver it to the contralateral vessel.

A second technique to secure and embolize the stent in the MPA is to place a second, longer stent telescoped into the embolized stent. The longer stent can be secured into a distal branch pulmonary while capturing and stabilizing the embolized stent in the proximal segment (Figure 12.17). This technique would risk jailing the contralateral pulmonary artery. Fortunately, jailing the contralateral pulmonary artery does not cause an obstruction to flow. However, it may be difficult to gain access into the jailed contralateral vessel in the future.

ANATOMIC BASED COMPLICATIONS

Jailing side branches

Jailing a side branch pulmonary artery can be inadvertent when a stent migrates distally or intentional when the stenotic segment is adjacent or straddles a side branch. We previously discussed the technique of simultaneous implantation of two crossing stents in the proximal right and left branch pulmonary arteries or at the lobar branches to avoid jailing of either branch and to permit future access. A study from Texas Children's Hospital of the first 100 stents placed into the pulmonary arteries showed 41 stents (34 patients) straddled the origin of 62 side branches, 79% (49/62) remained patent after stent implantation while 21% (13/62) were occluded. Factors associated with side branch occlusion included severity of stenosis of the stented vessel, stenosis at the origin of the side branch, acute angle of the side branch to stented vessel and small BSA.[10] The optimal situation is to implant a stent to treat a stenosis and not jail a side branch, but when that is not possible, the new open-cell Double-strut or Mega-LD stent may offer an alternate solution.[51,54,55] Bench testing shows that the 'open-cell' design of this stent allows passage and inflation of a balloon up to 12mm in diameter through the side of the stent to create an 8–9 × 11 mm in diameter opening (Figure 12.18).[51] If a side branch was indeed jailed, the stent would permit access for angioplasty or stenting of the side branch if indicated (Figure 12.19).

Vascular tears and aneurysms

Vascular tears and aneurysm formation have also reported for pulmonary artery stenting, both at initial implant as well as at redilation.[2–4,6,14,52–54,56–58] Predictive risk factors for this severe complication are not well defined except they are more commonly seen in patients with congenital branch pulmonary artery stenosis, which tend to be long segmented, severe in nature and highly resistant to dilation. Overdilation with high-pressure balloons increases this risk. General recommendations are to implant a stent using a balloon whose diameter is within 1–2 mm of the normal adjacent segment. In the highly resistant stenoses, leaving a small waist within the stent is acceptable. Data has shown that at follow up redilation, these residual waists can be further dilated using the same size

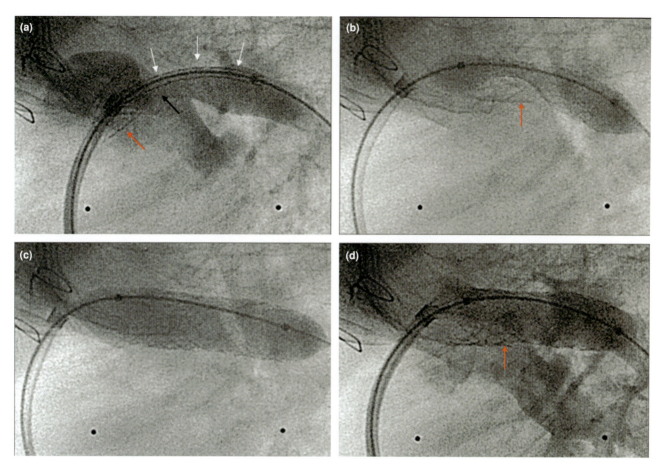

Figure 12.17   (A) LPA stent embolized into MPA (red arrow) during removal of balloon (without protection of sheath). A second longer stent (white arrows) is telescoped into embolized stent and positioned in LPA stenosis (black arrow). (B) Sheath used to push embolized stent (red arrow) as far against LPA stenosis as possible. Balloon inflation and partial expansion of second stent within embolized stent. (C) Full expansion of longer stent to relieve LPA stenosis and to stabilize embolized stent in MPA. (D) Post stent angiogram showing stable embolized stent (red arrow) and widely patent LPA. Notice first stent partially jails RPA orifice but there is good flow into RPA.

balloon and inflation pressure.[8] Perhaps the implanted stent has a 'softening effect' on the residual stenosis.

Stenting branch stenosis in the early post-operative period also carries high risk of vascular tears.[59,60] Intraoperative stenting may be the most appropriate choice of treatment. If a fresh suture line tears, the surgeon is in the best position to repair the tear. However, if there is intraoperative diameter measurements of the vessel at the time of the original repair and restenosis occurs in the early post-operative period, stenting in the cath lab can be performed using a balloon whose diameter is no larger than the diameter measured in the operating room. The assumption is that the circumference of the suture line is adequate to accommodate the circumference of the balloon used for the stent implant without suture dehiscence. A study from Miami Children's Hospital indicated that stenting of pulmonary arteries in the early post-operative period can be performed safely but requires a multidisciplinary approach involving the anesthesia and surgical services.[60]

Aneurysms can develop overtime following a small confined vascular tear due to high PA pressures usually found in patients with severe bilateral hypoplasia of the pulmonary arterial tree or multiple distal branch stenoses such as in William syndrome, Alagilles syndrome or pulmonary atresia following unifocalized aortopulmonary collaterals. Reports of coil occlusion or use of covered stent to obliterate the aneurysm or tears have been reported[4,56] (Figure 12.20). Occasionally, a vascular tear is noted following predilation and stent implantation can be used to 'tack down' the dissected intima (Figure 12.21). If the tear is large or uncontained, severe bleeding and hemoptysis can develop. When this occurs, a balloon can be inflated at the site of the tear to temporarily occlude the vessel while emergency surgery is initiated. However, since the site of bleeding is often difficult to control and repair, lobectomy is commonly performed. Even if the surgery is successful, death usually occurs due to loss of pulmonary parenchyma in the presence of already deficient and hypoplastic pulmonary

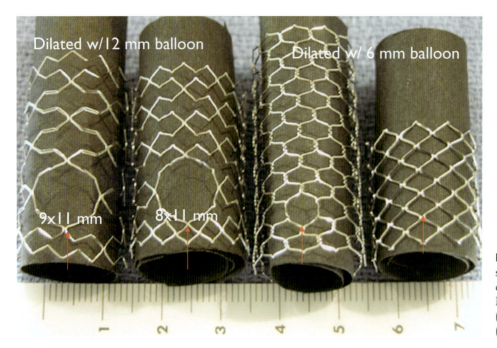

Figure 12.18 Comparison of side holes following balloon dilation: Doublestrut (9 x 11 mm), Mega-LD (8 x 11 mm), Genesis (minimal enlargement), Palmaz (no change in cell size).

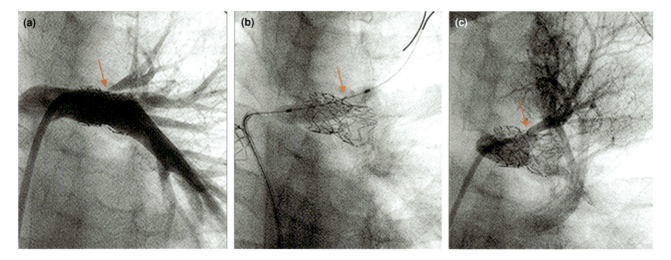

Figure 12.19 (A) LUL branch (red arrow) jailed by 'open-cell' Doublestrut stent previously implanted to treat proximal LPA stenosis which straddled the origin of the LUL. (B) Balloon dilation across side of stent (red arrow) into LUL. (C) Post dilation angiogram: improved caliber and flow to LUL (red arrow).

vascular bed. While a covered stent may be the most logical choice to treat this severe complication, there are no FDA approved covered stents for use in congenital heart disease to date.

OTHER COMPLICATIONS

Pulmonary thromboembolic events

Intracardiac or pulmonary thromboembolic events during the stent procedure have been reported.[2,4,9]

It is important to rule out any intracardiac thrombi prior to the stent procedure. This issue is probably more important in the Fontan patient or those with poor right ventricular function. During the procedure, full heparinization is recommended, especially when the large delivery sheath is inserted. In severe stenoses, this sheath may completely obstruct flow to the stenotic branch. Thrombi can also form within the large sheath during the procedure. If a long procedure is anticipated, frequent flushing of the sheath or use of a small continuous flush via a fluid line is recommended. ACT values should be kept at 220 or greater. Following stent implantation,

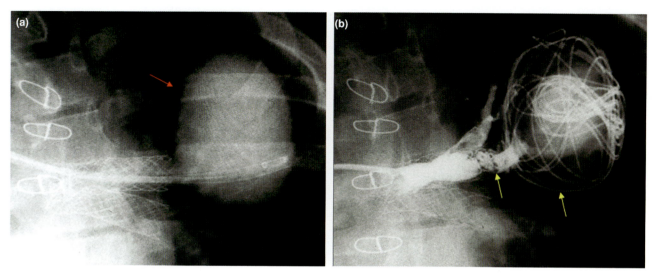

Figure 12.20   (A) Large aneurysm in distal LUL following redilation of LUL and LLL stents. (B) Following implantation of long coil in aneurysm and a Grifka sack (yellow arrows) in the distal branch, the aneurysm is occluded.

it has been a general practice to keep a patient on low dose aspirin for at least 6 months while the stent endothelializes. For other co-morbidities such as poor function or single ventricle, additional anti-platelet or anticoagulation therapy may be necessary.

Air embolism

Air embolism is a minor complication usually associated with introduction of air through the valve of the delivery sheath. This can occur when a catheter or wire is withdrawn rapidly out of the sheath. When blood cannot replace the space previously occupied by the retrieved catheter, air will be 'sucked into' the sheath from the valve. A continuous flush connected to the sideport of the sheath or placing the valve inside a bowl of saline will prevent air embolism.

Pulmonary edema

Pulmonary edema can be seen following successful angioplasty or stenting of severe branch stenosis, especially in the setting of combined hypoplastic lungbeds or multiple distal branch stenoses and elevated pulmonary pressures.[4,6,61] This phenomenon is due to significant reperfusion of a chronically underperfused lungbed and resolves over the next several days. Conservative management with respiratory support and diuretics is usually the treatment of choice.

LATE COMPLICATIONS

Restenosis

Follow-up studies have shown restenosis rates to be less than 10%[4,8,9,62] but tend to be higher in smaller patients.[9,17] Follow up angiography typically shows 1–2 mm of in-stent intimal growth. However, in regions of abrupt changes in diameter, such as in an overdilated stent, intimal hyperplasia may be noted, usually at the transition zone, resulting in a smooth luminal wall with a diameter equal to the smaller caliber of the adjacent unstented segment.[8,53] The causes of in-stent restenosis are unclear but it is thought to be due to local flow turbulence and shear stresses that result in intimal buildup. More commonly, restenosis is due to normal somatic growth of the child, resulting in a larger distal unstented pulmonary artery while the caliber of the stented segment remains unchanged. In both cases, redilation and further dilation has been shown to be highly successful, albeit occasionally requiring high-pressure balloons (Figure 12.22).[4,6,8,9,17,63] A recent 15-year follow up study from Texas Children's Hospital showed excellent long-term results in 52 patients. Available clinical data on 42 patients showed 39 (90%) patients to be asymptomatic (NYHA class of I or II) & 4 pts (10%) with NYHA class III symptoms. In that series, 35 patients had follow-up cath data, indicating need for further dilation due mostly to patient growth. Seven patients required surgery (conduit replacement and Fontan revision), but none for pulmonary artery stenosis (unpublished).

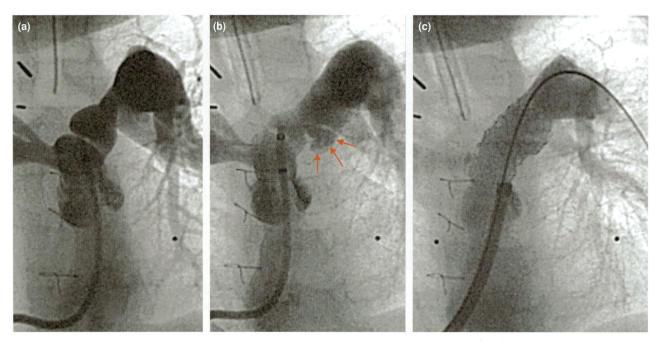

Figure 12.21   (A) Proximal LPA stenosis. (B) Intimal flap with small aneurysm (red arrow) noted after predilation which is tacked down by stent (C).

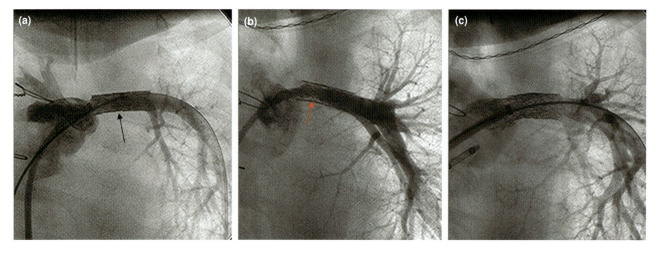

Figure 12.22   (A) Angiogram of initial LPA stent (6 mm diameter) (black arrow) implanted in 7 kg infant. Residual stenosis at the origin of LPA (red arrow) resulting in abrupt change in diameter from origin to stent. (B) Follow-up 9 months later: showed proximal in-stent restenosis due to intimal hyperplasia (red arrow). Note increase in growth of distal vessels and improved perfusion in spite of the restenosis. (C) Additional stent (yellow arrow) added to cover LPA ostia stenosis and further dilation with 8 mm balloon.

Stent fracture

Stent fracture has been reported in follow-up studies.[3, 4,6,64,65] Longitudinal fractures are more often found with the Palmaz stents while circumferential fractures have been seen in Genesis stents. These fractures can be subtle and not noticeable on plain chest x-ray. On fluoroscopic imaging, the fractured ends of the stent may be noted to 'flex' during the cardiac cycle. Angiography will usually show restenosis localized to this region. Overall, stent fractures are more commonly found in right ventricle to PA conduits.[66] Stent fractures in the branch pulmonary arteries are uncommon but when a stent is implanted in a pulmonary artery located behind a dilated ascending aorta, the pulsatile forces on the stent can cause a longitudinal

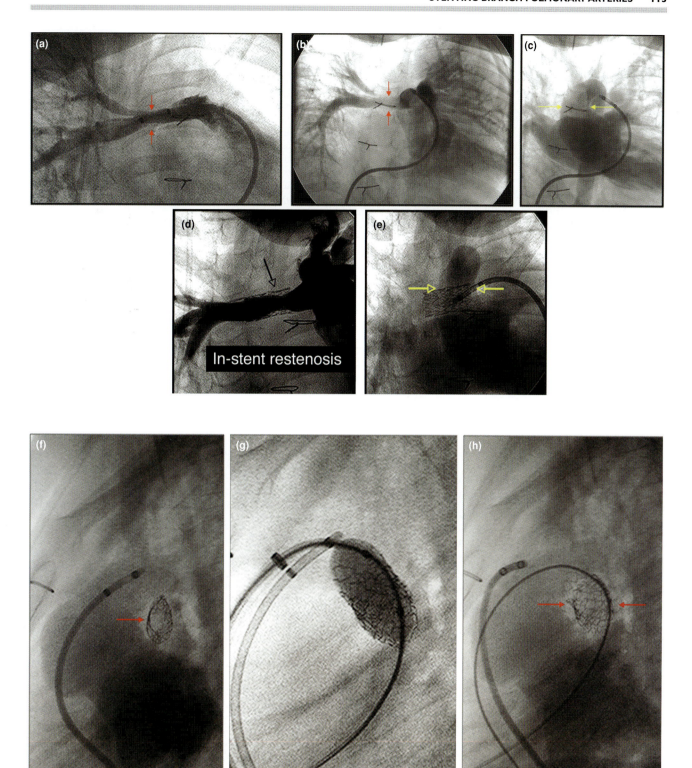

Figure 12.23 (A) RPA stenosis (red arrow). (B) MPA angiogram showing more flow to left lung. (C) On levophase, dilated ascending aorta (yellow arrows) is positioned in front of the proximal RPA stenosis. (D) At follow up cath following initial RPA stent implantation, in-stent restenosis is noted (black arrow). (E) Levophase again show dilated ascending aorta (yellow arrows) in front of the region of restenosis. (F) Lateral projection shows 'tear-drop' shaped stent (red arrows), highly suggestive of stent fracture, presumably due to the constant pulsatile compressive forces of the anterior ascending aorta. (G) Additional stent added to redilate stenosis and to add radial support in proximal RPA. (H) 'Tear-drop' shape stent returned to original round shape with second telescoped stent (red arrows).

fracture (Figure 12.23). Occasionally, further dilation can result in a longitudinal fracture. This is easily noted when the stent separate at the fracture site during balloon inflation. Restenosis due to fractured stents can be easily treated with a second stent implanted within the original stent for additional support.

SUMMARY

In summary, stenting of branch pulmonary artery stenosis requires careful attention to all the small details involved with the procedure. Careful measurements are needed for proper stent and balloon selection. Each phase, from stent delivery to balloon removal, should be done with great care and anticipation. Most of the limitations and potential complications can be overcome with the newer design stents and balloons, along with improved stent delivery techniques and careful advance planning. A complete implantation and exit strategy for this intervention, as well as any anticipated problems, should be well thought out before the start of each case. A full armamentarium of interventional supplies and retrieval devices should be ready and available in the catheterization laboratory. One should become very familiar with repositioning and retrieval techniques. Accurate measurements of vascular stenosis and the patient's anatomy should be performed prior to selection of the stent and balloon. Potential problems of all phases of the stent implantation should be anticipated and monitored. Surgical back-up should be readily available. Keep in mind that the little details of the procedure can often be the source of an initial adverse event, and, if managed improperly, can result in a major complication. Finally, if an adverse event does occur, the operator must remain calm and think. Seek another opinion if desired. As long as vital signs are stable, additional heparin should be given and a bail-out strategy should be mapped out. One can usually get out of trouble and avoid an emergency surgery.

REFERENCES

1. Mullins CE, O'Laughlin MP, Vick GW III et al. Implantation of balloon-expandable intravascular grafts by catheterization in pulmonary arteries and systemic veins. Circulation 1988; 77: 188–99.
2. O'Laughlin MP, Perry SB, Lock JE, Mullins CE. Use of endovascular stents in congenital heart disease. Circulation 1991; 83: 1923–39.
3. O'Laughlin MP, Slack MC, Grifka RG et al. Implantation and intermediate-term follow-up of stents in congenital heart disease. Circulation 1993; 88: 605–14.
4. Schaffer KM, Mullins CE, Grifka RG et al. Intravascular stents in congenital heart disease: Acute and long-term results from a large single-center experience. JACC 1998; 31: 661–7.
5. McMahon C, Grifka RG, El-Said H et al. 'Long-term outcome of pulmonary artery stent implant: A single center experience over 10 years'. Accepted in Cardiology in the Young for Nov/Dec, 2002.
6. McMahon CJ, El Said HG, Vincent JA et al. Refinements in the implantation of pulmonary arterial stents: impact on morbidity and mortality of the procedure over the last two decades. Cardiology in the Young 2002; 12: 445–52.
7. Hosking MK, Thomaidis C, Hamilton R et al. Clinical impact of balloon angioplasty for branch pulmonary arterial stenosis. Am J Cardiol 1992; 69: 1467–70.
8. Ing FF, Grifka RG, Nihill MR, Mullins CE. Repeat dilation of intravascular stents in congenital heart defects. Circulation 1995; 92: 893–7.
9. Fogelman R, Nykanen D, Smallhorn JF et al. Endovascular stents in the pulmonary circulation: clinical impact on management and medium-term follow-up. Circulation 1995; 92: 881–5.
10. McMahon WS, Mullins CE, Grifka RG et al. Fate of Pulmonary Artery Branch Vessels with Intravascular Stents. Circulation (Suppl) 1996; 94: I-57.
11. Stapleton G, Zellers TM, Mullins CE et al. Simultaneous implantation of 2 stents to treat bifurcation stenoses in pulmonary arteries: early and intermediate and long-term results. Cath Cardiovasc Interv 2007; 69(6): S89.
12. Ing, FF. Improving control and delivery of coils and stents and management of malpositioned coils and stents. Progress in Pediatric Cardiology 2001; 14: 13–25.
13. Ing, FF. Stents: what's available to the pediatric interventional cardiologist? Catheterization and Cardiovascular Interventions, 2002; 57: 374–86.
14. Forbes TJ et al. The Genesis stent: A new low-profile stent for use in infants, children, and adults with congenital heart disease. Catheter Cardiovasc Interv 2000; 59: 40–414.
15. Ing FF, Mathewson JW, Cocalis M, Perry J, Mullins CE. A new technique for implantation of large stents through small sheaths in infants and childrens with branch pulmonary artery stenoses. J Am Coll Cardiol (Supplement A) 2000; 35(2): 500A.
16. Ing FF, Perry JC, Mathewson JW et al. Percutaneous implantation of large stents for the treatment of infants with severe post-operative branch pulmonary artery stenoses. J Am Coll Cardiol (Supplement A) 2001; 37(2): 461A.
17. Frazer J, Bavier J, Ing FF. Pulmonary artery stents in infants and small children (<12 kg): short and mid-term results. Circulation (Supplement) 2005; 112: II649.
18. Zaidenweber CM, Kim DW, Vincent RN (2006) Right ventricular outflow tract and pulmonary artery stents in children under 18 months of age. Catheter Cardiovasc Interv 69: 23–7.
19. Ashwath R, Gruenstein D, Siwik E. Percutaneous Stent Placement in Children Weighing Less Than 10 Kilograms. Pediatric Cardiology 2007 Nov 29.
20. Ing FF. Delivery of stents to target lesions: techniques of intra-operative stent implantation and intra-operative angiograms. Pediatric Cardiology. 2005; 26: 260–6.
21. Mendelsohn AM, Bove eL, Lupinetti FM et al. Intraoperative and percutaneous stenting of congenital pulmonary artery and vein stenosis. Circulation 1993; 88: 210–17.
22. Mitropoulos FA, Laks H, Kapadia N, Plunkett M et al. Intraoperative pulmonary artery stenting: an alternative technique for the management of pulmonary artery stenosis. Ann Thorac Surg. 2007 Oct; 84(4): 1338–41; discussion 1342.
23. Bacha EA, Marshall AC, McElhinney DB, del Nido PJ. Expanding the hybrid concept in congenital heart surgery. Semin Thorac Cardiovasc Surg Pediatr Card Surg Annu. 2007; 146–50.
24. Hijazi ZM. Intraoperative intervention (hybrid surgery) and intervention in the immediate perioperative period. Catheter Cardiovasc Interv 2003 Sep; 60(1): 99–100.

25. Ungerleider RM, Johnston TA, O'Laughlin MP, Jaggers JJ, Gaskin PR. Intraoperative stents to rehabilitate severely stenotic pulmonary vessels. Ann Thorac Surg 2001 Feb; 71(2): 476–81.

26. Hirsch R. The hybrid cardiac catheterization laboratory for congenital heart disease: From conception to completion. Catheter Cardiovasc Interv 2007 Nov 1 [Epub ahead of print].

27. Ing FF, Fagan TE, Grifka RG et al. Reconstruction of stenotic or occluded iliofemoral veins and inferior vena cava using intravascular stents: re-establishing access for future cardiac catheterization and cardiac surgery. J Am Coll Cardiol 2001; 37: 251–7.

28. Ing FF. Recanalization techniques for vascular occlusions. In: 'Percutaneous interventions for congenital heart disease' Sievert H, Qureshi SA, Wilson N, Hijazi Z, eds. Alan Burgess, Taylor & Francis Medical Books. Informa Healthcare, UK, 2007.

29. Fraser JR, Murphy CL, Ing FF. Systemic venous stents in children: acute results and mid-term follow-up. Cath Cardiovasc Interv 2006; 67(5); 836–7.

30. Mullins CE. Chapter 4 'Vascular access: needle, wire, sheath/dilator and catheter introduction'. In: 'Cardiac Catheterization in Congenital Heart Disease', Blackwell Publishing Inc. 2006, MA, pp. 100–62.

31. Emmel M, Sreeram N, Pillekamp F, Boehm W, Brockmeier K. Transhepatic approach for catheter interventions in infants and children with congenital heart disease. Clin Res Cardiol 2006 Jun; 95(6): 329–33. Epub 2006 Apr 3.

32. Shim D, Lloyd TR, Cho KJ, Moorehead CP, Beekman RH 3rd. Transhepatic cardiac catheterization in children. Evaluation of efficacy and safety. Circulation 1995 Sep 15; 92(6): 1526–30.

33. Wallace MJ, Hovsepian DM, Balzer DT. Transhepatic venous access for diagnostic and interventional cardiovascular procedures. J Vasc Interv Radiol 1996 Jul-Aug; 7(4): 579–82.

34. Rhodes JF, Lane GK, Mesia CI et al. Cutting balloon angioplasty for children with small-vessel pulmonary artery stenoses. Catheter Cardiovasc Interv 2002 Jan; 55(1): 73–7.

35. Bergersen LJ, Perry SB, Lock JE. Effect of cutting balloon angioplasty on resistant pulmonary artery stenosis. Am J Cardiol 2003 Jan 15; 91(2): 185–9.

36. Bergersen L, Jenkins KJ, Gauvreau K, Lock JE. Follow-up results of Cutting Balloon angioplasty used to relieve stenoses in small pulmonary arteries. Cardiol Young 2005 Dec; 15(6): 605–10.

37. De Giovanni JV. Balloon angioplasty for branch pulmonary artery stenosis—cutting balloons. Catheter Cardiovasc Interv 2007 Feb 15; 69(3): 459–67. Review.

38. Mullins CE. Chapter 22 'Intravascular stents in congenital heart disease-general considerations, equipment.' In 'Cardiac Catheterization in Congenital Heart Disease.' Blackwell Publishing Inc. 2006, MA, pp. 537–96.

39. Stapleton G, Zellers TM, Mullins CE et al. Simultaneous implantation of 2 stents to treat bifurcation stenoses in pulmonary arteries: early, intermediate and long term results. Catheterization and Cardiovascular Interventions 2007; 69(6): S89.

40. Formigari R, Santoro G, Guccione P et al. Treatment of pulmonary artery stenosis after arterial switch operation: stent implantation vs. balloon angioplasty. Catheter Cardiovasc Interv 2000 Jun; 50(2): 207–11.

41. Ailawadi G, Lim DS, Peeler BB, Matsumoto AH, Dake MD. Traumatic ascending aortopulmonary window following pulmonary artery stent dilatation: therapy with aortic endovascular stent graft. Pediatr Cardiol 2007 Jul-Aug; 28(4): 305–8. Epub 2007 May 25.

42. Núñez M, Beleña J, Cabeza R, Beltrán M. Bronchial compression due to stent placement in pulmonary artery in a child with congenital heart disease. Paediatr Anaesth 2005 Dec; 15(12): 1137–9.

43. Preminger TJ, Lock JE, Perry SB. Traumatic aortopulmonary window as a complication of pulmonary artery balloon angioplasty: transcatheter occlusion with a covered stent. A case report. Cathet Cardiovasc Diagn 1994 Apr; 31(4): 286–9.

44. Carano N, Agnetti A, Tchana B, Squarcia A, Squarcia U. Descending thoracic aorta to left pulmonary artery fistula after stent implantation for acquired left pulmonary artery stenosis. J Interv Cardiol 2002 Oct; 15(5): 411–13.

45. Chau AKT, Leung MP. Management of branch pulmonary artery stenosis: balloon angioplasty or endovascular stenting. Clin Exp. Pharmacol Physiol 1997; 24: 960–2.

46. Schneider HE, Lindblade CL, Tamooka L, Ing FF. Management and outcome of balloon rupture during interventional catheterization in congenital heart disease. Catheterization and Cardiovascular Interventions 2004; 62: 139.

47. Hoyer MH et al. Transcatheter retrieval of an embolized Palmaz stent from the right ventricle of a child. Cathet Cardiovasc Diagn 1996; 39: 277–80.

48. Ing FF, Sauberli D. Chapter 30 'Basic Science of Cardiac Catheterization Laboratory Imaging In.': The Science and Practice of Pediatric Cardiology, 2nd ed. Editors, Garson A, Bricker JT, Risher DJ, Neish SR, eds Williams & Wilkins, MD, 1998, pp. 559–75.

49. Recto MR, Ing FF, Grifka RG, Nihill MR, Mullins CE. A technique to prevent newly implanted stent displacement during subsequent catheter and sheath manipulation. Catheterization and Cardiovascular Interventions 2000; 49: 297–300.

50. Sy A. Pulmonary infarction due to vascular stent migration. South Med J. 2006 Sep; 99(9): 1003–4.

51. Takao CM, Vepa SN, Connolly D, Mathewson J, Ing FF. Jailed Subclavian Artery after Stent Implantation for Coarctation of the Aorta: Midterm Results and Geometric Analysis of Stent Cells following Side Cell Dilation. Cathet Cardiovasc Interv 2006; 68(3): 485.

52. Hijazi ZM, Al-Fadley F, Geggel RL, Fulton DR et al. Stent implantation for relief of pulmonary artery stenosis: immediate and short-term results. Cathet Cardiovasc Diagn 1996; 38: 16–23.

53. Duke C, Rosenthal E, Qureshi SA. The efficacy and safety of stent redilatation in congenital heart disease. Heart. 2003 Aug; 89(8): 905–12.

54. Kreutzer J, Rome JJ. Open-cell design stents in congenital heart disease: a comparison of IntraStent vs. Palmaz stents. Catheter Cardiovasc Interv 2002 Jul; 56(3): 400–9.

55. Davenport J, Mullins CE, Ing FF. Mega LD, Max LD. Stents: a new generation of open cell design for treatment of congenital heart disease. Cathet Cardiovasc Interv 2007; 69(6): S9.

56. Preminger TJ, Lock JE, Perry SB. Traumatic aortopulmonary window as a complication of pulmonary artery balloon angioplasty: transcatheter occlusion with a covered stent. A case report. Cathet Cardiovasc Diagn. 1994 Apr; 31(4): 286–9.

57. Baker CM, MCGowan FX, Keane JF, Lock JE. Pulmonary artery trauma due to balloon dilation: Recognition, avoidance and management. 2000; 36: 1684–90.

58. Carano N, Agnetti A, Tchana B, Squarcia A, Squarcia U. Descending thoracic aorta to left pulmonary artery fistula after stent implantation for acquired left pulmonary artery stenosis. J Interv Cardiol 2002 Oct; 15(5): 411–13.

59. Rosales AM, Lock JE, Perry SB, Geggel RL. Interventional catheterization management of perioperative peripheral pulmonary stenosis: balloon angioplasty or endovascular stenting. Cathet Cardiovasc Interv 2002; 56: 272–7.

60. Zahn EM, Dobrolet NC, Nykanen DG et al. Interventional catheterization performed in the early postoperative period after congenital heart surgery in children. J Am Coll Cardiol 2004 Apr 7; 43(7): 1264–9.

61. Edwards BS, Lucas RV Jr, Lock JE, Edwards JE. Morphologic changes in the pulmonary arteries after percutaneous balloon angioplasty for pulmonary arterial stenosis. Circulation 1985; 71: 195–201.

62. McMahon et al. Redilation of endovascular stents in congenital heart disease: factors implicated in the development of restenosis and neointimal proliferation. J Am Coll Cardiol 2001; 38: 521–6.

63. Morrow WR et al. Re-expansion of balloon-expandable stents after growth. J Am Coll Cardiol 1993; 22: 2007–13.

64. Breinholt J, Nugent AW, Justino H, Mullins CE, Ing FF. Stent fractures in congenital heart disease.

65. Knirsch W, Haas NA, Lewin MA, Uhlemann F. Longitudinal stent fracture 11 months after implantation in the left pulmonary artery and successful management by a stent-in-stent maneuver. Catheter Cardiovasc Interv 2003 Jan; 58(1): 116–18.

66. Peng LF, McElhinney DB, Nugent AW et al. Endovascular stenting of obstructed right ventricle to pulmonary artery conduits: a 15 year experience. Circ 2006; 113(22): 2598–605.

13 Balloon aortic angioplasty

Dennis W Kim and Robert N Vincent

Since the initial report of balloon angioplasty of aortic coarctation by Lababidi in 1983,[1] treatment of this condition has evolved from a strictly surgical procedure to having multiple transcatheter-based options. As the techniques of balloon aortic angioplasty have matured, understanding of the potential as well as the pitfalls specific to balloon dilation of the aorta has also improved.

Efficacy of balloon angioplasty of aortic coarctation depends on many factors, including age at the time of initial intervention, whether the coarctation is native or postsurgical, and whether the coarctation is discrete or long segment/tubular. In addition, the location of the coarctation may also affect the results of balloon angioplasty. Coarctation may exist at many levels including the ascending, transverse, juxtaductal, early descending, as well as abdominal aorta. It is generally accepted that supravalvar aortic stenosis present in William's syndrome is not amenable to balloon angioplasty. While coarctation of the aorta is most commonly associated with a primary congenital process, secondary systemic diseases, such as fibromuscular dysplasia, Takayasu's arteritis, and other 'middle aortic syndromes' can also result in hemodynamically significant narrowing of the aorta.

It is becoming increasingly evident that the vascular properties of aortas affected by coarctation differ from normal aortic tissue. Regional differences seem to exist in the elastic properties of the aorta in coarctation which affect local compliance and distensibility.[2,3] Various genetic syndromes such as Turner syndrome are associated with a higher risk of spontaneous aortic dilation and dissection, likely due to alteration of aortic vascular properties;[4] this may pose an increased risk for complications with aortic angioplasty. Histologically, areas of coarctation demonstrate intimal recruitment of non-proliferative smooth muscle cells, and increased thickness of the extracellular matrix, that together create a widened subendothelial region, and some areas may have features of cystic medial necrosis.[5] Furthermore, differential gene expression for both cytoskeletal proteins as well as elements involved in the generation of oxidative stress has been demonstrated.[6,7] Not only may this play a role in the dilation mechanism during angioplasty, but it may also affect long-term success or failure of balloon aortic angioplasty.

The goal of successful aortic angioplasty is to increase lumen diameter and reduce the pressure gradient across the narrowed area (Figures 13.1–13.3). While lumen

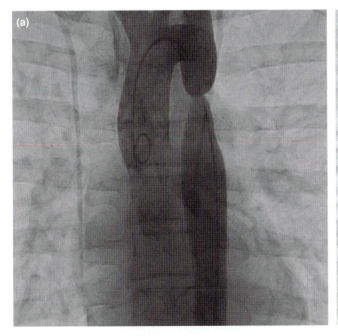
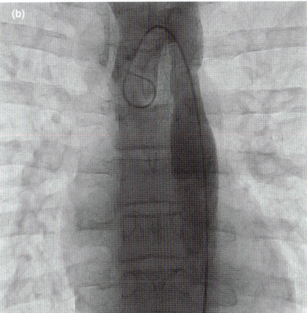

Figure 13.1 Native coarctation before (A) and after (B) balloon angioplasty.

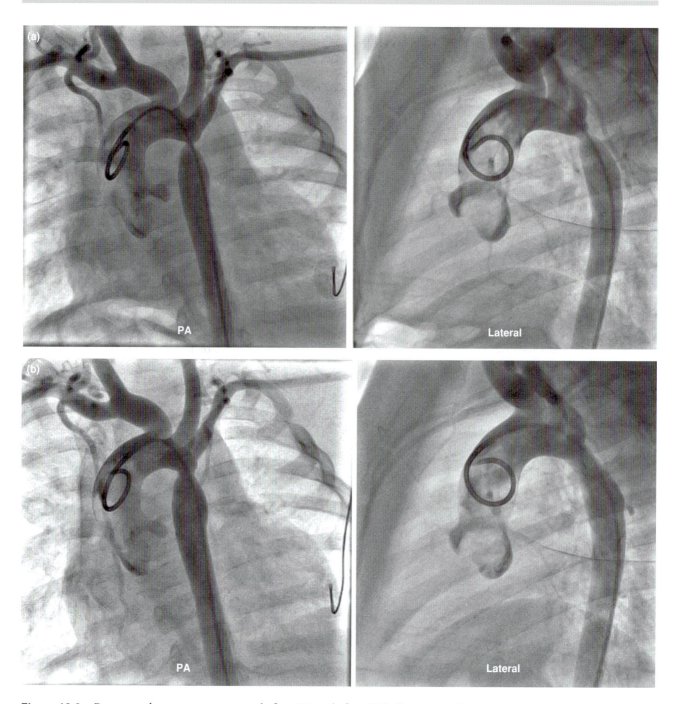

Figure 13.2 Postsurgical recurrent coarcation before (A) and after (B) balloon angioplasty.

diameter may provide a reference for the choice of initial dilation catheter diameter, it is generally not necessary for lumen diameter to achieve equivalent diameter compared to the pre- or postcoarctation segments in order to provide adequate gradient relief. Generally, reduction of gradient to less than 20 mmHg after intervention is felt to represent procedural success for isolated coarctation. In the setting of congenital heart disease representing single ventricle physiology, the goal of minimization of potential extraneous afterload alters this goal to less than 10 mmHg.

Immediate procedural success of balloon aortic angioplasty has been reported to approximate that of surgical repair.[8–10] However, the age at the time of

initial transcatheter intervention affects the technical success and incidence of potential complications, with improved long-term rates of success seen in older children rather than neonates or infants. Multiple reports have shown that balloon angioplasty in infants can be successful at improving lumen diameter and reducing the gradient across the coarctation site.[9–12] However, recurrence of coarctation is common, particularly in neonates and infants. Recoarctation rates after balloon angioplasty of native coarctation in neonates and infants have been reported to range between 25 and 83%.[8,12–15] Aneurysm rates after primary balloon aortic dilation have been reported to be as high as 20–35%, with some aneurysms initially detected more than 5 years after the

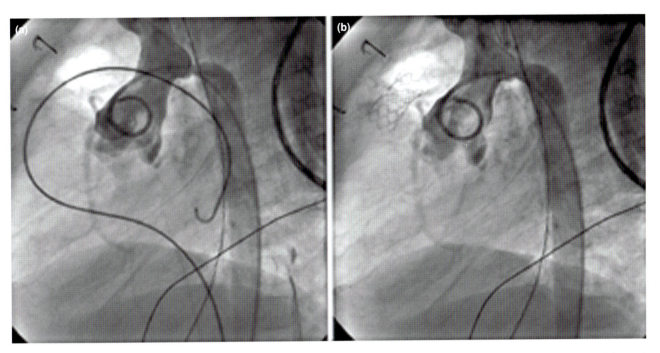

Figure 13.3   Recurrent coarctation after Norwood procedure before (A) and after (B) balloon angioplasty. Note additional stent placement in the RV–PA shunt in (B).

procedure.[10,13,14] This has given many interventionalists some pause in pursuing aortic dilation in neonates and infants. However, balloon angioplasty of recurrent coarctation after initial surgical repair does not have the same recurrence risk, making this the procedure of choice for initial reintervention after primary surgical repair, even in infants. Most likely this represents an ability to re-expand an area of surgical scarring rather than of abnormal native aortic and associated ductal tissue.

TECHNIQUE

Approach

As significant aortic complications can occur immediately in the catheterization lab as well as in the recovery period, it has been our general policy to admit patients for overnight observation after aortic interventions. The arterial sheaths used in these patients typically are larger than would be used in a diagnostic case and anticoagulation is maintained during the procedure, which potentially increases the possibility of bleeding at the access sites.

Most commonly, balloon aortic angioplasty is performed in a retrograde fashion from the femoral artery. The catheter course is generally straightforward to the area of coarctation and multiple sites of proximal (toward the aortic valve from the coarctation) wire position are possible. Care must be taken not to enter the femoral artery above the inguinal ligament as postprocedural bleeding from the arterial puncture site may be into the retroperitoneal space and can go unrecognized for some time.

In very small infants, including premature infants, even 'standard' sized sheaths may pose a significantly increased risk for femoral vascular injury. A carotid approach can be considered, though this typically requires familiarity with cut-down techniques. It would be rare to consider aortic angioplasty in an infant who continues to have availability of umbilical arterial access; however, as with neonatal aortic valve dilation, this approach is feasible.

In younger children who may continue to have patency of the atrial septum, or in older children/adults after transseptal puncture, an antegrade approach is possible. As this route is more circuitous, there may be some difficulty in the smooth passage of the dilation catheter over the guide wire. Additionally, careful attention should be made to wire position and mobility in order to avoid damage to the mitral valve apparatus. The use of a long sheath over the guide wire, while protecting the mitral valve apparatus from wire laceration, may cause hemodynamic instability due to the creation of mitral and/or aortic regurgitation. Antegrade balloon aortic angioplasty is a particularly attractive option for infants and young children with single ventricle anatomy, such as hypoplastic left heart syndrome after aortic arch reconstruction where the passage of the venous catheter to the aorta is relatively straightforward. This is true even if there is femoral venous obstruction requiring vascular access from the subclavian or jugular vein. Careful monitoring for signs of inadequate cardiac output is crucial as the wire and balloon may cause hemodynamically significant atrioventricular (AV) and aortic/neoaortic valve regurgitation and AV block. Wire placement, catheter exchanges, and angiography should proceed expeditiously. Additional invasive femoral arterial blood pressure monitoring should also be utilized. Not only does this provide continuous systemic blood pressure evaluation, it allows for simultaneous pre- and post-angioplasty blood pressure and gradient assessment.

Equipment

As with all angioplasty procedures, a variety of angioplasty catheter sizes and lengths are required. A reasonably stiff wire in a length that allows for catheter exchanges should be chosen to minimize balloon movement during inflation. Balloon length should be long enough to allow for some movement during inflation while allowing for complete angioplasty. As most areas of coarctation tend to be areas of high resistance to angioplasty, particularly in the setting of recurrent postoperative coarctation, a manometer-equipped inflation device should be used to achieve high pressure and to monitor inflation pressure. The inflation sequence should be fluoroscopically recorded to document the balloon inflation and residual balloon 'waist' at peak inflation. Exceeding maximum balloon inflation specifications should be discouraged as sudden balloon rupture may inflict additional damage to the vessel wall and may make balloon extraction difficult.

In older children and adults, there can be excessive movement of the catheter during inflation. When this occurs, slow inflation during balloon positioning until the balloon is 'caught' in the narrowed area, followed by rapid inflation, may allow for maintenance of balloon position. If catheter position cannot be maintained, temporary diminution of cardiac output during balloon inflation by rapid right ventricular pacing or intravenous adenosine bolus can be performed.

Maintenance of the wire position throughout the entire intervention is of the utmost importance. One should avoid recrossing the area of dilation with wires or catheters that are not placed over the initial guide wire. As successful angioplasty results in intimal disruption, unprotected catheter or wire passage across this area could result in further vessel damage or perforation. After dilation, an angiographic catheter such as the Multi-Track™ catheter, manufactured by NuMED (Hopkinton, NY) and distributed in the US by B Braun Medical, Inc, Bethlehem, PA, can be advanced over the guide wire to the area proximal to the dilation. This catheter allows for pull-back pressure recording as well as angiography without manipulating the initial wire position. Alternately, postangioplasty residual gradient can be assessed by catheter exchange over the guide wire into the ascending aorta after measurement of femoral arterial pressure via the side arm of the arterial sheath. If a direct pull back is required, the wire is exchanged for a much smaller caliber wire relative to catheter lumen diameter, followed by pull-back pressure recording using a Tuohy-Borst style 'Y' connector. If for whatever reason wire position is lost during the procedure and the area of dilation needs to be crossed, careful use of a 'J' tipped or floppy-tipped wire generally can be safely performed.

POTENTIAL COMPLICATIONS

Postprocedure hypertension

While postcoarctectomy syndrome is not common after catheter-based intervention for coarctation, hypertension can occur for a variety of reasons after transcatheter aortic intervention. Patient discomfort as well as pre-existing hypertension may play a role. Significant hypertension after aortic intervention should be immediately recognized and diligently treated in order to avoid further extension of vascular disruption beyond what was intended in the catheterization lab. Patient pain, both at the site of vascular access as well as due to aortic dilation, should be aggressively managed. Infiltration of the access sites with 0.25% Marcaine® bupivacaine at the conclusion of the procedure prior to sheath removal may allow for a longer local anesthetic effect than lidocaine. For those patients requiring aggressive antihypertensive treatment, esmolol infusion is an attractive therapy in this setting due to its quick onset of action as well as its short half life. However, continuous infusions such as esmolol or nicardipine typically require monitoring in the intensive care unit setting. Short-acting oral medications such as labetalol or hydralazine can also be used, as long as increased surveillance for continuing hypertension is maintained. New onset hypertension after aortic intervention is typically a transient phenomenon, with discontinuation of new antihypertensive therapy possible in most cases within the first 24 hours after the procedure.

Vascular injury

Femoral arterial injury after angioplasty has been described in 14–24% of patients undergoing balloon aortic angioplasty, although the development of lower profile dilation catheters has likely reduced this incidence in the modern era.[8,16] Retrograde balloon aortic angioplasty requires a larger femoral arterial sheath than otherwise would be used in diagnostic catheterization. Even in the setting of large sheath arterial access, manual compression is a reliable method for achieving hemostasis. A variety of active and passive vascular hemostasis products are available, although most of these products are not recommended for use in femoral entry sites greater than 8–9 French or in small children. Complications related to device-mediated arterial access site closure include improper device deployment, hematoma formation, pseudoaneurysm, vascular stenosis/obstruction, distal limb ischemia, as well as patient discomfort. No head to head comparisons between manual compression and the use of vascular closure systems for large sized arterial sheaths have been published. Nevertheless, one method deserves attention. The 'Preclose' method using the Perclose™ family of suture-based closure devices (Abbott Vascular, Abbott Park, IL) has become a popular alternative to manual compression for maintaining vascular hemostasis after aortic intervention in larger children and adults. In short, this method involves predeployment of the device sutures prior to large sheath introduction into the femoral artery. The sutures are left unsecured until after the intervention is completed. This method has been shown to be very successful in closing arteriotomy sites up to 24 French.[17]

In order to avoid possible femoral arterial injury, antegrade aortic angioplasty can be performed as previously discussed. However, even with this approach a small indwelling femoral catheter should be placed for pressure monitoring, and anticoagulation should be maintained.

Neurologic injury

Neurologic injury due to presumed thromboembolism is a major complication of aortic interventional procedures. Due to the proximities of catheter and wire position to the cerebral circulation, systemic anticoagulation measures should be used. When using heparin, an initial bolus of 100 IU/kg (maximum 5000 IU), is given, followed by hourly assessment of the activated clotting time (ACT) and repeat doses of 50 IU/kg in order to maintain an ACT in excess of 200–250 seconds. Bivalirudin, a newer direct thrombin inhibitor, is administered as an initial bolus dose, followed by a continuous infusion. The safety and efficacy of bivalirudin in pediatric patients are currently under investigation. Thromboembolic complications may be reduced if the guide wire tip is placed somewhere other than the carotid arteries. In addition to the potential of embolic complications, placement of the wire tip in the carotid artery out of the fluoroscopic view, along with movement of the wire with catheter manipulation, can lead to traumatic vascular damage and subsequent diminished cerebral perfusion via that vessel. Acute spinal cord infarction during balloon angioplasty is extremely rare.

Aortic dissection/rupture

Although rare, aortic dissection and rupture are the most feared immediate complications related to either primary balloon angioplasty or stenting of aortic coarctation. Dissection and/or rupture may occur during the procedure or in the postprocedure recovery period, making vigilant surveillance of patient status

imperative. Aortic angioplasty should not be performed unless there is blood available in the catheterization suite.

Selection of balloon sizes based on the diameter of coarctation largely has been relatively subjective, without detailed comparison of various methods. Methods described include balloon sizing to 200% of the area of coarctation, but not exceeding the dimension of the aorta at the level of the diaphragm,[8] within 2 mm of the diameter of the aorta at the level of the left subclavian artery but not greater than the diaphragmatic diameter,[18] the dimension of the diaphragmatic aorta irrespective of the dimension of the coarctation segment,[19] and the diameter of the uninvolved aorta proximal to the area of coarctation.[14] The diameter of the aorta at the level of the diaphragm is commonly much less than in the area just distal to the level of coarctation due to post-stenotic dilation. Likely, an initial balloon diameter of at least two times greater than the coarctation diameter is necessary to achieve reasonable results. If the area of coarctation is very tight, a balloon no more than 3–4 times the minimal diameter of the obstruction should be used initially, even if this is less than the proximal or distal aortic dimensions. Partial insertion and inflation of the balloon catheter into the subclavian or carotid arteries should be avoided to prevent accidental vascular disruption of these vessels during aortic angioplasty.

Exceeding the manufacturer's recommended maximum inflation pressure should be avoided as sudden balloon rupture may increase the risk of aortic wall damage. Extraction of a ruptured balloon may be very difficult, particularly in the setting of a transverse balloon tear. If the ruptured balloon cannot be removed through the sheath, one can pull it into the sheath as far as possible and then remove the sheath and catheter as a single unit, recognizing that this will enlarge the arteriotomy size and potentially significantly damage the vessel. Adequate hemostasis of the site will require a larger sheath. Maintaining the wire position continues to be important, though more difficult, in this setting. In the rare instance when the catheter cannot be removed, exchange with a larger sheath after separating the Luer connector tail of the catheter may allow for balloon extraction. Since a transverse balloon tear may result in an 'inverted umbrella' effect, it may be necessary to place a large sheath in the opposite femoral artery and snare the distal end of the catheter in order to remove it. In this case, the guide wire must be removed from its ideal position and the catheter shaft must be cut so that it can be pulled from the original sheath into the new one. Whenever balloon rupture is encountered, full inspection of the catheter must account for all fragments. As the balloon material is not radio-opaque, fluoroscopy is of little value in localizing missing balloon fragments. Intravascular filling defects may be seen by angiography suggestive of retained balloon fragments. Intravascular or transthoracic/abdominal ultrasound may help identify the lost material. Careful physical examination looking for peripheral pulse loss may help localize the retained fragment. Extraction of catheter fragments may be possible using a snare-type catheter or bioptome. If all else fails, surgical extraction can be considered.

Careful evaluation of the area of angioplasty after balloon dilation is mandatory after aortic intervention. Angiographically, areas of intimal disruption may commonly be seen. If significant intimal disruption is suspected based on the postangioplasty aortogram, any attempts for further dilation of the area of coarctation must proceed with extreme caution. Angiography alone may only detect 50% of intimal flaps and dissections created by balloon angioplasty that otherwise may be detectable with intravascular ultrasound.[20] It must be remembered, however, that the intent of vascular angioplasty is to intentionally create vascular wall injury in order to promote future remodeling and growth. Visualization of intimal disruption, either by angiography or using intravascular ultrasound, may be an indicator of procedural success in this regard.

For areas of coarctation that are resistant to standard balloon angioplasty, sequential angioplasty using peripheral cutting balloons (Boston Scientific, Natick, MA) to create the initial intimal disruption, followed by standard angioplasty, can be considered. Theoretically, the atherotomes of the cutting balloon should create a more controlled localized injury to the vessel wall, which can then be extended by the use of a larger, standard dilation balloon. The largest available cutting balloon is 8 mm in diameter, which may be smaller than the minimal aortic diameter in older patients. However, no published data exist regarding the immediate or long-term success of this technique.

If severe aortic wall injury or rupture is encountered, efficiency is of the utmost importance. Maintaining a calm environment will allow further procedures to occur more quickly and successfully. It is extremely important to maintain wire position across the angioplasty site until severe vascular injury or rupture is excluded. The cardiothoracic surgical service should be notified immediately. The lung fields should be carefully evaluated for developing hemothorax. If significant blood extravasation is suspected, the angioplasty balloon can be inflated in order to obstruct extravascular blood egress. If significant hemothorax develops, chest tube insertion should occur expeditiously. Drained blood can be autotransfused in addition to supplemental blood products or crystalloid in order to maintain vascular volume. It is crucial that large-bore IV access is available during aortic interventions.

Probably the best method for acutely containing extravascular hemorrhage after aortic disruption, while allowing for continuing blood flow below the area of damage, is placement of a covered stent. In the United States, options for balloon-expandable covered stenting for aortic use are limited. The NuMED ePTFE-covered CP stent (NuMED, Inc, Hopkinton, NY) is available outside of the United States and allows expansion from 8 to 24 mm. In smaller patients, placement of the Atrium iCAST (available in the US) or Advanta V12 (available outside of the US) encapsulated PTFE-covered stent (Atrium Medical Corp, Hudson, NH) could be considered. Achievable diameter with this stent is 5–12 mm. Due to the current unavailability of large-sized covered stents in the United States, many catheterization laboratories will construct hand made ePTFE covered stents strictly for emergency use. These hand made covered stents are either created in advance, sterilized, and kept in the catheterization lab for future use, or are made during the procedure prior to angioplasty in high-risk patients. If aortic rupture occurs, there is not enough time to create this stent for use. The technical details of balloon-expandable covered stent placement will not be covered here as they are addressed in other chapters. In the adult-sized patient, self-expanding covered nitinol stents such as the Gore TAG thoracic endoprosthesis (WL Gore, Flagstaff, AZ) can be considered for emergency use. This system is available in diameters from 26 to 40 mm but requires a 20–24 French arterial sheath for deployment. As opposed to interventional radiologists and vascular surgeons, most pediatric interventional cardiologists are not comfortably familiar with rapid deployment of these types of large, self-expanding, covered stents which can result in delay in treatment, or worse, inadequate deployment.

Aortic aneurysm

Aneurysm occurrence immediately after aortic dilation can be encountered (Figure 13.4A). Although of concern, small aneurysms may be very stable and may not progress. Evidence for progression of the aneurysm or increasing concern for stability of the vessel wall are indications for further intervention, whether by surgery or by further transcatheter methods. Covered-stent placement (Figure 13.4B) can result in therapeutically successful aneurysm exclusion. Aneurysm formation in the long term should be monitored diligently with intermittent chest radiographs, CT, MRI/MRA, or standard angiography. Continuing aneurysm surveillance should be performed indefinitely as some aneurysms may be initially detected more than 5 years after angioplasty.[14]

Complications in the recent era

Severe early complications of femoral arterial injury and aortic rupture are now rare due to continuing development of smaller profile catheters and careful

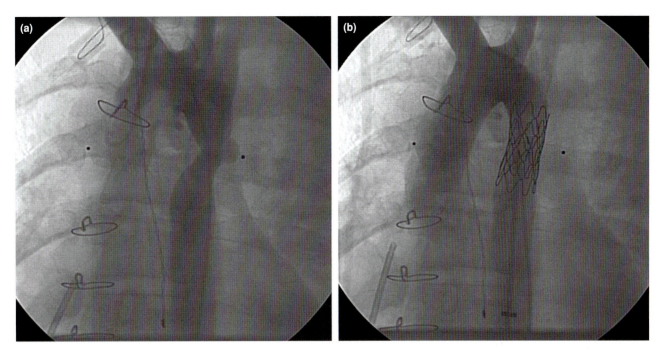

Figure 13.4   Aneurysm after balloon angioplasty (A) and aneurysm exculusion using a CP covered stent (B). Images courtesy of Dr Thomas Forbes.

avoidance of excessive overdilation of the aorta. Most recent complications relate to vascular tears and non-life-threatening aortic dissections and aneurysms. The Congenital Cardiovascular Interventional Study Consortium (CCISC) database identifies 50 recent patients having undergone balloon angioplasty for native or recurrent coarctation (Tom Forbes MD personal communication). Complications occurred in 3/27 patients with native coarctation (1 dissection and 2 aneurysms) and 4/23 patients with recurrent coarctation (1 dissection and aneurysm, 1 balloon rupture, 1 intimal-medial tear, and 1 intimal-medial tear and dissection).

CONCLUSION

As long as the potential pitfalls are understood, balloon angioplasty can be a useful technique in the treatment of aortic coarctation. While the incidence of aneurysm formation may be higher than with surgical correction, long-term success can be achieved in many patients. In most instances, aortic stenting in small children and infants necessitates further surgical intervention due to the inability of these stents to achieve full adult diameters. The ability to perform repeat angioplasty in these patients may make this an attractive option in this subset of patients. In the setting of postoperative recurrent coarctation, balloon angioplasty is the procedure of choice in most instances. Regardless of the age of initial balloon aortic angioplasty, careful surveillance for the development of aortic aneurysms is mandatory.

REFERENCES

1. Lababidi Z. Neonatal transluminal balloon coarctation angioplasty. Am Heart J 1983; 106(4 Pt 1): 752–3.
2. Xu J, Shiota T, Omoto R et al. Intravascular ultrasound assessment of regional aortic wall stiffness, distensibility, and compliance in patients with coarctation of the aorta. Am Heart J 1997; 134(1): 93–8.
3. Vogt M, Kuhn A, Baumgartner D et al. Impaired elastic properties of the ascending aorta in newborns before and early after successful coarctation repair: proof of a systemic vascular disease of the prestenotic arteries? Circulation 2005; 111(24): 3269–73.
4. Matura LA, Ho VB, Rosing DR, Bondy CA. Aortic dilatation and dissection in Turner syndrome. Circulation 2007; 116(15): 1663–70.
5. Jimenez M, Daret D, Choussat A, Bonnet J. Immunohistological and ultrastructural analysis of the intimal thickening in coarctation of human aorta. Cardiovasc Res 1999; 41(3): 737–45.
6. Vatta M, Chang AC, McMahon CJ. Altered expression of dystrophin within the thoracic aorta in coarctation. Cardiol Young 2005; 15(1): 73–4.
7. Vaziri ND, Ni Z. Expression of NOX-I, gp91phox, p47phox and P67phox in the aorta segments above and below coarctation. Biochim et Biophys Acta 2005; 1723(1–3): 321–7.
8. Rao PS, Galal O, Smith PA, Wilson AD. Five- to nine-year follow-up results of balloon angioplasty of native aortic coarctation in infants and children. J Am Coll Cardiol 1996; 27(2): 462–70.
9. Walhout RJ, Lekkerkerker JC, Oron GH, Bennink GB, Meijboom EJ. Comparison of surgical repair with balloon angioplasty for native coarctation in patients from 3 months to 16 years of age. Eur J Cardiothorac Surg 2004; 25(5): 722–7.
10. Rodes-Cabau J, Miro J, Dancea A et al. Comparison of surgical and transcatheter treatment for native coarctation of the aorta in patients > or = 1 year old. The Quebec Native Coarctation of the Aorta study. Am Heart J 2007; 154(1): 186–92.
11. Walhout RJ, Lekkerkerker JC, Ernst SM et al. Angioplasty for coarctation in different aged patients. Am Heart J 2002; 144(1): 180–6.
12. Rao PS, Chopra PS, Koscik R, Smith PA, Wilson AD. Surgical versus balloon therapy for aortic coarctation in infants < or = 3 months old. J Am Coll Cardiol 1994; 23(6): 1479–83.

13. Shaddy RE, Boucek MM, Sturtevant JE et al. Comparison of angioplasty and surgery for unoperated coarctation of the aorta. Circulation 1993; 87(3): 793–9.

14. Cowley CG, Orsmond GS, Feola P, McQuillan L, Shaddy RE. Long-term, randomized comparison of balloon angioplasty and surgery for native coarctation of the aorta in childhood. Circulation 2005; 111(25): 3453–6.

15. Fiore AC, Fischer LK, Schwartz T et al. Comparison of angioplasty and surgery for neonatal aortic coarctation. Ann Thorac Surg 2005; 80(5): 1659–64; discussion 64–5.

16. Yetman AT, Nykanen D, McCrindle BW et al. Balloon angioplasty of recurrent coarctation: a 12-year review. J Am Coll Cardiol 1997; 30(3): 811–16.

17. Lee WA, Brown MP, Nelson PR, Huber TS. Total percutaneous access for endovascular aortic aneurysm repair ('Preclose' technique). J Vasc Surg 2007; 45(6): 1095–101.

18. Ovaert C, McCrindle BW, Nykanen D et al. Balloon angioplasty of native coarctation: clinical outcomes and predictors of success. J Am Coll Cardiol 2000; 35(4): 988–96.

19. Maheshwari S, Bruckheimer E, Fahey JT, Hellenbrand WE. Balloon angioplasty of postsurgical recoarctation in infants: the risk of restenosis and long-term follow-up. J Am Coll Cardiol 2000; 35(1): 209–13.

20. Sohn S, Rothman A, Shiota T et al. Acute and follow-up intravascular ultrasound findings after balloon dilation of coarctation of the aorta. Circulation 1994; 90(1): 340–7.

14 Complications encountered in intravascular stent treatment for native and recurrent coarctation of the aorta

Thomas Forbes and Daniel R. Turner

INTRODUCTION

Intravascular stent treatment for coarctation of the aorta has been shown to be successful in 96–98% of patients.[1–4] In theory, stent dilation of coarctation is a straightforward procedure, but in reality this is one of the most technically demanding procedures performed in the catheterization laboratory.[1,3,5–7] This chapter focuses on complications encountered with this procedure, techniques used to avoid the complication, and methods used to overcome the complication should it occur. Adult issues will be briefly covered, although these will be more thoroughly covered in Chapter 33.

The most difficult aspect of this procedure is that the interventionalist may 'do everything right,' yet an unexpected and catastrophic outcome may result from the procedure. Fortunately, increased understanding of technical and anatomic issues has significantly decreased the complication rate associated with this procedure. In this chapter, complications will be divided into technical and aortic wall complications. Each section will be further subdivided into a discussion of the complication, methods used to avoid the complication, and treatments used to overcome the complication if it should be encountered.

BASIC PRINCIPLES IN STENTING COARCTATION OF THE AORTA

This information was obtained from the 40 institutions currently enroling patients on the coarctation study in the Congenital Cardiovascular Interventional Study Consortium (CCISC). The majority of these institutions are in the United States.

All institutions consider stenting native or recurrent coarctation of the aorta, regardless of the severity of narrowing. The majority (95%) would consider stent placement as the primary treatment in patients > 30 kg and balloon angioplasty the treatment of choice in patients < 30 kg. Some institutions (30%) consider stenting coarctation of the aorta in patients as small as 15 kg. No institution would consider primary stenting of coarctation in infants unless surgery was contraindicated. Location of the coarctation segment would not deter the majority of institutions from stent placement. Although all participants attempt to avoid overlapping a brachiocephalic vessel, 96% would consider partially overlapping a vessel if necessary to achieve a reasonable outcome.

Nearly 90% of the institutions use general anesthesia during the procedure and 98% hospitalize the patient overnight. The most commonly used balloons were the Balloon-in-Balloon (BIB – 58%), Z-Med (21%), and Cordis (16%) balloons. The Genesis-XD (44%), Intratherapeutic Mega (27%), and Palmaz XL (15%) were the most commonly used stents. The majority positioned the distal end of the wire either in the ascending aorta (51%) or the right subclavian artery (31%). Eight percent performed cardiac output controling measures (the majority used ventricular pacing) to decrease the likelihood of encountering stent migration.

TECHNICAL COMPLICATIONS: INCIDENCE AND ASSOCIATED FACTORS

In a multi-institutional retrospective review of 650 stents placed during 565 stent procedures, technical complications were encountered in 59 of 565 procedures (10.4%). The most common technical complication was stent migration, which occurred in 28/565 (4.5%) procedures. Balloon rupture occurred in 13/565 (2.3%) and cerebrovascular accident or peripheral embolic events occurred in 5/565 (0.8%) patients. Technical complications were more likely to occur in patients over the age of 40 years (24% vs 10.5%), patients not under general anesthesia (19.8 vs 5.8%), and those undergoing stent procedures prior to January 2002 (16.3 vs 6.1%) (Figure 14.1).[1]

Stent migration

The incidence of stent migration ranges from 4 to 10% during stent placement for coarctation of the

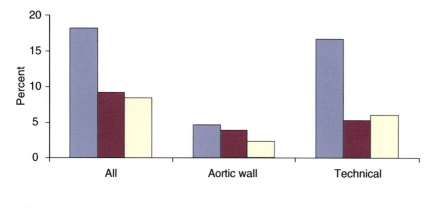

■ < Jan 2002 (*n* = 301)   ■ > Jan 2002 (*n* = 264)   □ Current CCISC (*n* = 147)

Figure 14.1 Trends of acute complications encountered in the performance of stent angioplasty for coarctation of the aorta. Complications have been broken down into all, technical, and aortic wall.

aorta.[1,8–10] In the current prospective CCISC experience as of September 2007, 7/147 (4.8%) patients had stent migration during initial deployment. In the multicenter retrospective review, stent migration occurred during 28 of 565 (5%) procedures. The most common cause of stent migration was use of a balloon catheter that was larger in diameter than the aortic diameter proximal to the coarctation site (> 2 mm). In addition, location of the coarctation segment nearer the transverse aortic arch also increased the likelihood of stent migration (Figure 14.2). The second most common cause for stent migration was attempting to place the stent in a pseudocoarctation segment, where the aortic obstruction was a fold within the wall rather than a true stenosis. Stent migration tended toward larger balloon diameters, where 18 of 28 (64%) stents were delivered on balloon catheters greater than or equal to 15 mm diameter.

Balloon rupture

Balloon rupture during initial stent deployment was encountered in 13/565 (2.3%) patients in the multi-institutional study.[1,4,10] Surprisingly, larger balloon size was not associated with rupture, with all types of balloons encountering this complication.[1] In the prospective CCISC database, there is a trend toward decreased balloon rupture when 'modern' balloons (BIB, Cordis Maxi Plus, and the Z-Med) are used (2/147 or 1.3% of patients). Additionally, the use of newer stents (Genesis-XD, eV3 Series, CP Platinum) may also play a role in decreased balloon rupture due to their rounded edges. One patient encountered a cerebrovascular event associated after balloon rupture in the transverse aortic arch;[1] therefore particular care must be taken to ensure the balloon is properly de-aired prior to use, especially when in proximity to the brachiocephalic vessels.

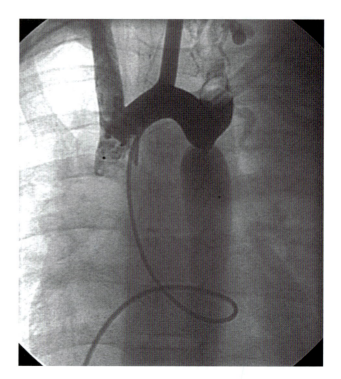

Figure 14.2 This coarctation segment is nearer to the transverse aortic arch (absence of the isthmic portion of the aortic arch), which increased the likelihood of encountering stent migration. Note the mild transverse aortic arch hypoplasia, with oversizing of the balloon catheter relative to the transverse aortic arch dimensions also playing a role in encountering stent migration.

Cerebrovascular events

Cerebrovascular/peripheral embolic events, some associated with technical complications, have been noted in multiple series (0.1–0.7%).[1,4,11] Cerebrovascular events have been associated with balloon rupture,[1] and during redilation of the stent crossing a brachiocephalic vessel.[11] In the CCISC multi-institutional experience,

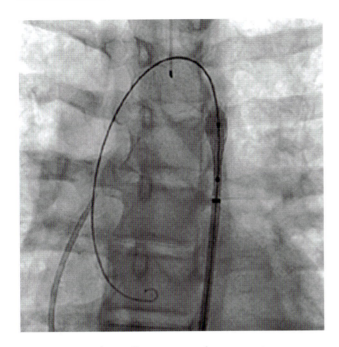

Figure 14.3   Slow inflation across the coarctation segment, with the sheath covering the proximal balloon catheter and near complete expansion of the distal stent.

4/565 patients encountered a cerebrovascular event. Although in 3 patients the etiology was not known, wire position within the brachiocephalic vessel was thought to be a possible contributing factor. Overall, the outcomes were encouraging, with 3/4 making complete recovery prior to discharge, while one patient had long-term mild residual deficits.[1]

PREVENTION OF TECHNICAL COMPLICATIONS

To decrease the likelihood of stent migration, adenosine infusion, rapid atrial/right ventricular pacing, and esmolol infusion have been used by some centers to decrease cardiac output and decrease the likelihood of distal balloon/stent migration.[12–14] During adenosine infusion, the stent is delivered during the brief period of complete heart block. With esmolol infusion, the stent is delivered after appropriate decrease in cardiac output and blood pressure due to β-blockade. Rapid atrial or ventricular pacing decreases cardiac output by decreasing diastolic filling time and therefore preload. For older children and adults, the goal is to decrease the systolic blood pressure by approximately 50%, usually at a paced rate of 210–250 beats/minute. Once this is achieved, the stent is deployed across the coarctation segment. In the CCISC prospective experience, atrial/ventricular pacing has encountered no stent migration in 44 patients, compared to 7/103 (6.8%) stent migrations in patients where pacing was not performed. Qureshi *et al.* advocated predilation of the

coarctation segment to assess both balloon expansion properties across the aortic arch and aortic wall compliance prior to stent deployment.[4] This technique, they feel, decreased the likelihood of encountering stent migration during initial deployment.

Another method that may decrease the likelihood of stent migration during initial deployment is slow inflation of the balloon in a distal to proximal fashion across the coarctation site. The long sheath is withdrawn so that the stent is exposed, with the proximal balloon remaining covered. The balloon is slowly inflated across the coarctation segment distal to proximal (Figure 14.3). Once the distal end of the stent is nearly completely expanded, the sheath is pulled off the proximal end and final dilation of the stent is performed. The theoretic benefit of this technique is that the sheath offers support to the balloon and stent during inflation and that gradual inflation of the distal balloon/stent unit decreases cardiac output gradually rather than suddenly across the coarctation segment. Using this technique, the authors have not encountered stent migration in 37 consecutive procedures.

FIXING THE COMPLICATION IF IT SHOULD OCCUR

During stent migration, the stent migrates distally to the mid thoracic or abdominal aorta. The safest treatment is to deploy the stent in the infrarenal aorta or iliac system if possible. Movement of a partially or fully expanded stent in the aorta can cause significant trauma to the aortic vessel wall. Snaring the distal end of the stent, thereby collapsing part of the stent onto the balloon catheter and readvancing it across the coarctation segment for final deployment, has been performed (Figure 14.4). This technique of 're-crimping' the distal end of the stent is difficult to perform with the open cell eV3 stent series due to malformation of the stent by the snare, and nearly impossible with the covered CP stent.

If a covered stent is being used for treatment of coarctation of the aorta, one must be cognizant of the size of the mid thoracic aorta. If the covered stent should migrate distally, and the mid thoracic aorta is greater than 20 mm in diameter, the covered stent may not be able to be deployed here. In this situation, the stent may be maneuvered past the abdominal aortic vessels into the infrarenal aorta, though this can be an exceedingly difficult and dangerous maneuver. If the stent is able to reach the size of the mid thoracic aorta, it may be safely deployed here, using an Atlas balloon or other large, non-compliant balloon catheter.

If the balloon ruptures proximally, the author has noted that partially covering the proximal part of the balloon with the sheath and aggressively injecting saline into the balloon catheter has achieved expansion of the distal balloon/stent complex, thereby anchoring the stent above the coarctation and preventing it from

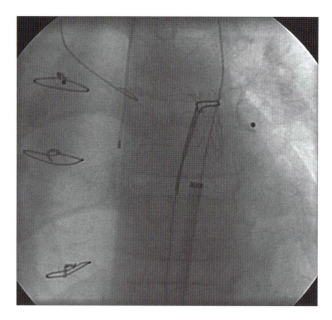

Figure 14.4 The Genesis stent was snared distally with a Microvena snare catheter, partially recrimping the stent back onto the balloon catheter. The stent could be adequately repositioned across the coarctation site, where final expansion was performed. This patient had mild coarctation of the aorta; this maneuver is exceedingly difficult, if not impossible, to perform in a patient with severe coarctation of the aorta.

distal migration. A second balloon catheter is then advanced across the partially deployed stent for final expansion. If the balloon ruptures distally, it may be difficult to generate enough pressure in the balloon catheter to allow for expansion of the distal stent, anchoring it across the coarctation segment. Some have advocated hooking the balloon to the power injector and injecting saline directly into the balloon catheter, thereby generating more pressure and expanding the stent (Cheatham JP, personal communication). This should be done with caution, as the high pressure may cause further rupture/fragmentation of the balloon catheter. Again, the importance of properly de-airing the balloon catheter needs to be stressed.

STENT OVERLAP OF A BRACHIOCEPHALIC VESSEL

This will be handled as a separate issue, as the majority of interventionalists would consider this not to be a complication. Out of 343 procedures where specific mention of whether or not stent overlap of a brachiocephalic vessel was made, 61 patients (17.8%) had either partial or complete overlap of one of the brachiocephalic vessels. No acute complications were encountered. Presently, with over 300 patient-years of follow-up, no cerebrovascular events or peripheral embolic events have been encountered.[1] This is consistent with the experience of others.[4,6] The only event

reported in a patient with brachiocephalic vessel overlap was during redilation of a stent that partially crossed the left subclavian artery.[11]

AORTIC WALL COMPLICATIONS: INCIDENCE AND ASSOCIATED FACTORS

Acute aortic wall complications, including intimal tears, dissections, and aortic wall rupture, occurred in 1–4% of procedures.[1–4,9,15,16] The definitions are as follows:

- an intimal tear is a filling defect within the vessel lumen
- dissection is extravasation of contrast outside the vessel lumen within the adventitial region
- an aneurysm is defined as the expansion of the aortic wall greater than 10% of the adjoining native lumen that was not present prior to stent placement
- aortic rupture is extravasation of contrast outside the vessel lumen and through the adventitial wall layer.

In the CCISC retrospective multi-institutional study, aortic wall complications were encountered in 22 of 565 (3.9%) patients. Aggressive present angioplasty (11.4 vs 3%) and age > 40 years were significantly associated with encountering aortic wall complications. Interestingly, acute aortic wall complications were not associated with the balloon:coarctation ratio.[1] Intimal tear was encountered in 8 of 565 (1.4%) patients. The majority of intimal tears occurred just proximal to the previously placed stent and were not associated with a technical complication. Aortic dissection (including aortic rupture) was observed in 9 out 565 procedures (4.6%). In 8 of the 9 procedures, no technical complications were encountered during stent deployment. Three patients had aortic rupture during stent deployment; one expired in the lab, one was successfully treated with covered stents, and a third suffered severe neurologic injury and subsequently expired 6 months later.[1] Aortic wall rupture has been mentioned in case reports also, each occurring in adult patients older than 19 years of age (the 19-year-old was a patient with Turner syndrome).[5,7,17–19] Thankfully, the incidence of encountering acute aortic wall injury appears to have decreased recently (Figure 14.1).

AVOIDANCE OF ACUTE AORTIC WALL INJURY

Currently, risk factors for developing aortic wall injury during intravascular stent placement are much better understood than how to avoid these complications. The best solution would be to use covered stents in all high-risk patients, although dissections have been reported with the use of covered stents as well.[18] Unfortunately, at this time in the United States, covered stents which reach 20–24 mm in diameter are not available. Covered stents are used in high-risk patients (adults, and patients with Turner syndrome) routinely in other countries.[15] Balloon compliance testing is advocated by some to assess aortic wall compliance.[4] A compliant balloon is inflated across the coarctation segment, inflated to 2–3 atmospheres of pressure. If there is a residual waist greater than 30% of the balloon diameter the aorta is considered to be non-compliant, and the patient is considered higher risk for the use of bare metal stent treatment for the coarctation segment. Recent imaging studies have been used to better assess aortic wall compliance utilizing systolic/diastolic dimensional or flow changes.[20–22] Unfortunately, the value of this information in the patient undergoing stent placement remains unknown. Finally, some have advocated the use of intravascular ultrasound to assess aortic wall calcifications prior to stent placement. Patients with aortic wall calcifications are considered higher risk for bare metal stent placement (Pedra CA and Cheatham JP, personal communication).

In the United States, the interventionalist is left to manually create a covered stent in the catheterization laboratory for the high-risk patient. The authors use a polytetrafluoroethylene (PTFE) material called Impra (Impra Corporation, Division of Bard Corporation of Arizona.). This material is able to be expanded to 5–6 times its normal diameter without tearing (Figure 14.5A and B). Therefore, 4 and 5 mm shunt tube grafts can be expanded reliably up to 20 and 25 mm diameter, respectively.[23,24]

The old adage 'an ounce of prevention is worth a pound of cure' is certainly true when dealing with aortic wall injuries. In high-risk patients, the authors no longer aim for angiographic success, but hemodynamic success. In our experience ($n = 61$), no patient has needed stent dilation greater than 20 mm final diameter to achieve an excellent hemodynamic outcome.

AVOIDANCE OF AORTIC WALL INJURY AT INTERMEDIATE FOLLOW-UP

Follow-up, utilizing integrated imaging (CT, MRI, or cardiac catheterization), has been poor. In the CCISC retrospective multi-institutional study, only 160 of 588 procedures (27%) had integrated imaging performed at follow-up, with 16 being a planned staged procedure, thus excluded from further analysis. Forty-one (28.5%) of the remaining 144 patients had abnormal imaging studies at 12-month median follow-up. Sixteen (11%) had significant neo-intimal build-up, 13 (9%) had aneurysm, 5 (3%) had dissection/intimal tear, and 6 (4.2%) had stent fracture (Figure 14.6).[25] Stent fractures have been observed in Palmaz, Genesis-XD, and CP bare metal stents.[2,25] In the Qureshi et al. series of 153 patients, 82 patients (54% of surviving

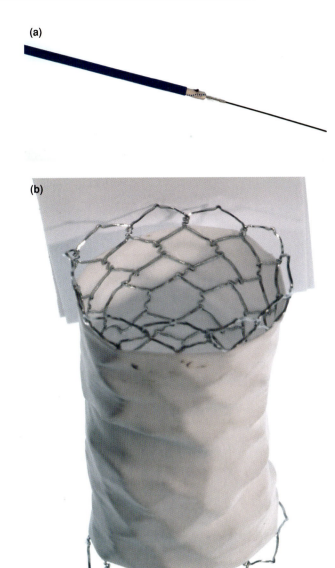

Figure 14.5 (A) Pre-expansion and (B) final expansion of a Genesis XD stent covered with Impra (PTFE) material. This stent can be deployed through a 14 French sheath, and expanded up to 20 mm final diameter.

patients) underwent integrated aortic arch imaging at a median of 2.8 years, with stent fractures occurring in 12/67 (18%) patients. New aneurysms were observed in 6% of patients, none requiring surgical reintervention.[4] With poor follow-up, it is difficult to comment on the true incidence of aortic wall complications, or who is at high risk for aortic wall injury at follow-up. Data from the CCISC retrospective multi-institutional study showed that exceeding a balloon:coarctation ratio of > 3.5 and aggressive present angioplasty increased the risk of an abnormal follow-up study, but more information is clearly needed.[25] We are now prospectively evaluating these patients in a more systematic fashion in order to better assess the incidence of encountering aortic wall complications.

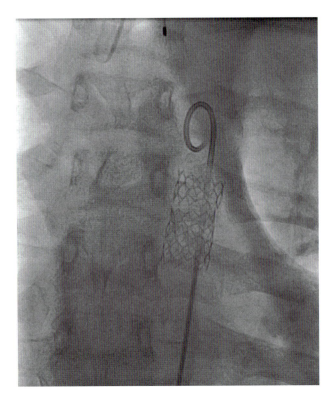

Figure 14.6   A fractured Genesis stent in a patient 2 years out from deployment. No further treatment was required, as the coarctation site remained expanded.

SUMMARY

Stent treatment of recurrent and native coarctation of the aorta remains a highly successful procedure with distinct technical challenges. Through improved understanding of this procedure, we have successfully decreased all types of complications (Figure 14.1). In the relatively near future, we will have a better understanding on how to approach the high risk patient with coarctation of the aorta and, more importantly, we will have the tools to overcome them if they should occur in the catheterization laboratory.

REFERENCES

1. Forbes TJ, Garekar S, Amin Z et al. Procedural results and acute complications in stenting native and recurrent coarctation of the aorta in patients over 4 years of age: a multi-institutional study. Cathet Cardiovasc Interven 2007; 70(2): 276–85.
2. Ledesma M, Jauregui R, Ceron CK et al. Stent fracture after stent therapy for aortic coarctation. J Invas Cardiol 2003; 15(12): 719–21.
3. Suarez de Lezo J, Pan M, Romero M et al. Immediate and follow-up findings after stent treatment for severe coarctation of aorta. Am J Cardiol 1999; 83(3): 400–6.
4. Qureshi AM, McElhinney DB, Lock JE et al. Acute and intermediate outcomes, and evaluation of injury to the aortic wall, as based on 15 years experience of implanting stents to treat aortic coarctation. Cardiol Young 2007; 17(3): 307–18.
5. Korkola SJ, Tchervenkov CI, Shum-Tim D, Roy N. Aortic rupture after stenting of a native coarctation in an adult. Ann Thorac Surg 2002; 74(3): 936.
6. Ebeid MR, Prieto LR, Latson LA. Use of balloon-expandable stents for coarctation of the aorta: initial results and intermediate-term follow-up. J Am Coll Cardiol 1997; 30(7): 1847–52.
7. Varma C, Benson LN, Butany J, McLaughlin PR. Aortic dissection after stent dilatation for coarctation of the aorta: a case report and literature review. Cathet Cardiovasc Interven 2003; 59(4): 528–35.
8. Hamdan MA, Maheshwari S, Fahey JT, Hellenbrand WE. Endovascular stents for coarctation of the aorta: initial results and intermediate-term follow-up. J Am Coll Cardiol 2001; 38(5): 1518–23.
9. Pedra CA, Fontes VF, Esteves CA et al. Stenting vs. balloon angioplasty for discrete unoperated coarctation of the aorta in adolescents and adults. Cathet Cardiovasc Interven 2005; 64(4): 495–506.
10. Harrison DA, McLaughlin PR, Lazzam C, Connelly M, Benson LN. Endovascular stents in the management of coarctation of the aorta in the adolescent and adult: one year follow up. Heart 2001; 85(5): 561–6.
11. Boshoff DE, Eyskens B, Gewillig M et al. Late redilation of a stent in the aorta crossing the subclavian artery complicated with a cerebellar infarction. Acta Cardiol 2007; 62(3): 295–7.
12. Sivaprakasam MC, Veldtman GR, Salmon AP et al. Esmolol-assisted balloon and stent angioplasty for aortic coarctation. Pediatr Cardiol 2006; 27(4): 460–4.
13. Kahn RA, Marin ML, Hollier L, Parsons R, Griepp R. Induction of ventricular fibrillation to facilitate endovascular stent graft repair of thoracic aortic aneurysms. Anesthesiology 1998; 88(2): 534–6.
14. De Giovanni JV, Edgar RA, Cranston A. Adenosine induced transient cardiac standstill in catheter interventional procedures for congenital heart disease. Heart 1998; 80(4): 330–3.
15. Pedra CA, Fontes VF, Esteves CA et al. Use of covered stents in the management of coarctation of the aorta. Pediatr Cardiol 2005; 26(4): 431–9.
16. Chessa M, Carrozza M, Butera G et al. Results and mid–long-term follow-up of stent implantation for native and recurrent coarctation of the aorta. Eur Heart J 2005; 26(24): 2728–32.
17. Panten RR, Harrison JK, Warner J, Grocott HP. Aortic dissection after angioplasty and stenting of an aortic coarctation: detection by intravascular ultrasonography but not transesophageal echocardiography. J Am Soc Echocardiogr 2001; 14(1): 73–6.
18. Collins N, Mahadevan V, Horlick E. Aortic rupture following a covered stent for coarctation: delayed recognition. Cathet Cardiovasc Interven 2006; 68(4): 653–5.
19. Fejzic Z, van Oort A. Fatal dissection of the descending aorta after implantation of a stent in a 19-year-old female with Turner's syndrome. Cardiol Young 2005; 15(5): 529–31.
20. Krug R, Boese JM, Schad LR. Determination of aortic compliance from magnetic resonance images using an automatic active contour model. Phys Med Biol 2003; 48(15): 2391–404.
21. Kuecherer HF, Just A, Kirchheim H. Evaluation of aortic compliance in humans. Am J Physiol Heart Circ Physiol 2000; 278(5): H1411–13.
22. Nurnberger J, Kribben A, Philipp T, Erbel R. [Arterial compliance (stiffness) as a marker of subclinical atherosclerosis]. Herz 2007; 32(5): 379–86.
23. Marston WA, Risley GL, Criado E et al. Mechanical characteristics of dilated polytetrafluoroethylene used for transluminally placed endovascular grafts. Ann Vasc Surg 1997; 11(1): 68–73.
24. Palmaz F, Sprague E, Palmaz JC. Physical properties of polytetrafluoroethylene bypass material after balloon dilation. J Vasc Interven Radiol 1996; 7(5): 657–63.
25. Forbes TJ, Moore P, Pedra CA et al. Intermediate follow-up following intravascular stenting for treatment of coarctation of the aorta. Cathet Cardiovasc Interven 2007; 70(4): 569–77.

15 Stenting the arterial duct

Dietmar Schranz

INTRODUCTION

Congenital heart diseases with duct-dependent circulation after birth are complex. Continued patency of the arterial duct (ductus arteriosus, DA) is essential in two major types of congenital heart disease: newborns with duct-dependent pulmonary blood flow who have a critically or totally obstructed ventricular-pulmonary connection, and neonates with duct-dependent systemic blood flow who require either a patent DA for the systemic circulation in total, which includes retrograde flow through the aortic arch for adequate coronary and cerebral blood flow, or to support partially the systemic blood flow in patients with multiple left heart obstructive lesions. Both duct-dependent systemic as well as pulmonary blood flow can be associated with a 'single ventricle,' as lacking two well-developed ventricles at birth, and also with a normal or borderline developed right or left ventricle with the option for biventricular repair. Blalock and Taussig[1] were the first to create a surgical shunt as an alternative to the arterial duct. The modified Blalock–Taussig shunt (mBTS) is still the most commonly created systemic-pulmonary shunt in neonates with cyanotic heart disease. Morbidity and mortality after mBTS are related to several factors including age, pulmonary artery diameter, and the baseline cardiac anatomy.[2,3] Norwood *et al.*[4] in 1981 reported the first experience in surgical reconstruction of the aortic arch combined with a modified Blalock–Taussig shunt. Such surgery in neonates, particularly in premature infants, can involve major complications, and despite improvements over the last decade both this and modified approaches still have significant mortality.[5–7] In the past, attempts have been made to alter the native DA in various ways to maintain its patency. Formalin infiltration, and even balloon angioplasty and thermal balloon dilatation have been investigated, but long-term patency was disappointing.[8–11] In 1991, the first experimental use of an intravascular stent to maintain ductal patency in an animal model was reported.[12,13]

Worldwide experience in stenting the DA in humans was quite limited in the last century.[14] Previous attempts to stent the neonatal duct in humans used early generation, rigid, bare stents, and relatively bulky, stiff wires, balloons, and sheaths, and frequently resulted in worsening cyanosis or shock, bleeding, vessel rupture, duct spasm, tissue prolapse, or acute thrombosis.[15–17] Additionally, incomplete covering of the duct was frequently followed by duct constriction, with inadequate pulmonary or systemic flow within hours or days after implantation. Some indications for duct stenting were performed without a conclusive follow-up strategy. Based on these experiences, it was concluded that, for the majority of patients, ductal stenting could not be recommended due to the procedure risk and short duration of palliation.[18] Duct stenting for newborns in duct-dependent pulmonary circulation was apostrophized 'a wanna-be' Blalock–Taussig.[19] By learning from these failures, and applying better patient selection criteria and preparation, using new techniques and better interventional access, and covering the complete length of the duct with current low-profile, flexible, premounted stents (with good scaffolding) or even self-expandable nitinol stents, the results of ductal stenting have been significantly improved. The 'new era' of duct stenting was started by the experience of Gerd Hausdorf and his team.[20] Meanwhile, duct stenting is used worldwide in various forms of duct-dependent congenital heart defects.[21–29] Duct stenting combined with bilateral banding as a percutaneous or intraoperative surgical–interventional hybrid approach has been developed and nowadays established as an alternative for the classical Norwood approach.[21,30–36]

In the context of the current knowledge and literature,[37] as well as based on our own experience of ductal stenting in more than 170 patients with duct-dependent systemic ($n = 115$) and pulmonary ($n = 59$) circulation, this chapter deals with the technical aspects, including risk stratification and possible pitfalls of ductal stenting, to maintain pulmonary and systemic circulation.

GENERAL PRINCIPLES

Ductal morphology

In the heart with a normal left-sided aortic arch, the arterial duct connects the junction of the pulmonary

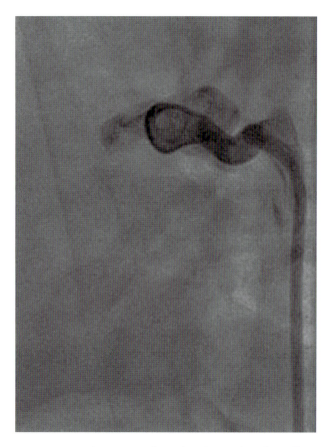

Figure 15.1   Angiogram through a 4 French right Judkins catheter placed into the junction of a short, straight ductus to descending aorta. A 0.014 inch coronary wire is advanced through the duct into the pulmonary artery.

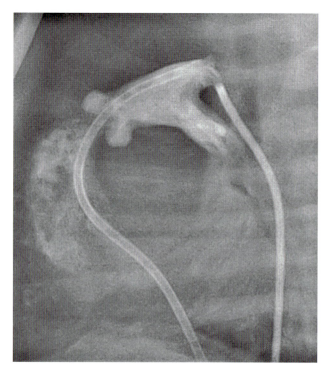

Figure 15.2   Angiogram through a 4 French right Judkins catheter advanced from the descending aorta, placed within a straight short duct, shows central pulmonary arteries and the pulmonary part of the ductus arteriosus after interventional valve perforation and gradual valvuloplasty in a newborn with pulmonary atresia (PAt) and intact ventricular septum (IVS). A 4 French multipurpose catheter is placed from the venous site in a 'kissing' position to the 4 French right Judkins catheter.

bifurcation with the left pulmonary artery to the descending aorta just distal to the origin of the left subclavian artery and has a short, straight course (Figure 15.1). Such ducts are also typically seen in patients who develop pulmonary stenosis or atresia late in fetal life, as it is seen in most cases of pulmonary atresia with intact ventricular septum (Figure 15.2). The arterial duct in neonates with severe right heart obstructive lesions early in fetal life has a very different anatomy: the duct in these patients is longer, much more tortuous in different planes, and mostly has a vertical origin from the aortic arch (Figure 15.3). The pulmonary trunk and pulmonary bifurcation may have a variable size; if not completely absent, the trunk is small to hypoplastic; flow characteristics or even ductal tissue in the wall of the pulmonary arteries can account for early or late stenosis of branch pulmonary arteries.

The duct can be left-sided, right-sided, or bilateral. When ipsilateral to the arch, the duct connects at the inner curve of the arch just distal of the ipsilateral subclavian artery (Figure 15.3); when the duct is contralateral to the arch it originates from the innominate or subclavian artery. The pulmonary arteries can be confluent or non-confluent (Figure 15.4).

In newborns with duct-dependent systemic circulation, the morphology of the duct was classified by Boucek et al.[31] into three types depending on the orientation from the vertical plane. Type 1 ductal anatomy with a leftward orientation was described in 65%, type 2, with a direct front-to-back duct orientation, was seen in almost 30% of the patients, type 3 ductal anatomy with a rightward axis was uncommon.

Cardiac catheterization

Considering ductal stenting as first-stage palliation, detailed diagnosis of the congenital heart disease has to be established by two-dimensional and Doppler echocardiography before cardiac catheterization. The patients must be categorized into either single-ventricle or two-ventricle physiology, and the duct morphology must be defined with its positioning in relation to the aortic arch. In addition, in patients with duct-dependent retrograde aortic arch flow, the junction of the duct with the descending aortic arch needs to be justified, and the presence of a significant aortic coarctation has to be determined, as well as the dimension of the ascending aorta and its connection to

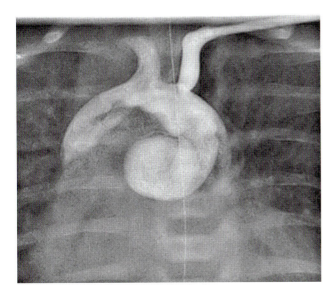

Figure 15.3 Aortogram through a 4 French sheath placed in the left subclavian artery advanced from the left axillary artery. A tortuous duct connects at the inner curve of the arch just distal of the ipsilateral subclavian artery.

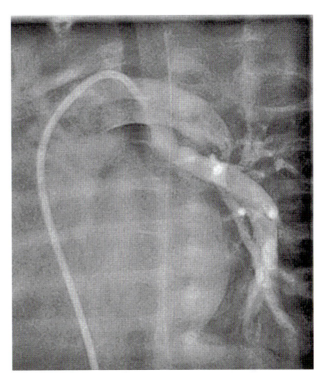

Figure 15.4 A unilateral left-sided duct is depicted by application of contrast medium through a 4 French right Judkins catheter.

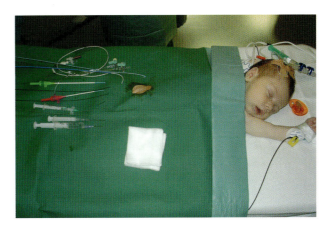

Figure 15.5 A newborn, with hypoplastic left heart complicated by endocardial fibroelastosis with duct-dependent systemic blood flow, prepared for percutaneous duct stenting. The patient is spontaneously breathing and sedated with diazepam and ketamine. Depicted are the usual used materials for puncture of the femoral artery and vein: local anesthesia syringe, 4 and 5 French Terumo introducer sheaths, multipurpose, right Judkins, and wedge-catheters, all in 4 French sizes. Prostaglandin E1 is still being infused by iv line at the head (the parents gave written consent for publishing the picture).

the transverse arch. In terms of the interventional risk, in patients with duct-dependent pulmonary circulation, a single or dual pulmonary blood supply, or even a separated pulmonary blood flow to both lungs, has to be known in advance to create a sufficient interventional strategy.

Depending on the institutional experience, procedures are performed under general anesthesia or conscious sedation. In the case of hemodynamically stable patients we prefer them to be spontaneously breathing, particularly those with duct-dependent systemic circulation (Figure 15.5). Diazepam (0.2–0.5 mg/kg) and ketamine (0.2–0.5 mg/kg) in repetitive small single doses are generally sufficient; where prostaglandin is still being infused, the first dose should be as low as possible to avoid apneas.

Prophylactic antibiotic treatment (cefazolin in most patients) is usually recommended. Attention to hemostasis during catheter and wire manipulation is extremely important. After creation of the vascular access and placement of the sheaths, intravenous heparin is routinely administered (50–100 U/kg as a single dose), and after successful stent placement heparin is given continuously in a dose of 300 U/kg over a minimum of 24 hours. Some centers use acetylsalicylic acid (ASA) in a dosage of 1–3–5 mg/kg/day for the long term, as long as stent patency is required. We do not give ASA as cyclo-oxygenase inhibitor routinely in any patient after duct stenting. Since the dose of clopidogrel for newborns is being evaluated, we give this drug in a dose of 0.2 mg/kg/day in newborns with duct-dependent pulmonary circulation, and in patients with duct-dependent systemic circulation only if there is an additional stent placed within the interatrial septum or at the site of aortic coarctation. However, the role of anticoagulation and antiplatelet therapy is still unclear and needs to be determined.

Management of prostaglandin infusion

The management of prostaglandin infusion depends on the morphology of the duct, and should be handled in context of the patient's actual pathophysiology and even of the experience and equipment in the cath lab. According to the current equipment available in our cath lab, we have changed our management of prostaglandin infusion within the last two years. Considering the safety of the patients with duct-dependent circulation, nowadays prostaglandin infusion is stopped immediately before cardiac catheterization or even after placement of the stent. The routinely used dose of prostaglandin infusion in patients with duct-dependent systemic circulation is 10 ng/kg/min. Higher doses are only used to reopen a narrowed duct. In patients with duct-dependent pulmonary blood flow, the routine dosage can be slightly higher (10–20 ng/kg/min) because a prostaglandin-induced decrease in pulmonary vascular resistance is mostly beneficial, in contrast to patients with duct-dependent systemic blood flow. However, a dose that provokes apnea in spontaneously breathing newborns should be avoided. Unfortunately, in many textbooks recommended dosages for prostaglandin E1 range from 50 to even 100 ng/kg/min, which in most patients is dangerous not only in consideration of side-effects such as apnea or fever, but also due to its hemodynamic effects in a spontaneously breathing 'healthy' newborn with duct-dependent systemic or pulmonary blood flow.

The management of prostaglandin therapy can be summarized as follows:

Duct-dependent pulmonary circulation. In patients with pulmonary atresia with intact ventricular septum, the duct is mostly short and straight, and ductal constriction is required in order to grip the stent at deployment. Ideally, the patient should arrive at the catheterization laboratory with the smallest acceptable size of the patent duct; if the duct has not constricted since birth, some constriction should be allowed by stopping the prostaglandin infusion for several hours, and restarting it if some constriction has occurred. In patients presenting after ductal constriction with cyanosis, prostaglandin can be stopped at the beginning of the procedure, or after the duct has been crossed with the guiding wire. In patients with pulmonary atresia and ventricular septum defect, no ductal constriction is required as this duct is long and tortuous. An access for reinitiating or increasing the dose of prostaglandin during the procedure should always be available; in case of acute constriction, local application of a small dose of prostaglandin (bolus from the continuous infusion) can be useful. Enhanced constriction during the procedure can be obtained by administering intravenous ibuprofen (10 mg/kg bolus). However, it has to be noted that the author has no personal experience with ibuprofen use for this purpose.

Duct dependent systemic circulation. Since self-expandable and balloon-expandable stents are available for stenting ducts with a diameter ranging between 5 and 9 mm, the infusion can be stopped immediately before the catheterization in most patients, or even after the stent has been implanted, as mentioned.

Vascular access

Access is usually obtained through a 5–6 French venous and/or 4–5 French arterial short or long sheath. In newborns with duct-dependent systemic circulation, femoral vein access is mostly adequate to advance a self-expandable stent (SinusRepo™, Optimed, Karlsruhe, Germany) through a 5 French short sheath (Terumo™) or a premounted balloon-expandable stent through a short 6 (7) French sheath (Terumo™) or 6 French long sheath (Cordis™). In elective cases with duct-dependent systemic circulation we recommend an additional femoral artery access by placing a 4 French sheath to facilitate percutaneous stent implantation (Figure 15.5) Modern self-expandable stents usable through a 5 French short sheath can also be used by a femoral artery access when it is needed in individual situations, such as in a right-deviated duct (Boucek Type 3).

Vascular access for duct stenting in newborns with duct-dependent pulmonary circulation depends on the position of the duct, the anatomic considerations of the congenital heart disease, and the technical equipment available. The duct that has a more common orientation, arising from the descending aorta, typically seen in patients with pulmonary atresia with intact ventricular septum, or arising from the subclavian artery, is retrogradely stented in most newborns via the femoral artery using a short 7 cm long 4 French sheath (Terumo™), a 25 cm long 4 French sheath (Terumo™), or even a 4 French long sheath (COOK™). For stenting a duct originating from the underside of the inner curve of the transverse aortic arch, axillary access at the same side just opposite to the duct insertion at the aortic arch is very useful. In most patients, a 4 French sheath can be placed after direct puncture of the axillary artery; surgical cut down is only rarely necessary (Figure 15.6). Alternatively, a long multipurpose catheter, cobra-shaped long sheath, or guiding catheter can be used from the femoral artery or venous access.

Materials

Catheter materials used in newborns for percutaneous duct stenting:

Duct-dependent systemic circulation (see also Figure 15.5):

- 4 French short sheath (Terumo) femoral artery access
- 5/6 French short sheath (Terumo) femoral venous access

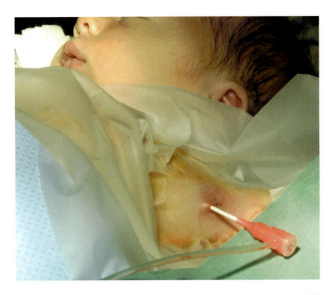

Figure 15.6 A 4 French Terumo sheath is placed in the left axillary artery as an access for duct stenting in a spontaneously breathing newborn with duct-dependent pulmonary circulation. The axillary artery is percutaneously punctured after intravenous analgo-sedation with diazepam and ketamine in small single dosages, and after infiltration of the axillary area by local anesthesia.

- Berman wedge catheter 4 French (transvenously)
- Multipurpose 4 French catheter (transarterial)
- Facultative:
    Berman angiographic catheter 4/5 French
    Pigtail catheters 4 French 0.035 inch lumen
    Judkins R 4 French, 0.035 inch lumen
    Long sheath 6 French (Cordis)
- 0.014 inch floppy guide wire (soft tip; stiff body)
- 0.035 inch guide wire (standard, Terumo)
- Stents:
    SinusRepo™
        7 mm width, lengths 12, 15, 18, 20 mm
        8, 9, 10 mm widths, lengths 18 or 20 mm
        introducer: 5 French short sheath
    Genesis™ (premounted)
        widths 7, 8, 9 mm
        lengths 12, 15, 18/19 mm

Duct-dependent pulmonary circulation:

- 4 French short sheath (Terumo) femoral, axillary artery access
- Cobra 4 French catheter (Terumo, Cordis)
- Facultative:
    Berman angiographic catheter 4 French
    Pigtail catheters 4 French 0.035 inch lumen
    Judkins R 4 French, 0.035 inch lumen
    Balloon-catheter 3 × 20 mm (Maverick™ Boston Scientific)
    Long sheath 4 French (Cook)

Guiding catheter 5 French (Launcher™, Medtronic)
- 0.014 inch floppy guide wire (soft, stiff)
- 0.035 inch guide wire
- Stents: Driver™(Medtronic), Liberte™ (Boston Scientific), 4 (3) mm widths, lengths 9, 12, 15, 18, 22, 24 mm

Choice of stents

When choosing a stent, important features are stent length, diameter, and design. The most distal parts of the duct appear to have a remarkable power to constrict, even when only a few millimeters are left unsupported. Therefore great care must be taken to cover the duct completely from the aortic end until well within the pulmonary trunk, without covering the orifice of the pulmonary arteries. Ideally, the complete duct should be covered by a single stent. In case of incomplete stenting or significant prolapse of tissue through the stent cells, an additional stent should be implanted to cover and open the whole duct. The *stent length* is thus chosen slightly longer than the length of the duct. Determining stent length is usually relatively easy in case of the short, straight duct, but it may be challenging in patients with long and tortuous ducts. In a tortuous vertical duct where the length is not exactly predictable, particularly when the advanced guiding wire will change the ductal shape, ductal stenting should be started at the pulmonary end to be sure that this part of the duct is covered at least. It is often superior to implant two short stents in a telescope technique than to have problems advancing too long a stent. *Stent diameter* will depend on the indication for ductal stenting (duct-dependent pulmonary flow: bilateral vs single lung, or duct-dependent systemic flow), the ductal length and anatomy, and of course the weight of the newborn. In our experience, in the case of most patients with duct-dependent pulmonary circulation, the ductus was stented with a diameter of 4 mm. In newborns with a duct-dependent systemic blood flow the most frequently used stent diameters were 7 and 8 mm, depending on the width of the duct and body weight. In general, the stent diameter is chosen to be 1–2 mm larger than the duct at its narrowest part.

DUCTAL STENTING TO MAINTAIN PULMONARY CIRCULATION

Technique in patients with dual pulmonary blood flow

In newborns with critical pulmonary stenosis or pulmonary atresia and intact ventricular septum, balloon valvuloplasty or perforation and gradual dilatation of the atretic pulmonary valve is generally performed as the initial treatment. If the patients become unacceptably cyanotic with discontinuation of prostaglandin E1, ductal stenting is a reasonable alternative to placement of a surgical shunt or continuation of prostaglandin infusion for days or weeks. The antegrade approach to stenting of the ductus from the femoral vein is preferable for such patients. An additional 4 French arterial catheter is helpful to facilitate accurate placement of the stent. Additionally, a 0.014 inch floppy-tipped guide wire, which is advanced through the duct, can be caught from the arterial site with a 5 mm snare, if necessary. A venous catheter (4 French Judkins, Cobra) is first advanced from the femoral vein, through the right ventricle, in the pulmonary artery, when a floppy 0.014 inch guide wire (preference BMW™, Guidant) is already advanced through the duct, and placed in the descending aorta. An additional excellent angiographic delineation of the length and diameter of the ductus is essential. It has to be underlined that the morphology of the arterial duct predicts the technical difficulty of stenting and the risk of restenosis and necessity for reintervention. As with any complex interventional procedure in neonates, biplane fluoroscopy is recommended. Angiography is typically performed in the lateral projection or lateral-cranial – left anterior oblique 30° and cranial 20–30° – projection (Figure 15.7). Contrast hand injections are usually performed through a transvenously placed right coronary guiding catheter, arterially placed multipurpose catheter, a long 4 French arterial sheath, or with a Berman angiographic catheter by balloon occlusion of the descending aorta below or proximal to the duct prior to wire placement through the duct. A useful landmark during the catheterization for the aortic end of the duct is the arterially advanced multipurpose catheter. Gentle technique should be utilized since spasm of the duct can be induced by any irritation. Flexible coronary stents, premounted on low-profile balloons, are used. Examples include the Driver™ stent (Medtronic, Minneapolis, MN, USA) and the Liberte™ stent (Boston Scientific, Natick, MA, USA). These stents can be implanted through a 5 French (transvenously) guiding catheter such as the Launcher™ (Medtronic), a 4 French (transarterial) 25 cm long sheath (Terumo), or a 4 French long sheath (Cook). However, an optimal premounted stent system is currently not available to stent an *unobstructed* vessel as seen in some ducts under continuous prostaglandin infusion. Not all balloons have satisfactory deflation behavior, and there is a risk of stent dislocation when retrieving the deflated balloon through the stented duct.

When positioning the stent, care should be taken to have a minimal protrusion in the pulmonary artery as well as the aorta. Some protrusion into the aorta is acceptable, as long as the other side of the aortic wall is not touched, as this might lead to a fixed obstruction with coarctation (Figure 15.8). Excessive protrusion can complicate future stent re-entry for redilation (if necessary). The stent should protrude slightly into the pulmonary trunk, but in a patient with pulmonary trunk, the stent should optimally be placed in direction to the bifurcation. It has to be mentioned that

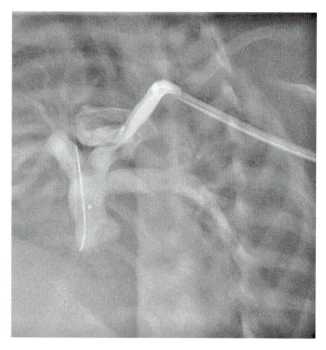

Figure 15.7 Angiogram through a 4 French Terumo sheath placed in the left-sided subclavian artery. Angiography is performed in the lateral-cranial – left anterior oblique 30° and cranial 20° – projection in a newborn with pulmonary atresia. Contrast injection performed by hand shows the subclavian artery, descending aortic arch, and opposite to the subclavian artery the torques duct, in which premounted coronary stent is still advanced directed by a floppy wire positioned to the pulmonary trunk.

creation of a short aorto-pulmonary communication larger than 4 mm has the potential to result in an excessive pulmonary run-off, particularly in newborns with relatively well developed pulmonary arteries, as seen in pulmonary atresia with intact ventricular septum. Typically, a stent with a length between 12 and 18 mm will be used in a mature neonate. In practice, the duct is stented to a diameter of 4 mm for a full-term baby. In babies weighing less than 2.5 kg, the stent diameter should not exceed 3–3.5 mm, especially if the ductal length is less than 10 mm.

However, the final stent lumen will not only depend on the stent diameter at implantation, but will also decrease within hours to days due to contraction of the vessel and tissue prolapse through the stent struts, and will further decrease within weeks to months due to endothelial hyperplasia or peal formation. This has to be considered and, on the other hand, an antifailure treatment should be prepared (i.e. a low-dose of β-blocker) due to increased pulmonary blood flow immediately after stent placement.

In rare cardiovascular malformation in which one pulmonary artery is not connected to the main pulmonary artery but arises from an arterial duct, stenting is an attractive alternative to a surgical shunt. Stent angioplasty enables the adaptation of shunt size to

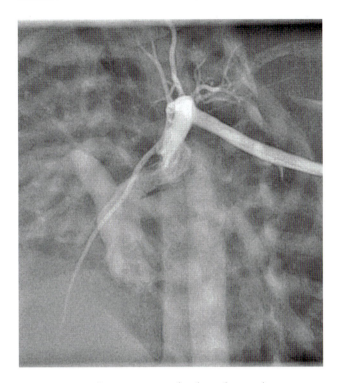

Figure 15.8 Angiogram in the lateral-cranial projection through the 4 French sheath after stent expansion in the same patient as in Figure 15.7.

pulmonary artery growth by serial stent dilations, whereby corrective surgery can be postponed beyond the age of 3 months until pulmonary artery resistance decreases. Stent diameter in a duct to a single lung however, should not be oversized: mostly 3–4 mm is recommended, depending on the duct length and weight of the baby. Larger stents can cause unilateral pulmonary overflow with the possibility of pulmonary hypertension, and can even cause significant steal from the systemic circulation inducing low cardiac output.

Technique in patients with completely ductal-dependent blood flow

The site of access depends on the congenital anomaly and the location of the ductus. Therefore, detailed diagnosis has to be established by two-dimensional and Doppler echocardiography for planning the interventional strategy. Aortic arch angiography, mainly in the anterior-posterior, lateral, and four-chamber views, has to be performed to evaluate the duct morphology and the state of the pulmonary arteries. In case of a 'normal' duct origin from the descending aorta, or even arising from the subclavian artery, the duct can be relatively easily engaged for guide wire anchoring with a 4 French Judkins right coronary or Cobra-shaped catheter. Retrograde duct stenting via the femoral artery is then the preferred access using a 4 French long sheath (Cook) or a 25 cm long 4 French sheath (Terumo).

When the duct has its origin from the underside, inner curve of the transverse aortic arch of the aortic arch as usual, femoral access is also feasible utilizing a 4 French pigtail catheter with its loop cut to give an 'inverted J' which can be used to engage the ductal ampulla. Alternatively, it may be possible to access the aorta antegrade from the femoral vein through the heart utilizing a right Judkins-shaped 5 French guiding catheter or 4 French long sheath (Figure 15.9a and b), but this route makes catheter control more difficult and may cause hemodynamic instability in small neonates by keeping the atrio-ventricular and semilunar valves open. However, in cases with a vertical duct, we prefer an access via the axillary artery route (Figure 15.8). Depending on the position of the duct at the inner curve of the aortic arch in relation to the subclavian arteries, the ipsi- or contralateral subclavian artery is used. Direct puncture of the axillary artery is preferred for placing a 4 French sheath (Terumo) within the subclavian artery. Contrast medium can easily be given by small hand injections through the sheath also during stent positioning. Placement of a floppy-tipped 0.014 inch coronary guide wire through the duct anchored in a distal pulmonary artery branch or looped in the main pulmonary artery is relatively easy by the axillary access using a 4 French Judkins or Cobra catheter for wire guiding.

However, any guide wire is very carefully maneuvered through such a duct. Particularly in this group of patients, the ductus tends to be longer, tortuous, and prompt to spasm with manipulation, so the procedure must be done very carefully. Duct stenting should be a minimally invasive alternative to surgical shunt placement, and it is not a must! A 0.014 inch high-torque floppy coronary wire is strongly recommended; thicker wires have a higher risk of spasm of the duct. This is an additional reason not to stop prostaglandin infusion before the wire or even the premounted stent has crossed the duct. If the duct shows any primary or acquired obstruction prior to stent placement, a trial to cross the duct with a 3 × 20 mm balloon catheter is recommended, and predilation with a 3 mm balloon might be necessary. If there is no chance of crossing the duct with such a balloon catheter, do not try to advance even a premounted stent, instead stop the intervention and send the patient to surgical shunt placement. However, a routine predilation with a balloon catheter is not further recommended. Additionally, the use of a long 4 French sheath, which was previously recommended to be advanced through the duct, is not necessary any longer, since exclusively premounted coronary stents are used for duct stenting. By avoiding this relatively traumatic manipulation, many severe complications of duct stenting are not seen any more. Particularly for stenting long tortuous ducts, the use of low-profile coronary stents with high longitudinal flexibility, high conformability, minimal foreshortening, and minimal recoil is highly beneficial. Stent diameters

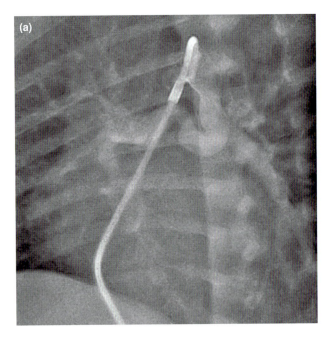

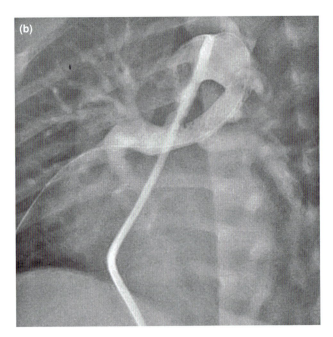

Figure 15.9 Angiogram performed by hand injection of contrast medium through a Judkins catheter depicts a vertical, tortuous duct at the inner curve of the aortic arch. Using a femoral venous access, a 4 French right Judkins catheter was advanced through the heart and placed in the aortic arch before (a) duct stenting. (b) The angiogram was performed through a 4 French long sheath (COOK) after stent placement; in context of the overestimated torque duct length, the utilized stent chosen was too long, but was uneventfully placed into the right pulmonary artery. The left pulmonary artery was perfused through the struts of the stent without negative sequelae for the left pulmonary vessel growth.

need to range from 3 to 5 mm and the lengths from 9 to 24 mm. In very long tortuous ducts, placement of two stents by a telescope technique is preferable to a trial with one too long premounted stent. Our experience is mostly with the Driver™ 4 mm coronary stent in different lengths. In this context, before stent placement is considered further, duct tortuosity and shape, the diameter at the duct's narrowest point (usually its insertion into the pulmonary artery), and its length have to be determined and measured by the angiographic data.

For selection of the correct stent length additional angiography is helpful when the guide wire is already placed, as the guide wire tends to straighten a tortuous duct. In case the duct preferentially perfuses one (left) side of the lung it seems to be better to advance the wire to the lesser perfused (right) lung. However, in most ducts the stent has to be implanted so that 2–3 mm of the stent protrude into the main pulmonary artery and the whole length of the ductus should be covered up to the ductal–aortic junction.

Patients with this type of duct frequently have a hypoplastic pulmonary trunk and a small bifurcation, with ductal tissue extending into the pulmonary arteries; this will result in stenosis early after discontinuation of prostaglandins. These patients were classically treated with bilateral shunts or a single shunt after plasty of the bifurcation on bypass. If stenting is chosen, the stent should preferably be advanced into the stenotic pulmonary artery, allowing perfusion of the

other lung through the stent struts, or alternatively have a stented duct to one lung, and a surgical shunt to the other lung, which avoids the need for surgical shunt creation by cardiopulmonary bypass. Despite all these techniques, some of the complex ducts with many turns remain very challenging and cannot be stented safely; this subgroup might remain the domain of surgical shunting.

Duct-dependent systemic circulation

For duct stenting in newborns with duct-dependent systemic circulation femoral venous access is the approach of choice (Figure 15.5). Placement of a femoral artery 4 French sheath serves both to monitor the blood pressure and for positioning of a multipurpose catheter in the duct–aortic junction. Angiographies performed by using an open ended 4 French wedge catheter positioned in the pulmonary trunk, and the multipurpose catheter placed in the descending aortic arch, allow a sufficient delineation of the duct morphology. The 90° lateral view and the 30° right anterior oblique view demonstrate the ductal anatomy very well; the right anterior oblique view particularly delineaties its junction with the distal aortic arch (Figure 15.10). This strategy reduces the interventional time for duct stenting dramatically, in addition to increasing the safety. It is no longer necessary to advance a Berman angiographic catheter by crossing

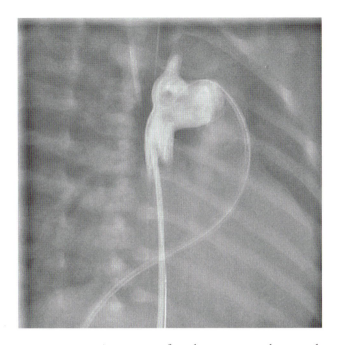

Figure 15.10 Angiogram of a duct in a newborn with hypoplastic left heart syndrome before duct stenting in the 30° right anterior oblique projection. The junction of the ductus arteriosus to the distal descending aortic arch is shown by hand injection of contrast medium through an arterially placed 4 French multipurpose catheter. A second multipurpose catheter was positioned in the duct and advanced transvenously by using a 0.014 inch floppy guide wire.

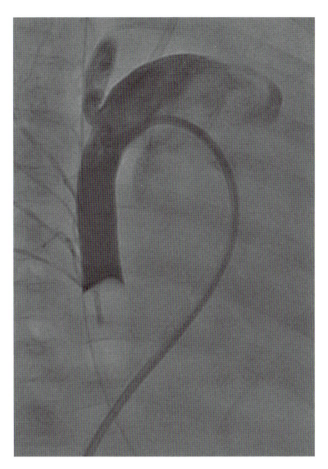

Figure 15.11 Angiogram of the duct to descending aorta junction by blocking the thoracic descending aorta during injection of contrast medium. A 4 French Berman angiography catheter was advanced from the femoral venous access by crossing the duct in the descending aorta.

the duct in the descending aorta to perform a balloon occlusion angiogram to profile the duct (Figure 15.11). Even a long sheath, previously used in a size of up to 7 French, is not routinely necessary any more for duct stenting, since modern balloon-expandable or self-expandable stents are available. In general, balloon-expandable stents are preferred if the advancement over the wire is comparable to the positioning of the self-expandable stents, and if the deflated balloon can be retrieved without the risk of the stent slipping in an unconstricted duct. Self-expandable stents, such as the nitinol SinusRepo™ stent (OptiMed, Karlsruhe, Germany), are therefore preferred for ductal stenting in large ducts without any constriction (Figure 15.12). Such stents can currently be advanced through a short 5 French venous sheath over a 0.014 inch guide wire. SinusRepo™ nitinol stents with a diameter of 7 mm are available in lengths of 12, 15, 18, and 20 mm. Self-expandable stents with a diameter of 8, 9, and 10 mm are commercially available in a length of 20 mm, and custom made in an additional length of 18 mm; a further advantage of the SinusRepo™ design is its 'anti-jump' mechanism, which allows stent retrieval after nearly 80% of stent expansion and facilitates repositioning if necessary. The diameter of the stents used is chosen to be at least 1–2 mm larger than the minimal ductal diameter, and even larger than the diameter of the

descending aorta. This last recommendation is of particular importance when stenting the duct of newborns with an interrupted aortic arch. This results in the implantation of stents with a diameter of 7 mm in most cases, particularly in newborns with a birth weight less than 2.5 kg, even in premature neonates less than 1.5 kg in weight. In patients where the ductal diameter measures 8–9 mm without any constriction, a 9 or 10 mm self-expandable stent should be implanted (also in patients with ductal aneurysms).

It is recommended that premounted Genesis™ stents (Cordis) should be used if some ductal constriction is seen either at the pulmonary or the aortic end. In an asymmetrically constricted duct a self-expandable stent may slip to the descending aorta or pulmonary trunk due to the nitinol material being still active after release. Genesis™ stents are available in lengths of 12, 15, 18, 19 and 20 mm, premounted on 7, 8, 9 or (10) mm balloons that can be advanced through a short 6 or 7 French venous sheath over a 0.035 inch guide wire. It is not necessary to advance through a long sheath because of the tightly fixed stent. Small injections of contrast medium through the

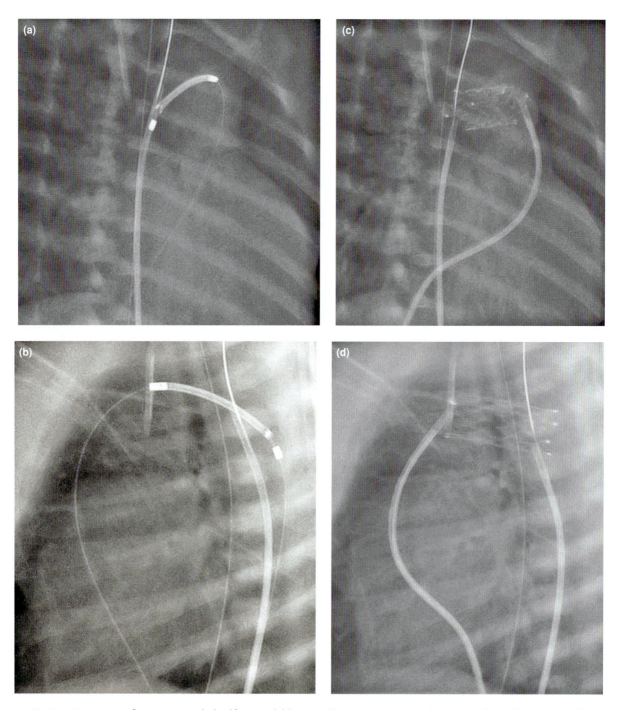

Figure 15.12 Depiction of a non-expanded self-expandable stent (SinusRepo™ nitinol stent) in the right anterior oblique 30° projection, guided by a 4 French multipurpose catheter placed in the descending aortic arch. The arterial catheter guided by a wire gives a landmark during duct stenting, and avoids overstenting of the descending aortic arch. (b) The 90° lateral view before releasing the self-expandable stent; the covered stent is advanced from the femoral venous access, guided by a 0.014 inch floppy wire. The lateral view is necessary to estimate the pulmonary part of the duct given by a landmark – here the central venous catheter is still in place; this view does not allow determination of the duct–aortic junction, as seen by the unpredictable relation of the arterial multipurpose catheter to the positioned stent. (c and d) The same projections as shown in (a) and (b), but after stent release.

arterially placed multipurpose catheter can be helpful in positioning the stent in the desired location (Figure 15.13).

Early in the experience of hybrid procedures, ductal stenting was mostly performed in advance of surgical bilateral banding. However, most centers now recommend that ductal stenting is done after banding due to the risk of stent dislocation during intraoperative manipulation; in the setting of a surgical–interventional hybrid procedure, the stent can be deployed through a direct arteriotomy of the pulmonary trunk through the sternotomy.[32]

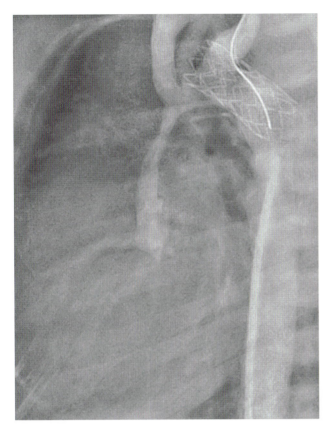

Figure 15.13 An expanded Genesis balloon-expandable stent is optimally placed within the duct in a newborn with hypoplastic left heart syndrome. Small injections of contrast medium through the arterially placed multipurpose catheter can be helpful in positioning the stent in the desired location.

CHECKLISTS TO AVOID COMPLICATIONS AND PITFALLS

Duct-dependent pulmonary circulation

1. Well-defined long-term therapeutical goal (biventricular or univentricular repair), and exactly planed strategy for the intervention of duct stenting.
2. Adequate vascular access in context of the duct origin from the aortic arch (vertical!).
3. Precise evaluation of the duct's morphology (tortuous, obstructed, or even unobstructed), exact determination of the duct length, the narrowest as well as the widest part, and precise evaluation of the pulmonary as well as the aortic–duct junction.
4. Optimal angle of the delivery sheath to the duct entrance; stable guide wire position by choosing a guide wire with a soft, but stable tip and a stiff, smooth gliding shaft, positioned perhaps with a wire loop distal in a pulmonary artery with prevalence to the side of the lung with the lowest blood flow.
5. Avoiding duct spasm by a gentle advance of the guide wire through a tortuous or even narrowed duct which is still being treated with a continuous prostaglandin E infusion.
6. Avoiding stent dislodgement during stent expansion by anticipation of an inhomogeneous duct lumen or even by careful retrieval of a non-optimal deflated balloon, particularly by stenting an unobstructed duct.
7. Anticipation of an immediate or late-onset pulmonary run-off due to an underestimated aorto-pulmonary shunt (stent) lumen in total in context of a dual or multiple lung supply, or in context of the neonatal physiology (persistent pulmonary hypertension postnatally, but with the tendency of a dramatic decrease days later).
8. Considering inhomogeneous lung perfusion by stenting a duct in a newborn with genuine or acquired pulmonary arterial stenosis.
9. Becoming aware of acute or chronic in-stent stenosis, or reconstriction of uncovered duct parts after discontinuation of the prostaglandin infusion or by an acute stent thrombosis.

Duct-dependent systemic circulation

1. Well defined long-term therapeutic goal and prepared strategy for the intervention.
2. Adequate vascular access using the femoral vein for placement of a 5 or 6 French sheath, and the femoral artery for placing a short 4 French sheath, particularly in an electively treated patient.
3. Precise evaluation of the duct's morphology by angiography in the right anterior oblique 30° projection and the 90° lateral projection (leftward, mesoverted, or rightward duct orientation); evaluation of an unrestricted duct or even a duct with a stenosis at the pulmonary, aortic, or mid duct part.
4. Exact determination of the duct length, the narrowest as well as the widest part, and precise evaluation of the duct–aortic junction; best by using a double catheter technique placed in the pulmonary trunk and within the descending aortic arch.
5. Choice of a self-expandable or balloon-expandable stent depending on the duct anatomy with or without obstruction.
6. Placement of a 0.014 inch stable guide wire with a soft, but stable tip and a stiff, smooth gliding shaft to advance a SinusRepo™ self-expandable stent from the venous access, or even a 0.035 inch guide wire to deploy a Genesis balloon-expandable

stent. In some cases, e.g. rightward stent or complex heart malformation, guide wire placement can also be obtained from the arterial side for duct stenting through the femoral artery (5 or 6 French short sheath)

7. Avoiding hemodynamic instability by indwelling/crossing a 4 French wedge catheter with an inflated balloon through the tricuspid valve and by gentle advancement of a 0.014 inch guide wire in the pulmonary trunk and through the duct in the descending aorta in most patients still treated with continuous prostaglandin E infusion. When the wire is correctly placed and the balloon catheter removed, the facility to advance a 4 French right Judkins or a 4 French multipurpose catheter through the tricuspid valve, right ventricular outflow tract, and the duct indicates the feasibility of the placement of a self-expandable or, even more importantly, of a premounted balloon-expandable stent without a long sheath covering.

8. Avoiding stent dislodgement during stent expansion by anticipating an inhomogeneous duct lumen or even by careful retrieval of a non-optimal deflated balloon, particularly by stenting an unobstructed duct with a balloon-expandable stent.

9. Anticipation of an immediate or late-onset obstruction of the duct caused by either an uncovered duct part or even an in-stent stenosis.

10. Becoming aware of acute and chronic stenosis, or reconstriction of uncovered duct parts after discontinuation of the prostaglandin infusion or by an acute stent thrombosis. The same is true in consideration of an early or late obstruction compromising a retrograde aortic arch perfusion.

CURRENT STATUS OF DUCTAL STENTING

Stenting of the ductus arteriosus for patients with either ductal-dependent systemic or pulmonary circulation is still not standard of care in most pediatric heart centers; but in some particularly experienced hands duct stenting has achieved a real role in the management of complex types of congenital heart disease.

The need for stenting the ductus in patients with left ventricular obstruction, i.e. hypoplastic left heart syndrome (HLHS), in our judgement implies that the patient will undergo the hybrid approach as an alternative to a classical Norwood procedure or even cardiac transplantation if an active cardiac transplantation program is established.

Ductal stenting in duct-dependent patients obviously still needs to be compared in a prospective randomized study with the standard surgical shunt. Therefore the interventional approach performed with the goal of being a minimally invasive alternative to a surgical shunt is currently not stressed as 'a must approach.'

Duct-dependent pulmonary circulation

The stented arterial duct fulfills its function as a surrogate for an aorto-pulmonary shunt, augmenting the pulmonary blood flow until a definitive surgical procedure can be performed or until the duct flow becomes redundant. In experienced hands, duct stenting seems to be feasible in about 80–90% of cases, the most challenging ducts being the long tortuous ducts in pulmonary atresia and ventricular septal defect. In addition, such a minimally invasive alternative may only be possible by using the currently best available materials and by choosing a variable arterial/venous access depending on the duct morphology and its position. Only then is this approach less invasive and offers the possibility of adapting to clinical needs in the individual patient compared to primary surgery. Compared to long-term prostaglandin infusion, early ductal stenting significantly shortens hospitalization and reduces treatment costs. The lumen of a stented duct appears to narrow faster than a surgical shunt. However, the stented duct can be redilated and restented, which allows titration of pulmonary flow to patient size and growth. Such redilation/restenting must obviously be considered when assessing the cost effectiveness of each strategy.

During follow-up no distortion of the pulmonary arteries has been seen and technical problems due to the stent are not encountered at subsequent surgeries, as the stent can easily be occluded by simple external compression.

Duct-dependent systemic circulation

Neonates with heart defects suitable for univentricular repair can benefit from this hybrid transcatheter surgical palliation, having the Norwood type of aortic reconstruction done beyond the neonatal period at the same time as the bidirectional superior caval anastomosis. Particularly in patients presenting with neonatal cardiogenic shock or other high-risk factors, percutaneous ductal stenting as part of this hybrid approach significantly improved early survival. In addition, patients with variants of the hypoplastic left heart complex, in whom the immediate postnatal decision regarding a uni- or biventricular approach is ambiguous, or who carry a high risk when biventricular repair is performed in the neonatal period, may have a major benefit from the strategy of primary hybrid transcatheter/surgical palliation·

In fact, there was and there still is room for further technical improvements for ductal stenting. However, since the use of the self-expandable Sinus-Repo™ nitinol-stents and the balloon-expandable Genesis™ stents for ductal stenting, the technique has really improved.

Considering the importance of a sufficient retrograde aortic perfusion (cerebral and coronary perfusion), patients with severe stenosis of the aortic isthmus may require either simultaneous stenting of the isthmus or creation of a 'reversed shunt' between the pulmonary trunk and the aortic arch at the time of the sternotomy for bilateral banding.

CONCLUSIONS AND PERSPECTIVES

Cognizant of the limitations of the current techniques used for duct stenting in duct-dependent pulmonary as well as systemic circulation, but recognizing also the improved features of stents and delivery systems, PDA stenting in neonates has already today become a reasonable alternative for initial palliation of complex heart disease. Duct stenting is an alternative to systemic to pulmonary shunts in securing pulmonary blood flow in duct-dependent cyanotic heart disease, and an alternative to a Norwood–Sano approach in newborns with hypoplastic left heart syndrome in securing systemic blood flow embedded in a surgical interventional hybrid approach.

The worldwide experience of ductal stenting in patients with either duct-dependent pulmonary or systemic circulation has significantly increased over the past years. In this context, these techniques deserve further evaluation.

However, in view of the rapid technical progress in the development of absorbable stents and the creation of new techniques for catheter-based drug deliveries, together with the extensive international exchange of interventional surgical experiences, PDA stenting has and will have a direct impact on improved results. Therefore, in future, this technique will be fully established as a minimally invasive approach to treat newborns with complex heart disease.

REFERENCES

1. Blalock A, Taussig H. The surgical treatment of malformations of the heart in which there is pulmonary stenosis or pulmonary atresia. JAMA 1945; 128: 189–202.
2. Fermanis GG, Ekangaki AK, Salmon AP et al. Twelve year experience with the modified Blalock–Taussig shunt in neonates. Eur J Cardiothorac Surg 1992; 6: 586–9.
3. Al Jubair KA, AlFagih MR, Jarallah AS et al. Results of 546 Blalock–Taussig shunts performed in 478 patients. Cardiol Young 1998; 8(4): 486–90.
4. Norwood WI, Lang P, Castaneda AR, Campell DN. Experience with operations for hypoplastic left heart syndrome. J Thorac Cardiovasc Surg 1981; 82: 511–19.
5. Griselli M, McGuirk S, Stümper O et al. Influence of surgical strategies on outcome after the Norwood procedure. J Thorac Cardiovasc Surg 2006; 131: 418–26.
6. Stasik CN, Goldberg CS, Bove EL, Devaney EJ, Ohye RG. Current outcomes and risk factors for the Norwood procedure. J Thorac Cardiovasc Surg 2006; 131: 412–17.
7. Ballweg JA, Dominguez TE, Ravishanker C et al. A contemporary comparison of the effect of shunt type in hypoplastic left heart syndrome on the hemodynamics and outcome at stage 2 reconstruction. J Thorac Cardiovasc Surg 2007; 134: 297–303.
8. Rudolph AM, Heymann MA, Fishman N, Lakier JB. Formalin infiltration of the ductus arteriosus: a method for palliation of infants with selected congenital cardiac lesions. N Engl J Med 1975; 292: 1263–8.
9. Lund G, Rysavy J, Cragg A et al. Long-term patency of the ductus arteriosus after balloon dilatation: an experimental study. Circulation 1984; 69: 772–4.
10. Walsh KP, Abrams SE, Arnold R. Arterial duct angioplasty as an adjunct to dilatation of the valve for critical pulmonary stenosis. Br Heart J 1993; 69: 260–2.
11. Radtke W, Anderson RR, Guerrero L, Heintzen PH. Creation of a palliative shunt by thermal balloon angioplasty of the ductus arteriosus. In: Proceedings of 26th Annual General Meeting of the Association of European Pediatric Cardiologist, Oslo, Norway, June 1990.
12. Moore JW, Kirby WC, Lovett EJ, O'Neill JT. Use of an intravascular prothesis (stent) to establish and maintain short-term patency of the ductus arteriosus in new born lambs. Cardiovasc Intervent Radiol 1991; 14: 299–301.
13. Coe JY, Olley PM. A novel method to maintain ductus arteriosus patency. J Am Coll Cardiol 1991; 18: 837–41.
14. Ruiz CE. Ductal stents in the management of congenital heart defects. Cathet Cardiovasc Intervent 2001; 53: 75–80.
15. Gibbs JL, Rothman MT, Rees MR et al. Stenting of the arterial duct: a new approach to palliation for pulmonary atresia. Br Heart J 1992; 67: 240–5.
16. Gibbs JL, Wren C, Watterson KG, Hunter S, Hamilton JRL. Stenting of the arterial duct combined with banding of the pulmonary arteries and atrial septectomy or septostomy: a new approach to palliation for the hypoplastic left heart syndrome. Br Heart J 1993; 69: 551–5.
17. Ruiz CE, Gamra H Zhang HP, Garcia EJ, Boucek MM. Brief report: stenting of the ductus arteriosus as a bridge to cardiac transplantation in infants with hypoplastic left-heart syndrome. N Engl J Med 1993; 328: 1605–8.
18. Gibbs JL, Uzun O, Blackburn MEC et al. Fate of the stented arterial duct. Circulation 1999; 99: 2621–5.
19. Ruiz CE, Bailey LL. Stenting the ductus arteriosus: a 'wannabe' Blalock–Taussig. Circulation 1999; 99: 2608–9.
20. Schneider M, Zartner P, Sidiropoulos A, Konertz W, Hausdorf G. Stent implantation of the arterial duct in newborns with duct-dependent circulation. Eur Heart J 1998; 19: 1401–9.
21. Akintuerk H, Michel-Behnke I, Valeske K et al. Stenting of the arterial duct and banding of the pulmonary arteries. Basis for combined Norwood stage I and II repair in hypoplastic left heart. Circulation 2002; 105: 1099–103.
22. Michel-Behnke I, Akitürck H, Marquardt I et al. Stenting of the ductus arteriosus and banding of the pulmonary arteries: basis for various surgical strategies in newborns with multiple left heart obstructive lesions. Heart 2003; 89(6): 645–50.
23. Michel-Behnke I, Akitürck H, Thul J et al. Stent implantation in the ductus arteriosus for pulmonary blood supply in congenital heart disease. Cathet Cardiovasc Interven 2004; 61(2): 242–52.
24. Gewillig M, Boshoff DE, Dens J, Mertens L, Benson LN. Stenting the neonatal arterial duct in duct-dependent pulmonary circulation: new techniques, better results. J Am Coll Cardiol 2004; 43: 107–12.
25. Alwi M, Choo KK, Latiff HA et al. Initial results and medium-term follow-up of stent implantation of patent ductus

arteriosus in duct-dependent pulmonary circulation. J Am Coll Cardiol 2004; 44(2): 438–45.

26. Alwi M, Kandavello G, Choo K et al. Risk factors for augmentation of the flow of blood to the lungs in pulmonary atresia with intact ventricular septum after radiofrequency valvotomy. Cardiol Young 2005; 15: 141–7.

27. Mahesh K, Kannan BR, Vaidyanathan B et al. Stenting the patent arterial duct to increase pulmonary blood flow. Ind Heart J 2005; 57(6): 704–8.

28. Santoro G, Bigazzi MC, Cainiello G et al. Transcatheter palliation of congenital heart disease with reduced pulmonary blood flow. Ital Heart J 2005; 6(1): 35–40.

29. Quereshi SA. Catheterization in neonates with pulmonary atresia with intact ventricular septum. Cathet Cardiovasc Interven 2006; 67(6): 924–31.

30. Bacha EA, Hijazi ZM, Cao QL et al. Hybrid pediatric cardiac surgery. Pediatr Cardiol 2005; 26: 315–22.

31. Boucek MM, Mashburn C, Kunz E, Chan KC. Ductal anatomy. A determinant of successful stenting in hypoplastic left heart syndrome. Pediatr Cardiol 2005; 26(2): 200–5.

32. Galantowicz M, Cheatham JP. Lessons learned from the development of a new hybrid strategy for the management of hypoplastic left heart syndrome. Pediatr Cardiol 2005; 26: 190–9.

33. Lim DS, Peeler BB, Matherne GP, Kron IL, Gutgesell HP. Risk-stratified approach to hybrid transcatheter-surgical palliation of hypoplasrtic left heart syndrome. Pediatr Cardiol 2006; 27: 91–5.

34. Bacha EA, Daves S, Hardin J et al. Single-ventricle palliation for high-risk neonates: the emergence of an alternative hybrid stage I strategy. J Thorac Cardiovasc Surg 2006; 131: 163–71.

35. Chan KC, Mashburn RN, Boucek MM. Initial transcatheter palliation of hypoplastic left heart syndrome. Cathet Cardiovasc Interven 2006; 68(5): 719–26.

36. Akintuerk H, Michel-Behnke I, Valeske K et al. Hybrid transcatheter-surgical palliation; basis for univentricular or biventricular repair, the Giessen experience. Pediatr Cardiol 2007; 28: 79–87.

37. Boshoff DE, Michel-Behnke I, Schranz D, Gewillig M. Stenting the neonatal duct. Expert Rev Cardiovasc Ther 2007; 5(5): 893–901.

16 Complications of transcatheter atrial septal defect closure

Christian Spies, Qi-Ling Cao, and Ziyad M Hijazi

INTRODUCTION

The Amplatzer® Septal Occluder (ASO) (AGA Medical Corporation, Plymouth, MN) is a self-expanding and self-centering occlusion device consisting of a Nitinol meshwork forming a left atrial disc, a self-centering stent, and a right atrial disc.[1] The ASO was the first device approved by the US Food and Drug Administration (FDA) for percutaneous closure of secundum atrial septal defects (ASDs). Due to its ease of transcatheter deployment and the effectiveness of shunt closure it has gained widespread acceptance among interventionalists. However, complications, both acute and chronic occur, which will be reviewed in this chapter.

Based on the diameter of the ASO's waist, there are different sizes available, ranging from 4 to 40 mm. A 6–12 French sheath is required for device deployment depending on the size of the device used. Eighty-one to 325 mg acetylsalicylic acid is started 2 days prior to the planned procedure and is given for 6 months following ASD closure. Clopidogrel is also given to adult patients on the day of procedure and is continued for 1 to 3 months. ASD closure is performed under fluoroscopic and echocardiographic guidance, using either transesophageal (TEE) or intracardiac (ICE) echocardiographic guidance. After placement of two 6 and 8 French sheaths in the right femoral vein (if TEE is used, only one sheath is needed) heparin is given and a full shunt run is performed. An angiogram in the hepatoclavicular projection with the catheter tip positioned in the right upper pulmonary vein is performed to profile the septum and the ASD. A sizing balloon is placed within the ASD in order to measure the 'stop-flow diameter.' If the defect has adequate rims (see below) a device 0–2 mm larger than the balloon stretched diameter is chosen. We now routinely deploy the ASO without balloon sizing. We usually choose a device about 20–30% larger than the two-dimensional size of the defect estimated by color Doppler. Following positioning of the delivery sheath in the left superior pulmonary vein, the ASO is introduced and deployed under echocardiographic and fluoroscopic guidance. After successful implantation, a secure position is confirmed by a pull-and-push maneuver (Minnesota wiggle) of the device. Further,

residual shunting and correct placement are assessed by echocardiography. The device is then released from the delivery system, and the final position is documented using echocardiography and fluoroscopy.

HOW TO AVOID COMPLICATIONS?

The first and probably most important part of avoiding complications is proper preselection of patients prior to attempting ASD closure. Aside from identifying the standard indications and contraindications for transcatheter ASD closure with the ASO (Table 16.1), a thorough evaluation of the size and rims of the defect, the number of defects, and of any combined potentially complicating anatomy is made by TEE by in adults. Transthoracic echocardiography in children is often sufficient for patient preselection. The perfect ASD for transcatheter closure is less than 20 mm in diameter with firm and adequate rims and a greater than 5 mm distance from the margins of important surrounding structures (mitral and tricuspid valves, inferior and superior vena cava, right upper pulmonary vein, and coronary sinus). In adults, ASDs up to 40 mm diameter can be closed effectively with the ASO. However, closure of very large ASDs frequently requires modifications of the standard deployment technique utilizing additional maneuvers in order to avoid prolapse of the left atrial disc through the ASD to the right atrium (Table 16.2).

Although firm and sufficiently large rims of an ASD are desirable, the interventionalist is frequently confronted with flimsy or deficient rims, making placement more difficult. A deficient anterior rim toward the aorta is not considered a contraindication for ASO placement. In a comparison of patients with sufficient rims with those without, defined as less than 5 mm, we were able to show that transcatheter closure of ASDs with small anterior, inferior, or posterior rims is feasible.[2] As long as there are three sufficient rims, the ASO seats well and effectively eliminates the shunt.

The most frequently encountered anatomic variant potentially complicating device deployment is an atrial septal aneurysm. Theoretically, atrial septal aneurysms can lead to a greater likelihood of residual shunting

Table 16.1 Indications and contraindications of ASD closure with the ASO.

Indications

1. Symptomatic or hemodynamically significant shunt (Qp/Qs > 1.5) and/or right ventricle volume overload as shown by transthoracic echocardiography
2. Patients with a small ASD and a history of paradoxical embolism resulting in either a stroke, transient ischemic attack, or peripheral embolism

Contraindications

1. Patients with an associated anomalous pulmonary venous drainage
2. Patients with a sinus venosus defect or primum ASD
3. A deficient rim (<5 mm) from the ASD to the superior or inferior vena cava, right upper or lower pulmonary vein, coronary sinus, mitral or tricuspid valve (a deficient anterior rim toward the aorta is not a contraindication for the ASO)
4. Associated other cardiac anomalies requiring surgical repair
5. Pulmonary vascular resistance of greater than 8 Woods units
6. Sepsis
7. Contraindication to antiplatelet therapy

and the risk of device embolization. Hence, most operators would choose a slightly larger device to stabilize the septum.

Other important structures to look out for during device closure are anomalous pulmonary venous drainage and a Chiari network. If there is a large Chiari network, care must be exercised not to entangle the delivery sheath and/or delivery cable through the network. Upon release of the device it is important to keep only a short distance between the tip of the delivery sheath and the ASO. Otherwise part of the Chiari network can get caught by the screw mechanism and the network fibers can get tangled around the delivery cable, making removal following ASO release difficult.

Necessary personnel and equipment involved in the procedure are of importance to achieve a successful outcome and to prevent complications. The interventional cardiologist needs to be familiar with echocardiography. Preferably, an experienced non-invasive cardiologist versed in congenital and structural heart disease should assist in image interpretation during the procedure. Finally, a fully equipped catheterization laboratory is mandatory with all equipment required for the standard procedure and possible complications (Table 16.3).

Table 16.2 Maneuvers to facilitate closure of very large atrial septal defects.

Maneuver	Description	Reference
Hausdorf sheath	The Hausdorf sheath (Cook, Bloomington, IN) is a specially designed long sheath with two posterior curves at its end, allowing for a better alignment of the left atrial disc parallel to the septum	22
Boosfeld sheath	This is a modified Mullins sheath with the creation of a bevel at the inner curvature, also allowing a more parallel alignment of the left atrial disc to the interatrial septum	23
Right upper pulmonary vein (RUPV) technique	The delivery sheath is placed in the RUPV and the left atrial disc is partially deployed. The sheath is then quickly retracted to deploy the remaining left disc; this results in the disc jumping into a location parallel to the septum	24
Left upper pulmonary vein (LUPV) technique	The delivery sheath is placed in the LUPV and the left atrial disc is partially deployed to create an 'American football'-like appearance. With further withdrawal of the sheath, the disc jumps parallel to the septum	25
Wahab technique	Following deployment of the left atrial disc, a long dilator is advanced into the left atrium, holding the superior anterior part of the left atrial disc to prevent it from prolapsing	26
Balloon-assisted technique	Similar to the dilator assisted method (Wahab technique), a balloon catheter is used following deployment of the left atrial disc to prevent its prolapse by holding the superior anterior part of the left atrial disc	27
Right Judkins catheter technique	The device (<16 mm) is advanced via an 8 French Judkins right catheter through a delivery sheath into the left atrium. Following removal of the sheath and deployment of the left disc, the assembly aligns to the septum	22

Table 16.3 List of equipment required for the ASD closure procedure.

- Full range of ASO devices
- ICE catheter or TEE probe
- 18 G access needle
- 6–8 French 11 cm sheaths
- 6–12 French Amplatzer delivery systems with sheaths
- 8–12 French Mullins sheaths
- 10–12 French Hausdorf sheaths
- 7 French balloon-tipped wedge catheter
- 7 French multipurpose (MP-A) diagnostic catheter
- 8 French JR 4.0 guide catheter (largest inner lumen: 0.098 inch).
- Regular J-tipped 0.035 inch 190 cm wire
- Amplatz super stiff 0.035 inch 260 cm wire
- Terumo glide wire 0.035 inch 190 cm
- Amplatzer 18, 24, and 34 mm sizing balloons
- Alternatively NuMED 20–40 mm sizing balloons
- Amplatzer exchange (rescue) system: 9 and 12 French
- Amplatz goose neck snares 5–25 mm diameter

COMPLICATIONS OF ATRIAL SEPTAL DEFECT CLOSURE USING THE ASO

In experienced hands, acute major complications are rare during transcatheter ASD closure. In the US multicenter pivotal trial that led to FDA approval of the ASO, the rate of major complications was 1.6% in the group of patients undergoing transcatheter ASD closure.[3] The rate of minor complications was 6.1%. In a large series of ASD closure by Chessa et al., using a patient population that underwent ASD closure with the ASO and the CardioSEAL®/STARFlex® device, the major complication rate was slightly higher at 2.6% (total complication rate 8.6%).[4] However, half of the complications were due to device embolization or malposition, and the authors noted that the majority of embolizations occurred with larger CardioSEAL/STARFlex devices, suggesting a device-related problem of these umbrella-like closure devices. Transcatheter ASD closure in small children also seems safe with the ASO with comparable complication rates, except for patients weighing less than 10 kg, when minor complications seem to be more common.[5] In comparison with open surgical ASD repair, complication rates of transcatheter ASD closure appear favorable. During the US multicenter trial of the ASO, the total complication rate in the surgical group was 24%, with major complications occurring in 5.4% of patients, compared to 7.2% total complications and 1.6% for major ones in the transcatheter ASD closure group.[3] In a large study, including 1284 open surgical and transcatheter ASD closure procedures, the complication rates were also favorable for the latter group, with 16% and 3.6% major complications, respectively.[6] Variation in the reported rates of major complications is mainly due to different definitions of 'major complications,' as for example some authors include all cases of device embolization in this group, while others only consider surgically retrieved embolized ASD occluders to be a major complication.

Device embolization

In an attempt to estimate the incidence of ASO embolizations, Levi and Moore surveyed AGA approved ASO proctors regarding their experience with device embolization.[7] They identified 21 device embolizations in 3824 procedures, translating into an incidence of 0.55%. Embolizations occurred almost exclusively in the periprocedural period, although two cases of ASO embolizations that occurred up to one year following defect closure have been reported.[4,8] According to Levi and Moore's report, most embolizations occurred into the right or left atrium and the great majority could be retrieved percutaneously (15 of 21 devices). The majority of embolizations were a function of either large defects or undersized devices, or occurred in patients with ASDs with inadequate rims. Mostly, the dislocated device did not cause hemodynamic compromise and snaring and percutaneous retrieval of the device could be attempted safely.

The first step in device retrieval is to move the ASO into a position where it will cause no harm. The delivery sheath should be exchanged for at least 2 French sizes larger than the delivery sheath used. We prefer rigid long Mullins sheaths. Using a Gooseneck snare (eV3, Plymouth, MN), the screw at the right atrial disc needs to be snared. In general, devices that embolize into the atria should be pulled into the inferior vena cava (IVC) inside a sheath. If the device embolizes into the left ventricle it should be moved back into the left atrium via a long sheath. Once the device is in a retrievable position the screw of the right atrial disc is snared and is pulled into the retrieval sheath. Perpendicular alignment of the micro screw of the right atrial disc to the orifice of the sheath is important. Once the screw of the ASO is within the sheath, the device is pulled forcefully into the sheath and externalized. For large devices (>34 mm), one may need at least a 16 French sheath or larger (Figures 16.1–16.4) to collapse the device inside the sheath.

Cardiac perforation and erosion

The most dreaded complication is cardiac perforation secondary to transcatheter ASD closure, resulting in pericardial effusion, tamponade, hemodynamic collapse, and possible death.[9] Two mechanisms of cardiac

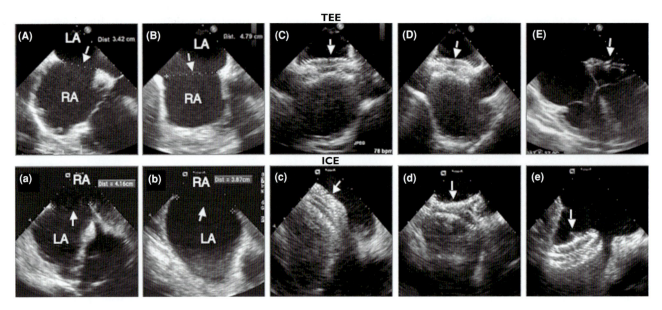

Figure 16.1 Echocardiographic images of a 28-year-old male patient with large secundum atrial septal defect (ASD). Top panel (A–E) Transesophageal echocardiographic (TEE) images. Bottom panel (a–e) Intracardiac echocardiographic images (ICE) during the closure procedure. (A, B, a, b) Different views demonstrating the large ASD (arrows) measuring at least 34–47 mm. (C, D, c, d) Postdeployment of a 38 mm Amplatzer Septal Occluder demonstrating good device position. (E, e) After the patient received DC cardioversion for atrial fibrillation, the device embolized to the left atrium (arrows). LA, left atrium; RA, right atrium.

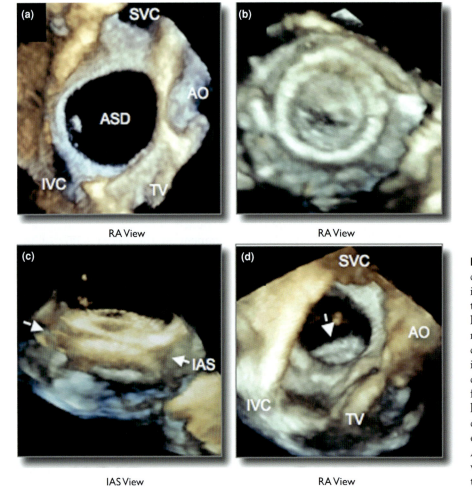

Figure 16.2 Corresponding three-dimensional TEE images of the patient in Figure 16.1. (A) En-face view from the right atrium (RA) demonstrating large ASD with somewhat deficient rims. (B) View demonstrating good device position and the presence of the interatrial septum between the two discs of the device (arrows). (C) View from the right atrium after the device has been released, demonstrating good device position. (D) After the device embolized to the left atrium (arrow). ASD, atrial septal defect; IVC, inferior vena cava; AO, aortic root; TV, tricuspid valve; IAS, interatrial septum.

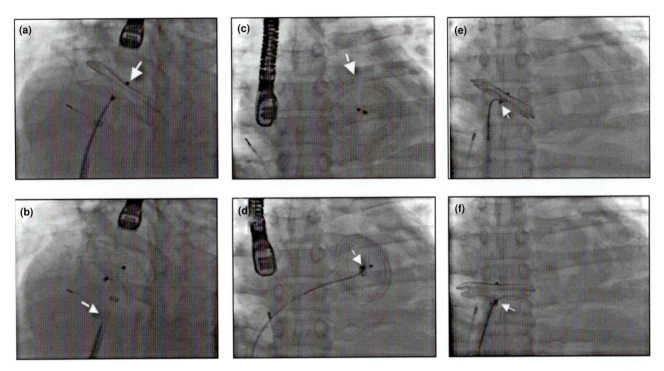

Figure 16.3   Corresponding fluoroscopic images of the patient in Figures 16.1 and 16.2, demonstrating device position and the embolization of the device. (A and B) Cine images in hepatoclavicular projection demonstrating good device closure (prerelease from cable) (A) and after the device has been detached from the cable (arrow) (B). (C–F) Cine images in straight frontal projection after the device has embolized. (C) Device (arrow) in the left atrium. (D) A 25 mm gooseneck snare captured the right atrial micro screw of the device (arrow). (E) The device was brought back to the right atrium using the snare (arrow). (F) An attempt to pull back the device inside a 14 French sheath (arrow) failed due to the angle between the micro screw and the sheath (arrow).

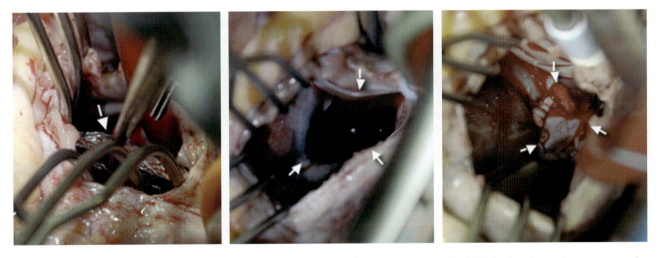

Figure 16.4   Corresponding intraoperative images in the patient shown in Figures 16.1–16.3. Left: After right atriotomy, the device is seen in the right atrium (arrow). Middle: The defect as seen by the surgeon (arrows). Right: After pericardial patch closure of the defect (arrows).

perforation need to be distinguished. First, perforation can occur during delivery of the device due to the device itself or other equipment used, such as guide wires or sheaths. Second, erosion of the device through the cardiac walls can lead to frank perforation and pericardial tamponade. The former complication can be avoided by careful technique and meticulous observation of the deployment process. The guide wire should be placed in the left upper pulmonary vein with its tip visible at all times. Care must be taken to avoid the left atrial appendage. The tip of the delivery sheath must be pulled back into the left atrium prior to deployment of the left atrial disc of the ASO; however, on occasions, deployment of the left disc inside the pulmonary vein (left or right upper) is needed to align the left atrial disc parallel to the septum. In such cases, extreme care should be exercised. Following these safety precautions, delivery-related perforations are exceedingly rare.[10]

Cardiac perforation due to erosion of the device itself into surrounding structures is a true concern of transcatheter ASD closure. Although estimated to occur at a rate of only 0.1% of all closure procedures, the potentially lethal consequences of this complication warrant close evaluation of its possible causes. A review of the AGA registry revealed 28 cases with the ASO device of hemodynamic compromise due to erosion, mainly manifested as pericardial tamponade.[11] Two-thirds of patients developed symptoms within 72 hours of the procedure, the longest interval between closure and erosion of the device was 3 years. The majority of patients underwent surgical drainage of the effusion with or without device removal or fistula repair. Almost 90% of the patients were found to have a deficient aortic rim or superior rim. The most common site of perforation was at the left atrial roof. Defect and device size was larger in the group of patients with device erosion compared to the FDA pivotal trial of the ASO. Further, the mean diameter of the device was 2 mm larger than the balloon-stretched defect in patients with complications compared to the FDA trial, where the mean difference was only 0.5 mm. The authors concluded that a deficient superior or anterior rim may increase the risk of atrial perforation. Oversizing of the device may further increase the risk. Hence, they recommended not to oversize devices in order to prevent embolization, especially since device embolization is a more benign complication compared to erosion. Among the list of further recommendations is the suggestion to perform an echocardiogram the day following the procedure. Even a trace amount of pericardial fluid should raise the suspicion for erosion and trigger further clinical observation. Any episode of chest pain, dyspnea, or syncope should be evaluated immediately with an echocardiogram. Surveillance echocardiograms should probably also be obtained every 1 to 2 years following transcatheter ASD closure.

Arrhythmias

Non-sustained supraventricular arrhythmia immediately following device closure is frequent, estimated to occur in 63% of patients as determined by a study utilizing ambulatory electrocardiographic monitoring.[12] More sustained arrhythmias, such as atrial fibrillation, atrial flutter, or other supraventricular tachycardias, are less common and are estimated to occur in 2.6 to 4.1% of procedures.[3,4] Considering the natural history of secundum ASDs, even if altered by defect closure, atrial arrhythmias are part of the disease process, and an expected finding.[13] Hence, to differentiate whether atrial arrhythmias during follow-up are related to device placement or

are a consequence of the underlying disease is impossible. Arrhythmias occurring in the periprocedural period, however, can be assumed to be due to the device.

Higher degree atrioventricular (AV) conduction blocks are rare, assumed to occur in less than 1% of cases. Suda et al. reported that 10 out of 162 patients (6.2%) presented with new-onset ($n = 9$) or aggravation of pre-existing ($n = 1$) AV block.[14] First-degree AV blocks were seen in 4, second-degree AV blocks in 4, and third-degree AV blocks were noted in 2 patients. Three of them occurred during the procedure, the remaining were noted 1 to 7 days later. All AV blocks resolved or improved spontaneously, with no recurrence at mid term follow-up. The authors noted that the occurrence of AV blocks was associated with the placement of large ASO devices.

Thrombus formation

Information about thrombus formation on devices used for closure of interatrial communications is limited, mainly because asymptomatic thrombi may be missed during routine physical examination except when surveillance echocardiography is performed. In the largest series evaluating this issue in 1000 patients status post ASD or patent foramen ovale closure, thrombi were seen in 20 patients (2%).[15] Thrombus formation was diagnosed at the 4-week follow-up echocardiogram in 14 patients, and in the remaining 6 patients later on. It is important to notice that the type of device had the biggest impact on the incidence of thrombus formation. While thrombus formation was noted in 5.7 and 7.1% of the STARFlex and Cardio SEAL devices, no thrombus was seen on Amplatzer occluders. Of note, 1 of 161 patients undergoing ASD closure with the HELEX device had evidence of thrombus formation (0.8%). The same dependence of thrombus formation on the type of occluder used has been confirmed by others, showing that the CardioSEAL device was more likely to have thrombus present during echocardiographic surveillance than the Amplatzer device.[16] The treatment of choice for manifest device-related thrombus is oral anticoagulation with warfarin. In the formerly quoted study of 1000 consecutive patients, 17 out of 20 were successfully treated with oral anticoagulation. In our own experience, dual antiplatelet therapy with acetylsalicylic acid and clopidogrel for the first few months has generally reduced the incidence of device-related thrombus formation even further.

Infection

Although a much dreaded complication of device closure of secundum ASDs, manifest bacterial infection of these implanted devices is exceedingly rare. A review of the literature reveals only two published, confirmed cases of infective endocarditis due to ASD occluder infection.[17,18] Nevertheless, despite the rare description of manifest infection, most interventionalists recommend endocarditis prophylaxis prior to invasive procedures for 6 to 12 months following device closure of ASDs. Theoretically, the occluder should be endothelialized after 6 to 8 months, making it an inert structure within the interatrial septum.

Headaches/migraine

About 5% of patients develop headaches/migraines following device closure of their atrial level shunt.[19] Despite thorough investigations, including CT scan of the brain and TEE to evaluate for thrombus formation on the left atrial disc, the etiology remains obscured. Over the last few years, we have added clopidogrel to the antiplatelet regimen. Since this practice was adopted, it is rare to have patients complain of such headaches.

Other possible complications during device placement

Extreme care must be exercised not to allow passage of air inside the delivery sheath. *Air embolism* usually manifests as transient ST-segment elevation. Fortunately, this normally does not result in clinical sequelae. In order to avoid air embolism, many operators now remove the dilator of the delivery sheath in the IVC and only cross the ASD into the left atrium with the sheath over the guide wire, after allowing generous back bleeding to de-air the sheath or while continuously flushing the side arm of the sheath.

Cobra-head formation refers to a condition when the left atrial disc maintains a high profile when deployed.[20] This may occur when the left atrial disc is opened against tissue in the left atrium, following difficulties loading the device and by twisting of the device during advancement through the sheath. If cobra-head formation occurs one should check the site of deployment; if appropriate, the device should be recaptured, removed, and inspected. If the cobra-head formation occurs outside the body it is recommended to use a different device. Of course, the device should not be released if it has a cobra-head appearance.

Another malformation of the ASO can occur if the device is too *oversized* in relation to the ASD. Under those circumstances, the atrial discs cannot fully flatten and their profile is increased, which may result in a mushroom-like appearance of the discs.[21] If such a bulging appearance of the ASO is noted, one should replace it with a smaller device. Lesser degrees of oversizing are tolerable, since with time the device gradually assumes a lower profile.

Once the ASO is deemed in optimal position it is released by counterclockwise rotation of the delivery cable. The *inability to release a deployed device* may be related to the fact that either the ASO is attached too firmly to the delivery cable or the device rotates in the defect while attempting to unscrew. The latter mechanism is more likely to occur in patent foramen ovale closures, since an ASD should be stented by the center portion of the device, granted the device is appropriately sized. In order to avoid difficulties in releasing the device from the delivery cable, it is generally recommended to attach the ASO to the delivery cable by clockwise rotation until resistance is encountered. The device should then be partially unscrewed by a 90° counterclock rotation. Management of either problem obviously requires removal of the device and subsequent reloading.

Recapturing of the device prior to release may be warranted if it is deemed in suboptimal position. The delivery sheaths usually have thin walls in order to allow the smallest access size possible. Consequently, upon recapturing the device, it may get kinked or damaged in an accordion-like fashion. In order to avoid this complication, the operator should hold the sheath at the groin with their left hand and with their right hand pull the delivery cable forcefully inside the sheath. If an accordion effect of the sheath occurs, one should use the Amplatzer exchange (rescue) system (AGA Medical Corporation, Plymouth, MN). First, the length of the delivery cable is extended by means of the rescue cable. Then the sheath can be removed or exchanged. Alternatively, the dilator of the rescue system can be advanced into the kinked delivery sheath until it reaches a few centimeters near the tip of the sheath. This strengthens the sheath and may allow the operator to pull back the device together with the dilator as a unit into the sheath.

Finally, impairment of mitral or tricuspid valve function as well as compromise of vena cava, pulmonary vein, and coronary sinus flow needs to be carefully assessed prior to release of the device. If any of these compromising features of the deployed device is recognized, it should be removed and a smaller device should be deployed.

REFERENCES

1. Masura J, Gavora P, Formanek A, Hijazi ZM. Transcatheter closure of secundum atrial septal defects using the new self-centering amplatzer septal occluder: initial human experience. Cathet Cardiovasc Diagn 1997; 42: 388–93.
2. Du ZD, Koenig P, Cao QL et al. Comparison of transcatheter closure of secundum atrial septal defect using the Amplatzer septal occluder associated with deficient versus sufficient rims. Am J Cardiol 2002; 90: 865–9.
3. Du ZD, Hijazi ZM, Kleinman CS, Silverman NH, Larntz K. Comparison between transcatheter and surgical closure of secundum atrial septal defect in children and adults: results of a multicenter nonrandomized trial. J Am Coll Cardiol 2002; 39: 1836–44.
4. Chessa M, Carminati M, Butera G et al. Early and late complications associated with transcatheter occlusion of secundum atrial septal defect. J Am Coll Cardiol 2002; 39: 1061–5.

5. Cardenas L, Panzer J, Boshoff D, Malekzadeh-Milani S, Ovaert C. Transcatheter closure of secundum atrial defect in small children. Cathet Cardiovasc Interven 2007; 69: 447–52.

6. Butera G, Carminati M, Chessa M et al. Percutaneous versus surgical closure of secundum atrial septal defect: comparison of early results and complications. Am Heart J 2006; 151: 228–34.

7. Levi DS, Moore JW. Embolization and retrieval of the Amplatzer septal occluder. Cathet Cardiovasc Interven 2004; 61: 543–7.

8. Verma PK, Thingnam SK, Sharma A et al. Delayed embolization of Amplatzer septal occluder device: an unknown entity – a case report. Angiology 2003; 54: 115–18.

9. Divekar A, Gaamangwe T, Shaikh N, Raabe M, Ducas J. Cardiac perforation after device closure of atrial septal defects with the Amplatzer septal occluder. J Am Coll Cardiol 2005; 45: 1213–18.

10. Spies C, Timmermanns I, Schrader R. Transcatheter closure of secundum atrial septal defects in adults with the Amplatzer septal occluder: intermediate and long-term results. Clin Res Cardiol 2007; 96: 340–6.

11. Amin Z, Hijazi ZM, Bass JL et al. Erosion of Amplatzer septal occluder device after closure of secundum atrial septal defects: review of registry of complications and recommendations to minimize future risk. Cathet Cardiovasc Interven 2004; 63: 496–502.

12. Hill SL, Berul CI, Patel HT et al. Early ECG abnormalities associated with transcatheter closure of atrial septal defects using the Amplatzer septal occluder. J Interven Card Electrophysiol 2000; 4: 469–74.

13. Gatzoulis MA, Freeman MA, Siu SC, Webb GD, Harris L. Atrial arrhythmia after surgical closure of atrial septal defects in adults. N Engl J Med 1999; 340: 839–46.

14. Suda K, Raboisson MJ, Piette E, Dahdah NS, Miro J. Reversible atrioventricular block associated with closure of atrial septal defects using the Amplatzer device. J Am Coll Cardiol 2004; 43: 1677–82.

15. Krumsdorf U, Ostermayer S, Billinger K et al. Incidence and clinical course of thrombus formation on atrial septal defect and patient foramen ovale closure devices in 1,000 consecutive patients. J Am Coll Cardiol 2004; 43: 302–9.

16. Anzai H, Child J, Natterson B et al. Incidence of thrombus formation on the CardioSEAL and the Amplatzer interatrial closure devices. Am J Cardiol 2004; 93: 426–31.

17. Balasundaram RP, Anandaraja S, Juneja R, Choudhary SK. Infective endocarditis following implantation of Amplatzer atrial septal occluder. Ind Heart J 2005; 57: 167–9.

18. Bullock AM, Menahem S, Wilkinson JL. Infective endocarditis on an occluder closing an atrial septal defect. Cardiol Young 1999; 9: 65–7.

19. Mortelmans K, Post M, Thijs V, Herroelen L, Budts W. The influence of percutaneous atrial septal defect closure on the occurrence of migraine. Eur Heart J 2005; 26: 1533–7.

20. Cooke JC, Gelman JS, Harper RW. Cobrahead malformation of the Amplatzer septal occluder device: an avoidable complication of percutaneous ASD closure. Cathet Cardiovasc Interven 2001; 52: 83–5.

21. Fischer G, Kramer HH, Stieh J, Harding P, Jung O. Transcatheter closure of secundum atrial septal defects with the new self-centering Amplatzer Septal Occluder. Eur Heart J 1999; 20: 541–9.

22. Fu YC, Cao QL, Hijazi ZM. Device closure of large atrial septal defects: technical considerations. J Cardiovasc Med (Hagerstown) 2007; 8: 30–3.

23. Spies C, Boosfeld C, Schrader R. A modified Cook sheath for closure of a large secundum atrial septal defect. Cathet Cardiovasc Interven 2007; 70: 286–9.

24. Berger F, Ewert P, Abdul-Khaliq H, Nurnberg JH, Lange PE. Percutaneous closure of large atrial septal defects with the Amplatzer Septal Occluder: technical overkill or recommendable alternative treatment? J Interven Cardiol 2001; 14: 63–7.

25. Varma C, Benson LN, Silversides C, Yip J, Warr MR et al. Outcomes and alternative techniques for device closure of the large secundum atrial septal defect. Cathet Cardiovasc Interven 2004; 61: 131–9.

26. Wahab HA, Bairam AR, Cao QL, Hijazi ZM. Novel technique to prevent prolapse of the Amplatzer septal occluder through large atrial septal defect. Cathet Cardiovasc Interven 2003; 60: 543–5.

27. Dalvi BV, Pinto RJ, Gupta A. New technique for device closure of large atrial septal defects. Cathet Cardiovasc Interven 2005; 64: 102–7.

17 Device closure of atrial septal defects using the HELEX device

Larry Latson

INTRODUCTION

The HELEX Septal Occluder (WL Gore and Associates, Flagstaff, AZ) device is a double-disk, non-self-centering, catheter-delivered occluder best suited for closure of small to moderate (less than or equal to 18 mm) atrial septal defects (ASDs).[1] It is also used widely around the world for closure of patent foramen ovale (PFO), but is not specifically approved for this indication in the United States.[2,3] The frame of the device is a single length of Nitinol wire which can be elongated over a central mandrel for catheter delivery. The frame is draped with an ultrathin expanded polytetrafluoroethylene (ePTFE) membrane which is also threaded over the central mandrel (Figure 17.1). When the device is correctly configured in the heart, the central mandrel is removed and a locking loop inside of the mandrel deploys. This loop assures a slightly variable, but reasonably close, approximation of the central portions of the two functional disks. The device is very flexible and its round shape has little potential for long-term trauma to the atrial walls or the aorta. A retrieval cord provides a flexible attachment to the right atrial eyelet of the device after release from all of the other delivery components. This cord allows a measure of control for removal of the device should the configuration or position be suboptimal after release from the mandrel.

Deployment of the HELEX device is an incremental process that requires more steps than most other ASD closure devices. The operator must become familiar with the basic design of the device and delivery system, and have a thorough understanding of how the major components are integrated and utilized to deliver the device. The basic steps for loading the device, and for deployment in the ASD, are outlined below, but a more detailed description and training course are available from the manufacturer.

TECHNIQUE OF ASD CLOSURE USING THE HELEX SEPTAL OCCLUDER

The HELEX Septal Occluder is packaged with all of the components connected and the device in its double-disk configuration at the end of the delivery system. The delivery system and device are held under water and the delivery catheter is first flushed to remove any air. The mandrel should be locked at its hub in the extended position (Figure 17.2). The device is loaded into the catheter, by simply pulling on the frame control (gray) catheter, which is attached to the right atrial eyelet by the retrieval cord. When the frame is nearly completely inside the catheter, the mandrel will begin to bend slightly (but must not be allowed to kink). The final step is to unlock the mandrel and pull the most distal portion of the frame, along with the mandrel, into the delivery catheter. The entire system should then be flushed again to be certain there is no air trapped inside the delivery catheter.

The HELEX delivery catheter is flexible, and can be directly advanced through a short 10 French sheath in the femoral vein, through the ASD, and into the left atrium. Alternatively, a guide wire can be placed in the left upper pulmonary vein using a standard end-hole catheter. This guide wire can be used to deliver the HELEX catheter as a monorail (13 French sheath in the femoral vein required), or for placement of a 10 French long transeptal style sheath into the left atrium. We generally reserve use of the guide wire techniques for guiding the catheter through a specific hole in patients with multiple ASDs, or occasionally through a tight PFO.

When the delivery catheter is in place in the mid left atrium, the left atrial disk is formed incrementally using a 'push, pinch, pull' sequence. The mandrel at this point is unlocked and several centimeters back from its locking hub on the delivery catheter. The gray-colored frame control catheter is pushed several centimeters. This also advances the mandrel until the mandrel is stopped at its locking hub. The frame control catheter is then pinched, to hold it in place, and the mandrel is pulled until the distal eyelet is close to the end of the delivery catheter on fluoroscopy. This process is repeated until the left atrial disk is fully deployed and configured. The entire system is then gently withdrawn until the left atrial disk is just touching the left atrial surface of the atrial septum.

The right atrial disk is then deployed. Several centimeters of the mandrel and frame are uncovered in the

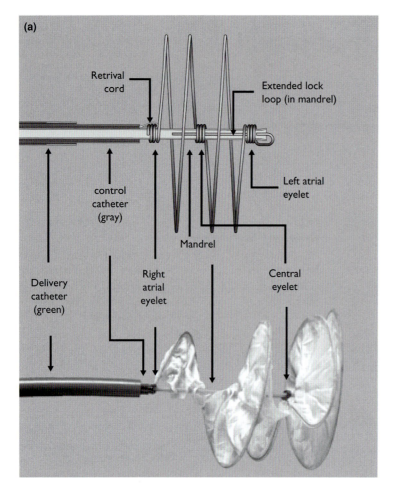

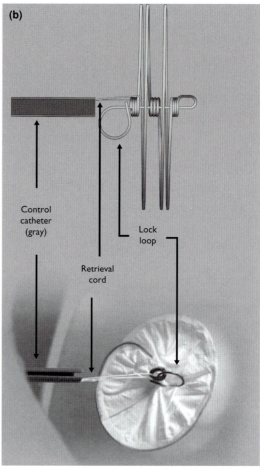

Figure 17.1 Diagram and photograph of the HELEX Septal Occluder in the deployed, but not released, configuration (A) and after release of the device from the mandrel (B). The diagrams emphasize the configuration of the wire frame and the photographs show the ePTFE covering draped over the frame and threaded through the mandrel (and the lock loop after the mandrel is removed). The retrieval cord has one end attached to the tip of the control catheter, is looped through the right atrial eyelet, and then exits the end of the delivery catheter. The retrieval cord is completely removed by withdrawing the delivery system from the body.

right atrium by holding the gray control catheter in place and withdrawing the (green) delivery catheter until the mandrel can be locked in place at its hub. Once the mandrel is locked to the delivery catheter, the gray-colored frame control catheter is simply advanced until it can be locked at its hub to form the right atrial disk in the right atrium. The device is now fully configured but still attached to the mandrel and to the retrieval cord. The position of the device should be checked fluoroscopically and echocardiographically. If there are any concerns about the device positioning, it can be withdrawn back into the delivery catheter in a manner identical to the initial loading process which was performed prior to insertion into the body.

If the device position and configuration are good, the device can be released from the delivery catheters. Before this release, it is important to remove the retrieval cord friction cap (red plug at the end of the gray frame control catheter) so the delivery catheter can move slightly away from the device after locking loop release. When the retrieval cord is free, the mandrel is withdrawn

briskly while using the gray-colored control catheter to maintain the device position. The locking loop deploys through a slit in the gray catheter when the mandrel is withdrawn. Some change in the position, orientation, and configuration of the device is normal as tension and angulation from the delivery system are released. At this point, the retrieval cord is still looped through the right atrial eyelet. If the device positioning and configuration are good, the retrieval cord is removed by simply withdrawing the gray-colored catheter (which has one end of the retrieval cord embedded in its tip) as far as it will easily move, and then withdrawing the entire delivery catheter system out of the body.

HOW NOT TO GET INTO TROUBLE WITH THE HELEX DEVICE: SKILLS AND EQUIPMENT NEEDED

The best ways to avoid trouble with deployment of the HELEX Septal Occluder are to fully understand

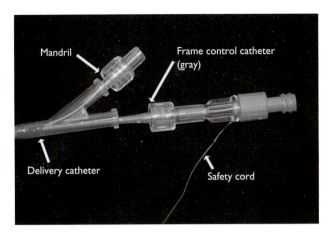

Figure 17.2 The proximal end of the delivery system of the HELEX Septal Occluder. The mandrel and its locking hub can be seen. The mandrel is shown unlocked and partially withdrawn. It is normally only pushed into the locked position during loading of the device into the catheter and as the right atrial disk is deployed. The control catheter is inside of the delivery catheter (green) and also is shown in its unlocked and slightly withdrawn position. The control catheter is normally only locked when the right atrial disk is fully deployed, and it is kept in the locked position as the occluder's lock loop is released by fully withdrawing the mandrel. The retrieval cord is seen as it exits the end of the control catheter. The friction cap holds the retrieval cord in place until the time for lock loop release.

the delivery of the device, understand the anatomic constraints that are important in device selection, and to be prepared to handle any untoward events. Deployment is briefly reviewed above. It is important to remember that the HELEX device is not very rigid. This is an advantage to the heart in the long run, but requires that the implanting physician maintain a gentle touch during deployment. The fine wire of the device is also not as radio-opaque as some other devices and may be difficult to visualize on fluoroscopy, especially in large patients. Intermittent short cineangiographic acquisitions will allow good visualization at important points in the delivery process. Perforations of the heart or pulmonary veins are extremely unlikely with this device because it is very soft. Nonetheless, care should be taken to configure the left atrial disk in the body of the left atrium, and not in the left atrial appendage or a pulmonary vein.

In general, the risk of an air or thrombotic embolus should be low with the standard HELEX delivery technique, since placement through a long sheath (which may have hidden pockets of air or blood) is not necessary. If it is elected to place the delivery catheter through a long sheath, then standard techniques to eliminate air and blood from the sheath should be carefully followed. Heparinization is recommended for all device delivery procedures. An activated clotting time (ACT) around 200–250 is our usual target, and patients are instructed to take an aspirin the day prior to the procedure.

Sizing of the ASD is important in many situations. Determination of the balloon occlusion or stop-flow diameter of an isolated single ASD is generally felt to be the preferred method of sizing.[4] It is important in our view to use a soft occlusion balloon that has a stated diameter of at least 1.5 (and preferably 2) times the estimated diameter of the defect. By using a large balloon, the waist in the balloon is clearly seen and flow is abolished well before the balloon is even fully inflated. This eliminates the risk of actually enlarging the defect by the process of sizing it. Review of the data from the initial trials of the HELEX indicated that a ratio of device diameter/balloon occlusion diameter greater than 2/1 resulted in no residual leaks and a 95% rate of clinical success.[5] This makes intuitive sense for a non-self-centering umbrella type device which can have its central connection move to an edge of an ASD rim and still cover the entire defect. Smaller device/balloon occlusion diameter ratios can be considered if the 2/1 ratio would require that a device be larger than the total length of the atrial septum. In smaller hearts, the device position will be constrained by the atrial chamber itself, and this prevents the device from moving far from the center of the septum. Because the device is not rigid, it can easily be pulled through the ASD during deployment when smaller device/balloon occlusion diameter ratios are attempted, so an especially gentle touch is required.

We have found that balloon sizing is not helpful or necessary for multiple small ASDs. In this situation, a central defect should be crossed and a large device – large enough to cover the adjacent defects – should be chosen. This will typically be significantly more than twice the diameter of the central defect. Similarly, balloon sizing is not important for device size selection for typical PFOs. Since a PFO is structurally more similar to a door that needs to be pulled to a closed position by the device, rather than a doorway that needs a complete covering, we would always use a relatively small device (15–25 mm) if the echocardiogram shows that the flap of the foramen nearly completely closes the opening in the resting state.

As with other ASD occlusion devices, the HELEX can be deployed with fluoroscopic guidance only, but use of adjunctive ultrasound guidance is strongly recommended. The most common adjunctive ultrasound technique currently is intracardiac echocardiography, since anesthesia for placement of a transesophageal echocardiographic probe can be avoided. Transesophageal or transthoracic echocardiography can also be utilized at the operator's preference.

Equipment and facilities should always be available for potential complications of any catheterization procedure. Although procedures are usually done with simple light sedation (unless transesophageal echocardiography is utilized), standard facilities for emergency airway management and management of catastrophic events should always be available. Equipment to handle device embolization should also be available for any occluder implantations. The HELEX device can be relatively easily captured with a large (20–30 mm) gooseneck snare. If any type of occluder device embolizes to the pulmonary artery (PA) or left ventricle (LV), we prefer to withdraw it as completely as possible into a long sheath in the main PA or LV, rather than try to pull it backwards through the tricuspid or mitral valve. We therefore recommend that long transeptal type sheaths at least 2–3 French sizes larger than the recommended delivery sheath size be on hand.

POSSIBLE COMPLICATIONS

The primary complications of transcatheter-delivered ASD devices are procedural. Major concerns with delivery of any ASD closure device include possibilities of anesthetic complications, femoral vessel damage, arrhythmias, air or thrombus embolization, and atrial wall or pulmonary vein perforation. Later complications of ASD devices include arrhythmias, thrombi on devices, infections, and erosions. These generic issues will not be discussed in detail. Specific difficulties of the HELEX device include achieving proper positioning during deployment, and handling an embolization of the device itself.

HOW TO MANAGE PROCEDURAL ISSUES OF HELEX SEPTAL OCCLUDER DELIVERY

The handling of a HELEX device which is poorly positioned or configured depends upon whether the device has been released from the mandrel. Prior to release from the mandrel, the device can simply be withdrawn back into the delivery catheter, and either exchanged for a different device or redeployed. If the left atrial disk appears to be abnormally deformed, it is possible that the device has been partially deployed in a pulmonary vein or a left atrial appendage. The device is flexible enough that it is unlikely to cause damage to these structures. Gentle traction on the entire system may allow the device to move into the body of the left atrium and then against the atrial septum.

As with all catheter ASD device delivery systems, precise device positioning can be a challenge. During normal deployment, one would prefer that there be a mechanism to pull the deployed LA disk directly toward the right atrium (RA) with the device parallel to the atrial septum. However, from the femoral venous approach, withdrawal of the delivery catheter results in the system moving toward the feet more than in the ideal direction from left to right. When it is possible to use a HELEX device to balloon occlusion diameter ratio of 2/1 or more as recommended (or when closing a PFO or multiple small ASDs), there is sufficient size of the device to achieve good positioning relatively easily. Slight to moderate tension can be applied to the device without the anterior-cephalad

portion of the left atrial disk prolapsing into the right atrium. If the length of the atrial septum is insufficient to allow the use of a device at least twice the diameter of the ASD, then it may be more difficult to achieve proper alignment. Echocardiography is utilized to detect when the cephalad portion of the disk first begins to contact the atrial septum. A straight lateral fluoroscopic view aids in insuring that the orientation of the device is reasonably parallel to the atrial septum. In very difficult cases, we have found that the use of a modified delivery sheath to adjust the angle and place of initial contact of the left atrial disk with the atrial septum has been useful for the HELEX as well as other ASD devices.[6] When the left atrial disk is lightly against the atrial septum, care must be taken to avoid any change in position as the right atrial disk is configured. Before release of the mandrel, the device should be carefully inspected fluoroscopically and with ultrasound to insure that all portions of the device are on the correct sides of the atrial septum (Figure 17.3). The central eyelet should be in the plane of the septum and a double layer of material should be seen over approximately one-third of the perimeter of the device on each side of the septum.

Once adequate placement and configuration of the device is confirmed, the mandrel is withdrawn to release the locking loop. This removes any tension or angulation caused by the stiffer components of the delivery system from the device, and it is normal for the device to move slightly and to become less compact as the central eyelets separate slightly. In many cases, this change in orientation may reduce the appearance of small leaks seen prior to release. In some cases, however, the change in orientation may demonstrate significantly larger leaks or abnormally wide separation between the left and right atrial disks. These types of adverse findings upon release of the device are most common with large devices in relatively small hearts. If the diameter of the device is close to, or exceeds, the approximate length of the atrial septum (best measured in echocardiographic apical views), the disks of the device will be pushed apart by the shape of the atrial walls. In these situations, one may see flow between the two disks from the superior vena cava (SVC) or IVC. If the defect is closed by the left atrial disk and the right atrial disk is stable, this condition is acceptable and may not require any specific treatment. However, if flow from the great veins causes excessive motion of the right atrial disk, if there is poor closure of the ASD by the left atrial disk, or if there is clear contact with the mitral or tricuspid valves against the frame of the device, the device should be removed. At this point the device is still attached to the (gray) control catheter by the retrieval cord through the right atrial eyelet, and can be removed without additional equipment.

To remove a deployed device with the retrieval cord, the first step is to pull on the free end of the retrieval cord so that the control catheter is snug against the right atrial eyelet. The red friction cap is then applied

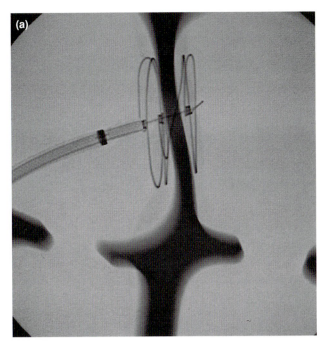

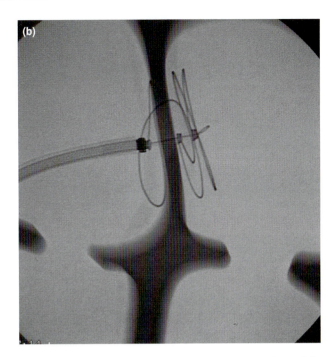

Figure 17.3 Fluroscopic images of the HELEX device deployed in suboptimal positions in an ASD model. In (A), the middle eyelet and a small portion of the LA disk are seen to the right side of the septum. In (B), the middle eyelet and a small portion of the RA disk are seen in the LA.

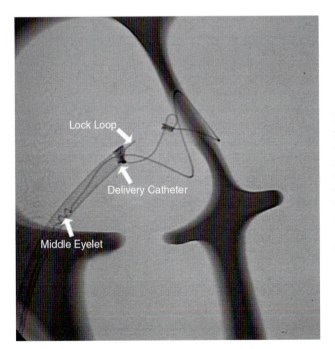

Figure 17.4 Fluroscopic image of the HELEX device during retrieval after the lock loop has been deployed. The delivery catheter has been advanced too close to the device to allow straightening of the lock loop. The tip of the catheter is being deformed and the middle eyelet is being straightened by tension on the control catheter. The delivery catheter should be withdrawn slightly if these signs are seen. When the LA disk comes through the ASD, the entire system should be withdrawn into the IVC or femoral vein. The smaller vessels will stop the LA disk so that tension can again be applied to straighten the lock loop. The device is soft and has not apparently damaged the veins when pulled down as far as possible during retrievals. Completing the retrieval with the device as far down as possible also means that the straightened proximal portion of the device will be out of the body should the retrieval cord break.

to the end of the catheter to prevent the retrieval cord from slipping during withdrawal. Once the retrieval cord is positioned and fastened, gentle traction on the entire system will pull the right atrial eyelet. With continued tension, one will see the locking loop straighten and will see and feel the locking loop alternately straighten and curl back somewhat as the small perforations in the ePTFE of the right atrial disk come off of the locking loop. Once the right atrial eyelet has come off of the locking loop, we generally recommend gently advancing the delivery catheter slightly and pulling on the gray-colored catheter to pull the locking loop and the right atrial frame inside of the delivery catheter. It is important, however, not to advance the delivery catheter too close to the locking loop, as the catheter can prevent the loop from straightening and allowing the material to come off of the locking loop (Figure 17.4). The middle eyelet of the device must be pulled off of the locking loop before attempting to withdraw this eyelet into the delivery catheter. Some manipulation of

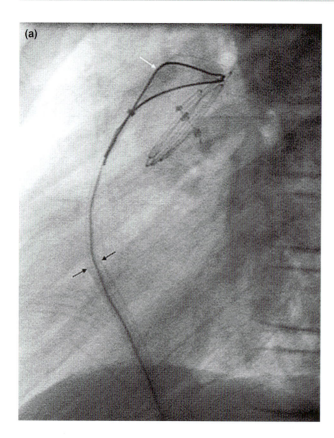

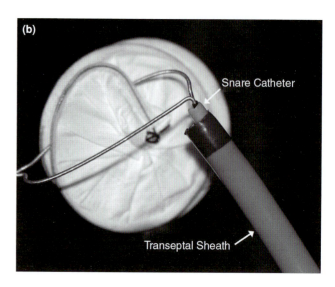

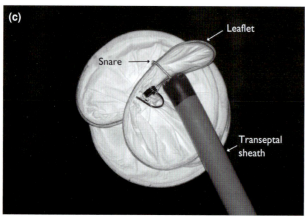

Figure 17.5 (A) Fluroscopic image of a HELEX Septal Occluder which has embolized to the main pulmonary artery. A snare (white arrow) is being manipulated through a long 11 French sheath (black arrows) placed in the main pulmonary artery. The snare only needs to be manipulated between the layers of the closest disk and then tightened to provide a means of removing the device into the sheath. (B) Photograph of snare relatively easily maneuvered between the overlapping portions of one disk of the HELEX occluder. (C) Photograph of snare through a 10 French transseptal sheath in a good position to retrieve a 25 mm HELEX occluder. If the snare is positioned closer to the center of the device, there is more bulk as the device is first withdrawn into the sheath. A larger sheath (11 or 12 French) and more accurate placement of the snare lessen the amount of tension required to remove the device.

the catheter may be required to successfully 'coax' the middle eyelet into the tip of the delivery catheter.

At some point, the device will pull through the ASD. When this occurs, we recommend withdrawing the entire system gently as far as possible into the IVC or even into the femoral vein. The reason for this is two-fold. In order to pull the ePTFE off of the lock loop and straighten the frame so that it can be withdrawn into the delivery catheter, some tension is necessary. The lowest tension is required if the entire system is withdrawn until the left atrial disk will remain in position as tension is applied to the gray control catheter. Secondly, the closer the retrieval occurs to the femoral sheath, the safer the position in case the retrieval cord should break. If the retrieval cord should

break with the device in the heart or a large IVC, the occluder may embolize. If the cord breaks when some of the straightened device is already out to the body, the delivery catheter can be clamped near the skin with a hemostat (to hold the exteriorized part of the device within the delivery catheter) and the entire system withdrawn out of the femoral sheath.

The HELEX device is relatively soft and embolizations can occur, especially if the device is undersized. Embolizations that have occurred have generally been asymptomatic and discovered incidentally. Because the device frame is relatively easily deformed, it can be grasped anywhere around the perimeter and pulled into an adequate sized sheath. The easiest and most reliable method to grasp a portion of the device is with a medium to large diameter catheter snare (25 to 30 mm) (Figure 17.5). To insure that the device can be withdrawn completely into the sheath, we recommend that the snare be delivered through an 11 or 12 French long transeptal sheath that has been advanced to the embolized device. We have found that a snare can generally be easily manipulated so that the loop will catch just the outer layer of the overlapping portion of either disk. The snare can then be tightened, and used to withdraw the device into the long sheath. There is less bulk to the initial part of the retrieved device if the leaflet can be snared at its mid section instead of at the center of the device. Some manipulation may be required if the eyelets tend to catch at the end of the sheath. If this should occur, tension needs to be slightly released and the sheath rotated as tension is reapplied.

SUMMARY

The HELEX Septal Occluder is a double-disk, non-self-centering catheter-delivered septal occlusion device. It takes some practice and initial thought to fully understand how to deliver the device. Once the delivery is mastered, we prefer this device for small to moderate sized septal defects, especially in young children. The retrieval features of the delivery system and the fact that this device has never caused a perforation are reassuring factors. The device is also excellent for closing multiple ASDs, since the device can be delivered through the most central defect and spread out to cover the additional holes. Proper sizing should result in few complications. Should a device embolize, or for any reason need to be retrieved after release from the delivery system, the occluder can almost always be relatively easily captured and removed in the catheterization laboratory, without the need to send the patient to surgery.

REFERENCES

1. Zahn EM, Wilson N, Cutright W, Latson LA. Development and testing of the Helex septal occluder, a new expanded polytetra-fluoroethylene atrial septal defect occlusion system. Circulation 2001; 104(6): 711–16.
2. Post MC, Van Deyk K, Budts W. Percutaneous closure of a patent foramen ovale: single-centre experience using different types of devices and mid-term outcome. Acta Cardiol 2005; 60(5): 515–19.
3. Krumsdorf U, Ostermayer S, Billinger K et al. Incidence and clinical course of thrombus formation on atrial septal defect and patient foramen ovale closure devices in 1,000 consecutive patients. J Am Coll Cardiol 2004; 43(2): 302–9.
4. Carlson KM, Justino H, O'Brien RE et al. Transcatheter atrial septal defect closure: modified balloon sizing technique to avoid overstretching the defect and oversizing the Amplatzer septal occluder. Cathet Cardiovasc Interven 2005; 66(3): 390–6.
5. Latson LA, Jones TK, Jacobson J, Zahn E, Rhodes JF. Analysis of factors related to successful transcatheter closure of secundum atrial septal defects using the HELEX septal occluder. Am Heart J 2006; 151(5): 1136. e7–1136. ell.
6. Kutty S, Asnes JD, Srinath G et al. Use of a straight, side-hole delivery sheath for improved delivery of Amplatzer ASD occluder. Cathet Cardiovasc Interven 2007; 69(1): 15–20.

18 Device closure of atrial septal defects using the CardioSEAL/STARFlex devices

Phillip Moore

TECHNIQUE INVOLVED IN THE MANAGEMENT OF AN ATRIAL SEPTAL DEFECT

An atrial septal defect (ASD) results in left to right shunting with resultant right heart volume overload, increased pulmonary flow, increased pulmonary vascular shear stress, and, in up to 25% of patients, the development of pulmonary hypertension in young to middle adult years.[1,2] The vast majority of patients are diagnosed in childhood on routine physical examination due to an audible pulmonary flow murmur associated with the increased volume through the pulmonary valve. Approximately 3–5% will have symptoms in childhood of increased respiratory effort, frequent respiratory infections, and even failure to thrive, even as early as a few months.[3] More commonly, symptoms develop in young to middle adult years as insidious mild exercise intolerance. Some adult patients will present with atrial arrhythmias due to right atrium (RA) dilation, most typically PACs but occasionally atrial flutter or fibrillation. Paradoxical embolus-related stroke or TIA is a precipitating event for some. Many adult patients are diagnosed incidentally when evaluated for palpitations or chest pains unrelated to the ASD.

Once an ASD has been diagnosed a complete transthoracic echocardiogram should be performed to evaluate the suitability of device closure. This includes specific attention to the pulmonary vein drainage as well as the size and location of the defect, including tissue rims to the AV valves, inferior vena cava (IVC), right pulmonary veins, aortic valve, and roof of the atrium. If the transthoracic study is inadequate to delineate these structures then transesophageal echo should be performed. The CardioSEAL/STARFlex device system is effective at closing defects of 22 mm diameter (balloon occlusion) if all rims are present, and ≤20 mm diameter if there is absence of the aortic knob rim. A device to occlusion diameter of >2:1 is preferred. Patients with inadequate AV valve, IVC, atrial roof, and pulmonary vein rims can not be effectively closed with the CardioSEAL/STARFlex devices. If patients have a history of frequent palpitations a 24-hour Holter moniter should be performed prior

to device closure. If an accessory pathway tachycardia exists, and ablation may be beneficial, it should be performed prior to closure of the septal defect for ease of access to the left atrium.

Preprocedural evaluation includes a CBC with differential and type and screen for children with the addition of lytes, BUN, Cr, PT, PTT, INR, and glucose for adults. Patients begin 81 mg aspirin (5 mg/kg if <16 kg) daily 3 days before the procedure. The catheterization is performed as an outpatient procedure for the majority, with admission the morning of the procedure and discharge 6 hours after completion. The procedures are performed under moderate conscious sedation. Fluoroscopic and echocardiographic guidance are used for ASD assessment and device positioning. If patients are < 4 years of age transthoracic echo usually suffices; older patients require an additional venous sheath for intracardiac echocardiography. Some operators still prefer general anesthesia with transesophageal echocardiography.

The CardioSEAL/STARFlex device system consists of the device and the delivery catheter system. The device comprises two metal MP35N frameworks, each covered by a polyester fabric patch and, in the case of the STARFlex device, a Nitinol centering spring (Figure 18.1). From the proximal umbrella frame a pin extends at 90° to the device for attachment to the delivery catheter system. The Nitinol microsprings are attached between the two frameworks at the umbrella tips to align the device centrally within the defect. The devices come in sizes of 17, 23, 28, 33, and 40 mm diameter. The delivery system consists of a loading tube that facilitates folding of the umbrellas flat with attachment to the delivery catheter/cable (Figure 18.2). The handle on the delivery catheter has a button slide that opens the forceps tip of the cable that locks onto the pin on the proximal frame of the device. A slot in the forceps tip allows free movement of the device independent of the cable to facilitate alignment with the atrial septum. Once the device is loaded into the loading tube and attached to the delivery catheter, the loading tube is inserted through the back bleed valve of the long sheath and the device advanced through the long sheath by pushing the delivery catheter.

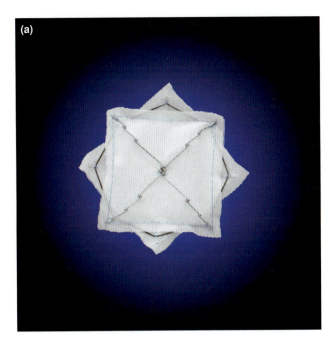

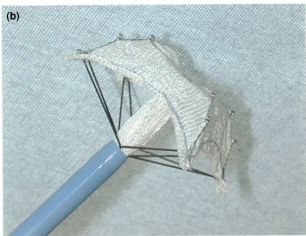

Figure 18.1   STARFlex device: (a) front view; (b) side view as distal umbrella emerges from the delivery sheath, exposing the Nitinol self-centering microsprings.

HOW NOT TO GET INTO TROUBLE WITH THE CardioSEAL/STARFlex DEVICES: SKILLS AND EQUIPMENT NEEDED

Sheath placement

Like all ASD device closure procedures, the Cardio SEAL/STARFlex device delivery system requires a relatively large sheath, 10 or 11 French, in the left atrium. Care must be taken with initial venous access and catheter wire manipulation to minimize vascular injury. A directional catheter such as a multipurpose or JR4 makes it easy to advance a soft-tipped straight or J-tip wire to the left upper pulmonary vein. A stiff 0.035 inch wire is then placed to facilitate test balloon occlusion and positioning of the large delivery sheath. The most common risk by far is thrombus or air introduction into the left atrium (LA) during sheath/device

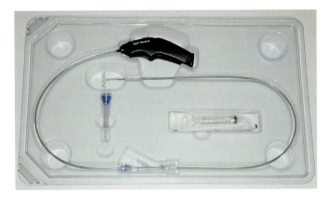

Figure 18.2   STARFlex device and delivery system.

placement, so attention to an appropriate activated clotting time (ACT) >250 seconds, with adequate iv heparin and aggressive flushing of the long sheath with heparinized saline, is imperative. Continuous flushing of the sheath and dilator with heparinized saline through a removable side arm back bleed valve is recommended both during sheath advancement to the LA as well as during dilator and wire removal. Another approach is to clear the sheath of all clot and air in the RA, then advance the sheath independently across the ASD into the LA. This works well as long as the ASD is large, but care must be taken to avoid tissue injury as this is a relatively stiff sheath system due to the size.

Device sizing

The CardioSEAL device should be twice the balloon occlusion diameter, whereas the STARFlex device with the self-centering springs can be sized smaller, to 1.8 times, if needed. If the defect has limited anterior superior rims then increasing device size, if the total LA size is large enough, is helpful to prevent a prolapse 3–5 arm split. If balloon sizing is not used, carefully evaluate all dimensions of the ASD as most are oval and some can be quite complex 'C' shaped defects. The device must be at least twice the largest diameter. A larger device may also be needed if there are multiple defects or a fenestrated septum. A careful understanding of the atrial septal anatomy with assessment for multiple defects is critical before choosing the device size. The tips of the umbrella on this device may catch or prolapse into an additional defect or small fenestration, leading to device malposition. Test balloon occlusion of the ASD with color Doppler assessment will clarify any other defects prior to choosing a device.

Device loading

The device and loader should be well flushed. Care must be taken when loading the device to prevent damage to the device tips and shoulder joints by retracting too hard into the loader. Similarly, the device tips should be fully in the loader as the device is advanced into the sheath to prevent damage. Constant flushing during loading of the device will minimize the risk of air embolus. When advancing the device through the sheath, if significant resistance is met evaluate the sheath with fluoroscopy. A kinked sheath can be difficult to traverse with a loaded device and may result in distal umbrella damage. Remove the device and straighten the sheath with reinsertion of the dilator or, if necessary, replacement of the sheath.

Device delivery

For small defects in large patients open the distal umbrella in the mid LA away from the pulmonary veins and roof of the atrium. If the defect is relatively large and the patient small then open the distal umbrella deep in the LA near the mouth of the left upper pulmonary vein, taking care not get trapped in the vein or distort the umbrella against the roof, atrial appendage, or back wall. The entire system is then withdrawn to the septum.

As with many devices, the most challenging aspect is the correct positioning of the superior anterior edge of the distal umbrella. There is a tendency for prolapse through the defect as the LA umbrella is withdrawn towards the septum due to the relative planes of the IVC, device, and septum. The problem has been dramatically improved with improved flexibility in the delivery pin–cable connector, and with the self-centering springs of the STARFlex device, although prolapse remains a significant issue in patients with absent anterior superior rims or very large defects. Tricks to avoid this problem include clockwise rotation of the delivery sheath to drive the tip posterior and rightward in the LA. Another approach is to place the tip of the delivery sheath in the right upper pulmonary vein, delivering the tips of the distal umbrella in the vein origin then quickly withdrawing the sheath to open the RA umbrella. If positioned correctly, the RA umbrella opening will free the distal umbrella from the mouth of the vein, positioning it correctly. An easier approach is to shape the delivery sheath with a posterior rightward bend, available commercially (Hausdorf-Lock Atrial Sheath, Cook, Inc, Bloomington, IN). The key to insure proper positioning is good echocardiographic imaging in the parasternal short axis and subcostal sagittal planes to assess the superior septal–device interface. If a leak is present over the superior anterior aspect of the left atrial umbrella there should be concern about arm tip prolapse.

This device, more than some others, needs to be delivered with the central pin slightly into the LA for optimal positioning. Once the center pin is within 5 mm of the septal plane, the device is held in place and the sheath is withdrawn to release the right atrial umbrella, being careful not to put tension on the device. Remember the RA arms of the device will sweep from the sheath tip near the RA–IVC junction toward the septum, capturing the RA side of the septum. The most common mistake, by far, of positioning this device is too much tension toward the RA during the RA arm release, resulting in LA arm tip prolapse through the defect into the RA. Poor expansion of the right atrial umbrella may either be restriction by IVC or Eustachian valve tissue, or improper flexion of the right atrial umbrella shoulder joints. Echo evaluation can help decipher the cause. Both can usually be overcome by advancing the delivery sheath over the cable to the right atrial umbrella arm shoulder joints and gently coaxing them to fully open. If a device arm is caught on Eustachian valve tissue it can be gently grabbed with a snare or tip deflecting wire from a separate IJ approach and pulled off the Eustachian valve tissue.

Repositioning/recapture

The CardioSEAL/STARFlex device system does not have the ability to reposition or recapture the device intact after delivery of the proximal right atrial umbrella. Once opened, the distal umbrella can be fully recaptured and redeployed. However, once the proximal umbrella is deployed, the entire device can be recaptured and removed from the body safely, but the device cannot be reused at that point. If both umbrellas have been deployed but the device has not been released, still connected with the forceps–pin delivery cable, then simply retract the device into the large sheath by advancing the sheath over the RA umbrella. It is best to do this maneuver with the device free in the RA so as not to trap any tissue in the device or sheath with retraction. The device will not pull completely into the sheath, but both umbrellas will invert and retract, usually up to the elbow joints, with only a small funnel-shaped portion of the umbrella extending out of the tip of the sheath. The entire system can then be carefully withdrawn through the IVC, iliac, and femoral veins out of the body. A small incision in the skin and subcutaneous tissue facilitates removal that can at times require some force with the larger devices. In experienced hands, it is not necessary to dissect out the vein for direct removal and, in fact, this tends to complicate removal substantially. A set of sterile cut-down instruments should be available in the cath lab. Back loading a larger, short sheath (2 French sizes larger than the long delivery sheath, 12 or 14 French) at the time of placement of the long sheath will allow complete removal of the protruding device inside this larger, short sheath, adding extra protection of the femoral vein during removal. A trick to preserving femoral access at that site is to slip a small 0.018 inch straight wire in the femoral sheath next to the delivery catheter and maintain it in the vein as the device, delivery catheter, and sheath are removed. This allows replacement with another sheath to control bleeding and assess for vascular damage.

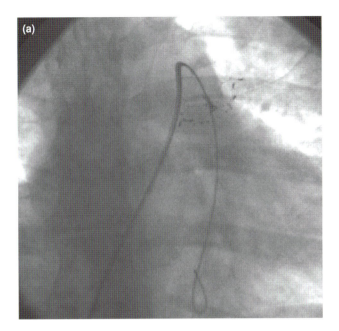

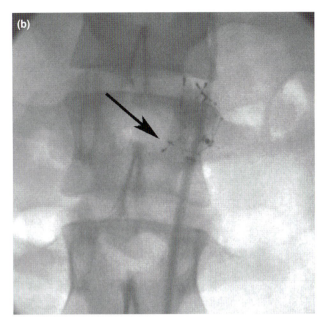

Figure 18.3 Embolized device: (a) through the right heart to the proximal left pulmonary artery (LPA); (b) through the left heart to the abdominal descending aorta. The arrow identifies the frame arm tip protruding into the right renal artery.

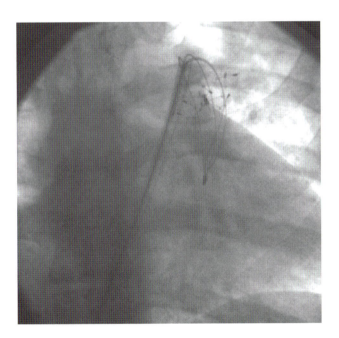

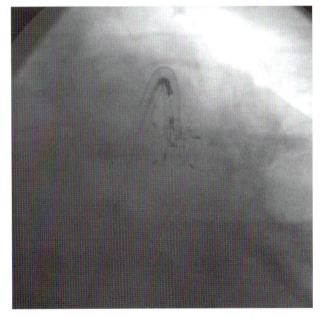

Figure 18.4 Basket in the LPA capturing an embolized device.

Figure 18.5 Device crushed and retracted into the sheath up to the elbow joints of the frame.

If the device has already been released and needs to be recaptured then the process is more extensive. If the RA pin can be loop snared, then theoretically the device could be recaptured as described above. The pin can be successfully snared but the loop snare will slip off the pin during retraction into a large sheath. The arms of the umbrella are quite easy to snare, but then retracting the device into the sheath is problematic. The loop snare should be used to position the embolized device in a safe large vascular space such as the RA, central pulmonary arteries, or aorta if possible (Figure 18.3). Use the largest sheath possible (14 or 16 French for the large

devices) with a basket retrieval device. The basket easily captures the device (Figure 18.4), and with retraction into the sheath, partial release, repositioning of the basket, recapture, and retraction into the sheath the device can be crushed to fit mostly into the sheath (Figure 18.5). The system is then carefully retracted to the femoral vein and removed from the body as described above. If there is significant protrusion of the device from the tip of the long sheath, evaluation of the tricuspid valve with echococardiography is prudent during withdrawal through the heart to prevent entanglement with the tricuspid valve chordae.

Table 18.1

Author	Nugent et al.[15]	Post et al.[4]	Butera et al.[5]	Chessa et al.[7]	Carminati et al.[9]	Carminati et al.[16]	
Year	2006	2006	2004	2002	2001	2000	**Total**
n	72	26	121	159	117	334	**829**
Median age (years)	11.6	46	21	—	17	12	
ASD diameter (mm)	14	16	14	—	15	15	
Success (%)	93	85	95	96	97	93	**94.2**
Major complications							
Embolization							
Early	2	1	5	6	4	13	**3.4%**
Late	0	1	0	0	0	1	**0.24%**
Vessel injury	0	0	1	1	0	—	**0.4%**
Effusion/perforation	1	1	0	0	0	0	**0.24%**
Thrombus	0	—	—	0	—	0	**0**
Minor complications							
Malposition	15	2	10	5	1	1	**4.1%**
Arrhythmia	4	—	1	0	—	0	**0.6%**
Arm fracture	25	—	—	—	15	20	**11.5%**
6 month leak	2	—	12	—	11	69	**14.9%**

POSSIBLE COMPLICATIONS

Possible complications with the device are similar to those with other ASD closure devices, and some have been mentioned above within the context of procedural details. Table 18.1 details those complications reported in the literature and their frequency.[4-10] Severe complications including death, stroke, and bleeding requiring transfusion, have not been reported.

Major complications

Embolization

The most common major complication is device embolization, with the need for non-emergent surgical removal and defect closure occurring in < 4% of implants. This risk is significantly increased with defects over 18 mm in diameter, especially if there is absent anterior superior or posterior superior rim. Most typically, the device will embolize to the RA then get pumped with blood flow through the tricuspid and pulmonary valves into the central pulmonary arteries. There are reports of entanglement with the tricuspid valve or entrapment in trabeculations of the RV, but these are extremely rare. Obstruction to flow has not been reported as the device takes the position of least resistance, sideways in a vessel, allowing unobstructed flow around either side of the device. If the device embolizes to the LA, it will usually be pumped through the LV and into the aorta, and lodge in the thoracic or abdominal descending aorta in older patients, and the transverse arch in small children. Care must be taken during device recapture to prevent vessel injury from manipulation of the wire frame.

Vascular injury

Significant femoral vein vascular injury complications that have been reported include retroperitoneal hematoma during vascular entry and femoral/iliac vein damage during retrieval of an embolized device. These have been reported in less than 0.5% of patients and have resolved either spontaneously or with surgical repair. AV valve injury secondary to embolized device retrieval requiring surgical repair has been reported,

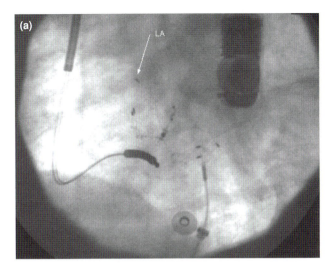

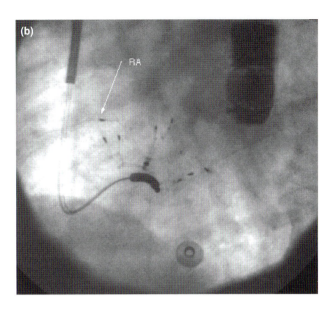

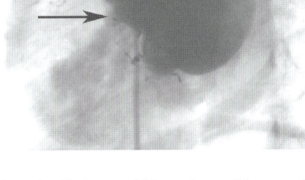

Figure 18.6 Left atrium (LA) arm prolapse through defect with limited superior anterior aortic knob rim (3-5 split). (a) 40 mm CardioSEAL device immediately after release with all LA arms positioned appropriately, including the superior arm (arrow). (b) Seconds later the superior anterior LA arm prolapsed through the defect into the RA (arrow). The device then embolized to the left pulmonary artery. (c) 23 mm CardioSEAL 4 years after implant with a residual leak at the site of superior LA arm prolapse (3-5 split).

but should be avoidable with careful retrieval techniques.[11]

Cardiac perforation/pericardial effusion

Cardiac perforation early by the tip of an umbrella has occurred, resulting in hemopericardium, although it is extremely rare and seems related to extreme oversizing of the device. Pericardial effusion early without sequelae has been reported in less than 0.3% of implants. The etiology is hemopericardium through a small self-sealing perforation in some and serosanguinous inflammatory reaction in others. The mechanism for the inflammatory reaction has not been elucidated. Late cardiac perforation or erosion with this device has not been reported.

Thrombus

Although not reported in the literature of Cardio SEAL/STARFlex ASD closure, this author has had 2/250 implants develop late thrombus, both resulting in surgical removal. In mixed ASD and patent foremen ovale (PFO) closure series with this device the incidence of thrombus ranges from 1 to 4%.[12,13] Because of the low incidence specific risk factors have not been

identified, although it is important to note that nearly all reports occurred early in the device use, before combination antiplatelet medical treatment was commonly in use postprocedure.

Minor complications

Procedural intravascular air or thrombus

This common minor complication, reported in up to 5% of device deliveries, is due to the large sheath required in the left atrium, but is completely preventable with careful attention to detail. Continuous heparanized saline infusion and regular clearing of the sheath can abolish this complication. Air released in the LA typically goes to the anterior right sinus and into the right coronary artery, resulting in mild chest pain and transient ST-T wave elevation,[14,15] although ventricular tachycardia and TIA have occurred rarely.

Malposition

Malposition of the device occurs in approximately 4% of implants and may result in embolization, as noted above, although most commonly it results in only poor device apposition and residual leak. The most common form of malposition is prolapse of the superior anterior LA umbrella arm tip through the defect into the RA. This malposition has been termed a '5-3 split,' since five arms end on the RA side and only three on the LA side (Figure 18.6). This is preventable in most cases with careful device size selection and optimal positioning with skilled echocardiographic support. Risk factors for malposition include undersized device, oversized device, and absence of adequate rim tissue, the most common being the superior anterior aortic knob rim. Malposition can occur if the device is oversized for the atrium with an inability of full expansion of either the LA or RA umbrellas. Inadvertent contact with the Eustachian valve in the RA may prevent appropriate expansion of the RA umbrella. Damage to the shoulder joints of the device during loading may result in poor umbrella apposition on release (Figure 18.7).

Arrhythmia

Atrial tachycardia, including atrial fibrillation, atrial flutter, and supraventricular re-entrant tachycardia have been reported during device placement in less than 1% of patients. These arrhythmias are responsive to appropriate medical cardioversion management. There is a report of device embolization immediately after cardioversion, although this is extremely rare.

Arm fractures

Arm fractures have plagued the CardioSEAL/STAR Flex device system from its conception as the Lock Clamshell device. Modifications in the frame have reduced the incidence over the years substantially,[15] but fractures still occur in over 10% (Figure 18.8). Device size is the critical contributing factor, with the majority of fractures in the larger sized devices (33 and 40 mm) and only a few in sizes 28 mm and less. Fractures do not appear to cause sequelae, with only a few case reports of thrombus formation in the area of a fracture. Some argue this tendency of the frame to fracture is a desirable characteristic to prevent late perforations or erosions when excessive stress develops between the device frame and cardiac tissue.

Residual leak

The 6-month residual leak rate remains modestly high for this device at approximately 15%. For the most part, these are hemodynamically insignificant oval-shaped leaks at the edge of the device, often associated with an arm malposition (Figure 18.9). Repeat interventional or surgical closure is rarely required for these

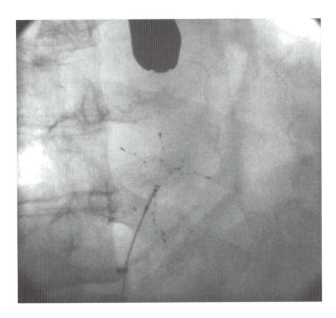

Figure 18.7 Poor right atrium arm apposition prior to release due to oversized device with shoulder joint injury during delivery.

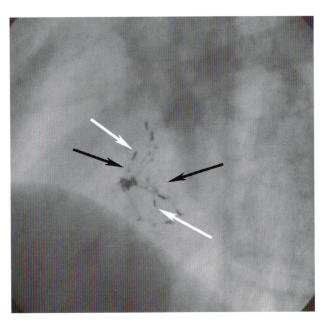

Figure 18.8 Lateral angiogram 6 months after device placement showing two RA arm fractures, both at the elbow joint. Black arrows point to broken elbow joints, white arrows to distal tips of the displaced fractured arms.

leaks, ranging from 0 to 1.5%. The rate of residual leaks and need for repeat intervention has decreased significantly with the STARFlex device as compared to the CardioSEAL.[15,16] As one might expect, increasing defect size and lack of adequate rim tissue are the main risk factors for a residual leak.

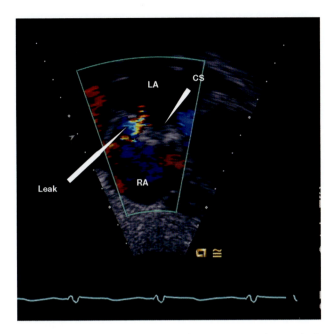

Figure 18.9 Echocardiogram showing a moderate leak 6 months after CardioSEAL (CS) device placement with 3-5 split positioning.

HOW TO MANAGE COMPLICATIONS

Many of the techniques to avoid complications have been discussed above. How to address complications once they have occurred is described below.

Embolization/malposition

Minimizing the risk of embolization is the cornerstone of management. Choose an appropriate sized device for the test occlusion diameter, at least 1.8 times and preferably 2 times the size, if total septal length allows. Remember to be generous with the device size if there is absence of the superior anterior defect rim. Use echocardiographic guidance, both parasternal short axis and subcostal sagittal (if transthoracic) views, as well as angiographic guidance, LAO 65° with 10° cranial angulation, to insure the superior LA arm tip does not prolapse into the RA. Deliver the RA umbrella when the center point of the device is still several mm into the LA. Facilitate capture and retrieval of the device by preloading a short 12 French sheath on the long 10 French delivery sheath. This can be advanced into the femoral vein over the long 10 French sheath if needed to remove a crushed embolized device from the femoral vein to minimize injury.

Once a device is embolized and mobile in the circulation, rapidly advance a directional catheter such as a JR4 over a directional wire to the device. Replace the wire with a 10 mm snare so the device can be quickly captured and kept in a safe location, preferably in the RA or the central pulmonary arteries. Once the device is controlled in a stable position, the long sheath is advanced to the device and the directional snare system replaced with a large wire basket retrievable system. The basket is closed and released on the embolized device until it is crushed and adequately withdrawn into the sheath up to the elbow joints of the umbrella (Figure 18.5). At this point the long sheath with the captured, crushed device is carefully withdrawn with constant steady pull through the pulmonary valve, RV, tricuspid valve, and down the IVC to the femoral vein. If at any time there is significant resistance, retraction should stop and the tip of the sheath/device area should be assessed with echo and fluoroscopy. A contrast injection through the side arm of the long sheath is often not possible, so additional access from the opposite femoral vein should be obtained for angiography if needed. This second sheath is definitely needed if the device cannot easily be withdrawn into the femoral vein. A directional catheter with a 10 or 15 mm snare can be advanced from the second access vessel and used to further crush the tip of the device extruding from the long sheath. If not successful, a larger sheath can be placed in the second access vessel and the device removed through this approach.

Removal from the vessel and from the body is facilitated by a small 2 cm incision through the skin and subcutaneous tissue. Do not dissect out the vein completely unless absolutely necessary. Supportive tissue around the vessel is very helpful to allow removal by steady pressure without rupturing the vessel. As the device emerges from the vessel a pair of forceps can be used to free the device from subcutaneous tissue. Maintain wire access in the femoral vessel if possible. This is done by sticking the vein a few centimeters inferior to the long sheath entrance site and advancing a small 0.018 inch straight wire along the side of the original long sheath into the IVC. After removal of the long sheath with the device, a new long sheath can be placed over the retained inferior wire, both to give new access to proceed with additional device placement and to create hemostasis at the initial puncture site.

Vascular injury

Vascular injury associated with ASD device closure is either due to stenosis or thrombosis associated with the large sheath in the femoral iliac vein or dissection of the vein related to removal of a partially collapsed device. Surgical repair is always a possible fallback option, although successful management of the vascular injury should be possible with interventional techniques. A key to success is maintaining wire position through the area of injured vessel throughout the process. Small, soft-tipped 0.014 inch wires and microglide hydrophilic catheters should be used to prevent additional injury. Access to the injured femoral or iliac vein can be achieved through separate sheath placement in the contralateral vessel or, if the injury is high in the iliac vein, through separate inferior femoral access. A gentle hand angiogram in both the PA and lateral projection should be performed using a 'Y' connector through a 0.038 inch lumen microglide catheter with a 0.014 inch wire across the area of injury. If there is extravasation, then a covered stent should be used, sized 2 to 3 mm larger than the surrounding non-injured vein diameter. If there is no extravasation but obstruction to flow, a determination of thrombus vs intimal flap must be made. If there is thrombus then an appropriate sized clot removal system, such as AngioJet (Possis, Medical Inc, Minneapolis, MN) should be used to remove thrombus, then reassess with a repeat angiogram. A peripheral bare metal stent can be used at this point to optimize the chance of long-term patency. Medical treatment with combination antiplatelet therapy is recommended for 6 months, at which time Doppler evaluation of the vessels should be performed.

Cardiac perforation/pericardial effusion

Presumably cardiac perforation and pericardial effusion associated with the CardioSEAL/STARFlex device system are due to acute puncture of the atrial free wall with a procedural wire or the tip of an oversized umbrella. Late perforation has not been reported. Presumably, arm frame fracture reduces excessive stress on an umbrella arm tip poised to perforate the myocardial free wall late. Malposition of the device, such as occurs with entanglement in the Eustachian valve, may predispose to perforation. The occurrence is rare, less than 0.5%, and most cases can be managed conservatively with observation or pericardial drainage. If the effusion persists, then surgical device removal with repair is necessary. These small device tip perforations appear to seal spontaneously, although careful observation including daily echocardiograms is warranted. The incidence is too low to determine risk factors, but an oversized device for the total atrial size and malposition of the device at the time of release are most likely. Careful sizing of the device, including a measure of total septal length in small patients, should minimize this complication.

Thrombus

Late thrombus on this device is rare, mostly reported in young adults, many of whom were not compliant with postprocedure antiplatelet medications. The presumed mechanism is blood stasis in pockets of poor device apposition to the atrial wall. A second mechanism is endocardial irritation at the site of an umbrella tip. There are case reports of non-thrombus endocardial hyperplasia/fibrosis at an umbrella tip mistaken for thrombus on echo. Prevention is the optimal

strategy, with appropriate sizing of the device and strict adherence to antiplatelet medications postimplant. Aspirin 81 mg with 75 mg of clopidogrel daily for 6 months after implant is recommended. Screening echoes at 1 and 6 months should be performed to evaluate for thrombus.

If thrombus is found on the device, it can be managed by aggressive medical therapy with iv heparin and conversion to oral Coumadin® (warfarin). Once the thrombus size is seen to decrease by echocardiographic evaluation, the patient can be managed as an outpatient. If the thrombus is unresponsive to medical therapy, or is large, mobile, and attached to the left atrial umbrella, surgical removal is warranted.

Procedural air/thrombus

Thrombus associated with the large sheaths required in the left atrium during device delivery can result in myocardial infarction (MI), TIA, or stroke. Fortunately this is a preventable complication with aggressive anticoagulation of the patient during the procedure and frequent flushing of the sheath with heparinized saline (2 units heparin per cc normal saline) before, during, and after device placement. Some operators prefer continuous infusion while others use frequent intermittent flushing. The patient's ACT should be kept at >250 seconds throughout the procedure using bolus iv heparin 100 units/kg to a maximum of 4000 units, with repeat ACT every 20 minutes, and repeat dosing of heparin as needed. If a clot is noted by echocardiography associated with the sheath or attached device, the entire system should be withdrawn to the right atrium, the sheath cleared, and then replaced with a new sheath over a wire. The ACT should be checked and additional heparin given prior to repositioning the sheath in the left atrium.

Because this device, like others currently available, requires loading of the device into an open large sheath, introduction of air during the device delivery process is quite common. To reduce this risk the operator should continuously flush the system during loading, or load the device under saline in a large tub. If the ASD is large the delivery sheath can be positioned in the RA, and the device advanced to the tip of the sheath, thereby releasing any air in the system in the right heart. The sheath/device system is then advanced across the defect into the LA for delivery, minimizing left-sided air embolus risk.

Arrhythmia

Atrial flutter or fibrillation is uncommon but does occasionally occur during implantation due to catheter/device atrial wall stimulation. Because the majority of patients have otherwise normal hearts they tolerate the tachycardia without significant hemodynamic instability. Careful attention to the ACT and heparinization when this occurs is warranted. If the patient is stable, continuing the procedure with delivery of the device is most appropriate. Although cardioversion immediately is an option, further manipulation of catheters and the device in the atrium may restart the tachycardia. Complete the device placement, release the device, and finish postplacement hemodynamic assessment, then cardiovert (0.5 to 1 joule/kg with biphasic defibrillator) at the end of the procedure. Although device embolization immediately after cardioversion has been reported, cardioversion with the device is quite safe. Antiarrhythmic medication in the acute setting is rarely needed as recurrence after the procedure is rare.

Late development of atrial flutter or fibrillation has been reported in up to 7% of adult patients with the CardioSEAL/STARFlex device system.[17] The rate is highest in adults who get PFO closure, and has not been reported in children. The etiology of late atrial arrhythmia is not known, although the mechanism is presumed to be the development of non, slow, and normal conduction areas as endocardium covers the device. Treatment with antiarrhythmic medicines such as β-blockers or amiodarone has been very effective. At 6 to 9 months postplacement the device is completely covered with endocardium and the arrhythmia substrate no longer present, so medication can be discontinued. Remember, however, that some patients present with non-specific symptoms such as mild palpitations at the time of ASD diagnosis, and in some patients these symptoms may be the first presentation of paroxsysmal atrial flutter unrelated to the device. In that situation the device may exacerbate an underlying atrial flutter substrate that may not resolve with coverage of the device, with the need for ongoing antiarrhythmics.

Arm fracture

Arm fractures continue to be an issue with this device system, although the incidence has decreased dramatically with the STARFlex device as compared to earlier systems.[15] Clearly size of device is critical, with fractures rare in 28 mm or smaller devices. Late complications associated with device fracture are extremely rare, with only local irritation granuloma development and significant residual leak having been reported. Screening X-ray is recommended at 6 months to evaluate for arm fracture. Fluoroscopy in the RAO caudal and LAO cranial projections should be performed if there is any question of a fracture. Treatment is not required, but long-term follow-up is appropriate to insure no late granuloma, leak, or thrombus formation. The question of long-term aspirin for patients with arm fracture and poor umbrella atrial wall apposition has been raised. The incidence is too low for clinical data to guide therapy in this situation, but many operators recommend long-term low-dose aspirin to reduce the potential risk of late thrombosis.

Residual leaks

Residual leak is present in 15% of patients at 6 months, but few of these cases are clinically significant. At UCSF between 1997 and 2002, 3 of 261 patients (1.1%) treated with CardioSEAL/STARFlex devices required repeat intervention for a significant residual leak. All patients had a second device placed successfully with complete closure. Because ongoing endocardial coverage can reduce the size of residual defects up to several years conservative observation for at least 12 months is recommended. The decision to intervene is based on RV size remaining > the 95th percentile. If the residual leak size is getting smaller over time, then continued observation is warranted. Additional device placement has been without difficulties in our experience. The only consideration is that if the residual defect is due to a 3-5 arm split of the superior left atrial umbrella through the defect as it extends toward the SVC, an internal jugular approach for second device delivery is preferred.

REFERENCES

1. Engelfriet P, Meijboom F, Boersma E, Tijssen J, Mulder B. Repaired and open atrial septal defects type II in adulthood: an epidemiological study of a large European cohort. Int J Cardiol Jun 21 2007.
2. Engelfriet PM, Duffels MG, Moller T et al. Pulmonary arterial hypertension in adults born with a heart septal defect: the Euro Heart Survey on adult congenital heart disease. Heart (Br Card Soc) 2007; 93(6): 682–7.
3. Lammers A, Hager A, Eicken A et al. Need for closure of secundum atrial septal defect in infancy. J Thorac Cardiovasc Surg 2005; 129(6): 1353–7.
4. Post MC, Suttorp MJ, Jaarsma W, Plokker HW. Comparison of outcome and complications using different types of devices for percutaneous closure of a secundum atrial septal defect in adults: a single-center experience. Cathet Cardiovasc Interven 2006; 67(3): 438–43.
5. Butera G, Carminati M, Chessa M et al. CardioSEAL/STARflex versus Amplatzer devices for percutaneous closure of small to moderate (up to 18 mm) atrial septal defects. Am Heart J 2004; 148(3): 507–10.
6. Anzai H, Child J, Natterson B et al. Incidence of thrombus formation on the CardioSEAL and the Amplatzer interatrial closure devices. Am J Cardiol 2004; 93(4): 426–31.
7. Chessa M, Carminati M, Butera G et al. Early and late complications associated with transcatheter occlusion of secundum atrial septal defect. J Am Coll Cardiol 2002; 39(6): 1061–5.
8. Pinto FF, Sousa L, Fragata J. Late cardiac tamponade after transcatheter closure of atrial septal defect with Cardioseal device. Cardiol Young 2001; 11(2): 233–5.
9. Carminati M, Chessa M, Butera G et al. Transcatheter closure of atrial septal defects with the STARFlex device: early results and follow-up. J Interven Cardiol 2001; 14(3): 319–24.
10. Pedra CA, Pihkala J, Lee KJ et al. Transcatheter closure of atrial septal defects using the Cardio-Seal implant. Heart (Br Card Soc) 2000; 84(3): 320–6.

11. Berdat PA, Chatterjee T, Pfammatter JP et al. Surgical management of complications after transcatheter closure of an atrial septal defect or patent foramen ovale. J Thorac Cardiovasc Surg 2000; 120(6): 1034–9.

12. Varma C, Benson LN, Warr MR et al. Clinical outcomes of patent foramen ovale closure for paradoxical emboli without echocardiographic guidance. Cathet Cardiovasc Interven 2004; 62(4): 519–25.

13. Krumsdorf U, Ostermayer S, Billinger K et al. Incidence and clinical course of thrombus formation on atrial septal defect and patient foramen ovale closure devices in 1,000 consecutive patients. J Am Coll Cardiol 2004; 43(2): 302–9.

14. Beitzke A, Schuchlenz H, Gamillscheg A, Stein JI, Wendelin G. Catheter closure of the persistent foramen ovale: mid-term results in 162 patients. J Interven Cardiol 2001; 14(2): 223–9.

15. Nugent AW, Britt A, Gauvreau K et al. Device closure rates of simple atrial septal defects optimized by the STARFlex device. J Am Coll Cardiol 2006; 48(3): 538–44.

16. Carminati M, Giusti S, Hausdorf G et al. A European multi-centric experience using the CardioSEal and Starflex double umbrella devices to close interatrial communications holes within the oval fossa. Cardiol Young 2000; 10(5): 519–26.

17. Alaeddini J, Feghali G, Jenkins S et al. Frequency of atrial tachyarrhythmias following transcatheter closure of patent foramen ovale. J Invas Cardiol 2006; 18(8): 365–8.

19 Potential complications of transcatheter closure of ventricular septal defects using the PFM NitOcclud VSD Coil

Trong-Phi Lê, Rainer Kozlik-Feldmann, Horst Sievert

Transcatheter closure of ventricular septal defects (VSDs) is a very complex procedure. It has a greater potential for a wide range of complications that are common to all extensive intracardiac manipulations. There are more intracardiac manipulations and a higher complexity of manipulations, with the multiple exchanges of wires, sheaths, catheters, snares, and devices, than with any other interventional procedure. The avoidance of complications is the best guarantee against complications. This includes best possible monitoring of patients during the procedure, a good choice of catheter materials, a cool head, a delicate hand, and – last but not least – the readiness to abandon the procedure in insecure or uncertain situations.

The shape (Figure 19.1) of the PFM VSD coil (PFM Company, Cologne, Germany) is much more flexible than that of the Amplatzer Occluder (AGA Medical, Golden Valley, MN). This flexibility of its design and shape allows a better adaptation of the coils to the anatomy of the individual defect. This is reflected in the fact that VSD closure using the coils, unlike the Amplatzer Occluder, has led to no significant arrhythmic disorders.[1–4] The application of coils demands, however, appreciable clinical experience, and highly skilled operators. In general, the preparation for closure procedures with coils is comparable with that of the application of umbrella-like implantations.

The preparation for a VSD closure – before the coil deployment itself can begin – must entail several steps. First, complications can even occur in this preparation phase, which may aggravate the procedure from the very start, and in some cases even prevent the coil implantation. In the preparation phase it is important to take an angiogram of the left ventricle with the best profile of the defect. This not only serves to depict the size of the VSD, but also determines the plausibility of 'crossing' the defect. It should be kept in mind that, even in this preparation phase, severe heart rhythm disorders can be evoked – even atrioventricular (AV) block. Injuries of the right coronary artery can especially ensue in cases of membranous defects. Repetitive passages of the aortic valve with the guide wire or catheter can sometimes lead to injury of the aortic valve.

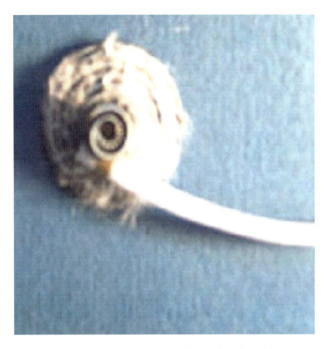

Figure 19.1 The PFM VSD coil. The distal coil loops are reinforced and covered with Decron® fibers. The proximal loops are reversed and without fibers.

If the defect cannot be visualized clearly, and the right heart is significantly contrasted on the left ventricular angiocardiogram, the defect could be much larger than measured using echocardiography. Based on our experience, such a defect could be of oval shape, and on echocardiogram only the smaller diameter can be imaged. In such cases we recommend balloon sizing to determine the exact defect size.

For the delivery of a coil to a muscular ventricular septal defect, an arterio-venous loop is not absolutely necessary, because the defect could directly be crossed from the right ventricle in the majority of cases. A perimembranous ventricular septal defect can sometimes be directly crossed from the right ventricular side. However, a through-and-through wire is, very often necessary to initially cross a perimembranous defect and/or to position the delivery catheter/sheath across the defect from the right to the left ventricle for a venous delivery.

Once the defect has been successfully crossed, the next step is to conduct the guide wire into the right ventricle in such a way as to not interfere with the moderator band or the tricuspid valve apparatus. We remind the reader at this point that the operator should thus choose his guide wire with an appropriate size and bend wisely. We favor catching it in the pulmonary artery, because if the guide wire reaches the right atrium or the vena cava there is no way of ensuring that it does not interfere with the tricuspid valve apparatus. In order to catch the guide wire in the pulmonary artery, we recommend that an open snare should lie waiting in the trunk of the pulmonary artery in advance. If a 6 French end-hole balloon catheter is used to enter the pulmonary artery from the venous side, the risk of interference with the tricuspid valve can be reduced. The lumen of such a catheter should be large enough to accommodate up to a 15 mm snare. For the creation of the arteriovenous circuit it is important that an appropriate length of the guide wire should be chosen for the patient to be treated. Its distal end should be sufficiently stable so that it does not break off when it is snared.

In creating an arteriovenous circuit it should be insured that no loops are found in the right ventricle or atrium. A curving course within the right heart is often an expression of the fact that certain heart structures such as the moderator band or the tricuspid valve apparatus have been influenced by the guide wire, forming a possible source of interference or entanglement later in the procedure. In such cases it is advisable to repeat the guide wire catching maneuver.

When the arteriovenous circuit has been established, a 6 French long sheath can be advanced from the venous side into position. We recommend that the ends of the arterial catheter and the dilator of the long sheath should meet ('kissing') in the vena cava inferior. In order to insure this we recommend securing the guide wire at the hub of the arterial catheter as well as the long sheath with a clamp.

The distal diameter of the chosen coil should be at least double the size of the effective diameter of the VSD measured on the right ventricular side, and about 1–2 mm larger than the VSD diameter from its left ventricular opening. Estimation of the VSD size is more difficult when the defect is associated with an aneurysmal septum, especially in the setting of complex shaped VSDs with more than one opening into the right ventricle. In this case, only the left ventricular diameter of the aneurysm is used when selecting coils. Closure of a perimembranous VSD with a well developed aneurysm does not require a rim to the aortic valve. The selected coil should fit into the aneurysm without protruding into the left ventricular outflow tract. The coil could be displaced or even embolize towards the left heart if more than two distal coil loops protrude into the left ventricle.[5]

Prior to introducing the coil delivery catheter, the long sheath must be aspirated and flushed to ensure no thrombi are inadvertently pushed into the patient's circulation. It is advisable to have the tip of the delivery catheter at least 1 cm away from the tip of the sheath, since the tension on the relatively stiff sheath can often distort the original anatomy of the defect. It is particularly important for passage of the configured coil through the aortic valve and adaptation of the coil into the defect. Apart from the last two loops, all the other loops of the coil are deployed in the ascending aorta. Thereafter, the entire system (i.e., delivery catheter and long sheath) is gently pulled back across the aortic valve and positioned into the left ventricular outflow tract. When the coil is pulled back into the VSD, it usually adapts itself to the configuration of the defect. Very slight backward movement of the sheath and the delivery catheter during adaptation of the coil is necessary to prevent pulling the device through the defect.

Upon passage of the ascending aorta into the left ventricle, the employed coil can, in some cases, become entangled in the aortic valve. In such cases it is very important to advance the tip of the long sheath to the left ventricular side, allowing an easier advancement of the delivery catheter to free the coil from the aortic valve. Two scenarios are feasible at this point. First, the delivery catheter with the configured coil is pushed back into the ascending aorta. A new attempt, i.e. new passage of the coil from the ascending aorta to the left ventricle, can be made. Second, the delivery catheter with the configured coil could fall or tip into the left ventricle. In such a case the coil can be carefully manipulated into the defect.

If the diameter of the coil exceeds 70% of the diameter of the ascending aorta, the likelihood that it could become entangled in the aortic valve is relatively high. In such cases, the configuration of only four distal loops in the ascending aorta could reduce the risk. The remaining distal loops could be constituted in the left ventricular outflow tract. The other option is, similar to the employment of AGA Amplatzer Occluders, the placement of the tip of the long sheath in the left ventricular outflow tract. The coil is then unraveled as close to the septum as possible. Care should be taken to insure that the coil is kept away from the apparatus of the mitral valve. During deployment of the proximal loops of the coil on the right ventricular side the tip of the long sheath is kept close to the septum, so as to avoid interference of the coil loops with the tricuspid valve.

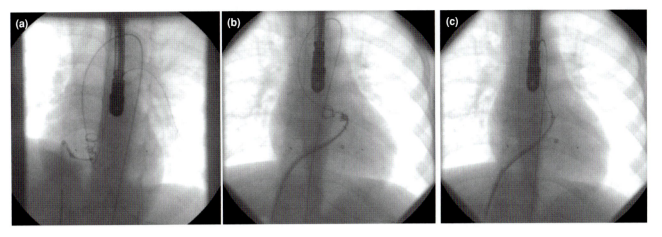

Figure 19.2   Removal of an improperly deployed coil using a snare. Crossing of VSD using a guide wire (a). Snaring of the proximal end of the coil (b). Coil being pulled into long sheath (b). Coil completely retrieved (c).

If the coil must be retrieved it is recommended to first pull the delivery catheter together with the configured coil into the long sheath. Once within the lumen of the long sheath, the coil is favorably extended such that its retrieval is more dependable. If, upon retrieval, resistance is felt, then the operator should be convinced that the coil is not snagged at the tip of the catheter. If this is suspected, a careful manipulation of the catheter should be attempted in order to release the snag and retrieve the coil successfully. The use of too much force on the coil can lead to its premature detachment.

If necessary, the delivery catheter containing the device could be withdrawn completely and the sheath repositioned, and/or a different size device and/or approach utilized. The coil can be repositioned even after it has been entirely opened by withdrawing the device completely back into the catheter. If the catheter and the sheath can be readvanced further into the defect, the same device can be redeployed in the more favorable position. If the delivery catheter, with the contained device, cannot be readvanced on its own, the device is withdrawn into the catheter and the sheath. Both should then be repositioned and the procedure started anew.

Postimplantation angiography and echocardiography are used to insure that there is no interference with or distortion of the aortic valve. Ten minutes after the coil placement, a large-volume left ventricular angiocardiogram is performed to verify the exact position of the coil and the degree of closure of the defect. Often there will be a 'smoke-like' leak through the fibers of the coil at this stage. This type of residual leak closes over a short time. If, on the other hand, there is a relatively large and/or a jet-like leak, the residual leak tends to persist.

We recommend closing a significant residual shunt after follow-up at 6 months. The approach to the residual leak is the same as for the original defect. There is almost no risk of dislodging the original device with further manipulation through and/or around it. The second coil is implanted with a similar technique to the first coil. The loops of the second coil are usually positioned inside the cone of the first device. Once the additional coil has been implanted, the same process of reassessment is carried out.

Occasionally during positioning of the coil across the VSD, too many loops are delivered on the right ventricular side. These additional loops could interfere with the tricuspid valve apparatus and may lead to residual shunting. This is best dealt with by pulling the coil back into the delivery catheter whilst simultaneously pushing the delivery catheter across the VSD back into the left ventricular outflow tract. The implantation can then be reattempted.

If the delivery catheter cannot be advanced into the left ventricular outflow tract, the coil must be retrieved via the catheter. If it is not possible to pull the coil completely back into the delivery catheter, it should be pulled back along with the delivery catheter inside the long sheath. If the coil is prematurely released from the delivery system while it is in a suboptimal position, it does not usually embolize into the right ventricle, as the stiff distal loops will hold it in position. In this case, the VSD should be recrossed in a retrograde fashion and a new guide wire circuit is re-established. A long sheath is carefully positioned next to the proximal end of the coil. Next, a snare catheter is also advanced along the long sheath with the guidance of the wire circuit. The coil is snared from its right ventricular end and then pulled back into the long sheath (Figure 19.2). It is essential that, during this maneuver, the coil is not positioned too deep into the right ventricle, as it could become entangled with the tricuspid valve apparatus.

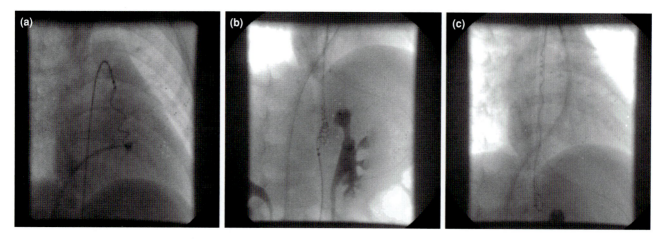

Figure 19.3 Removal of an improperly deployed coil using a snare. (a) Snaring of the distal end of the coil. (b) Coil being pulled into the long sheath after being snared at its proximal end, using a second snare. The distal end is still held with the first snare. (c) Coil completely retrieved into the long sheath.

A poorly positioned coil in the VSD can also be dealt with by snaring it at its distal end and pulling it back into the descending aorta. With the help of a larger arterial long sheath, the coil can be safely retrieved. Alternatively, after accessing the contralateral femoral artery, a guide wire circuit can be established as described before. A long sheath is then positioned from the venous side across the VSD into the descending aorta. The coil can then be retrieved with a snare transvenously (Figure 19.3).

Coil embolization to the branch pulmonary arteries could happen. Of 126 patients who underwent VSD closure using the PFM VSD coil, device embolization into the pulmonary artery occurred in only one case. This event, however, does not usually lead to hemodynamic instability. The largest possible long sheath should be introduced into the corresponding pulmonary artery. A 10 to 15 mm snare should be used to grasp the coil at its proximal end. The coil should be captured into the long sheath in the pulmonary artery to prevent the coil loops being entangled in the tricuspid valve apparatus.

Being an implant with fibers, the PFM VSD coil can cause hemolysis, especially in cases in which significant residual shunts are in place. However, hemolysis is a rare complication in our series. It occurred in four cases, in which only one required surgical removal of the device

due to a significant fall in hemoglobin. The remaining three cases resolved spontaneously within 5 days.

ACKNOWLEDGMENT

The authors wish to thank Dr Franz Freudenthal for his invaluable technical support.

REFERENCES

1. Lê TP, Freudenthal F, Sievert H et al. Transcatheter occlusion of subaortic ventricular septal defect using a nitinol coil (NitOcclud); initial clinical results. Circulation 2001; 104: SII 593.
2. Lê TP. Closure of VSD-PFM coil. In: Sievert H, Wilson N, Qureshi SA, Hijazi ZM, eds. Percutaneous Interventions for Congenital Heart Disease. London: Informa Healthcare, 2007.
3. Fu YC, Bass J, Amin Z, Radtke W, Cheatham JP et al. Transcatheter closure of perimembranous ventricular septal defects using the new Amplatzer membranous VSD occluder: results of the U.S. phase I trial. J Am Coll Cardiol 2006; 47(2): 319–25.
4. Carminati M. Transcatheter treatment of congenital and postinfarction ventricular septal defects: Preliminary Results of a European Multicenter Study. 8th International Workshop on Catheter Interventions in Congenital and Structural Heart Disease, Frankfurt, Germany, 16–19 June 2005.
5. Kotthoff S, Lê TP, Debus V et al. Late coil displacement after interventional closure of a perimembranous ventricular septal defect: a case report. Cathet Cardiovasc Interven 2005; 66(2): 273–6.

20 Device closure of ventricular septal defects (percutaneous and hybrid) using the Amplatzer VSD devices

Karim Diab, Qi-Ling Cao, and Ziyad M Hijazi

Ventricular septal defects (VSDs) represent the most common congenital heart disease and account for approximately 20–30% of all congenital cardiac malformations.[1] Perimembranous VSDs (PmVSDs) involve the membranous portion of the ventricular septum and represent approximately 70–80% of all VSDs. On the other hand, Muscular VSDs (mVSDs) are located entirely in the muscular septum and account for approximately 10–15% of all VSDs. These latter defects can be further classified in order of frequency into apical, mid septal, anterior, and posterior defects. In addition, they can be either solitary or multiple ('Swiss cheese' VSDs). Patients with VSDs who show evidence of left atrial and ventricular volume overload require closure of these defects in order to prevent the development of pulmonary hypertension, ventricular dilatation, aortic regurgitation, double-chambered right ventricle, and endocarditis.[2] Surgical closure of these defects is currently widely acceptable but is still associated with significant morbidity, especially in the case of the muscular type. This includes the potential risk for complete heart block, chylothorax, phrenic nerve injury, wound infection, neurologic sequelae of cardiopulmonary bypass, and a thoracotomy scar.[3–7] Patients with mVSDs, in particular, also present a significant challenge to the surgeon. Various surgical approaches have been attempted to close these defects: right ventriculotomy tends to provide suboptimal exposure due to the heavy right ventricle (RV) trabeculations, while left ventriculotomy has been associated with significant ventricular dysfunction.[8] In addition, the rate of residual defects remains significant after surgical repair. Hence, with the availability of new effective occluders, device closure of both mVSDs and PmVSDs is a promising alternative to surgery.

In this chapter, we review the techniques of device closure of mVSDs and PmVSDs using the percutaneous approach and, in the case of mVSDs, the perventricular or hybrid approach, with an emphasis on the potential complications that may be encountered during catheter closure, how to avoid such complications, and possible solutions.

PRECATHERERIZATION EVALUATION AND PATIENT SELECTION

Transthoracic (TTE) and/or transesophageal (TEE) echocardiography is essential for the correct diagnosis of the location and number of VSDs and the relationship of the VSD to important structures, such as the tricuspid and mitral valves, and the moderator band. Currently, only mVSDs and PmVSDs are eligible for device closure. In the case of PmVSDs, it is also important to measure the rim between the defect and the aortic valve when considering eligibility for device closure. This rim needs to be at least 2 mm when using the Amplatzer Membranous VSD Occluder, and at least 6 to 8 mm when using the other devices available.

The weight of the patient is also an important consideration when contemplating device closure. Currently, we consider patients to be candidates for percutaneous VSD device closure when they weigh at least 5.0 kg and 8 to 10 kg for mVSDs and PmVSDs, respectively. Otherwise, the perventricular approach should be the method of choice for patients with mVSDs.

THE AMPLATZER DEVICES

The Amplatzer Muscular VSD Occluder device

In the United States, there are currently two devices available for transcatheter closure of mVSDs. The Cardio-SEAL device (NMT, Boston, MA) is a modification of the Clamshell device, and is approved by the Food and Drug Administration (FDA) for mVSD closure in patients who are at high risk for surgical closure. Unlike this device, the Amplatzer Muscular VSD Occluder (AGA Medical, Plymouth, MN), is designed specifically for the muscular septum. It was initially reported by Amin et al. in 1999[9] and first used in humans by Thanapoulos et al. in 1999.[10] It is made of 0.004–0.005 inch Nitinol wire with polyester mesh.

The self-expandable discs are connected via a central waist, the diameter of which determines the size of the device. The waist is 7 mm long and the two discs are 4 mm larger than the connecting waist. The device is available in sizes ranging from 4 to 18 mm in 2 mm increments, and it requires a 6–9 French delivery sheath, depending on the device size used. This device gained FDA approval at the end of 2007.

The PmVSD device

The relatively new Amplatzer Membranous VSD Occluder device (AGA Medical) is specifically designed for the membranous septum. Like the mVSD device, it is a self-expandable double-disc device made of Nitinol wire mesh. Unlike the former, however, the connecting waist is shorter (1.5 mm long), to minimize the risk of interference with the tricuspid valve. In addition, the left ventricle (LV) disc is asymmetric: its aortic end is 0.5 mm larger than the waist to prevent interference with the aortic valve, while the other end is 5.5 mm longer to provide secure anchorage. The right ventricle (RV) disc, on the other hand, is 2 mm larger than the waist at both sides. The device is currently available in sizes ranging from 4 to 18 mm in 2 mm increments (recently, the manufacturer introduced odd-numbered sizes). The sheath for the device is curved 180° to help direct its tip toward the LV apex when across the VSD. This sheath is available in three different sizes: 7 French (for 4–8 mm devices), 8 French (for 10–12 mm devices), and 9 French (for 14–18 mm devices).

CLOSURE PROTOCOL

Percutaneous closure protocol

The protocols for mVSD and PmVSD device closure are similar in many respects. Thus, the steps are herein outlined for both procedures, while differences are mentioned when they exist. The procedure is typically performed under general anesthesia with TEE guidance. In the case of mVSDs, TEE can be optional when dealing with a single defect, but is essential when multiple or Swiss cheese mVSDs are present, as it helps to determine the size and location of the different defects and helps to monitor the atrioventricular (AV) valves throughout the procedure. For PmVSDs, the use of TTE or intracardiac echocardiography (ICE) can allow the procedure to be performed under conscious sedation in older patients.

Prior to the procedure, it is essential to ensure the presence of a competent echocardiographer with experience in TEE. This echocardiographer will work very closely with the interventionalist in obtaining the correct views needed to ensure a successful procedure. Access is obtained in both the femoral artery and vein.

In case of mVSDs located in the mid, posterior, or apical septum, access should also be obtained from the right internal jugular vein.

Heparin is given at 100 units/kg to achieve an activated clotting time of greater than 250 seconds at the time of device deployment. Routine right and left heart catheterization is performed to assess the degree of shunting and evaluate the pulmonary vascular resistance. Angiography is then performed to define the location, size, and number of VSDs present: for mVSDs, this is done in the hepatoclavicular view (35° LAO/35° cranial); for PmVSD, it is done in the long axial oblique view (60° LAO/20° cranial). Detailed evaluation of the defect, AV valves, and any associated anomalies is done by TEE, focusing on the papillary muscles, moderator band, and chordae tendinea. The AV valves are interrogated for baseline regurgitation and tissue rims, and distances from the aortic, tricuspid, and mitral valves are also measured to determine adequacy for device closure. The VSD is measured in different planes including the frontal 4-chamber and basal short-axis views. The appropriate device is chosen to be 1–2 mm larger than the VSD size as determined by TEE and angiographic evaluation (maximal size at end-diastole).

After a full evaluation has been done, the next step is to cross the VSD. The usual approach is to cross from the LV side, either retrograde (our preferred method) or, in case of mVSDs, via the transseptal approach using a 4–5 French end-hole catheter (Judkins right, or Cobra). On occasion, floating a balloon-tipped catheter in the LV will facilitate crossing the VSD. A soft-tipped 0.035 inch glide wire (Terumo, Japan) is then advanced through this catheter to the VSD. Usually, the guide wire will be advanced to the branch pulmonary arteries. The catheter is advanced over the guide wire to the branch pulmonary artery. This wire is then removed and a softer exchange length guide wire (Noodle wire from AGA) or a regular stiffness wire from Cook is advanced to the tip of this catheter in the pulmonary artery. This wire is snared from there using the proper size gooseneck (10–25 mm loop) snare, and exteriorized from either the right internal jugular vein or the femoral vein, depending on the location of the VSD as mentioned above. It is worth noting that, if the mVSD is large, one might consider crossing the VSD from the RV side. However, it is important to make sure that the wire/catheter does not go through the trabeculations of the RV.

Once the arteriovenous wire loop is formed, the next step will be the advancement of the proper size delivery sheath over the venous side of the wire all the way to the LV or ascending aorta. Once the tip of the sheath is in the LV/ascending aorta, the dilator and wire are removed slowly, making sure that the sheath itself is in the left side of the heart. Once the sheath position is confirmed by angiography and/or echocardiography, the proper size device is screwed to the cable and loaded under water seal to eliminate any air bubbles. It is important here to note a critical step when securing the PmVSD device to the cable. Unlike the mVSD device, the PmVSD device has a pusher catheter with a metal capsule at its end to help identify the position of the device as it has asymmetric disks. Thus, it is critical that the operator aligns the flat part of the screw in the device to the flat part of the capsule at the end of the pusher catheter. This ensures that, when deploying the LV disk, the flat part of the device is deployed underneath the aortic valve. This can be easily confirmed by fluoroscopy that shows the platinum marker on the LV disk pointing toward the patient's feet.

Once the device is loaded, it is advanced under continuous fluoroscopic guidance until it approaches the tip of the sheath. The LV disk is then deployed in the mid LV cavity for mVSD by slowly retracting the sheath over the delivery cable. For PmVSD, the sheath is slowly pulled back away from the apex until it reaches the outflow tract; the LV disk is then deployed between the anterior mitral valve leaflet and the LV outflow tract. Then the entire assembly is pulled towards the septum under both fluoroscopy and TEE guidance. An angiogram can be performed using the pigtail catheter positioned in the LV. This will delineate the position of the ventricular septum. Further retraction of the sheath over the cable will deploy the waist and the right ventricular disk in the respective positions. Again, TEE and angiography should be performed prior to device release. This is important to assess the device position, the function of the AV valves, and the presence of any residual VSD. Once correct device position is ensured, the device can be released by counterclockwise rotation of the pin vise at the end of the cable. In case of the PmVSD device, prior to release, one should make sure that the capsule and the flat part of the microscrew are disengaged from each other. After the device has been released, final assessment of the end result is crucial. This includes detailed echocardiographic assessment as well as angiography in the LV. If the mVSD is solitary, sheaths are removed and hemostasis is achieved, otherwise the same steps are repeated to close a second or third mVSD.

Patients routinely receive a dose of an appropriate antibiotic (commonly cephazolin at 20 mg/kg) during the catheterization procedure, and two further doses at 8-hour intervals. Patients are kept overnight and the following morning a TTE is performed to assess device position and any potential complication. Patients are discharged home on 81 mg aspirin per day for 6 months, and are instructed to receive subacute bacterial endocarditis (SBE) prophylaxis when needed until the device is endothelialized (6–12 months) if there is no residual shunt.

Perventricular mVSD closure protocol

The perventricular or hybrid approach is particularly advantageous when mVSDs are encountered in small infants (<5 kg), patients with poor vascular access, and patients with other associated cardiac lesions requiring concomitant surgical repair. The latter group includes, for example, neonates with coarctation of the aorta and a large mVSD, where this approach provides a one-stage repair. This procedure was initially reported in a baby by Amin et al. in 1998.[11] It can be performed in the catheterization laboratory to allow the additional use of fluoroscopy, unless additional surgical repair is required. A major advantage of this technique is that it is completely performed off-pump without cardiopulmonary bypass (CPB), unlike the surgical techniques for closure of mVSDs. In the event where other surgical interventions are required for associated lesions, the mVSD is then closed first prior to initiation of CPB.

Typically, the heart is approached via a median sternotomy or a subxyphoid minimally invasive incision without sternotomy. The surgeon and the echocardiographer determine the best location for puncturing the RV free wall by having the surgeon softly tap on the RV free wall under TEE guidance using a clamp or the fingers. The location should be chosen away from the papillary muscles and moderator band, but perpendicular to the septum. The surgeon then places a 5.0 polypropelene purse-string suture at the chosen location. An 18 G needle is used to puncture the RV free wall. A 0.035 inch short guide wire is then passed through the needle and manipulated into the LV cavity across the mVSD. The needle is then removed while keeping the wire positioned in the LV. A 7–10 French short introducer sheath (8–13 cm), depending on the size of the device chosen, is then fed over the wire with its dilator and advanced into the LV cavity. With the help of continuous TEE monitoring, it is essential to ensure that the dilator is not advanced too deep into the LV as it could perforate the LV free wall. The dilator is then removed and the sheath tip kept in the LV mid cavity. As with the percutaneous approach, the VSD device is chosen and loaded onto the delivery cable under water seal to prevent any air bubbles. The device is then advanced inside the delivery sheath under TEE guidance until it reaches the tip of the sheath. The LV disc is then deployed in the LV mid cavity by gentle retraction of the sheath over the cable. The whole cable/delivery sheath system is then pulled toward the ventricular septum. The sheath is then further retracted off the cable to deploy the connecting waist and then the RV disc. Continuous TEE monitoring is of extreme importance to confirm device position. If this is satisfactory, the device is released by counterclockwise rotation of the cable using the pin vise. A complete TEE study is then performed to confirm device placement, assess for any residual shunting, and evaluate for valve regurgitation that might have been induced by the device. The same procedure can be repeated in case of multiple mVSDs. If the patient has other associated cardiac malformations requiring surgical repair, CPB is then initiated. If mVSD was the only lesion, the chest is closed and postoperative care is carried out similar to that with the percutaneous closure protocol.

Results of the perventricular closure technique have been very encouraging despite the small number of clinical studies available in the literature using this approach.[12-14] No significant complications were reported with this technique except for a few related to the surgical intervention (e.g. mediastinitis). This technique is currently being used only for mVSD closure, though studies have been attempted using a similar approach on an animal model with PmVSDs.[15]

HOW NOT TO GET INTO TROUBLE: SKILLS AND EQUIPMENT NEEDED

In order to avoid complications during the closure procedure, the most important step is planning the procedure itself, which is largely based on the echocardiographic (TTE and TEE) evaluation of the defect and associated structures. This step is done as part of the precatheterization evaluation as well as during the actual procedure. This is of paramount importance as it helps in the selection of the appropriate patients for device closure (e.g. defect size and location, distance from various valve structures) and in deciding the most appropriate access (e.g. femoral and/or internal jugular).

The equipment needed includes that usually used for performing a routine right and left heart catheterization. The equipment specifically required for VSD device closure includes 4–5 French Judkins right catheters of various curves; one should make sure that gooseneck snares of various sizes are available (ev3, Plymouth, MN). Exchange-length soft wires and kink-resistant delivery sheaths of all sizes (7–10 French) must be available. The manufacturer recommends that the new delivery sheath (TorqVue, AGA Medical Corporation, Plymouth, MN) be used since it is kink resistant. From our experience, the Mullins type sheath can also do the same job (Cook, Inc, Bloomington, IN). However, for device retrieval one would need a larger delivery sheath (up to 14–16 French). Terumo glide wires of various thicknesses (0.018–0.35 inch), and exchange-length guide wires, for various device sizes (4–18 mm), should be all present in the catheterization laboratory prior to the puncture of the femoral/jugular vessels. Selecting an oversized or undersized device may result in complications.

As the VSD closure procedure is significantly complex, operator experience is key to avoiding potential complications. Due to the extensive manipulation of wires, catheters, and sheaths compared to other interventional catheterization procedures, meticulous handling of the equipment is essential in order to avoid getting into trouble during the VSD closure procedure.

First, it is important to avoid any air or clots in the system, as in any other catheterization intervention.

Air or clot embolism should be a preventable complication by being vigilant in periodically clearing all equipment used of clots or air bubbles. As the VSD closure procedure can be a lengthy one, it is important also to keep routinely checking the activated clotting time, keeping it more than 250 seconds at the time of device deployment.

Second, as significantly large sheaths are used in this procedure, it is important to avoid vascular complications as these sheaths can potentially cause damage to the access vessels. This is done by advancing the sheaths slowly and under fluoroscopic guidance, and by not forcing them through when resistance is encountered. This is true when the arteriovenous wire loop is formed and the delivery sheath is advanced from the venous side to the LV side. On occasions, the loop becomes trapped under trabeculations and forcing the delivery sheath may result in tearing a chordae or a papillary muscle. If resistance is significant, one should abort this step and cross the defect again.

Third, as the procedure involves the use of multiple wires, catheters, and large sheaths across cardiac valves, it is important to prevent any damage to such valves. This is done by using soft wires and avoiding forcing any wires across the valves. As mentioned previously, internal jugular venous access can be advantageous in the case of mid, posterior, or apical mVSDs. When crossing these defects with a stiff wire to position the sheath in the LV cavity, the wire can stent the aortic and tricuspid valves open and can thus cause significant hypotension, even without damaging the valves per se. To prevent such a complication, we avoid using extra-stiff wires and we try to minimize the time the wires are across the valve as much as possible.

The large delivery sheath needed can also occasionally damage the valves as well. Therefore, if any resistance is met, or if any increase in valvular regurgitation is noted on echocardiography, the sheath should be slowly removed and repositioned as it could be entangled in the valve leaflets or valve chordae. It is important to emphasize that the snaring step should be performed in the branch pulmonary arteries or the superior vena cava away from the valve chordae in order to prevent such complications.

Fourth, the VSD devices themselves can cause potential complications. It is important to use the appropriate device size and avoid oversizing by relying on the appropriate measurements obtained by TEE and angiography. The device disks can potentially interfere with the valve function (Figures 20.1 and 20.2). This can be prevented by choosing the right device size and checking the device position prior to release, making sure it is not impinging on the leaflets or catching the valve chordae. It is essential to measure the rim separating the defect from the aortic valve to confirm that the defect is amenable for device closure in case of PmVSDs. Perforation of the right aortic valve cusp has been reported after PmVSD device closure, especially

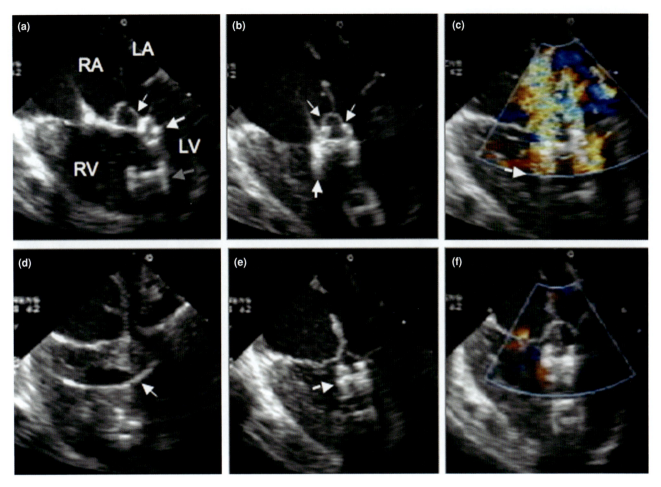

Figure 20.1 TEE images in a 7-month old infant, 7.3 kg in weight, with transposition and ventricular septal defects (three), status postpulmonary artery banding undergoing percutaneous closure of the defects prior to surgical correction of the transposition. (A) Four-chamber view showing the first deployed 6 mm Amplatzer muscular VSD device (gray arrow) and the left disc of the second device (arrow) in the left ventricle. Note the mitral valve leaflet (short arrow) is between septum and disc. (B) Both discs have been deployed, but not released, showing both mitral and tricuspid leaflets were caught (arrows). (C) Color Doppler prior to release of the device (arrow) demonstrating significant mitral and tricuspid valve regurgitation. (D) The device was captured and the defect was crossed again (arrow). (E) Device in good position (arrow) with no interference with any valvular structure. (F) Final color Doppler demonstrating no mitral regurgitation and trivial tricuspid regurgitation. LA, left atrium; LV, left ventricle; RA, right atrium; RV, right ventricle.

with devices other than the Amplatzer device.[16] It is important as well to closely follow up these patients postprocedure for any valvular regurgitation.

When crossing the VSD from the right side (in case of a large mVSD) care should be exercised not to go through the RV trabeculations. When the heavy RV trabeculations prevent the RV disk of the device from expanding completely, we sometimes use the PDA Amplatzer occluder device.[17] This mushroom-shaped device fits well in the mVSD and avoids the RV trabeculations, and can thus be helpful in such cases.

It is possible, though very rare, that the device embolizes after release (Figure 20.3). The main way to prevent such a serious complication is to carefully evaluate the device position by TEE and angiography prior to releasing it from the cable.

POSSIBLE COMPLICATIONS AND HOW TO MANAGE THEM

The aim of the operator should really be to plan to prevent any potential complication from taking place during the closure procedure. In the event that such complications do occur, however, the operator should be ready to handle them and the catheterization laboratory should have the appropriate equipment required.

Complications related to VSD device closure can be divided into those that occur acutely during the procedure and those that are encountered on long-term follow-up. To date, the rates of these complications compare well with those associated with surgical repair. The immediate and mid term results of the US registry involving 14 tertiary referral centers on device closure of

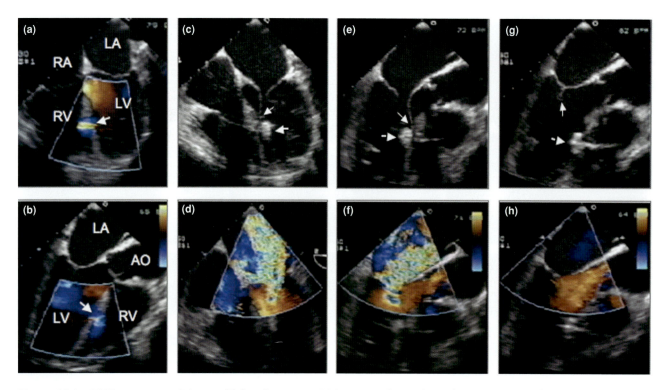

Figure 20.2   TEE images in a 54-year-old female patient, 58 kg in weight, with moderate size muscular VSD (10 mm). (A and B) Four-chamber and long-axis views with color Doppler showing the defect (arrow). Four-chamber view without (C) and with (D) Color Doppler showing the left disc (arrow) of a 12 mm Amplatzer Muscular VSD device was deployed. Note, the anterior mitral valve leaflet (arrow) was caught between disc and septum, and the resultant severe mitral regurgitation. (E and F) Long-axis view without and with color Doppler showing the leaflet and the mitral regurgitation. (G and H) The disc was recaptured and redeployed away from the leaflet, resulting in good position with no regurgitation.

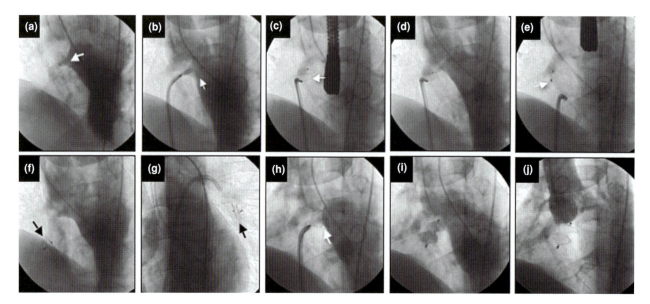

Figure 20.3   Cine fluoroscopic images in long axial oblique projection in a 27-year-male with 6 mm perimembranous VSD and Qp:Qs of 1.8:1. (A) Left ventricle angiogram showing the defect (arrow). (B–E) Steps of implantation of a 10 mm Amplatzer Membranous VSD device (arrows). (F and G) The device embolized to the right ventricle and finally to the left pulmonary artery. (H) A 14 mm device was implanted after the first device had been recaptured. (I) Repeat left ventricle angiogram showing good device position and minimal residual shunt through the device. (J) Aortogram showing good device position and no aortic insufficiency.

mVSD with the Amplatzer device reported major complications in 10.7% of patients.[18] This rate significantly improved with better experience with this technique. The rate of major complications reported in later studies ranged from 0 to 3.3%, with a mean of 2.8% from the data pooled from the available literature.[19–22] No significant major complications have been reported in the clinical studies involving the perventricular approach.[12–14] Similarly, the rate of major complications reported in PmVSD closure studies improved with better familiarity

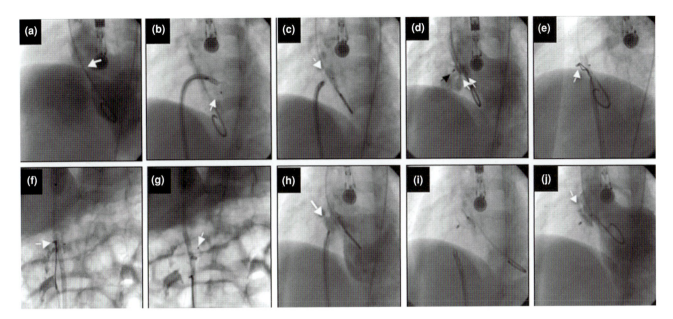

Figure 20.4 Cine fluoroscopic images in a 6.5-year-old male with 7 mm perimembranous VSD. (A) Angiogram in the left ventricle demonstrating the VSD (arrow). (B and C) Implantation of an 8 mm Amplatzer device (arrow). (D) Left ventricle angiogram demonstrating both discs in the left ventricle side (arrows); only the microscrew (black arrow) is in the right ventricle side of the defect. (E) The microscrew of the device was snared (arrow). (F and G) Device removed using a larger sheath (arrows). (H–J) Implantation of a new 12 mm device appropriately. Note final angiogram showing the right ventricle disc on the right side of the defect (arrow).

with the use of the Amplatzer Membranous VSD Occluder device. These rates range from 0 to 5% in different studies, with an average rate from pooled data in the literature of 1.2%.[23–29] It is important to note that a weight <5.0 kg and <10 kg was found to significantly correlate with an increased incidence of procedure- or device-related complications with the percutaneous approach for mVSD and PmVSD closure, respectively.[18,23] It is also worth noting that deployment of multiple devices across the muscular septum was not associated with increased risk for complications.[14]

Two major complications are device embolization and cardiac perforation. Embolization of the device can occur if the device is released prematurely or in the improper position (Figures 20.3 and 20.4). The device can then embolize to the LV, ascending aorta, RV, or pulmonary arteries. In order to avoid such a complication, we routinely evaluate the device position by TEE, as well as by performing an LV angiogram prior to releasing the device (Figure 20.4). In the event that such a complication occurs, however, it is essential to have available the appropriate tools in order to attempt to retrieve the device percutaneously. This includes larger sheaths (e.g. Mullins long sheath), gooseneck snares, and biopsy forceps. A larger sheath needs to be placed first, then one can attempt to catch the device with either a snare or a biopsy forceps, and exteriorize it through the larger sheath (Figure 20.4). One should never pull a device through cardiac structures unfolded, since this may result in significant damage to the structures. If this fails, then surgical back-up should be available in the institution for emergency retrieval. Cardiac perforation has also been rarely reported, especially during the initial trials of VSD device closure. It is important to

position the delivery sheath in the LV cavity not too close to the LV free wall while delivering the device. This prevents potential perforation of the LV free wall during device delivery. Meticulous use of wires and catheters should allow avoidance of this serious complication as well. With the perventricular technique, this complication is possible when the sheath and its dilator are being advanced into the LV across the mVSD. The dilator is stiff enough to puncture the LV if it is pushed too far into the LV, even if it is being advanced over a guide wire! Therefore, it is essential to keep the tip away from the LV free wall by monitoring its position with TEE.

Vascular complications, namely thromboses, have been reported but are rare. It is important as mentioned above to keep an activated clotting time above 250 seconds. In case this complication occurs, usual treatment with heparin infusion or recombinant tissue plasminogen activator factor is sometimes successful in revascularizing the vessel. Obviously, this complication is avoided in the perventricular approach.

Hemolysis has been rarely reported with VSD device closure.[30] This rare complication occurs if there is residual shunting as the device sits between two chambers with a high pressure difference across them. This can be prevented by using the appropriate device size (avoiding undersizing) and by appropriately positioning the device. In addition, one possible way to minimize this complication is to soak the device in 10–15 cc of the patient's blood rather than in saline. This is done for about 15–20 minutes, then the device is loaded under blood and flushed with 5 cc of blood. This may increase the chance of complete closure and clotting around the device. In the event that hemolysis is encountered, the patient should be monitored and treated medically as

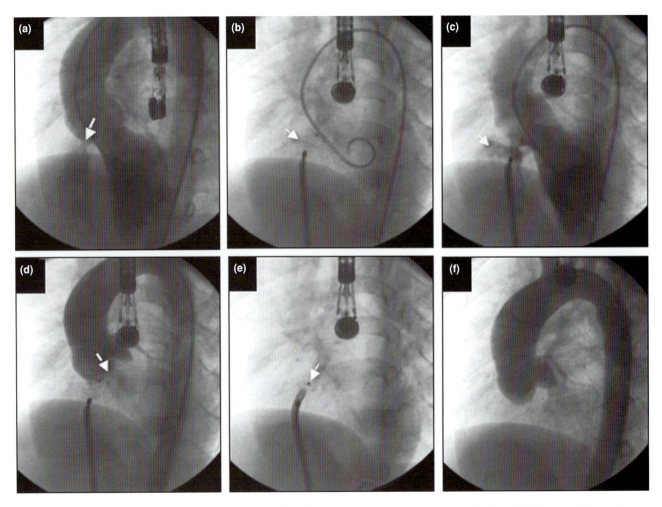

Figure 20.5 Cine fluoroscopic images in a 6-year-old male with 4.7 mm perimembranous VSD. (A) Left ventricle angiogram showing the VSD (arrow). (B and C) Device deployment showing good position (arrows). (D) Aortogram prior to device release demonstrating increased aortic insufficiency (arrow). (E) Device was recaptured. (F) Final aortogram after the device was removed showing no aortic insufficiency.

the residual shunt tends to decrease on follow-up. If hemolysis is so significant that medical management is not sufficient, the residual shunt should be closed by implanting another device if possible, or the device should be removed and the defect closed surgically.

Valvular regurgitation is a serious potential complication. It can involve the tricuspid, mitral, or aortic valve, and can result from the manipulation of wires and catheters as described above or, more seriously, from the impingement of the device on the valve apparatus (Figure 20.5). In case of PmVSD, the proximity of the PmVSD device to the aortic valve can result in significant insufficiency. Therefore, it is essential to monitor valve function by TEE and angiography prior to device release. In most cases, valve regurgitation is usually not hemodynamically significant and patients can be followed up medically as the degree of regurgitation tends to decrease with time. However, if the device causes significant valvular regurgitation postrelease (as when it is impinging on the valve apparatus), it should be removed surgically. In the VSD phase I trial for device closure of PmVSDs using the

Amplatzer Membranous VSD Occluder, new trivial and mild aortic regurgitation developed in 15.6% and 9% of patients, respectively.[29] This decreased on follow-up as many of the cases were transient and related to crossing the aortic valve with wires during the catheterization procedure.

Pericardial effusion is another preventable complication when meticulous care is used in manipulating wires and catheters. It is a very rare complication and it has not been reported postdevice implantation. Management of this complication, when it occurs, is through draining the effusion as usual when significantly large.

Complications involving the conduction system are particularly concerning and can potentially be serious. Most of the rhythm complications are transient and are due to catheter manipulation and device deployment. There are, however, cases of more permanent rhythm disturbances with device closure. Persistent right bundle branch block (BBB) has been reported in 2.7% of cases after mVSD device closure, and in about 6% of cases after device closure for PmVSDs.[29] Rhythm and conduction complications, especially the development of complete heart block, are more concerning with the PmVSD device as the occluder is positioned very close to the atrioventricular conduction tissue. Complete heart block has been reported with both mVSD and PmVSD device closure, though it is extremely rare with mVSDs.[30] The incidence of complete heart block after PmVSD closure with the Amplatzer Membranous VSD Occluder has been reported in 0–3.7% of cases in different studies.[24–26,28,31] The average rate of complete heart block needing pacemaker implantation after PmVSD device closure from pooled data from the literature is 1%.[19] Development of complete heart block in patients with PmVSD is rare if the patient's age is over 6 years (personal experience). Therefore, currently, we do not recommend using the Amplatzer Membranous VSD device in patients who are younger than this, unless surgical repair is not an option or carries more risk.

For patients with mVSDs, the incidence of these rhythm complications still compares well to the reported rates of 4% and 0–2.3% of right BBB and complete heart block, respectively, after surgical closure of VSDs.[32,33] It is most likely that the device might disturb the conduction system due to direct traumatic compression. It is possible, however, that the device also induces an inflammatory reaction that results in scarring around the conduction tissue. Thus, it is advisable to treat those patients who do develop acute complete heart block postdevice closure of their VSDs with high-dose aspirin and steroids, as some reports documented resolution of this complication with this empiric therapy.[34] It is essential, however, that if prolonged complete heart block is noted during the procedure prior to device release, that the device be removed and possibly the procedure be aborted. It is important to note that this complication can occur early (within a few days) or late (several months) after the closure procedure.[35] Thus, it is crucial to monitor patients undergoing VSD device closure, particularly PmVSD closure, for rhythm and conduction abnormalities on a long-term basis.

In the current era, device closure of VSDs is safe, effective, and provides a promising alternative to surgery. The percutaneous approach is highly effective for closing mVSDs (over 5 kg of weight) and PmVSDs (over age 6 years), and the perventricular technique provides a more feasible approach for closing mVSDs in small infants. It is certain that, with increasing operator experience with these procedures, major complications should be completely prevented. Further experience with the perventricular technique might expand the application of this beneficial approach to closure of PmVSDs.

REFERENCES

1. Rudolph AM. Ventricular septal defects. In: Rudolph AM, ed. Congenital Diseases of the Heart: Clinical-Physiological Considerations, 2nd edn. Armonk, NY: Futura Publishing Company, 2001: 197–244.

2. Kidd L, Driscoll DJ, Gersony WM et al. Second natural history study of congenital heart defects: results of treatment of patients with ventricular septal defects. Circulation 1993; 87(Suppl 1): I38–51.

3. Kirklin JW, Barrett-Boyes BG. Ventricular sepatal defect. In: Kirklin JW, Barrett-Boyes BG, eds. Cardiac Surgery, 2nd edn. New York, NY: Churchill Livingstone, 1993: 749–824.

4. Yeager SB, Freed MD, Keane JF, Norwood WI, Castaneda AR. Primary surgical closure of ventricular septal defect in the first year of life: results in 128 infants. J Am Coll Cardiol 1984; 3: 1269–76.

5. Zhao J, Li J, Wei X, Zhao B, Sun W. Tricuspid valve detachment in closure of congenital ventricular septal defect. Tex Heart Inst J 2003; 30: 38–41.

6. Gaynor JW, O'Brien JE Jr, Rychik J et al. Outcome following tricuspid valve detachment for ventricular septal defects closure. Eur J Cardiothorac Surg 2001; 19: 279–82.

7. Kitagawa T, Durham LA III, Mosca RS, Bove EL. Techniques and results in the management of multiple ventricular septal defects. J Thorac Cardiovasc Surg 1998; 115: 848–56.

8. Seddio F, Reddy VM, McElhinney DB et al. Multiple ventricular septal defects: how and when should they be repaired? J Thorac Cardiovasc Surg 1999; 117: 134–9.

9. Amin Z, Gu X, Berry JM et al. New device for closure of muscular ventricular septal defects in a canine model. Circulation 1999; 100: 320–8.

10. Thanopoulos BD, Tsaousis GS, Konstadopoulou GN, Zarayelyan AG. Transcatheter closure of muscular ventricular septal defects with the Amplatzer ventricular septal defect occluder: initial clinical applications in children. J Am Coll Cardiol 1999; 33: 1395–9.

11. Amin Z, Berry JM, Foker JE, Rocchini AP, Bass JL. Intraoperative closure of muscular ventricular septal defect in a canine model and application of the technique in a baby. J Thorac Cardiovasc Surg 1998; 115: 1374–6.

12. Bacha EA, Cao QL, Starr JP et al. Perventricular device closure of muscular ventricular septal defects on the beating heart: technique and results. J Thorac Cardiovasc Surg 2003; 126: 1718–23.

13. Bacha EA, Cao QL, Galantowicz ME et al. Multicenter experience with perventricular device closure of muscular ventricular septal defects. Pediatr Cardiol 2005; 26: 169–75.

14. Diab KA, Cao QL, Mora BN, Hijazi ZM. Device closure of muscular ventricular septal defects in infants less than one year of age using the Amplatzer devices: feasibility and outcome. Cathet Cardiovasc Interven 2007; 70: 90–7.

15. Amin Z, Woo R, Danford DA et al. Robotically assisted perventricular closure of perimembranous ventricular septal defects: preliminary results in Yucatan pigs. J Thorac Cardiovasc Surg 2006; 131: 427–32.

16. Vogel M, Rigby ML, Shore D. Perforation of the right aortic valve cusp: complication of ventricular septal defect closure with a modified Rashkind umbrella. Pediatr Cardiol 1996; 17: 416–18.

17. Diab KA, Hijazi ZM, Cao QL, Bacha EA. A truly hybrid approach to perventricular closure of multiple muscular ventricular septal defects. J Thorac Cardiovasc Surg 2005; 130: 892–3.

18. Holzer R, Balzer D, Cao QL, Lock K, Hijazi ZM. Amplatzer Muscular Ventricular Septal Defect Investigators. Device closure of muscular ventricular septal defects using the Amplatzer muscular ventricular septal defect occluder: immediate and mid-term results of a US registry. J Am Coll Cardiol 2004; 43: 1257–63.

19. Butera G, Chessa M, Carminati M. Percutaneous closure of ventricular septal defects, state of the art. J Cardiovasc Med (Hagerstown) 2007; 8: 39–45.

20. Thanopoulos BD, Rigby ML. Outcome of transcatheter closure of muscular ventricular septal defects with the Amplatzer ventricular septal defect occluder. Heart 2005; 91: 513–16.

21. Arora R, Trehan V, Thakur AK et al. Transcatheter closure of congenital muscular ventricular septal defect. J Interven Cardiol 2004; 17: 109–15.

22. Carminati M, Butera G, Chessa M et al. Transcatheter closure of congenital ventricular septal defects with Amplatzer occluders. Am J Cardiol 2005; 96(12A): 52–8L.

23. Holzer R, de Giovanni J, Walsh KP et al. Transcatheter closure of perimembranous ventricular septal defects using the Amplatzer membranous VSD occluder: immediate and midterm results of an international registry. Cathet Cardiovasc Interven 2006; 68: 620–8.

24. Hijazi ZM, Hakim F, Hawaleh AA et al. Catheter closure of perimembranous ventricular septal defects using the new Amplatzer membranous VSD occluder: initial clinical experience. Cathet Cardiovasc Interven 2002; 56: 508–15.

25. Bass JL, Kalra GS, Arora R et al. Initial human experience with the Amplatzer perimembranous ventricular septal occluder device. Cathet Cardiovasc Interven 2003; 58: 238–45.

26. Thanopoulos BD, Tsaousis GS, Karanasios E, Eleftherakis NG, Paphitis C. Transcatheter closure of a perimembranous ventricular septal defect with the Amplatzer asymmetric ventricular septal defect occluder: preliminary experience in children. Heart 2003; 89: 918–22.

27. Arora R, Trehan V, Kumar A, Kalra GS, Nigam M. Transcatheter closure of congenital ventricular septal defects. Experience with various devices. J Interven Cardiol 2003; 16: 83–91.

28. Pedra AC, Pedra SRF, Esteves CA et al. Percutaneous closure of perimembranous ventricular septal defects with the Amplatzer device: technical and morphological considerations. Cathet Cardiovasc Interven 2004; 61:403–10.

29. Fu YC, Bass J, Amin Z et al. Transcatheter closure of perimembranous ventricular septal defects using the new Amplatzer membranous VSD occluder: results of the US phase I trial. J Am Coll Cardiol 2006; 47: 319–25.

30. Carminati M, Butera G, Chessa M et al. for the Investigators of the European VSD Registry. Transcatheter closure of congenital ventricular septal defects: results of the European Registry. Eur Heart J 2007; 28: 2361–8.

31. Masura J, Gao W, Gavora P et al. Percutaneous closure of perimembranous ventricular septal defects with the eccentric Amplatzer device: multicenter follow-up study. Pediatr Cardiol 2005; 26: 216–19.

32. Bol-Raap G, Weerheim J, Kappetein AP, Witsenburg M, Bogers AJ. Follow-up after surgical closure of congenital ventricular septal defect. Eur J Cardiothorac Surg 2003; 24: 511–15.

33. Zhao J, Li J, Wei X, Zhao B, Sun W. Tricuspid valve detachment in closure of congenital ventricular septal defect. Tex Heart Inst J 2003; 30: 38–41.

34. Yip WC, Zimmerman F, Hijazi ZM. Heart block and empirical therapy after transcatheter closure of perimembranous ventricular septal defect. Cathet Cardiovasc Interven 2005; 66: 436–41.

35. Butera G, Massimo C, Mario C. Late complete atriovenous block after percutaneous closure of a perimembranous ventricular septal defect. Cathet Cardiovasc Interven 2006; 67: 938–41.

21 Occlusion of the patent arterial duct

Ralf J Holzer and John P Cheatham

TECHNIQUE

Transcatheter closure of the patent ductus arteriosus (PDA) was first introduced by Porstmann and colleagues in 1968.[1] While the device was cumbersome to use and required a large arterial cannulation, it set the stage for subsequent device developments, such as the Rashkind device in the late 1970s.[2–4] At present, the only device approved specifically for the closure of the patent arterial duct is the Amplatzer® Duct Occluder (ADO), which was introduced in 1997.[5] The device is mushroom-shaped and made of 0.005 inch Nitinol wire mesh, with Dacron fabric incorporated into the retention disc as well as the skirt of the device (Figure 21.1).

Prior to the introduction of the ADO, detachable as well as controlled-release coils were used to occlude the majority of PDAs, irrespective of size or shape. However, at the present time, coil occlusion is virtually exclusively reserved for the occlusion of very small PDAs. The Nit-Occlud PDA Occlusion System (pfm AG, Cologne, Germany) (Figure 21.2), which was introduced in 2001, is a suitable alternative to the ADO for medium sized PDAs, and is presently undergoing clinical evaluation in the US. A variety of additional devices have been used for PDA occlusion, such as the Amplatzer Muscular VSD Occluder,[6] the Amplatzer Septal Occluder,[7] the buttoned device,[8] the Amplatzer Vascular Plug,[9] and the Gianturco-Grifka Vascular Occlusion Device (GGVOD).[10–12] The techniques referred to in this chapter are focused mainly on the ADO as well as the detachable Flipper coil (Cook, Bloomington, IN).

PDA occlusion can be performed under deep sedation or general endotracheal anesthesia, depending on patient age and preference of patient and/or parents. The transcatheter evaluation should include a basic left- and right-heart catheterization. Care should be taken to avoid inadvertently entering the PDA before angiographic evaluation can be completed, as this may trigger ductal spasm, thereby rendering any obtained angiographic measurements inaccurate. An aortogram is the most important evaluation of the PDA, and is obtained by placing an angiographic catheter (such as a pigtail catheter) just underneath the ductal ampulla, using biplane imaging with standard lateral projection as well as 30° right anterior oblique (RAO) projection. The imaging planes may have to be altered slightly in

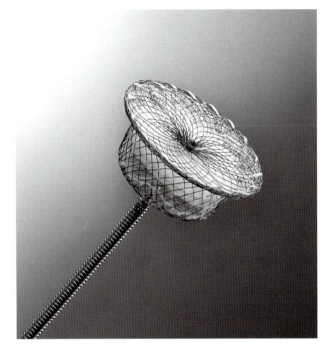

Figure 21.1 Amplatzer® Duct Occluder, image provided by AGA Medical Corporation (AGA Medical, Golden Valley, MN).

each individual patient to best profile the PDA. Measurements should be obtained at the pulmonary arterial end and the aortic end, as well as for the total length of the PDA. The type of device or coil that is chosen for any specific PDA occlusion does not only depend on the size of the PDA, but also its shape. The majority of PDAs are classically cone-shaped (type A), while rarer varieties include PDAs that are short with a narrow aortic end (type B), tubular (type C), having multiple constrictions (type D), or elongated conical with a distant constriction (type E).[13]

Coil occlusion of the PDA can be performed using either an antegrade or retrograde approach. The antegrade approach is usually preferable, as it allows angiographic confirmation of adequate coil placement, and effective occlusion prior to release of the coil. However, in very small PDAs it may not always be possible to cross the PDA antegradely (Figure 21.3). The most frequently used coil for occlusion of very small PDAs is the detachable Flipper coil, which is a

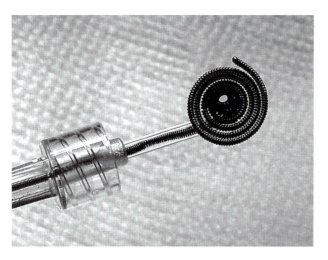

Figure 21.2 Nit-Occlud PDA Occlusion System. The image shows the aortic spiral disc with the device still attached to the delivery system.

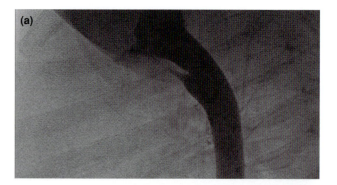

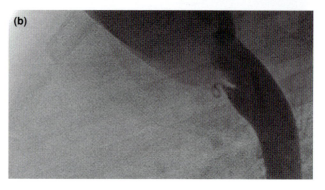

Figure 21.3 Small type A PDA in a 16-month-old male infant, measuring 0.5 mm at the pulmonary arterial end. The PDA was closed retrogradely using a 3 mm * 3 loop Flipper coil. (A) Prior to closure; (B) postclosure.

variation of the standard 0.035 inch Gianturco coil. It has the distinct advantage of a controlled-release mechanism, but has less thrombogenic Dacron fibers than the standard Gianturco coil.[12]

The diameter of the chosen coil should be about twice the size of the pulmonary end of the PDA and the length of the coil should be chosen depending on the length of the PDA as well as the size of the aortic ampulla. The coil is deployed so as to place about 0.5–1 loop distal to the pulmonary arterial end, with the remainder of the loops being placed in the ductal ampulla. Delivery of Flipper coils is technically fairly easy, and the controlled-release mechanism allows an extra safety margin to prevent inadvertent coil embolization. If the coil position appears to be suboptimal, the coil can be recaptured and redeployed into a more appropriate position. While, in the past, a variety of techniques have been used to allow placement of the standard Gianturco coil (with its increased filament when compared to the Flipper coil) in a more controlled fashion, as well as specific techniques used to place multiple coils, these techniques are rarely used today, because most larger PDA varieties can be safely and more effectively occluded using the ADO. As such, these techniques are not further discussed in this section. The Flipper coil is usually adequate to occlude those PDAs that are very small. In the rare event of a residual shunt after coil placement, despite allowing sufficient time for clotting to occur, attempts should be made to place additional coils until complete closure has been achieved. Additional coils are usually placed retrogradely, taking the utmost care not to dislodge the originally placed coil when advancing the wire and delivery catheter.

Occlusion of the PDA using the ADO requires an antegrade approach (Figure 21.4). The detailed technique has been described by Masura and colleagues.[5]

The device size is chosen so that the pulmonary end of the skirt is about 2 mm larger than the size of the PDA at the narrowest pulmonary arterial end. The PDA is crossed antegradely, which is most easily facilitated using a V18 wire (Boston Scientific, Boston, MA), which frequently advances directly across the PDA. Depending on the size of the delivery sheath, either the V18 wire or an exchange length 0.035 inch wire can be used to track the delivery sheath into the descending aorta.

On occasion, especially with a tortuous PDA, crossing the PDA antegradely may be difficult. In this case, the PDA can be crossed retrogradely and then a 0.035 inch standard exchange length wire can be snared in the main pulmonary artery (MPA) using an appropriately sized Gooseneck snare (Microvena Corporation, White Bear Lake, MN), thereby allowing establishment of an arteriovenous loop.

The tip of the delivery sheath is positioned in the lower descending aorta and, once the wire is removed, the device is loaded and then advanced until it reaches the tip of the delivery sheath. At this point the whole assembly is gradually withdrawn, beginning to deploy the aortic retention disc when a position just in the mid portion of the descending aorta, opposite to the PDA insertion, is reached. The initial angiographic recording is used as a roadmap during the deployment process, with the anterior end of the trachea and its

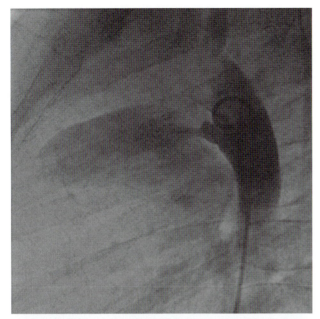

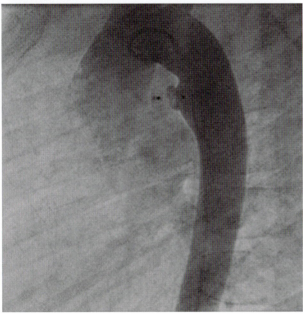

Figure 21.4 Nine-year-old female with a medium sized PDA who underwent PDA occlusion using an Amplatzer Duct Occluder. (Top) Before closure; (Bottom) after closure.

relation to the PDA being the most important reference point. Once the retention disc is deployed the whole assembly is withdrawn into the mouth of the aortic ductal ampulla, at which point the skirt is deployed. In a PDA with atypical morphology, or in smaller infants, it may be necessary to deploy at least part of the retention disc within the duct itself, thereby limiting the amount of aortic protrusion that is created by the retention disc.

Once the device is deployed a repeat aortogram is performed, carefully evaluating for the presence of any residual shunt around the device, and for any

significant protrusion into the descending aorta. Whenever concern exists about potential obstruction of flow to the left pulmonary artery, an angiography can be performed (LAO projection) through the delivery sheath using a Touhy Borst adapter. An aortogram is repeated after release of the device, and final pressure recordings are obtained in the ascending as well as the descending aorta.

HOW NOT TO GET INTO TROUBLE

With the devices available today, closure of the standard PDA in a child should have virtually zero mortality and extremely minimal morbidity.

Essential for successful closure of a PDA is a well profiled angiographic evaluation using accurate calibration methods. It cannot be emphasized strongly enough how important it is to avoid inducing ductal spasm through unnecessary catheter manipulation during the initial hemodynamic evaluation. For the baseline hemodynamic evaluation, a balloon-tipped wedge catheter should be advanced directly into a distal branch pulmonary artery position, and then a quick withdrawal pressure recording obtained, limiting the time the catheter remains inside the MPA. Baseline gradients to both branch pulmonary arteries, especially the LPA, are helpful to subsequently identify potential obstructions caused by the device itself, but these gradients can be readily obtained after the angiographic evaluation. Choosing a device or coil size based on the angiographic appearance of a PDA in spasm can lead to gross underestimation of the PDA size, with the potential risk of subsequent device embolization (Figure 21.5). Coil embolization has been one of the most frequent complications prior to introduction of the ADO, but this complication can be virtually eliminated if coils are exclusively used in very small PDAs.

In small infants it is important to attempt to reduce the risk of the device causing a degree of obstruction to flow to the LPA or aorta. At the aortic end, this risk can be reduced by partially deploying the retention disc within the PDA itself, thereby limiting the amount of protrusion into the descending aorta. However, in short PDAs this may not be feasible, because of the risk of the device protruding too much at the pulmonary arterial end. Therefore, in small infants with a fairly short duct, it is extremely important to be very conservative when choosing the initial device size. While this may occasionally mean having to recapture a deployed device if angiographic evaluation documents some residual shunt around the device, this is in itself does not cause any harm to the patient.

In large PDAs in adult patients, determining the accurate angiographic size may be difficult. As such, balloon sizing may be of benefit, which can be most

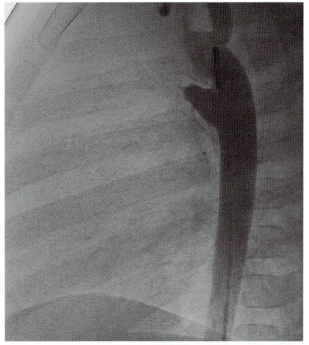

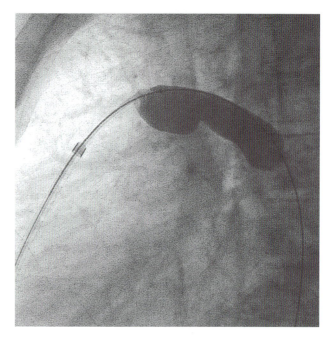

Figure 21.6   Large pulmonary-hypertensive type A PDA in a 20-year-old female. Balloon sizing was undertaking using a 20 mm * 5 cm Tyshak II balloon, measuring 13.4 mm at the pulmonary arterial end. The PDA was subsequently closed using an 18 mm Amplatzer Muscular VSD Occluder.

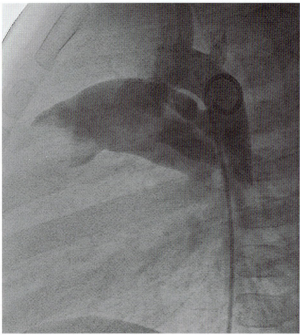

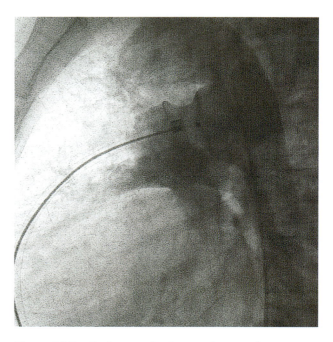

Figure 21.5   Thirteen-month-old female infant undergoing transcatheter PDA occlusion. Catheter manipulation induced ductal spasm. (Top) Initial aortogram documenting the PDA in spasm. (Bottom) Aortogram after a considerable wait, documenting a moderate tubular-type PDA.

Figure 21.7   Occlusion of a large pulmonary-hypertensive type A PDA in a 20-year-old female. The image demonstrates an 18 mm Amplatzer Muscular VSD Occluder prior to release. On follow-up there was no echocardiographic evidence of any residual shunting across the PDA.

readily performed by inflating a non-compliant balloon with a low pressure towards the pulmonary arterial end of the PDA and then gradually pulling it back through the PDA under cine recording (Figure 21.6), allowing it to milk through the duct, rather than using any significant inflation pressure to expand the PDA, which should be avoided. In the same group of patients, specifically when the duct morphology is

more tubular, the Amplatzer Muscular VSD Occluder may be the more appropriate device[6] (Figure 21.7), especially as the size of the ADO is limited to 12/10 mm in the US.

(a)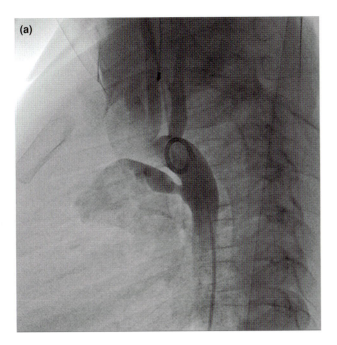

(b)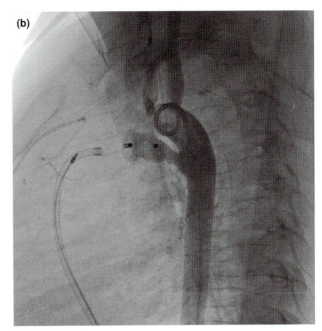

Figure 21.8   Moderate tubular-type PDA, with the largest central portion measuring about 5.6 mm in diameter. Occlusion was performed using a 10 mm Amplatzer Vascular Plug. On follow-up there was no echocardiographic evidence of a residual shunt. (A) Prior to occlusion; (B) postocclusion.

When deploying the ADO, one should avoid exerting too much tension on the cable and delivery sheath. This tension will not only pull the ADO into the duct, but at the same time may pull the duct and aorta slightly anterior. When the device is subsequently released, the sudden loss of tension may lead to a forceful backdrop of the device towards the aorta, which may change the device position slightly and can create a higher degree of aortic protrusion than anticipated from the initial angiography, especially in small infants.

The ADO is a less suitable device for the more tubular type PDA, especially if the largest diameter is seen in the central portion of the PDA. In these circumstances, attempts have been made to use the cylindrical Amplatzer Vascular Plug[9,14] (Figure 21.8). However, caution has to be applied for this indication, because the lack of Dacron fabric in these devices may prevent complete occlusion in moderate sized high-flow PDAs, as was demonstrated in a patient with a type C PDA.[15–17] Whether the modified Amplatzer Vascular Plug II may be more suitable for this purpose remains to be seen, but initial case experiences are promising (Figure 21.9).

Whenever possible, an antegrade approach should be used for coil deployment across a PDA, as this facilitates an angiographic evaluation prior to release of the coil. Residual shunts or coil–PDA size discrepancies can then be identified at a time when the coil is still easily retrievable, thereby allowing a choice to be made between a larger diameter coil or ADO. This is a clear advantage to placing a second coil which, if not performed carefully, can be associated with coil migration, malposition, or embolization of the first coil (usually to the pulmonary artery).

COMPLICATIONS

Results of PDA closure using the ADO have generally been favorable. Pass and colleagues reported the results of a multicenter US trial which enrolled 484 patients with a median age of 1.8 years between 1999 and 2002.[18] Rates of complete closure were as high as 99.7% at 1-year follow-up, which has also been confirmed during a recent long-term follow-up study by Masura and colleagues.[19] While the original US multicenter trial reported major complications in 2.3%, with the overall rate of adverse events being 4.8%, this is likely a reflection of the learning curve that was seen after this device was introduced in the US.[18] In contrast, the more recent study by Masura and colleagues reported a 0% incidence of major adverse events after PDA closure.[19] Major morbidity and mortality should remain close to zero percent, considering the very minimal risk a small to medium sized pressure restrictive PDA is expected to pose to the affected individual. Rare complications that have been described include partial occlusion of the LPA, aortic obstruction, as well as device embolization.[18,20–22] Vascular complications and/or blood loss requiring transfusion were reported in 18/484 (0.3%) patients during the initial US multicenter trial.[18] Hemolysis secondary to a residual shunt has been observed after coil as well as device closure of a PDA in about 0.5% of patients.[22–24]

With the availability of the ADO, adverse events related to PDA coil occlusion have become extremely

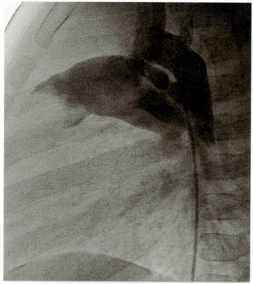

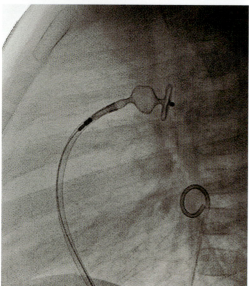

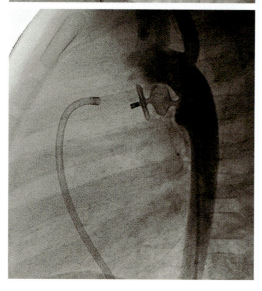

Figure 21.9 Thirteen-month-old female infant undergoing transcatheter PDA occlusion. (Top) Moderate tubular type PDA. (Middle) Deployment of a 10 mm Amplatzer Vascular Plug II. (Bottom) Aortogram after release of the device documenting excellent device position and no residual shunt.

rare. In 1999, preceding the introduction of the ADO, Patel and colleagues reported their experience of PDA coil occlusion in 149 patients,[25] with a rate of complete closure of 97%. The study further documented zero mortality and very low morbidity. Coil migration or embolization during the procedure was seen in 6 patients (4%), and it has been well documented that attempts to occlude larger PDAs are associated with an increased risk of coil embolization, being as high as 16% in PDAs with a diameter in excess of 4 mm.[26] However, the availability of the ADO has virtually eliminated the need to use coils in PDAs other than those of very small size. Inadvertent coil or device embolization should today be expected to occur in less then 1% of cases, if full use is made of all available devices and techniques.

HOW TO MANAGE COMPLICATIONS

With the rarity of complications occurring after PDA closure, management strategies have mainly focused on the retrieval of malpositioned or embolized devices or coils, as well as the closure of residual shunts, which in addition to the continued need for endocarditis prophylaxis, are a potential hazard for inducing intravascular hemolysis.

The need to retrieve embolized coils should be extremely rare, especially if the angiographic evaluation was accurate and a controlled-release Flipper coil is being deployed using an antegrade approach. Most frequently, a coil may be partially dislodged protruding out of the pulmonary arterial end of the duct, while attempting to place a secondary coil. In this case, a Gooseneck snare (Microvena Corporation, White Bear Lake, MN) is placed in the MPA and, in most circumstances, the coil can easily be snared using biplane fluoroscopic guidance. If the coil embolizes towards a pulmonary arterial branch, retrieval using a snaring technique is usually feasible. However, care has to be taken not to push the coil further distally when advancing the snare and snare catheter. The use of a biopsy forceps to grab an end of the coil should be avoided due to the increased risk of causing injury to the vessel wall. If all attempts at retrieving the coil fail, then the coil should be pushed as distally as possible, so that only a very small side branch of the pulmonary vasculature remains occluded.

Embolized ADOs are more difficult to retrieve compared to other Amplatzer devices or coils, as a result of the recess of the microscrew into the device itself. Therefore, unless the microscrew does not recess into the ADO, the device can only be snared circumferentially. For that purpose, a delivery sheath at least 4 French sizes larger than the one used to deploy the ADO should be used for device retrieval. In small children, device retrieval should be attempted antegradely to avoid the need for a large arterial cannulation.

However, a catheter advanced retrogradely may aid in positioning the ADO within the aorta, so it is more amenable for retrieval using a snaring technique. Late-recognized device embolization after the procedure is usually an indication for surgical retrieval, as the device will be firmly adherent to adjacent vasculature.[21]

Residual shunts should be considered a major complication after transcatheter PDA closure. They not only fail to abolish the risk of bacterial endocarditis, but can also be associated with intravascular hemolysis.[24] Attempting to occlude a small hemodynamically insignificant PDA without achieving complete closure represents a clear procedural failure. If a residual shunt is encountered after coil occlusion, the operator should either place an additional coil using a careful retrograde approach, or retrieve the originally placed coil and deploy an appropriately sized ADO instead. Residual shunts through the device after placement of an ADO are rare, but can be treated successfully by placing small platinum coils within the wire cage of the device.[22]

REFERENCES

1. Porstmann W, Wierny L, Warnke H. [Closure of ductus arteriosus persistens without thoracotomy. 2] Fortschr Geb Rontgenstr Nuklearmed 1968; 109: 133–48.

2. Rashkind WJ, Cuaso CC. Transcatheter closure of patent ductus arteriosus; successful use in a 3.5 kilogram infant. Pediatr Cardiol 1979; 1: 3–7.

3. Rashkind WJ, Mullins CE, Hellenbrand WE, Tait MA. Nonsurgical closure of patent ductus arteriosus: clinical application of the Rashkind PDA Occluder System. Circulation 1987; 75: 583–92.

4. Rashkind WJ. Therapeutic interventional procedures in congenital heart disease. Radiol Diagnost 1987; 28(4): 449–60.

5. Masura J, Walsh KP, Thanopoulous B et al. Catheter closure of moderate- to large-sized patent ductus arteriosus using the new Amplatzer Duct Occluder: immediate and short-term results. J Am Coll Cardiol 1998; 31(4): 878–82.

6. Demkow M, Ruzyllo W, Siudalska H, Kepka C. Transcatheter closure of a 16 mm hypertensive patent ductus arteriosus with the Amplatzer Muscular VSD Occluder. Cathet Cardiovasc Interven 2001; 52(3): 359–62.

7. Pedra CA, Sanches SA, Fontes VF. Percutaneous occlusion of the patent ductus arteriosus with the Amplatzer device for atrial septal defects. J Invas Cardiol 2003; 15(7): 413–17.

8. Rao PS, Sideris EB, Haddad J et al. Transcatheter occlusion of patent ductus arteriosus with adjustable buttoned device. Initial clinical experience. Circulation 1993; 88(3): 1119–26.

9. Holzer R, Cao QL, Sandhu S, Hijazi ZM. The Amplatzer Vascular Plug – an addition to our interventional armantarium. Pediatr Cardiol Today 2004; 2(6): 6–8.

10. Hoyer MH, Leon RA, Fricker FJ. Transcatheter closure of modified Blalock–Taussig shunt with Gianturco–Grifka Vascular Occlusion Device. [see comment] Cathet Cardiovasc Interven 1999; 48(4): 365–7.

11. Ebeid MR, Gaymes CH, Smith JC, Braden DS, Joransen JA. Gianturco–Grifka vascular occlusion device for closure of patent ductus arteriosus. Am J Cardiol 2001; 87: 657–60.

12. Mullins CE. Cardiac Catheterization in Congenital Heart Disease. Malden: Blackwell, 2006.

13. Krichenko A, Benson LN, Burrows P et al. Angiographic classification of the isolated, persistently patent ductus arteriosus and implications for percutaneous catheter occlusion. Am J Cardiol 1989; 63: 877–80.

14. Hoyer MH. Novel use of the Amplatzer plug for closure of a patent ductus arteriosus.[see comment] Cathet Cardiovasc Interven 2005; 65(4): 577–80.

15. Hill SL, Hijazi ZM, Hellenbrand WE, Cheatham JP. Evaluation of the AMPLATZER vascular plug for embolization of peripheral vascular malformations associated with congenital heart disease. Cathet Cardiovasc Interven 2006; 67(1): 113–19.

16. Cheatham JP. Not so fast with that Novel use: does AVP = PDA? [comment] Cathet Cardiovasc Interven 2005; 65(4): 581–3.

17. Javois AJ, Husayni TS, Thoele D, Van Bergen AH. Inadvertent stenting of patent ductus arteriosus with Amplatzer Vascular Plug. Cathet Cardiovasc Interven 2006; 67: 485–9.

18. Pass RH, Hijazi Z, Hsu DT, Lewis V, Hellenbrand WE. Multicenter USA Amplatzer patent ductus arteriosus occlusion device trial: initial and one-year results. J Am Coll Cardiol 2004; 44(3): 513–9.

19. Masura J, Tittel P, Gavora P, Podnar T. Long-term outcome of transcatheter patent ductus arteriosus closure using Amplatzer duct occluders. Am Heart J 2006; 151: 755.

20. Shahabuddin S, Atiq M, Hamid M, Amanullah M. Surgical removal of an embolised patent ductus arteriosus amplatzer occluding device in a 4-year-old girl. [see comment] Interact Cardiovasc Thorac Surg 2007; 6: 572–3.

21. McMullan DM, Moulick A, Jonas RA. Late embolization of Amplatzer patent ductus arteriosus occlusion device with thoracic aorta embedment. Ann Thorac Surg 2007; 83: 1177–9.

22. Joseph G, Mandalay A, Zacharias TU, George B. Severe intravascular hemolysis after transcatheter closure of a large patent ductus arteriosus using the Amplatzer duct occluder: successful resolution by intradevice coil deployment. Cathet Cardiovasc Interven 2002; 55: 245–9.

23. Anil SR, Sivakumar K, Philip AK, Francis E, Kumar RK. Clinical course and management strategies for hemolysis after transcatheter closure of patent arterial ducts. Cathet Cardiovasc Interven 2003; 59: 538–43.

24. Henry G, Danilowicz D, Verma R. Severe hemolysis following partial coil-occlusion of patent ductus arteriosus. [see comment] Cathet Cardiovasc Diagn 1996; 39(4): 410–12.

25. Patel HT, Cao QL, Rhodes J, Hijazi ZM. Long-term outcome of transcatheter coil closure of small to large patent ductus arteriosus. Cathet Cardiovasc Interven 1999; 47(4): 457–61.

26. Hijazi ZM, Geggel RL. Transcatheter closure of large patent ductus arteriosus (> or = 4 mm) with multiple Gianturco coils: immediate and mid-term results. Heart 1996; 76(6): 536–40.

22 Closure of coronary artery fistulas

Zahid Amin

INTRODUCTION

Coronary artery fistulas (CAFs) (also known as coronary arteriovenous malformations) are a communication between the coronary artery and a segment of the systemic (artery or vein) or the pulmonary artery (including the coronary sinus) or any of the four cardiac chambers of the heart. If the connection is to one or multiple chambers of the heart, it is termed a coronary-cameral fistula.

A CAF was described by Krause in 1865.[1] A pathologic description of a CAF was first given in 1908 by Maude Abbott. It was almost 40 years later that the first report of surgical closure of a fistula was reported by Bjork and Craaford, in a patient whose preoperative diagnosis was patent ductus arteriosus.

CAF is a rare anomaly, and the majority of them are benign in nature and do not cause hemodynamic issues. Clinical examination is consistent with a continuous murmur heard over the precordium, mimicking patent ductus arteriosus. The timing and quality of the murmur are dependent upon the drainage site of the fistula.

In some patients, CAFs can cause symptoms. The symptoms depend upon the size of the fistulous communication. Some patients exhibit signs of congestive heart failure after birth. These patients have large communication to the right ventricle or pulmonary artery with significant left to right shunt, left ventricle volume overload, and perhaps coronary steal. In others, the communication becomes more evident later in life, with symptoms of vague chest pain.

PATHOPHYSIOLOGY

Myocardial stealing, resulting in a reduction in myocardial blood flow distal to the fistulous connection, is the main mechanism causing symptoms and other changes in the coronary artery. In an effort to attempt to compensate for the coronary steal, the size of the coronary artery enlarges over time. The coronary artery becomes tortuous with further dilation, and may even become aneurysmal. These changes increase the risk of rupture, side branch obstruction, ulceration, atheroma, and calcium deposition. Depending upon the size of the fistulous connection, and the resistance of the drainage vessel or chamber, patients may be completely asymptomatic or, rarely, in congestive heart failure. For example, if the drainage is to the right ventricle or the pulmonary artery, significant high left to right shunt will result in congestive heart failure in early infancy, necessitating closure.

COMPLICATIONS OF UNTREATED CAF

If left untreated, the risk of complications increases with age. Below the age of 20 years the risk is 11%, and above the age of 20 the risk increases to 35%.[2] Congestive heart failure with large fistulas, myocardial infarction or ischemia because of coronary steal, arrhythmias, infectious endocarditis, aneurysm formation, rupture, and death may occur in untreated patients.

Primary symptoms of untreated fistulas are dyspnea, palpitations, angina, and occasionally syncope.

TREATMENT

The CAF can be treated surgically or by using transcatheter techniques. Closure, however, is controversial in asymptomatic patients.[3] This chapter will address results and complications related to transcatheter and surgical treatment of the CAF.

The first transcatheter closure of a CAF was reported in 1983.[4] Since then, there have been an array of case reports and several studies published where the transcatheter technique has been utilized.[5–11] This approach is frequently a complicated intervention and hence complications are subject to happen during and after closure of the fistula. A brief overview of the procedure is warranted, so that the explanation and timing of the complications can be addressed later in this chapter.

After the diagnosis has been established by physical examination, EKG, echocardiogram, multidetector row computed tomography, and other techniques, the patient is taken to the cardiac catheterization laboratory for selective coronary angiography, which is the most definitive way to confirm the diagnosis. Angiography outlines the detailed anatomy of the size and origin of the fistula, the course of the fistula, the presence and number of stenoses in the fistulous tract, the exact drainage site, the number of feeder vessels, and the drainage sites. Angiography also helps the decision as to which tools (coils, devices) should be used, whether to use the antegrade or the retrograde route, and whether an arteriovenous loop will be helpful, if it can be formed, for closure of the fistula.

The therapeutic goal of treatment is complete obliteration of the fistula without compromising the normal coronary blood flow or obstruction of side branches. Hence, the ideal location to close the CAF is as distal (close to the drainage point) as possible. The distal closure has several advantages; it will prevent occlusion of side branches, it will occlude all connections if multiple vessels were draining into the communication, it usually has a smaller caliber when compared to the proximal fistula and hence larger coils/devices will not have to be used, and it is the site that is accessible via the retrograde route, rather easily.

For effective closure with emphasis on minimizing the complications, the operator should be experienced and well versed in coronary artery anatomy and closure techniques, and the catheterization laboratory should be well equipped with various size guiding catheters, especially for children (JL 1, 1.2, 2, 2.5 curves). These catheters are not readily available as they are custom made. All types of micro catheters (tracker); coils (detachable, Nestor, Gianturco, etc.); devices (Amplatzer PDA, muscular VSD, Vascular Plugs I and II); retrieval catheters and snares. The coronary artery fistulas, ideally, should be closed in the pediatric cardiac catheterization laboratory, with the availability of and/or expert opinion of an adult interventionalist. The adult interventionalists are better versed in coronary artery anatomy and intervention than pediatric interventionalists. An array of catheters, microcatheters for co-axial techniques to reach distal areas of the fistula, coils, and micro-coils; devices (Amplatzer PDA devices, Plugs and Muscular VSD closure devices) should be available.

Coronary angiography in multiple plains should be performed to delineate the origin, course, drainage site(s), and the number of feeder vessels. Once the course of the fistula has been established, a trial of balloon occlusion of the fistula (as distal as possible) for 20 to 30 minutes with close monitoring of the EKG and rhythm, and evaluation of regional wall motion abnormality by transesophageal echocardiography is recommended in all patients. We recommend performing another set of coronary angiograms during balloon occlusion; this is very helpful in delineating side branches from the coronary arteries that are usually not seen well while the fistulous connection is draining freely. Rarely, we have used dobutamine stress echocardiography to further ensure that no regional wall motion abnormality is present when the fistula is occluded. These maneuvers are helpful, but do not guarantee that there will not be any ischemia after the fistula is closed, especially if the coil or the device migrates proximally during or after deployment.

Depending upon the location of the drainage, the accessibility, length, and tortuosity of the fistula, and the type of device needed to occlude the fistula, the decision is made whether to create an arteriovenous loop, and whether to proceed via the retrograde or antegrade approaches. Once the fistula is occluded, repeat coronary angiography is recommended to ascertain that the fistula is closed, and to evaluate the precise position of the coils/devices used.

COMPLICATIONS

Surgical

The surgical closure of a CAF carries a low risk of morbidity and mortality. The defect is approached via median sternotomy, and a cardiopulmonary bypass may be required. Acute myocardial infarction, stroke, transient ischemic attack, arrhythmias, a risk of recurrence in patients with multiple feeders, and death have all been reported with this technique.[12–14]

Transcatheter

The complication rate of transcatheter closure is comparable to surgical closure,[5,8,11] with the advantage that no sternotomy or cardiopulmonary bypass is required. The complication rate may even be lower in experienced hands, and in institutions where this procedure is performed more commonly than in others. The very few patients who need the procedure, in addition to the rarity of the defect, make this procedure more risk prone.

The complications can be divided into intraprocedure and postprocedure complications. The intraprocedure complications may relate to catheters and wires positioned in the circuitous routes of the fistula, which may result in coronary spasm, arrhythmias, injury leading to intimal dissection, and thrombosis. The availability of nitroglycerin in the laboratory is crucial to treat any coronary artery spasm. Perforation of the fistula or the coronary artery has also been described. Complications may also occur due to coil or device migration proximally, resulting in obstruction of the side branches and muscle infarction. If the coils or devices embolize into the systemic circulation, the catheterization procedure is even more prolonged, as it requires removal of the inappropriately placed coils/devices.

Postprocedure complications consist of myocardial infarction, thrombosis[9] of the fistulous connection with extension into the coronary artery (Figures 22.1 and 22.2), and recanalization of the fistula that may require another catheterization procedure. The persistence of leakage after the intervention is problematic.

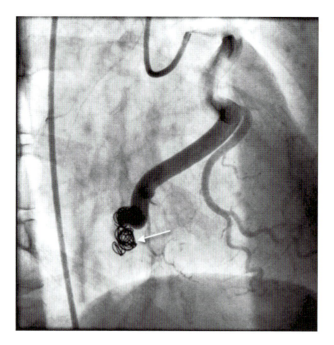

Figure 22.1   This patient had a large fistulous connection that was effectively occluded with the help of multiple coils (white arrow). The patient suffered from myocardial infarction a few days later (see Figure 22.2).

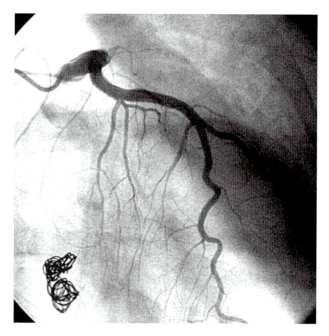

Figure 22.2   A selective coronary angiogram revealed complete occlusion of the circumflex artery (with permission).

POSTINTERVENTION STRATEGY

Once the fistula has been occluded, it is highly recommended to observe the patient overnight. An echocardiogram, chest X-ray, and 12 lead EKG should be performed the next morning prior to discharge. These tests help to evaluate the function, device/coil position, and rhythm of the patient prior to discharge. An anticoagulation regimen should be instituted the day of the procedure. If the fistula is large, we recommend aspirin (325 mg) and clopidogrel (75 mg) per day for a period of 6 months minimum.

REFERENCES

1. Krause W. Ueber den Ursprung einer accessorischen A. Coronaria Cordis aus der A. pulmonalis. Z Rationele Med 1865; 24: 225.
2. Liberthson R, Sagan K, Berkober K, Weintraub R, Levine FH. Congenital coronary artery fistula. Report of 13 patients, review of literature and delineation of management. Circulation 1979; 59(5): 849–54.
3. Sherwood MC, Rockenmacher S, Colan SD, Geva T. Prognostic significance of clinically silent coronary artery fistulas. Am J Cardiol 1999; 83: 407–11.
4. Reidy JF, Sowton E, Ross DN. Transcatheter occlusion of coronary artery to bronchial anastomosis by detachable balloon combined with coronary angioplasty. Br Heart J 1983; 49(3): 284–7.
5. Sunder KR, Balakrishnan KG, Tharakan JA et al. Coronary artery fistula in children and adults: a review of 25 cases with long-term observation. Int J Cardiol 2007; 3; 58(1): 47–53.
6. Fletcher S, Awadallah S, Amin Z. Extension of transcatheter coil occlusion to the treatment of complex coronary artery fistulas. J Interven Cardiol 2003; 16: 165–9.
7. Reidy JF, Anjos RT, Qureshi SA, Tynan M. Transcatheter embolization in the treatment of coronary artery fistula. J Am Coll Cardiol 1991; 18: 187–92.
8. Mcmahon CJ, Nihill MR, Mullins CE, Grifka RG. Coronary artery fistula: management and intermediate-term outcome after transcatheter coil occlusion. Tex Heart Inst J 2001; 28(1): 21–5.
9. Kharouf R, Cao QL, Hijazi ZM. Transcatheter closure of coronary artery fistula complicated by myocardial infarction. J Invas Cardiol 2007; 19: E146–9.
10. Qureshi SA, Reidy JF, Alwi MB et al. Use of interlocking detachable coils in embolization of coronary artery fistulas. Am J Cardiol 1996; 78: 110–13.
11. Armsby LR, Keane JF, Sherwood MC et al. Management of coronary artery fistulae. Patient selection and results of transcatheter closure. J Am Coll Cardiol 2002; 39(6): 1026–32.
12. Urrutia-S CO, Falaschi G, Ott DA, Cooley DA. Surgical management of 56 patients with congenital coronary artery fistulas. Ann Thorac Surg 1978; 35: 300–7.
13. Mavroudis C, Backer CL, Rocchini AP, Muster AJ, Gevitz M. Coronary artery fistula in infants and children: surgical review and discussion of coil embolization. Ann Thorac Surg 1997; 63: 1235–42.
14. Correl T, Tkebuchava T, Jenni R, Arbenz U, Turna M. Congenital coronary fistula in children and adults. Diagnosis, surgical technique and result. Cardiology 1996; 87(4): 325–30.

23 Complications of catheter-based interventions for pulmonary arteriovenous malformations

John T Fahey MD, Jeffrey S Pollak MD, and Robert I White MD

INTRODUCTION

Pulmonary arteriovenous malformations are abnormal vessels in which there is a direct connection from the pulmonary arterial circulation to the pulmonary venous circulation without an intervening capillary bed. These abnormal communications have been given various names including pulmonary arteriovenous fistulas, pulmonary arteriovenous aneurysms, hemangiomas of the lung, pulmonary telangiectasias, pulmonary hamartomas, and pulmonary arteriovenous malformations.[1–5] Only the term pulmonary arteriovenous malformation (PAVM) will be used here.

PAVMs provide a direct capillary-free communication between the pulmonary and systemic circulations with three major clinical consequences: (1) pulmonary arterial blood passing through these right-to-left shunts can not be oxygenated, leading to systemic hypoxemia, (2) the absence of the normal filtering of the pulmonary capillary bed allows particulate matter (air bubbles or clots) to reach the systemic circulation (paradoxical embolism) with potential clinical sequelae in the cerebral circulation (transient ischemic attack, stroke, brain abscess) or other circulations, and (3) these abnormal vessels may rupture into the bronchus (hemoptysis) or the pleural cavity (hemothorax).

The vast majority of PAVMs are congenital, with approximately 70% of patients having hereditary hemorrhagic telangiectasia (HHT).[4,6] However, with more extensive screening of patients with PAVMs, the incidence of HHT is probably closer to 80–90%.[5,7] The remaining congenital PAVMs are idiopathic lesions not associated with any underlying condition. Approximately 10% of PAVMs are acquired. These have been reported with hepatic cirrhosis (hepatopulmonary syndrome), trauma, mitral stenosis, Fanconi's syndrome, and bronchiectasis.[5,8–11] In addition, approximately 20% of patients with congenital heart disease who receive a Glenn shunt (superior vena cava to right pulmonary artery) will develop PAVMs.[12,13]

As 70 to 90% of patients who will be referred for transcatheter embolization of PAVMs will have HHT, it is mandatory that the interventionalist be thoroughly familiar with HHT, its presentation, multisystem involvement, and complications. A comprehensive review of this subject is beyond the scope of this chapter, but it has recently been reviewed.[12–15] Briefly, HHT is a genetic disorder of blood vessels. Also known as Rendu–Osler–Weber syndrome, HHT is a condition that is transmitted in an autosomal dominant pattern, and is characterized by arteriovenous malformations (AVMs) in the skin, mucous membranes, and visceral organs. Mild to moderate epistaxis is the most common symptom of HHT. To permit a high degree of clinical suspicion, recent international diagnostic criteria have been developed based on the four criteria of spontaneous recurrent epistaxis, mucocutaneous telangiectasia, visceral involvement (including PAVMs, and hepatic, cerebral, or spinal AVM), and an affected first-degree relative.[16] Approximately 50% of HHT patients have an AVM of the brain, lung, or liver, or a combination of two or three.[17–19] At least 30% of HHT patients have PAVMs.[19,20] About 10% of patients with HHT die prematurely or are disabled due to their vascular malformations. The focus of this chapter will be congenital PAVMs and we will discuss HHT predominantly as it relates to PAVMs and their management.

CLINICAL MANIFESTATIONS OF PAVM

Up to 55% of PAVMs are asymptomatic.[4,8] Only about 10% of cases are identified in infancy or childhood, with a gradual increase in the incidence through the fifth and sixth decades. Symptoms related to the PAVMs most commonly present between the fourth and sixth decades and are usually attributable to the right-to-left shunting.[4,5,12,21] The most common complaint in symptomatic patients with PAVMs is epistaxis, caused by bleeding from mucosal telangiectases, and reflects the high incidence of HHT in these patients.[4,5,12–16] Dyspnea is the second most common complaint in patients with PAVMs, particularly in those with large or diffuse PAVMs. Dyspnea is seen in almost all patients who have associated cyanosis, clubbing, easy fatigability, or polycythemia. Dyspnea and cyanosis are worse with exertion and exercise.[4,8,15,22,23] Hemoptysis and hemothorax occur in roughly 10% of patients.[24,25] PAVMs may enlarge during pregnancy and fatal hemorrhage from maternal PAVMs has been described.[26,27]

The most common serious symptoms in adults and children are ischemic stroke, transient ischemic

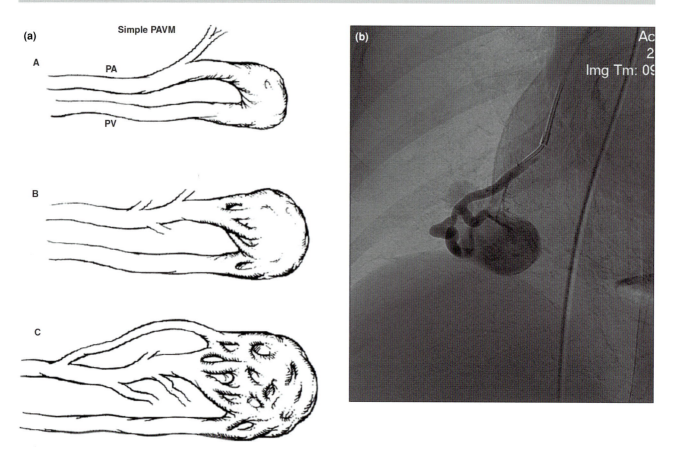

Figure 23.1 (A) Diagrams of the types of simple PAVM. In the simple PAVM, the artery to the PAVM may consist of a single branch (A), multiple branches (B), or multiple branches with a much more proximal branch arising from the same segmental artery (C). (B) Angiogram of a simple PAVM corresponding to simple PAVM type C. Modified from reference 34.

attack, or brain abscess.[4,5,12,13,28–31] Long-term follow-up studies in patients with untreated PAVMs were reviewed by Gossage and Kanj.[4] They estimated that the incidence of stroke was 11.4% and of brain abscess was 6.8%. Some reports have estimated that 25% of patients with PAVMs experience transient ischemic attacks or stroke as the initial presentation of a PAVM.[4,5,28–31]

It is usually considered that the incidence of symptoms is higher in patients with multiple PAVMs rather than a single PAVM. In a study from the Mayo Clinic, symptoms were present in 37% of patients with a single PAVM and in 59% of patients with bilateral PAVMs.[21] In addition, patients with diffuse PAVMs are almost always symptomatic.[4,32] This will be addressed further in the next section.

CLASSIFICATION AND DISTRIBUTION OF PAVMS

A classification of PAVMs based on segmental pulmonary artery anatomy was proposed by White *et al.* in 1983.[33] PAVMs can be classified as either simple or complex. In the initial classification, the simple type was defined as having a single segmental artery and draining vein. The complex type of PAVM was defined as having two or more arteries supplying the PAVM and one or two draining veins. Based on computed tomography (CT) findings, this classification has been modified subsequently.[34] A simple PAVM has single or multiple feeding arteries originating from a single segmental artery (Figure 23.1). Conversely, in complex PAVMs, feeding arteries always originate from two or more segmental arteries (Figure 23.2). Simple PAVMs usually account for 80 to 90% of PAVMs, but both simple and complex PAVMs are frequently seen in the same patient. In approximately 5% of patients with simple and/or complex PAVMs, a diffuse pattern of PAVMs is present. White *et al.* have described diffuse PAVMs when almost all segmental arteries have small PAVMs arising from segmental branches (Figure 23.3).[32,33] Patients with diffuse PAVMs usually have a more severe clinical presentation with exercise intolerance and profound cyanosis, and are also at higher risk of neurologic complications.[32]

PAVMs may be single or multiple. The incidence of single PAVMs ranges from 42 to 74%.[5,10,33–37] The majority of PAVMs (53 to 70%) are located in the lower lobes, with the left lower lobe being the most common, followed by the right lower lobe, left upper

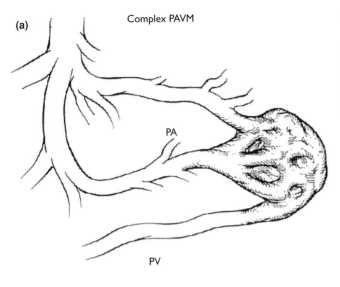

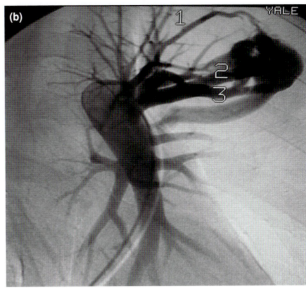

Figure 23.2   (A) Diagram of a complex PAVM. The complex variety is always supplied by two or more segmental arteries. (B) Angiogram of a complex PAVM. PA, pulmonary artery; PV, pulmonary vein. Modified from reference 34.

lobe, right middle lobe, and right upper lobe.[4,5] A review of the pathologic anatomy in 350 patients with PAVM found that 75% of patients had unilateral disease, 36% had multiple lesions, and half of those with multiple lesions had bilateral PAVM. In this review, PAVM involved the pleura in 81% and were totally subpleural in 21%, an important consideration for postembolization complications, as will be discussed later.[35]

Typically, an aneurysmal sac will exist at the arteriovenous connection, commonly a single one for simple lesions with one or two feeder arteries and more likely a plexiform, septate, or multichanneled one for lesions with multiple feeder vessels (Figure 23.1B). These sacs may be quite large and are usually thin walled.[35,38,39]

INDICATIONS FOR EMBOLIZATION AND PATIENT SELECTION

Indications for treatment of PAVMs include three broad categories: prevention of hemorrhage, improvement of hypoxemia in patients with exercise intolerance, and, most importantly, prevention of the complications associated with paradoxical embolism. Exercise intolerance consisting of dyspnea and fatigue is difficult to quantify, since most patients tolerate the hypoxemia quite well. In most centers, the primary indication for embolization of PAVMs is prevention of neurologic complications.

Since 1985, it has been recognized that patients with PAVM and a feeding artery of 3 mm in diameter or greater are susceptible to paradoxical embolus and TIA or stroke.[28] This is a threshold size for paradoxical embolus of bland thrombus, but smaller PAVMs have

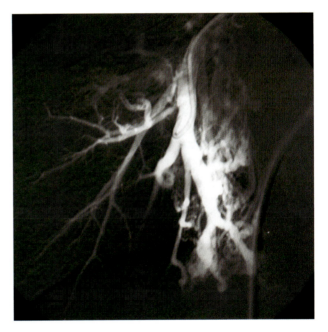

Figure 23.3   Right pulmonary angiogram showing diffuse involvement of the posterior and medial segment arteries.

been associated with brain abscess and much larger PAVMs with pulmonary hemorrhage. In general, it is our goal to occlude all PAVMs with arteries of 3 mm or larger, and to follow closely all patients with treated PAVMs as well as those with small PAVMs. The same criteria are used for children and adolescents, and these patients can be safely embolized.[31] The 3 mm diameter measurement is performed from non-contrast CT or pulmonary angiography and is at the site where the artery is of uniform diameter, preferably as close to the aneurysmal sac as possible. There is no correlation between the size of the aneursymal sac and paradoxical embolus, although large sacs are often present in patients with pulmonary hemorrhage.[4,7,28,30,34,40]

Special consideration should be given to women of childbearing age who have PAVMs. They should be informed that PAVMs may enlarge during pregnancy and fatal hemorrhage from maternal PAVMs has been reported. Most cases of PAVM deterioration occur during the second or third trimester. Semi-urgent embolization is performed in the later part of the second or early third trimester for patients with large PAVMs. In these unusual situations, diagnostic angiography is limited and procedure time carefully monitored in order to limit fetal and maternal radiation exposure. The option of treatment of PAVMs before pregnancy should be discussed with these women.[4, 25–27,41]

The roughly 5% of PAVM patients with diffuse PAVMs deserve special consideration. These patients have very small and numerous PAVMs and the criterion of a 3 mm feeder artery does not apply (Figure 23.3). Subsegmental embolization may be indicated in order to raise O_2 saturations to a level compatible with a productive life.[32] Interventions for diffuse PAVMs will be discussed later.

Finally, emergent embolization of PAVMs in patients with life-threatening complications such as pulmonary hemorrhage, hemothorax, or hemoptysis should be evaluated on a case by case basis.

TREATMENT OPTIONS AND GOALS OF THERAPY

The current preferred treatment for PAVMs consists of embolization using coils or other intravascular devices. Before 1977, surgical resection (including vascular ligation, local resection, segmentectomy, lobectomy, and pneumonectomy) was the only method of treatment.[2,4,42–45] Perioperative mortality ranged from 0 to 9%. In postoperative follow-up, the recurrence rate was 0 to 10%. Thus the disadvantages of surgery are the morbidity associated with a thoracotomy, the potential loss of normal pulmonary parenchyma surrounding the PAVM, particularly in the case of lobectomy or segmentectomy, and the long hospital stay. The first successful case of embolization of PAVMs was reported by Porstmann in 1977.[46] Since that time, embolization has become the first line of treatment and surgery is rarely indicated, since embolization results in permanent occlusion of PAVMs in a vast majority of patients with minimal complications in experienced hands.[4,5]

The goal of treatment is complete occlusion of all segmental arteries to the PAVM, with minimal or no loss of normal lung perfusion. Partial occlusion is not acceptable as the recanalization rate is unacceptably high. As the sac of the PAVM is very thin-walled, coils and devices should not protrude into the sac, except in rare circumstances, as will be discussed below.

CATHETERIZATION, EMBOLIZATION, AND PREVENTION OF PROCEDURAL COMPLICATIONS

Preparation

Most catheterizations and embolizations in adults may be performed with conscious sedation. General anesthesia is usually necessary in children and adolescents. The patient's history must be thoroughly reviewed with the anesthesiologist or nurse administering anesthesia or conscious sedation, especially if the patient has HHT. Prior history of stroke or brain abscess is important as some agents may lower seizure threshold. A history of severe nose bleeds or pulmonary hemorrhage due to AVM is important, especially if passing a nasogastric tube or orotracheal tube. The risk of air embolus when starting an intravenous line or administering medications must be reinforced. Continuous monitoring of ECG, O_2 saturation, and blood pressure is performed.

Techniques of catheterization

An indwelling 7 French sheath is placed in either the right or left femoral vein using sterile technique and connected to a heparinized flush solution, being careful to clear the connecting tubing of all air. The pulmonary artery is accessed using a pigtail catheter or other angiographic catheter. It is essential that the pulmonary artery pressure be measured in all patients. Most patients with PAVM have low pressures due to the low-resistance shunts from the PAVM. However, there is an important subset of patients with HHT who have pulmonary hypertension where pressures may approach systemic levels.[4,43,47–49] Special considerations for PAVMs in this setting are important and will be discussed under Special Considerations below, as embolization may not be indicated in some cases.

Patients should be fully heparinized for all procedures. Diagnostic angiography in multiple planes is performed in both lungs. The goal is to confirm the CT findings and, most importantly, to determine the morphology of the artery (or arteries) as it enters the sac, its length, and diameter.[33,34,50] Complex PAVMs are present in 10% of patients and all feeder arteries must be identified. High-flow feeder arteries less than 2.5 cm in length require special techniques for closing the PAVM, and will also be discussed later under Special Considerations.

Following the diagnostic angiogram, the angiographic catheter is exchanged for an 80/100 cm coaxial guide system with an outer 7 French 80 cm guide catheter and inner 5 French catheter (Figure 23.4). The development of 7 French guide catheters (Lumax, Cook) has greatly simplified access to PAVMs and increased stability of catheters when introducing pushable fibered coils. Guide catheters stabilize one's position proximally in the feeding artery, in order to provide a controlled and precise delivery of coils through a coaxially placed 5 French catheter, either 5 French multipurpose catheters (Cook), or angled 'J' catheters (Terumo). For the right middle lobe or lingula, a Judkins 5 French left coronary catheter (cordis) is passed through the 7 French guide catheter. Once entry into the right middle lobe or lingula is performed with the Judkins catheter, the guide catheter is advanced over the 5 French coronary catheter. Then the coronary catheter is removed and 5 French Polyethyelene Cook or Terumo catheter is used to place the coils in the feeding artery. Selective catheter positioning is achieved by advancing the catheter either directly or over a wire. Once a segmental artery has been cannulated, it is mandatory to aspirate blood through the catheter to prevent air or clot injections. If blood return is not obtained during aspiration, the catheter must be gently removed. It should be pulled back slowly, with the hub of the catheter under saline in a bowl to avoid air entry due to a vacuum effect. This 'underwater' technique should also be used for exchange of wires to prevent air aspiration.[34,50]

Once the 4 or 5 French catheter is positioned with free flow, the 7 French guide catheter is advanced or adjusted in position over the inner catheter in order to secure a stable position in the feeding artery (Figure 23.4). Hand injected angiograms in multiple projections are essential before selecting the technique and placement of occlusion devices. The view that profiles the entry of the artery into the aneurysmal sac, connecting the artery to the vein, is the view of choice for performing the occlusion.

Occlusion techniques and devices

Embolization needs to be carried out with devices large enough to occlude the feeding artery securely. In the first case reported by Porstmann in 1977, the PAVM was embolized using hand-made steel coils.[46] White et al. performed most of the early cases using different types of detachable balloon systems.[51] These devices, initially developed for neurovascular and cardiovascular large-vessel occlusion, are no longer available in most countries.[52] Balloons had the advantage of providing total cross-sectional occlusion, and recanalization was a rare event.[51,52] Experience with detachable balloons as well as newer occlusion devices, like the Amplatzer devices and vascular plugs and the Gianturco–Grifka vascular occlusion device, suggested

that cross-sectional occlusion should be the goal for embolotherapy for PAVMs.[53–55]

Most groups today favor the use of coils as the primary embolization agent and these techniques will be discussed in detail. Initially, only stainless steel coils such as the Gianturco–Anderson–Wallace were available. More recently, fibered and non-fibered variants of soft platinum coils have become available. The choice of a coil of correct size is critical. If too small, the coil may pass through the venous portion of the PAVM to the systemic circulation, with disastrous consequences.[34] If too large a coil is chosen, the coil may elongate, leading to recanalization, or cause occlusion of more proximal normal pulmonary artery branches and pulmonary infarction.[34,56,57] After placement of the first coil, additional coils must be positioned until blood flow to the PAVM has ceased. Packing of smaller coils in the center of the first placed coil is mandatory to obtain complete cross-sectional occlusion and prevent recanalization. If the number of coils is not sufficient, recanalization may also occur due to insufficient thrombus formation. While sac embolization is not felt to be necessary, as will be discussed below, the coils should be placed in the feeding artery as close to the sac as is safely possible to prevent persistent perfusion or reperfusion of a distal segment of artery leading to the PAVM.

The role of venous sac embolization remains unclear. We try to avoid placing coils into the sac due to the thin wall of the sac and the potential for erosion. In fact, the sac routinely involutes following occlusion of the feeding artery alone. Further, occluding the aneurysmal sac of the PAVM removes one of the most important anatomic signs of successful treatment, i.e. sac involution. In our experience, venous sac closure is necessary in less than 1% of PAVMs when the artery to the PAVM is short (less than 2 cm) and has high flow or uneven diameter, and there is a high risk of coil embolization.[58–61] These high-risk cases will be discussed below.

Experience with follow-up angiograms of patients treated for PAVMs showed that, when high-flow PAVMs were treated with pushable fibered coils, deployment of only one or two coils often produced a temporary occlusion which recanalized over time (Figure 23.4). It was soon appreciated that initial deployment of the first one or two coils was associated with elongation of the coil and spasm of the feeder artery. In other words, elongation of the coil during placement through an endhole catheter was not always associated with long-term occlusion.[39,56,57] The elongation of the pushable fibered coils can be avoided using coaxial catheters as described above. By advancing the coil through the inner 4 or 5 French catheter while holding the outer guide catheter stable in the artery prevents coil elongation.

Another benefit of using guide catheters and the improved control they provided when placing

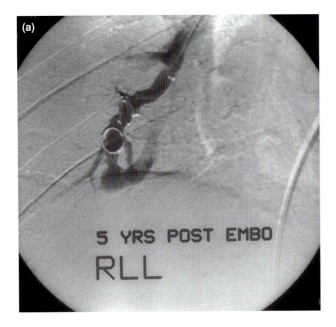

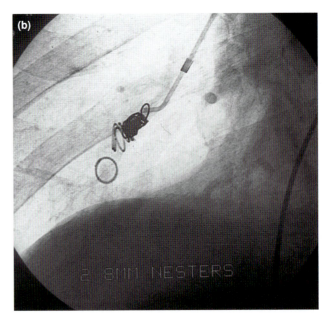

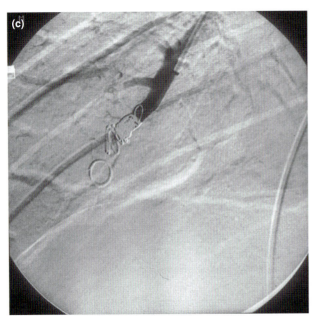

Figure 23.4 (A) Angiogram 5 years after attempted coil closure of a simple PAVM. There had been recanalization and the pulmonary malformation is still present. (B) Dense packing of two 8 mm Nester coils placed just proximal to the recanalized coils, producing cross-sectional occlusion. (C) Final angiogram showing complete occlusion.

pushable coils was the realization that we could anchor the first 2 cm of a long coil in a side branch close to the aneurysmal sac. Thus, by 'anchoring' the coil, we avoided any chance of coil migration and deployment of the remainder of the coil could be controlled.[39,62] The anchor coil is chosen with a diameter 2 mm larger than the feeding artery. The 'anchor technique' has been very useful in avoiding paradoxical embolization of the coil through the PAVM, is used whenever possible, and is used to occlude more than 50% of the PAVMs in our laboratory (Figures 23.5 and 23.6). The anchor branch is chosen as close to the aneurysmal sac as possible. This prevents unnecessary occlusion of normal branches, since a distal branch is usually sacrificed by whatever

occlusion technique is utilized. Once the anchoring coil is placed, additional coils are placed as needed to obtain complete cross-sectional occlusion of the feeder artery.

In very high flow fistulas with large arteries, or if no anchoring vessel is available, we have utilized a 'scaffold technique' (Figure 23.7). This technique is used to achieve a stable matrix in order to avoid migration. By first deploying high radial force, fibered stainless steel coils, a 'scaffold' is formed and the completion of the cross-sectional occlusion is produced with smaller coils which are 'weaved' into the interstices of the 'endoskeleton.' The first, high radial force coils placed to form the scaffold are oversized by 2 mm, i.e. for a 10 mm feeding artery, 12 mm diameter stainless steel

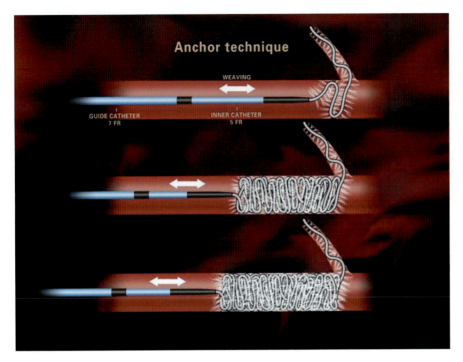

Figure 23.5 The 'anchor' technique. This technique provides safe and distal occlusion. Diagrammatically, the guide catheter is placed in the artery to be occluded and a 5 French inner catheter is advanced into a side branch next to the site requiring occlusion. At least 2 cm of the anchoring coil is advanced into the side branch. The rest of the coil is then deployed just proximal to that side branch and additional coils are packed so that cross-sectional occlusion is obtained.

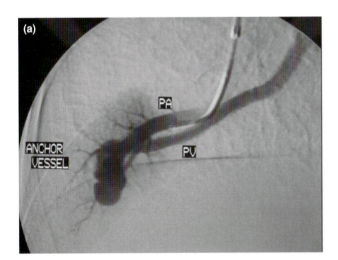

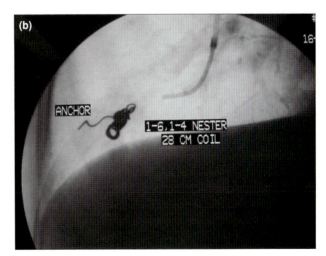

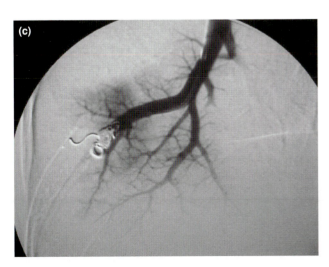

Figure 23.6 (A) Pulmonary angiogram showing a PAVM of the right lower lobe. A number of distal side branches are demonstrated immediately proximal to the aneurysmal sac and fistula. (B) The inner 5 French catheter was advanced into a side branch and 2 cm of the first coil was deployed. The 5 French catheter was then retracted and the remaining coil was packed into a tight coil mass. One additional coil was also packed into the previously placed coil. (C) The final angiogram demonstrates a very distal occlusion immediately adjacent to the sac with preservation of most of the normal branches. Note, the support or 'purchase' of the guiding catheter is critical to allow packing of the coil into a tight occlusion mass without elongation of the coil.

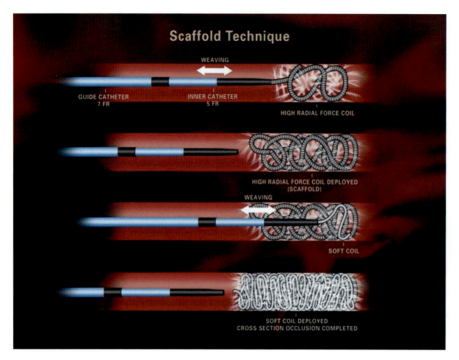

Figure 23.7   Diagram of the 'scaffold' technique. This technique is used for high-flow vessels when there is no 'anchor' vessel. Initially, a high radial force coil, with a diameter 2 mm larger than the artery being occluded, is placed to create a scaffold. Several additional high radial force coils may be placed and the occlusion is completed using softer Nester coils to tightly pack within the scaffold or 'endoskeleton.'

coils are placed first. Then several small diameter high radial force coils are placed as well into the endoskeleton, followed by several softer coils, until cross-sectional occlusion is obtained.[39,62]

In large feeder arteries, 12 mm or larger in diameter, the first scaffolding coils may be place through a balloon occlusion catheter (Boston Scientific).[59,62] The balloon-tipped catheter is placed into the feeder artery over a guide wire and inflated more proximally in the artery to stop flow. The wire is removed. The first coils are placed through the lumen of the balloon catheter. Once a scaffold is formed using two or three high radial force coils, the balloon is slowly deflated and removed. A coaxial guide system is substituted and the embolization is completed by packing additional coils as just described. The majority of PAVMs can be successfully coiled using either the anchor technique or the scaffold technique.

After embolization of the feeder artery or arteries by any of the above techniques, segmental and lobar angiography should be performed to assess for adequate occlusion and any accessory feeding vessels that might also require embolization. Patients are generally not hospitalized overnight.

High-risk cases requiring special considerations

Short (< 2 cm) feeder arteries

In our experience, coils are difficult to place in short arteries. This is one of the rare times that it is necessary to occlude the aneurysmal sac of the PAVM. Because the aneurysm of the PAVM is thin-walled, it is predisposed to injury by guide wires and coils. With this approach, the short artery is selectively entered and an occlusion balloon catheter is placed over a guide wire and inflated to occlude flow, as just described.[59] The guide wire is removed and replaced with a microcatheter (Target Therapeutics or Cordis), and advanced through the lumen of the balloon catheter over a 0.014 inch guide wire into the aneurysm. Microcoils equivalent to the diameter of the aneurysm and exceeding the diameter of the draining pulmonary vein are placed. These coils are generally referred to as vein of Galen or complex helical coils (Target Therapeutics). Several coils larger than the draining vein must be placed until a large matrix is established that will trap smaller coils without letting them enter the draining vein. To achieve complete occlusion of a large aneurysm, up to 40–50 coils may be required.

Patients with pulmonary hypertension

There are two subsets of patients with HHT who may have associated pulmonary hypertension.[4,5,47–49] Adult HHT patients with significant liver AVMs may have pulmonary artery systolic pressures exceeding 40 to 50 mmHg.[63] In addition, in HHT type 2 there is a subset of patients with primary pulmonary hypertension.[18,63] Elimination of the low-resistance PAVMs in this setting may lead to worsening pulmonary hypertension. It is our practice to balloon occlude the artery for about 30 minutes while monitoring the pulmonary artery pressure through a separately placed venous catheter. If the pulmonary pressure elevates with balloon occlusion, we do not embolize the PAVM.

Patients with diffuse PAVMs

As mentioned previously, about 5% of patients with PAVMs will have diffuse lesions.[7,32,65,66] These patients in general have very small and numerous PAVMs and are particularly prone to recurrent infections. We feel that subsegmental embolization may be indicated in selected patients in order to raise O_2 saturations to a level compatible with productive life. These patients are best seen in an HHT center with a large experience of treating PAVM, since methods for managing diffuse PAVM are undergoing re-evaluation.

COMPLICATIONS DURING CATHETERIZATION AND FOLLOW-UP

A thorough knowledge of reported complications (1) during catheterization and embolization therapy and (2) following the catheterization is mandatory before proceeding with any catheterization, in order to minimize or hopefully eliminate these complications. This knowledge is also important to fully inform the patients prior to the procedure as to what they may experience following the intervention.

Complications during the procedure

To our knowledge, no periprocedural mortality has been reported with embolization of PAVMs and complications have in general been infrequent and self-limited.[4] Air embolization during the procedure has been reported in up to 4.8% of procedures and is the most common intraprocedural complication.[5,7,50,52,67–69] This is probably more common when occluding small (3 to 4 mm) PAVMs.[67] Air accidentally passing into the coronary arteries produces angina with associated ST segment changes on the ECG or bradycardia, and usually resolves within 15 minutes. Air entering the cerebral circulation may cause transient ischemic attack symptoms including perioral and limb paresthesias or expressive aphasia and, like angina, these usually clear within 15 minutes. Careful flushing of catheters, observation for backbleeding, and removal of wires 'underwater' should largely eliminate this complication. In addition, filling the catheter with contrast between coils allows the interventionalist to detect residual air left in the catheter after withdrawing a pusher wire and before pushing the next coil.

Device migration with paradoxical embolization occurs in about 1% of embolization attempts, mainly with coils.[7,50,51,57,68–70] None of the reported migrations has resulted in permanent disability. Coil migration is more likely to occur in cases with large (> 8 mm) or high-flow PAVMs and during the learning curve of the interventionalist. These migrations will require additional intervention using intravascular retrieval devices.

Complications including stroke, seizures, and hemopericardium have been reported.[45,68,70] Coil migration can also be largely eliminated using coaxial catheters, along with the anchoring and scaffolding techniques previously described.

Complications following the procedure

Pleuritic chest pain occurring 3 to 7 days following the embolization procedure is the most frequent complication encountered in up to 15% of treated patients.[4,5,7,50,52,57,67–71] The incidence seems to be higher in large PAVMs, as it was seen in 31% of patients who had occlusion of PAVMs with feeding vessels greater than 8 mm.[67] It is thought that this pleuritic pain is due to irritation of the visceral pleura by thrombosis of the sac, and reflects the high incidence of PAVMs involving the pleura, as mentioned above. In patients with bilateral PAVM it is our preference to treat one lung at a time, starting with the most involved lung. Occluding PAVM in both lungs at a single session almost guarantees that the patient will experience pleurisy, which may be bilateral and contributes to anxiety and fear of additional procedures. We much prefer to bring the patient back 4 to 6 weeks later to complete the embolization of the less involved lung and to perform angiography of the first lung, to assure complete occlusion. All patients are instructed about pleurisy when they leave the hospital. Management of the pleurisy is usually easily accomplished by administration of ibuprofen for 48 hours after the procedure and hospitalization is rarely required. Antibiotics are not prescribed for patients experiencing pleurisy as we are not aware of infection being reported associated with the pleuritic episode.

A more significant event is delayed pleurisy, which occurs in less than 1% of patients about 4 to 6 weeks postembolization.[34] It may start explosively with high fever and pleuritic pain. It is thought that this is due to delayed thrombosis of the aneurysmal sac. In addition to fluids and ibuprofen, we have administered a short course of azithromycin empirically for this delayed form of pleurisy. All patients recovered without intervention.

Pleural effusion has been reported in up to 12% of patients and is usually small and self-limited.[50] Pulmonary infarction has been observed in about 3% of patients and most likely was related to occlusion of normal pulmonary arterial branches during the occlusion.[7,33,57,69,71] Now that very distal occlusions are possible by controlled anchoring of the coils immediately adjacent to the sac, we expect the incidence of this complication to be much decreased. A cerebral infarction occurring one week after coil embolization of a single PAVM without coil migration has been reported.[72] This was presumably due to clot migration from the embolized PAVM partially reperfused via a previously embolized feeding pulmonary artery and a bronchial artery.

Follow-up

All patients with treated PAVM should be evaluated at the treatment center at 6 to 12 months after treatment. Even in experienced centers, up to 7% of patients will have reperfusion of treated PAVMs.[39] In addition, in recent studies, 20% of untreated PAVMs enlarged.[39,68,73] Major neurologic complications after embolization have been reported, including cerebral abscess, transient ischemic attack, and stroke related to reperfused treated PAVM or new PAVM.[7,50,68,71]

Although follow-up evaluation of patients is clearly necessary, the precise method of follow-up is not agreed upon. Imaging follow-up of treated patients in conjunction with clinical and physiologic evaluation should be performed in order to document involution or reperfusion of embolized PAVMs, as well as to detect growth or enlargement of small PAVMs. In one study of patients who underwent embolization of large PAVMs, 91% of treated PAVMs disappeared on chest radiograph at a mean follow-up of 4 years.[67] In another large study, follow-up with CT scan one or more years after embolization showed that 96% of treated PAVMs had involution of the sac with a residual scar or marked reduction in the size of the sac.[74] This phenomenon is believed to be the result of thrombosis and retraction of the aneurysmal sac following embolization. It is likely that a combination of clinical evaluation, physiologic testing (including upright and supine oximetry), and CT imaging is the best algorithm.

Reperfusion of previously embolized PAVMs may be due to several mechanisms and has recently been reviewed.[52] Recanalization through coils is the most common mechanism. This is typically in the setting of coils that did not create a dense occlusive plug of metal in the vessel (Figure 23.4). Small accessory branches to the PAVM may be missed during the initial embolization or recruitment of initially normal branches adjacent to the PAVM may occur. In addition, bronchial and other systemic artery collateral flow into the pulmonary artery beyond the level of embolization may lead to recanalization. It is not known if these systemic collaterals place patients at risk for future hemoptysis.

SUMMARY AND CONCLUSIONS

Although transcatheter embolization is a safe and effective treatment in the management of children and adults with congenital or acquired PAVMs, complications can occur both during and remote from the procedure. Many of the complications can be eliminated or reduced significantly with improved techniques. Complete angiography in both lungs prior to any attempt at embolization is mandatory in order to identify all feeder vessels to a PAVM, their diameter, and length. This determines the occlusion strategy.

From a technical point of view, air embolism during the procedure can be eliminated using proper safeguards as outlined above. Coil migration can be largely eliminated using the anchor or scaffolding techniques in addition to the coaxial catheter system for catheter stabilization during coil implantation. It is important to perform the embolization with coils placed as distally as possible in the feeding artery to a PAVM close to the venous sac. This avoids the occlusion of branches to normal lung and reduces the rate of reperfusion and the risk of pleurisy or pulmonary infarction. Dense packing of coils to achieve complete cross-sectional occlusion is the best method to provide long-term occlusion. There are other devices (like the Amplatcer plug) that are available to occlude PAVMs. Follow-up studies are necessary to determine the incidence of reperfusion before they can be routinely used.

In patients with localized PAVMs, whether simple or complex, prevention of subsequent neurologic complications can be achieved in almost all cases if all PAVMs are occluded. Conversely, in patients with diffuse PAVMs, multiple procedures will be necessary to improve the profound hypoxia, decrease the risks of neurologic events, and obtain an acceptable quality of life for the patient. Long-term follow-up of all patients is mandatory to document aneursym retraction and to detect reperfusion of treated lesions and/or growth of small PAVMs before they reach the threshold size for neurologic emboli.

REFERENCES

1. Sloan RD, Cooley RN. Congenital pulmonary arteriovenous aneursym. AJR 1953; 70: 183–210.
2. Stringer CJ, Stanley AL, Bates RC. Pulmonary arteriovenous fistulas. Am J Surg 1955; 899: 1054–80.
3. Le Roux. Pulmonary hamartomas. Thorax 1964; 19: 236–43.
4. Gossage JR, Kanj G. State of the art: pulmonary arteriovenous malformations. Am J Resp Crit Care Med 1998; 158: 643–77.
5. Khursid I, Downie GH. Pulmonary arteriovenous malformations. Postgrad Med J 2002; 78: 191–7.
6. Sluiter-Eringa H, Orie NG, Sluiter HJ. Pulmonary arteriovenous fistula: diagnosis and prognosis in noncompliant patients. Am Rev Resp Dis 1969; 100: 177–88.
7. White RI, Lynch-Nylan A, Terry P et al. Pulmonary arteriovenous malformations: technique and transcatheter embolotherapy. Radiology 1988; 169: 663–9.
8. Burke CM, Safai C, Nelson DP, Raffin TA. Pulmonary arteriovenous malformations: a critical update. Am Rev Resp Dis 1986; 134: 334–9.
9. Lange PA, Stoller JK. The hepatopulmonary syndrome. Ann Intern Med 1995; 122; 521–9.
10. Prager RL, Laws KH, Bender HW. Arteriovenous fistula of the lung. Ann Thorac Surg 1983; 36: 231–5.
11. Taxman RM, Halloran MJ, Parker BM. Multiple arteriovenous malformations in association with Fanconi's syndrome. Chest 1973; 64: 118–20.
12. Guttmacher AE, Marchuk DA, White RI. Hereditary hemorrhagic telangiectasia. N Engl J Med 1995; 333: 918–24.
13. Shovlin CL, Hugues JM. Hereditary hemorrhagic telangiectasia. N Engl J Med 1996; 334: 33–332.

14. Cottin V, Plauchi H, Bayle J et al. Pulmonary arteriovenous malformations in patients with hereditary hemorrhagic telangiectasia. Am J Respir Crit Care 2004; 169: 994–1000.

15. Begbie ME, Wallace GM, Shovlin CL. Hereditary hemorrhagic telangiectasia (Osler–Weber–Rendu syndrome): a view from the 21st century. Postgrad Med J 2003; 79: 18–24.

16. Shovlin CL, Guttmacher AE, Buscarini E et al. Diagnostic criteria for hereditary hemorrhagic telangiectasia. Am J Med Genet 2000; 91: 66–7.

17. Fullbright RK, Chaloupka JC, Puttman CM et al. Imaging of hereditary hemorrhagic telangiectasia: prevalence and spectrum of cerebrovascular malformations. Am J Neuroradiol 1998; 19: 477–84.

18. Garcia-Tsao G, Korzenik JR, Young L et al. Liver disease in patients with hereditary hemorrhagic telangiectasia. N Engl J Med 2000; 343(13): 931–6.

19. Kjeldsen AD, Oxhoj H, Andersen PE et al. Pulmonary arteriovenous malformations: screening procedures and pulmonary angiography in patients with hereditary hemorrhagic telangiectasia. Chest 1999; 116: 432–9.

20. Haitjema T, Disch F, Overtoom TT, Westermann CJ, Lammers JW. Screening family members of patients with hereditary hemorrhagic telangiectasia. Am J Med 1995; 99(5): 519–24.

21. Swanson KL, Prakash UBS, Stanson AW. Pulmonary arteriovenous fistulas: Mayo Clinic experience. Mayo Clin Proc 1999; 74: 671–80.

22. Chilvers ER, Whyte MK, Jackson DJ, Allison DJ, Hughes JM. Effect of percutaneous transcatheter embolization on pulmonary function, right-to-left shunt, and arterial oxygenation in patients with pulmonary arteriovenous malformations. Am Rev Resp Dis 1990; 142: 420–5.

23. Pennington DW, Gold RL, Gordon RL et al. Treatment of pulmonary arteriovenous malformations by therapeutic embolization: rest and exercise physiology in eight patients. Am Rev Resp Dis 1992; 145: 1047–1051.

24. Adebgoyega PA, Youh G, Adesokan A. Recurrent massive hemothorax in Rendu–Osler–Weber. South Med J 1996; 89: 1193–6.

25. Ference BA, Shannon TM, White RI et al. Life-threatening pulmonary hemorrhage with pulmonary arteriovenous malformations and hereditary hemorrhagic telangiectasia. Chest 1994; 106: 1387–90.

26. Shovlin CL, Winstock AR, Peters AM, Jackson JE, Hughes JM. Medical complications of pregnancy in hereditary haemorrhagic telangiectasia. QJM 1995; 88(12): 879–87.

27. Gershon AS, Faughnan ME, Chon KS et al. Transcatheter embolotherapy of maternal pulmonary arteriovenous malformations during pregnancy. Chest 2001; 119(2): 470–7.

28. Hewes RC, Auster M, White RI. Cerebral embolism – first manifestation of pulmonary arteriovenous malformation in patients with hereditary hemorrhagic telangiectasia. Cardiovasc Interven Radiol 1985; 8(3): 151–5.

29. Maher CO, Piepgras DG, Brown RD, Friedman JA, Pollock BE. Cerebrovascular manifestations in 321 cases of hereditary hemorrhagic telangiectasia. Stroke 2001; 32: 877–82.

30. Moussouttas M, Fayad P, Rosenblatt M et al. Pulmonary arteriovenous malformations: cerebral ischemia and neurologic manifestations. Neurology 2000; 55: 959–64.

31. Faughnan M, Thabet A, Mei-Zahav M et al. Pulmonary arteriovenous malformations in children: outcomes of transcatheter embolotherapy. J Pediatr 2004; 145(6): 826–31,

32. Faughnan ME, Lui YW, Wirth JA et al. Diffuse pulmonary arteriovenous malformations: characteristics and prognosis. Chest 2000; 117: 31–3.

33. White RI, Mitchell SE, Barth KH et al. Angioarchitecture of pulmonary arteriovenous malformations: an important consideration before embolotherapy. AJR 1983; 140: 681–6.

34. White RI, Pollack JS, Wirth JA. Pulmonary arteriovenous malformations: diagnosis and transcatheter embolotherapy. J Vasc Interven Radiol 1996; 7: 787–804.

35. Bosher LH, Blake DA, Byrd BR. An analysis of the pathologic anatomy of pulmonary arteriovenous aneurysms with particular reference to the applicability of local excision. Surgery 1959; 45: 91–104.

36. Dines DE, Deward JB, Berantz PE. Pulmonary arteriovenous fistula. Mayo Clin Proc 1983; 58: 176–81.

37. Remy J, Remy-Jardin M, Giraud F, Wattinne L. Angioarchitecture of pulmonary arteriovenous malformations: clinical utility of three-dimensional helical CT. Radiology 1994; 191: 657–64.

38. Anabtawi IN, Ellison RG, Ellison LT. Pulmonary arteriovenous aneurysms and fistulas: anatomical variations, embryology, and classification. Ann Thorac Surg 1965; 1: 277–85.

39. Pollak JS, Saluja S, Thabet A et al. Clinical and anatomic outcomes after embolotherapy of pulmonary arteriovenous malformations. J Vasc Interven Radiol 2006; 17(1): 35–45.

40. White RI. Pulmonary arteriovenous malformations: how do we diagnose them and why is it important to do so? Radiology 1992; 182: 633–5.

41. Gamon RB, Miksa AK, Keller FS. Osler–Weber–Rendu disease and pulmonary arteriovenous fistulas. Deterioration and embolotherapy during pregnancy. Chest 1990; 98: 1522–4.

42. Sluiter-Eringa H, Orie NG, Sluiter HJ. Pulmonary arteriovenous fistula: diagnosis and prognosis in noncompliant patients. Am Rev Resp Dis 1969; 100: 177–88.

43. Dines DE, Arms RA, Bernatz PE, Gomes MR. Pulmonary arteriovenous fistulas. Mayo Clin Proc 1974; 49: 460–5.

44. Hugues JM, Allison DJ. Pulmonary arteriovenous malformations: the radiologist replaces the surgeon. Clin Radiol 1990; 41: 297–8.

45. Puskas JD, Allen MS, Moncure AC et al. Pulmonary arteriovenous malformations: therapeutic options. Ann Thorac Surg 1993; 56: 253–8.

46. Porstmann W. Therapeutic embolization of arteriovenous fistula by catheter technique. In: Kelop O, ed. Current Concepts in Pediatric Radiology 1977. Berlin: Springer, 23–31.

47. Sapru RP, Hutchison DC, Hall JI. Pulmonary hypertension in patients with pulmonary arteriovenous fistulae. Br Heart J 1969; 31: 559–69.

48. Sperling DC, Cheitlin M, Sullivan RW, Smith A. Pulmonary arteriovenous fistulas with pulmonary hypertension. Chest 1977; 71: 753–7.

49. Rodan BA, Godwin JD, Chen JT, Ravin CE. Worsening pulmonary hypertension after resection of arteriovenous fistula. AJR 1981; 137: 864–6.

50. Mager JJ, Overtoom TT, Blauw H, Lammers JW, Westermann CJ. Embolotherapy of pulmonary arteriovenous malformations long-term results in 112 patients. J Vasc Interven Radiol 2004; 15(5): 451–6.

51. White RI, Barth KH, Kaufman SL, de Caprio V, Strandberg JD. Therapeutic embolization with detachable balloons. Cardiovasc Intervent Radiol 1980; 3: 229–41.

52. Pollak JS, Egglin TK, Rosenblatt MM, Dickey MM, White RI. Clinical results of transvenous systemic embolotherapy with a neuroradiologic detachable balloon. Radiology 1994; 191: 477–82.

53. Cil B, Canyigit M, Ozkan OS, Pamuk GA, Dogan R. Bilateral multiple pulmonary arteriovenous malformations: endovascular treatment with the Amplatzer vascular plug. J Vasc Interven Radiol 2006; 17: 141–5.

54. Bialkowski J, Zabal C, Szkutnik et al. Percutaneous interventional closure of large pulmonary arterivenous fistulas with the Amplatzer duct occluder. Am J Cardiol 2005; 96: 127–9.

55. Ebeid MR, Braden DS, Gaymes CH, Joransen JA. Closure of a large pulmonary arteriovenous malformation using multiple Gianturco–Grifka vascular occlusion devices. Cathet Cardiovasc Interven 2000; 49: 426–9.

56. Lacombe P, LaGrange C, El-Hajjam M, Chinet T, Pelage JP. Reperfusion of complex large pulmonary arteriovenous malformations after embolization: report of three cases. Cardiovasc Interven Radiol 2005; 28: 30–5.

57. Remy-Jardin M, Wattinne L, Remy J. Transcatheter occlusion of pulmonary arterial circulation and collateral supply: failures, incidents, and complications. Radiology 1991; 180: 699–705.

58. Takahashi K, Tanimura K, Honda M et al. Venous sac of pulmonary arteriovenous malformation: preliminary experience using interlocking detachable coils. Cardiovasc Interven Radiol 1999; 22: 210–13.

59. Tal MG, Saluja S, Henderson KJ, White RI. Vein of Galen technique for occluding the aneurysmal sac of pulmonary arteriovenous malformations. J Vasc Interven Radiol 2002; 13: 1261–4.

60. Coley SC, Jackson JE. Venous sac embolization of pulmonary arteriovenous malformations in two patients. AJR 1996; 167: 452–4.

61. Dinkel HP, Triller J. Pulmonary arteriovenous malformations: embolotherapy with superselective coaxial catheter placement and filling of venous sac with Gugllielmi detachable coils. Radiology 2002; 223: 709–14.

62. Pelage J-P, Lacombe P, White RI, Pollak JS. Pulmonary Arteriovenous Malformations. Vascular Embolotherapy: A Comprehensive Approach, J Golzarian, S Sun, MJ Sharafuddin, Eds: Berlin, Germany: Springer: 279–96.

63. Bernard G, Mion F, Henry L, Plauchi H, Paliard P. Hepatic involvement in Hereditary hemorrhagic telangiectasia. Clinical, Radiological, and Hemodynamic Studies of all 11 Cases.

64. Harrison RE, Flanagan JA, Sankelo M et al. Molecular and functional analysis identifies ALK-1 as the predominant cause of pulmonary hypertension related to hereditary haemorrhagic telangiectasia. J Med Genet 2003; 40(12): 865–71. (Erratum in: J Med Genet 2004; 41(7): 576.)

65. Hales MR. Multiple small arteriovenous fistuae of the lung. Am J Pathol 1956; 32; 927–43.

66. Shapiro JL, Stillwell PC, Levien MG et al. Diffuse pulmonary arteriovenous malformations (angiodysplasia with unusual histologic features): case report and review of the literature. Pediatr Pulmon 1996; 21; 255–61.

67. Lee DW, White RI Jr, Egglin TK et al. Embolotherapy of large pulmonary arteriovenous malformations – long term results. Ann Thorac Surg 1997; 64: 930–40.

68. Dutton JA, Jackson JE, Hughes JM et al. Pulmonary arteriovenous malformations: results of treatment with coil embolization in 53 patients. AJR 1995; 165(5): 1119–25.

69. Terry PB, White RI, Barth KH, Kaufman SL, Mitchell SE. Pulmonary arteriovenous malformations. Physiologic observations and results of therapeutic balloon embolization. N Engl J Med 1983; 308: 1197–200

70. Haitjema T, Overtoom TT, Westermann CJ, Lammers JW. Embolisation of pulmonary arteriovenous malformations: results and follow-up in 32 patients. Thorax 1995; 50: 719–23.

71. Hartnell GG, Jackson JE, Allison DJ. Coil embolization of pulmonary arteriovenous malformations. Cardiovasc Interven Radiol 1990; 13: 347–50.

72. Mager JJ, Overtoom TT, Mauser HW, Westermann CJ. Early cerebral infarction after embolotherapy of a pulmonary arteriovenous malformation (letter). J Vasc Interven Radiol 2001; 12: 122–3.

73. Andersen PE, Kjeldsen AD. Clinical and radiological long-term follow-up after embolization of pulmonary arteriovenous malformations. Cardiovasc Interven Radiol 2006; 29(1): 70–4.

74. Remy J, Remy-Jardin M, Wattinne L et al. Pulmonary arteriovenous malformations: evaluation with CT of the chest before and after treatment. Radiology 1992; 182: 809–16.

24 Atrial septal defect device closure

Nicholas J Collins and Eric M Horlick

Secundum atrial septal defects (ASDs) are a common congenital abnormality and are amongst the most common congenital heart defects to present in adulthood. The development of transcatheter strategies for treatment of interatrial defects has allowed for effective closure of ASDs; these therapies offer advantages in terms of morbidity, hospital length of stay, and anesthesia duration compared to surgical closure,[1–7] with earlier hemodynamic improvement compared to surgical intervention.[8] The effectiveness of these devices has been demonstrated in both adult patients,[9] including those greater than 40 years of age,[10] as well as pediatric populations.[11] As such, percutaneous ASD closure has become the preferred treatment option in cases where it is feasible.

A number of different devices have been developed and successfully used for this indication. Earlier generation devices using a clamshell or double umbrella design were limited by an increased incidence of residual shunts and an increased risk of embolization, particularly when closing large defects. The development of the Amplatzer® Septal Occluder (AGA, Golden Valley, CA) was a significant advance; this Nitinol double disc device with a self-centering waist has demonstrated low thrombogenicity, ease of use, and excellent results in short- and long-term follow-up. Alternate occluder designs with demonstrated efficacy include the CardioSEAL and STARFlex double umbrella devices (Nitinol Medical Technical, Inc [NMT], Boston. MA), the AngelWings ASD occluder,[12] and the HELEX septal occluder (WL Gore & Associates, Flagstaff, AZ).[5,12]

Percutaneous device closure has thus clearly evolved since initial descriptions. The development of a self-centering device with a waist, as opposed to a thin connecting stem, has improved efficacy, in terms of residual shunts, and safety, with the likelihood of embolization reduced. Also, the ability to potentially retract the device after deployment, but before release, has increased the ease and safety of use. Smaller sheath sizes for device delivery reduce the risk of vascular trauma, and the advance of intracardiac echocardiography, with suitability again demonstrated in various age groups, obviates the need for general anesthesia.[13,14] Future refinements may include the manufacture of devices from bioabsorbable compounds, which may have the advantage of eliminating the need for a redundant synthetic implant after endothelialization. Recently, encouraging preliminary data from the use of a bioabsorbable ASD occluder have been reported

using the BioSTAR closure device (NMT, Boston, MA),[15,16] noting only a small number of patients have been treated with this technology.

Despite these advances and accompanying enthusiasm for transcatheter device closure of interatrial defects, a number of well recognized complications have been observed. Such complications may occur early during the periprocedural period, or manifest late, reinforcing the need for ongoing surveillance of these patients. As with all invasive diagnostic and therapeutic interventions, adequate training and preparation on behalf of the operator is essential.

TECHNIQUES OF PERCUTANEOUS ASD DEVICE CLOSURE

Preprocedure assessment

Ensuring that a patient is appropriate for percutaneous device closure of an ASD requires clinical assessment, with adjunctive use of various imaging modalities. The indication for ASD closure is evidence of hemodynamically significant volume overload of the right ventricle (RV) complicating left to right shunting. Clinically, this may present as effort intolerance, arrhythmia, or abnormalities on physical examination. Traditionally, confirmation of the presence of significant volume overload has been based on an increased pulmonary to systemic flow ratio (Qp:Qs > 1.5:1) obtained by cardiac catheterization. With modern imaging modalities, however, invasive assessment is infrequently required before proceeding to percutaneous closure.

Adequate echocardiography is an essential component of assessment in determining the suitability of a defect for transcatheter intervention. Echocardiography defines the nature of the interatrial defect, noting that ostium primum and sinus venosus defects remain unsuitable for percutaneous closure. Ensuring that the tissue rims at the margin of the defect are adequate for device deployment is important in terms of minimizing the risk of subsequent device embolization or device erosion. A margin of 5 mm from the defect margin to the atrioventricular valves, pulmonary veins, and coronary sinus is recommended.[2] Large ASDs (> 20 mm) rarely have a 5 mm aortic margin and this should not be considered a contraindication to device closure. Finally, echocardiography is critical in ensuring that there is no anomalous

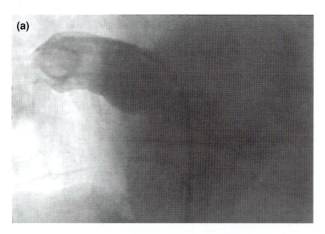

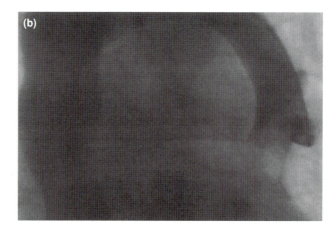

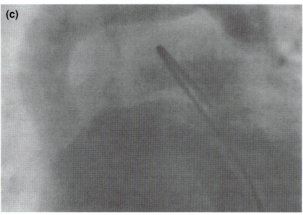

Figure 24.1 The spectrum of partial anomalous pulmonary venous drainage found in adults with secundum atrial septal defects. (a) Partial anomalous right lung drainage; (b) total left lung anomalous pulmonary venous drainage; (c) partial left lung anomalous venous drainage that went undetected at the time of ASD closure. In follow-up the patient had residual pulmonary hypertension and RV volume overload. She is awaiting surgery. When the SVC saturation is over 80% or the left upper pulmonary vein cannot be entered there should be a high index of suspicion for anomalous total or partial left lung pulmonary venous drainage.

pulmonary venous drainage. While anomalous pulmonary artery drainage is typically associated with sinus venosus defects (> 90%), partial anomalous pulmonary venous drainage has been associated with 2% of secundum defects[17] (Figure 24.1). Echocardiography is limited in its ability to define RV volume owing to the non-geometric shape of the chamber. Magnetic resonance imaging can most accurately define the presence and severity of right ventricular dilatation, an important marker of hemodynamically significant left to right shunting, as well as confirm normal pulmonary venous return. This may be especially helpful in cases where there are inconsistencies between defect size and the perception of right ventricular size as judged by echo. Gated computed tomography can provide similar information, but is less attractive given the radiation dose required for these studies at present. Elevation of pulmonary vascular resistance (> 8 Woods units) is considered a relative contraindication for closure, with defect occlusion then a potential precipitant for right heart failure. With current improvements in medical therapy for pulmonary hypertension, patients previously considered unsuitable for device closure may be reassessed after a period of treatment with pulmonary vasodilators.

Procedural considerations

Independent of the device utilized for ASD closure, the same basic principles of transcatheter closure apply.

Typically, femoral venous access is utilized; however, closure from other access sites, such as the internal jugular vein or the transhepatic route, has been performed. These access sites may be especially attractive in cases where femoral venous access is problematic (Figure 24.2), or when an azygous continuation of the inferior vena cava is present. In adult patients, the delivery sheath of the Amplatzer device is not sufficiently long to permit device delivery via an azygous continuation.

Before transcatheter device closure, patients are anticoagulated with unfractionated heparin and antibiotic prophylaxis is administered. The defect is crossed using the operator's choice of catheter (e.g. Gensini [Medtronic, Danvers, MA], Cobra [Cordis, Johnson and Johnson Company, Warren, NJ], Multipurpose [Cordis, Johnson and Johnson Company, Warren, NJ]). Confirmation of catheter position in the pulmonary veins is important to prevent accidental device release within the left atrial appendage which may be associated with perforation. This may be done using angiography, also potentially necessary for calibration for subsequent balloon sizing, or echocardiography. Once positioned within the left upper pulmonary vein, the initial catheter may be changed over an exchange length wire for a sizing balloon. We have found using an extra stiff exchange length wire an advantage in terms of stability for balloon sizing. Some operators alternatively prefer to base device sizing decisions solely on echocardiographic imaging. After accurate sizing of the defect, the delivery sheath is then

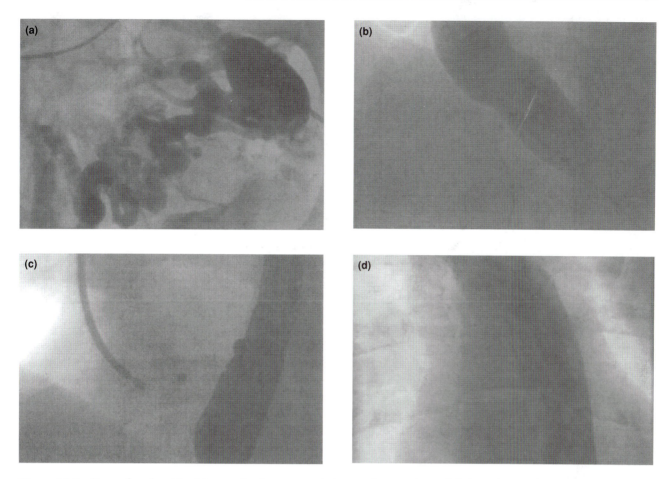

Figure 24.2   Young female with a history of pulmonary embolism and an atrial septal defect who was found to have occluded/recanalized iliacs and inferior vena cava. A device closure was carried out from the internal jugular approach. A second patient, a young female, with an azygous continuation that was discovered at the time of an attempted transfemoral ASD implant closure. The procedure was completed from the internal jugular approach using TEE guidance.

exchanged over the wire and positioned in the left atrium. The device can then be loaded following meticulous de-airing of the apparatus to prevent systemic air embolization. The left atrial disc is released first, with the entire system (closure device and delivery sheath) then gently pulled toward the interatrial septum. Under echocardiographic guidance, the device waist and right atrial disc are then released in sequence, with the discs now positioned on either side of the septum, thus closing the defect. Before device release, a secure device position can be grossly assessed by gentle forward and backward movement on the delivery cable (the so-called 'Minnesota Wiggle').

The need for adequate imaging during the procedure cannot be overemphasized, and should be obtained by intracardiac echocardiography or transesophageal echocardiography (Figure 24.3). Intracardiac echocardiography has the advantage of avoiding general anesthesia[13] (required in most centers for transesophageal echocardiography) and associated complications including aspiration and oropharyngeal trauma.[11] The large caliber of present intracardiac echo probes (8 or 10 French) limits the applicability of this technology to the pediatric population; however, it has been successfully utilized in

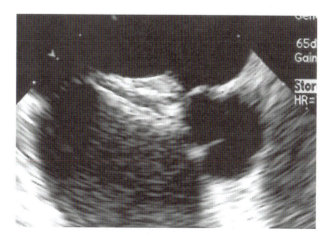

Figure 24.3   Intracardiac echo image of a fully deployed Amplatzer septal occluder.

patients less than 15 kg.[14] Echocardiography assists in defect sizing, excluding the presence of additional defects, confirming adequate defect closure after device deployment, and ensuring that adjacent structures, such as the atrioventricular valves, vena cavae, and pulmonary veins, are not impinged upon.

Adequate device sizing is critically important in optimizing the results of transcatheter ASD closure. The importance of accurate defect sizing is reflected both in terms of preventing undersizing and the inherent risks of embolization, but also with regard to the prevention of device erosion, which is another potentially catastrophic complication of device implantation.

Methods of ASD sizing have focused upon the use of sizing balloons to occlude the defect, with echocardiography confirming the absence of residual flow and additional defects. Most operators base device selection on the balloon diameter at which flow across the defect, as assessed by echocardiography, is stopped. Following calibration, a device 1–2 mm greater than the stretched balloon diameter is typically used. Using the stretched size or upsizing more than 2 mm greater than the *stop flow* size may result in oversizing,[18] which in turn may predispose to erosion. Irrespective of technique, ensuring a stable balloon position is important to allow for accurate estimation of defect size. This may be difficult with large defects, with the sizing balloon tending to prolapse into the right atrium; this may be overcome by advancing the balloon through a delivery sheath to stabilize the balloon position.[19] Alternate mechanisms of sizing large defects where sizing balloon stability is unsatisfactory include echocardiographic assessment of defect dimensions, although inaccuracy in measurement using this method has been described. In cases where echocardiography alone is utilized, an ASD occluder 30–40% greater than the echocardiographic assessment of the defect is used.[20] Although thought to be potentially safer than the balloon sizing method, there are no data to support this position. Finally, in cases where device sizing is clearly inadequate due to large defect size and difficulties in obtaining appropriate sizing balloon position encountered, surgery should be considered, rather than proceeding with device implantation based on inaccurate defect assessment. Additional complications of balloon sizing include septal tearing,[21,22] which may necessitate the implantation of a larger ASD device or, alternatively, potentially render the patient unsuitable for percutaneous closure. This phenomenon is often difficult to avoid in highly aneurysmal and thin septa.

It is important to note that the tendency to oversize devices to prevent embolization may predispose to device erosion (see below), as well as preventing normal device deployment.[2,18] Deployment of the Amplatzer Septal Occluder in cases following oversizing may result in the left atrial disc taking on a mushroom shape.[2,23] This may occur when the device waist is more than 4 mm greater than the stretched balloon measurement.[2] This appearance, when present, reflects constriction of the device waist. The Cobra deformity, often seen after the device has rotated in the delivery system, may be overcome by redeploying or replacing the device.

Following device deployment, systematic echocardiographic assessment should then be performed to insure device stability, assess tissue margins, and

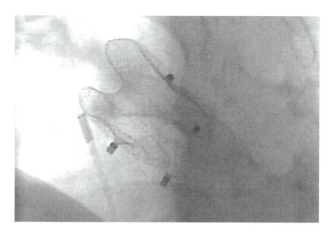

Figure 24.4 Interdigitating devices in a patient with multiple atrial septal defects.

exclude impingement on adjacent structures. Imaging will also exclude residual interatrial defects or remaining hemodynamically significant shunts. While small residual defects may not require further closure, the presence of a significant defect may require implantation of a larger device or insertion of a second device. While the implantation of multiple devices is now well described,[20] a number of technical considerations merit discussion. If possible, anticipating the need for multiple devices may permit multiple sites of vascular access prior to systemic anticoagulation and the associated increased risk of bleeding. Use of multiple access sites to allow simultaneous delivery of ASD closure devices, while increasing expense, has not been demonstrated to increase the risk of vascular complications.[20] Crossing additional defects with a catheter may be problematic; occasionally, use of a Judkins' right diagnostic coronary catheter may be useful. It may be helpful to repeat a Qp:Qs determination after the first device is placed to confirm that a second device is necessary before proceeding. We suggest balloon sizing all residual defects that may be significant at the time of the index procedure to assist in future management, regardless of whether the placement of a second device is planned immediately or to be delayed. Positioning of the second device across the interatrial septum before releasing the first device is recommended.[24] In terms of device placement, we aim to 'interdigitate' the discs of the devices, such that the discs of one device do not entrap both discs of the other (Figure 24.4). However, upon release of the devices they may not remain interdigitated and will take up a neutral position governed by septal redundancy. We also partially release each device before completely detaching the delivery cables; this reduces the amount of stored tension on each device and may prevent excessive movement after device release which may predispose to embolization.

Following every procedure, but, in particular, those involving small patients, it is important to ensure that the closure device has not impaired the function of other structures. Occlusion of the pulmonary veins and superior vena cava, as well as preventing normal atrioventricular valve apparatus function, has resulted in either abandoned procedures or subsequent surgical device removal.[2] This is an exceptionally rare occurrence in adult patients. This, too, can be anticipated by adequate preprocedural assessment. As mentioned, in all defects a distance of greater than 5 mm from the defect margin to the atrioventricular valves is recommended.[2,20] This is particularly relevant in anterior and inferior defects when device closure is more likely to encroach on these structures.

COMPLICATIONS OF PERCUTANEOUS ATRIAL SEPTAL DEFECT CLOSURE

The majority of events complicating ASD closure tend to occur early, either during the procedure itself, such as device embolization, or during the early postprocedural period (e.g. arrhythmia). The incidence of complications during hospitalization in the early experience of device closure was up to 8.6%, including device malposition and embolization, vascular injury, and arrhythmia.[25] As our experience with this technology has developed, recognition of additional late complications has emerged, in particular, late device erosion.

With progressive experience in this area, a number of device-related factors have been identified as associated with adverse outcomes. Similarly, various patient and operator characteristics have been recognized as risk factors for specific complications. As our appreciation and understanding of these complications has evolved, so too has their subsequent management as experience with this therapeutic modality increases.

Device embolization

Device embolization is a very infrequent event complicating percutaneous ASD closure. The incidence of embolization is unclear, with reported rates of 0.5% in procedures performed by experienced operators in the context of prospective studies. Indeed, the incidence may be higher among less experienced operators. It is interesting that current trends support adoption of the generally accepted principle that devices should not be oversized. Erosion rates have fallen modestly at the expense of a small increase in the rate of embolization.

Embolization of devices is more likely to occur in the early periprocedural course following closure; however late embolization is reported. In these published cases, late embolization was associated with strenuous activity, and embolization was into the pulmonary artery, rather than systemic circulation. This is similar to early embolization, with the most common site of embolization being the pulmonary artery.[25–27] Of note, these devices when retrieved were noted to have extensive endothelialization, reflecting that this alone is insufficient to prevent embolization, and adequate device support at the time of implantation therefore remains important for long-term prevention of embolic events.

A number of factors predisposing to embolization have been recognized in both adult and pediatric populations, with mechanisms of device retrieval also well described.

Certain anatomic features of the ASD and surrounding tissues are recognized as predisposing to device embolization. These include large defects, thus requiring larger occluder devices, deficient tissue rims, and mobile or 'floppy' septa. In particular, inadequate or deficient inferior rims may result in an increased risk of device embolization. A deficient aortic rim is most commonly encountered, typically resulting in the left atrial disc prolapsing into the right atrium during device deployment. The relatively large left atrial disc may prolapse, leading to both early and late embolization.[2] This has been overcome by a technique of flaring or splaying the atrial discs of a slightly oversized Amplatzer device at the aortic margin to capture aortic tissue.[28] While utilizing the aorta, rather than the deficient aortic rim of the interatrial septum, may permit adequate device placement, this needs to be balanced against the subsequent, albeit low, risk of erosion. In cases where there is a tendency of the device to prolapse at the aortic rim, modifications to the sheath design can assist device placement. Cutting the inner curvature at the tip of the delivery sheath creates a bevelled tip which may permit Amplatzer device placement.[29] A bevelled sheath tip prevents the tendency of the left atrial disc to prolapse into the right atrium by aligning the left atrial disc parallel to the interatrial septum. This can overcome the difficulty of device prolapse at the aortic margin and allow for adequate tissue capture, insuring a stable position for device deployment. The Hausdorf sheath (Cook, Bloomington, IN) has been similarly advocated in this situation.

Many operators will test device stability by pushing and pulling on the delivery cable to determine if the device is likely to prolapse into the atria ('Minnesota wiggle'). Interestingly, excess mobility after implant is also likely to predispose to subsequent embolization, with redundant, 'floppy' tissue margins presumably allowing for excessive movement and providing inadequate device support.

That larger devices and larger defects have been associated with an increased risk of embolization reflects the inherent limitations of closure of large defects, including inadequate balloon sizing and deficient tissue margins. The arms of large double umbrella type occlusion devices are felt to be inadequate to stabilize the device to prevent embolization, and the Amplatzer device is favored for larger defects.[26] Previous reports of embolization rates complicating the Amplatzer device of up to 4.4% in defects greater than 25 mm have been described.[30] However, a recently published series

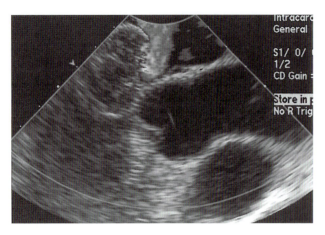

Figure 24.5 An embolized ASD device seen entrapped in the left ventricular outflow tract on intracardiac echo imaging. The device was initially placed alongside a larger Amplatzer septal occluder to close a residual defect. When we attempted to release the larger occlude after releasing the embolized device a significant amount of torque built up in the cable, distorting the septum and resulting in embolization of the smaller device. We suggest an initial partial release of both devices to avoid this problem. The device was successfully retrieved percutaneously.

reporting the safety and efficacy of closure of defects using the Amplatzer device in adults up to 40 mm demonstrated in experienced hands there is not a significantly higher incidence of device embolization.[31]

Retrieval of embolized ASD occlusion devices is potentially complex, due to the device structure and the anatomic milieu in which embolized devices may find themselves (Figure 24.5). Certainly, surgical retrieval is commonly employed due to these difficulties, particularly in the case of pulmonary artery embolization. Death has not been reported as a consequence of device embolization. Ideally, if percutaneous methods of device retrieval can be employed, then surgery, and the concomitant morbidity, can be avoided. Caution should, however, be advocated for complex retrievals, especially those where a device has embolized into the left ventricle. A low-risk surgical procedure is perhaps preferable to injury of critical intracardiac structures, such as left-sided valves, in the process of retrieving an embolized device.

Initial steps in device retrieval should focus on mobilizing the device from within the cardiac chambers into the vascular tree. It is helpful to upsize the sheath to 14–16 French for larger devices. It may be helpful to *preclose* (see below) these accesses should the situation allow, to improve hemostasis and reduce the risks of complication later. In cases of embolization into the atria or right ventricle, the use of various snares or bioptomes, either in the right-sided chambers or across the ASD into the left atrium, may allow for withdrawal of the device to the inferior vena cava. In cases where the device has embolized into the left ventricle, ventricular ectopy or left ventricular outflow obstruction

may result in significant hemodynamic sequelae, and removal into the aorta is desirable. A pigtail catheter may be used to cross the aortic valve and then 'drag' the device into the aorta. As moving the device across the atrioventricular valves may produce valvular damage, efforts should be made to avoid this maneuver; however, in cases of right ventricular embolization, this is unavoidable.

Once the embolized device is positioned within either the inferior vena cava or aorta, efforts can then focus upon removing the device from the circulation. Various available devices suitable for retrieval include gooseneck[25] and loop snares, as well as bioptomes. Retrieval of the Amplatzer ASD occluder is particularly problematic; its design is such that the only method of percutaneous removal is by screwing the cable back into the hub, or catching the screw hub on the right atrial disc with a snare. This difficult task can be facilitated by stabilizing the device within the circulation with a catheter, thus preventing excessive motion while attempting to snare the screw hub. In examples where the device is located within the inferior vena cava, a sheath in the superior vena cava to stabilize the device with a catheter may be useful.[32]

Once captured, the remaining challenge is to then remove the snared device from the circulation. In this setting, the sheath size is important to allow device and bioptome removal; the sheath size should be at least two French sizes greater than the delivery sheath to permit removal. A 'notch' in the sheath may further facilitate device extraction.[32]

Given the obvious difficulties in percutaneous removal, prevention of embolization by employment of meticulous technique and optimal echocardiographic imaging at the time of device deployment is critical. Avoidance of strenuous exercise has also been recommended to prevent late device embolization.[33]

Device erosion

Of the recognized complications of percutaneous interatrial defect closure, cardiac erosion and perforation remain potentially catastrophic, with awareness of the potential precipitants, presentation, and management being essential for operators undertaking this procedure. Fortunately, device erosion is an uncommon complication, but may be associated with pericardial effusion, cardiac tamponade, the need for urgent cardiac surgery, and death. Clinical manifestations typically relate to hemopericardium; however, fistula development has also been described.[34]

The incidence of device erosion, as mentioned, is low. The incidence of erosion complicating use of the Amplatzer septal occluder is 0.1% based on cases reported by physicians to the manufacturing company;[18] it is conceivable that additional cases of erosion have occurred in the absence of subsequent notification.

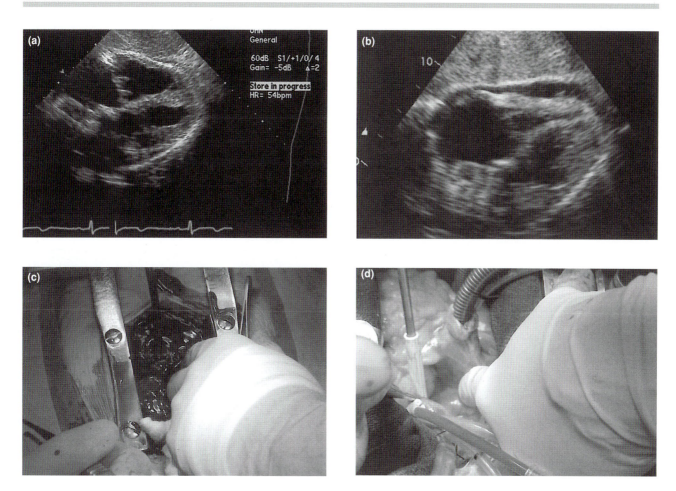

Figure 24.6   (A) Still frame from a transthoracic echo in the subcostal view taken as a routine at 8:30 am the morning after an ASD closure. (B) Image from the patient 3 hours later, demonstrating an increase in pericardial fluid. As the patient was preparing to leave hospital she experienced chest pain, prompting a repeat urgent echo. (C) At operative repair she was found to have a blood-filled pericardium. (D) An erosion through the roof of the left atrium and a laceration of the overlying aorta.

A more reasonable estimate is probably 0.3–0.4% of cases. Regardless, the overall event rate is clearly low, with the hope that recognition of those factors which may predispose to erosion will lead to a further reduction in events.

The clinical presentation of device erosion typically relates to the effects of hemopericardium. Patients may present with shortness of breath and chest pain, with more dramatic presentations, such as hemodynamic collapse and death, also reported. Sudden death occurring during follow-up was described during the early published series. In retrospect, sudden death may be related to device erosion; however, the possibility of arrhythmia as a contributor should not be ignored.[18]

Pericardial effusion during the ASD closure procedure has been reported to complicate guide wire perforation[18,25] and opening of the device in the pulmonary vein;[2] however, most cases of hemopericardium are believed to complicate erosion. In the case of double umbrella devices, pericardial effusion is believed to be the result of perforation by the metallic arms of the device; direct trauma of this nature is unlikely to be the cause complicating the use of the Amplatzer device due

to the atraumatic, rounded margins. The mechanism of device erosion in these cases is believed to be the consequence of transmission of compressive forces from the ASD occlusion device during the cardiac cycle to the sites of device contact.[35] The reduction in atrial size after device closure may then accentuate the contact between the occluder and adjacent tissues.[18] The aorta and the atria are the most common sites of perforation,[35] with erosions typically occurring at the dome of either the left or right atria, which may then extend to involve the aorta in about 50% of cases[18] (Figure 24.6). An insufficient superior and aortic rim favors a device position whereby the device margins are adjacent to the atrial roof and ascending aorta. Fistula complicating ASD closure seems to occur when the aortic rim alone is deficient, resulting in communication between the left atrium and aortic root[18,36] (Figure 24.7). While surgical correction is standard treatment for fistula repair, percutaneous device closure of such fistulae is reported.[34]

Erosion complicating Amplatzer ASD closure may occur during the index hospital admission in approximately 20% of cases.[35] Therefore, the vast majority of

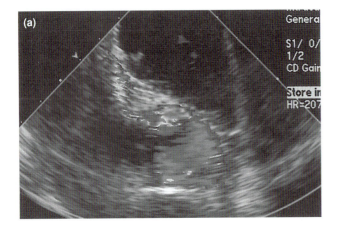

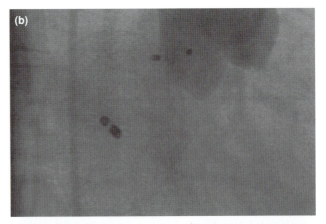

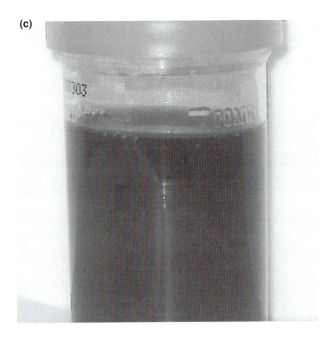

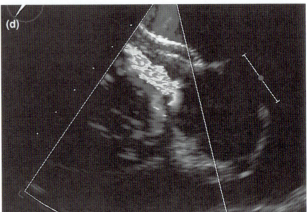

Figure 24.7 (A) Intracardiac echo image of an aorta to left atrial fistula. (B) A 4 mm Amplatzer septal occluder was used to close this fistula – the patient has been asymptomatic in 3-year follow-up. (C) A urine sample from a second patient who presented 3 weeks after ASD closure with atrial fibrillation to an outside hospital. Twenty-four hours after DC cardioversion the patient developed hemoglobinuria and a brisk intravascular hemolysis; an aorto-atrial fistula was demonstrated on TEE (D). He underwent an uneventful surgical repair.

cases occur after discharge, with examples occurring up to 3 years after implant. Careful review of reported cases has identified a number of contributors to erosion, with associated important implications in terms of implantation technique.

Device oversizing is the most commonly identified contributor to device erosion. In a previous registry review, patients experiencing subsequent adverse events were more likely to have a larger device size to ASD diameter ratio. Based on these findings, it has been recommended that deliberate oversizing of the ASD device by more than 2 mm greater than the stretched balloon diameter be avoided. An alternate method based on the diameter at which the sizing balloon occludes flow has therefore been proposed as a method of avoiding oversizing (stop flow size). Deliberate oversizing, aside from minimizing the risk of embolization, has also been employed to overcome the problem of deficient aortic rims, as mentioned previously. This is reflected in data demonstrating that deficient aortic rims having been

identified in almost 90% of reported series of erosions.[18] This may, in fact, be a marker of larger defects. Thus, the anatomic location of these defects and the tendency to oversize devices to successfully position occlusion devices combine to make defects with deficient aortic rims higher risk for erosion.

Once a diagnosis of erosion is made, urgent surgical intervention is indicated. Although pericardiocentesis may be performed for hemodynamic collapse, this may result in a potentially unstable situation of increased pericardial bleeding, necessitating aspiration of pericardial blood and immediate reinfusion through large-bore intravenous access. Emergent surgery is preferable. At the time of surgery, the atrial roof and adjacent aorta should be carefully explored for evidence of erosion. Cardiac surgeons who rarely see this type of complication need to be informed of the need to carefully inspect these areas, as this situation is quite dissimilar from a pacemaker or angioplasty guide wire perforation, for example. Approximately 50% of device erosions include an aortic injury that may be missed without careful exploration. Of note, in cases where the device has not been removed, there have been no reports of recurrence.[18]

All patients should undergo surveillance echocardiography within 24 hours of the procedure, with patients demonstrating evidence of pericardial effusion closely followed. Other patients who warrant more intensive follow-up include those with a significantly larger closure device than the native ASD diameter and those with evidence of device deformation after implantation. We routinely perform transthoracic echocardiography at 2 months postprocedure to exclude residual left to right shunting and document the presence of effusion. However, the frequency of, and requirement for, ongoing surveillance echocardiography is difficult to define given the unpredictable nature and timing of erosion.[18] We suggest yearly surveillance echocardiograms for the first 5 years postclosure. It is important to inform patients of the possibility of this complication and to encourage early presentation when symptoms referable to erosion develop. Prompt investigation and management when the diagnosis is considered are then critical.

Arrhythmia

Transient arrhythmia is common, occurring in up to 13% of patients undergoing percutaneous device closure of an ASD.[26] The propensity to arrhythmia complicating device closure does, however, compare favorably with surgery in comparative trials.[3] The early postprocedure period may be accompanied by frequent atrial ectopy and occasional non-sustained supraventricular tachycardia. These arrhythmias may occur both immediately after device implantation and during follow-up of patients undergoing transcatheter ASD closure. Many patients have symptomatic relief with early institution of a β-blocker.

The development or worsening of atrioventricular (AV) block during device insertion may occur in approximately 6–7% of patients, with second or third degree heart block seen in less than 4%.[37] Risk factors identified for the development of AV block include large defect size and larger shunt ratios. AV block tends to be transient in nature, with the risk of hemodynamic compromise and need for pacemaker insertion low.[1,38,39] Again, avoidance of oversizing is thus important in reducing the risk of AV block, with careful attention to rhythm observed during follow-up.

Development of atrial tachyarrhythmias following device closure is more likely in adults and those who have a history of such arrhythmias. Holter monitoring in pediatric patients undergoing percutaneous device closure has demonstrated an infrequent incidence of arrhythmia, with benign findings of infrequent atrial and ventricular ectopy noted.[40] While ASD closure has been demonstrated to be protective against arrhythmia in adults, patients with pre-existing atrial fibrillation or atrial flutter are prone to recurrence of their arrhythmia. Atrial flutter has been reported as complicating both adult and pediatric patients following device closure.[2] There is a low rate of atrial arrhythmia in those without an associated antecedent history. Early tachyarrhythmia is seen in up to 6% of patients without a prior history of arrhythmia, with this incidence reducing to approximately 1% in these patients at one year.[41] We systematically refer patients with a history of atrial fibrillation or flutter for consideration of ablative therapy prior to closure. Should a left atrial source of arrhythmia be noted, the decision to proceed with an ablation prior to closure should be undertaken in discussion with the patient.

While sudden death after transcatheter device closure has been reported,[25] this is more likely associated with the consequences of device erosion, pericardial effusion, and tamponade. Arrhythmic death after device closure has been suggested based on autopsy exclusion of pericardial effusion in the context of unexplained sudden death.

Thrombus formation

Thrombus formation on interatrial defect closure devices has been reported in up to 2.5% of cases in some series, with an increased incidence seen in various device types (7.15% in CardioSEAL).[42] This variable incidence reflects that the choice of device may influence thrombotic risk, with the lowest reported incidence noted in Amplatzer devices. This is attributed to the lack of exposed thrombogenic material on the Amplatzer device. This contrasts with the exposed arms on the CardioSEAL, STARFlex, and PFO-star devices.[43] It is anticipated that thrombus formation will complicate interatrial defect closure less commonly with newer generation devices.

Detection of thrombus complicating device implantation may occur during surveillance transthoracic echocardiography and is in many cases asymptomatic. In patients with embolic phenomena after device implantation, transthoracic echocardiography may be inadequate to detect small thrombi. Transesophageal echocardiography is superior for imaging the interatrial septum and interatrial occlusion devices, and detecting the presence of thrombus.[42] In addition, transesophageal echocardiography may also detect residual interatrial defects, which may predispose to paradoxical embolism. Many centers in Europe continue to perform routine transesophageal echocardiography 4 weeks and 6 months following device implantation.

Those risk factors which have been recognized for the development of subsequent device thrombosis include atrial fibrillation and the presence of a persistent atrial septal aneurysm. In terms of adjunctive pharmacotherapy, the use of anticoagulation does not influence the likelihood of device thrombus, and in fact, warfarin use

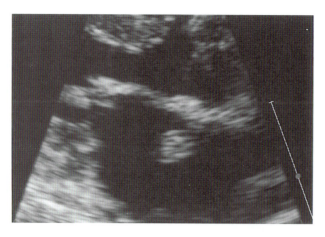

Figure 24.8 A mobile pedunculated thrombus in the left atrium attached to a CardioSEAL device. The patient was non-compliant with her dual antiplatelet therapy. The echo was performed when she presented for routine follow-up 2 months postprocedure and was asymptomatic. The thrombus completely resolved after 6 months of warfarin.

is associated with a higher incidence of residual shunt during follow-up. This is presumed to relate to inhibition of the usual healing process following device closure, which in the Amplatzer device depends upon the thrombogenicity of the polyester material within the retention discs. In contrast, the use of combination therapy with aspirin and clopidogrel has been shown to be associated with a lower risk of device thrombosis without impacting upon closure rates.[42,43]

Additional considerations in the evaluation of a patient with evidence of device thrombosis are exclusion of an underlying prothrombotic disorder (particularly relevant in patients referred for interatrial defect closure for previous stroke), and non-compliance with antiplatelet therapy (Figure 24.8).

While thrombus formation is uncommon, particularly on the Amplatzer ASD Occluder, even late thrombus has been described after discontinuation of antiplatelet treatment. This reflects that endothelialization remains incomplete after several months and, when in association with predisposing conditions, such as infection, thrombus formation may occur.[25]

Management options of device thrombosis are limited. While surgical removal of the device has been successfully employed, a trial of medical therapy with anticoagulation is acceptable. In one published series, patients with device thrombosis were treated with warfarin, with thrombus resolving in 85% of cases over a period of 4 weeks to 6 months.[42]

Vascular

Vascular complications remain a constant issue in percutaneous diagnostic and interventional procedures, with transcatheter ASD closure no exception. Although percutaneous ASD closure requires only venous access,

a large number of vascular complications have been described. Given the young age and small stature of some patients undergoing ASD closure, vascular access can be problematic. Recognition of these complications when they do occur is important and early treatment clearly desirable.

Published series have documented hematoma, iliac vein dissection, and deep venous thrombosis complicating femoral venous access.[1,6,25] Arteriovenous fistulae are also described, with a reported frequency of up to 2% when using a single access site exclusively, even when closing multiple defects.[24] It is important not to place a large sheath when there has been even a suspicion of passing through a branch of the femoral artery to enter the vein. This will almost certainly result in an arteriovenous fistula. Care should be taken to abduct and externally rotate the leg before cannulation is attempted. Retroperitoneal hemorrhage is also described, complicating laceration of a femoral artery branch.[2,6] When suspected, retroperitoneal hemorrhage should be treated with prompt fluid resuscitation; therapy should not be delayed while awaiting imaging confirmation of bleeding. In patients anticoagulated undergoing percutaneous coronary intervention, the mortality rate is not insignificant, with treatment delay a factor in adverse outcomes.[44] While this represents a different patient population, the principles of management are similar. Prompt reversal of anticoagulation, fluid and blood replacement, and timely surgical intervention, if rarely required, are the key issues in early management. Routine use of protamine to reverse anticoagulation may be associated with an increased tendency to thrombus formation during follow-up in patients on aspirin, and clopidogrel prophylaxis,[42] however, should not be withheld in patients with active hemorrhage.

Femoral venous access complications may be potentially minimized with the use of suture-mediated hemostasis devices.[45] These may be employed for closure of venous access sites after congenital interventions with excellent hemostasis rates and low rates of complications. We routinely *preclose* femoral vein access sites with suture-mediated hemostasis devices which are initially positioned immediately once vascular access is obtained. The procedure is then performed in the standard fashion, with the sutures finally secured at the completion of the procedure.

Air embolization

Air embolization is an infrequent complication of percutaneous device closure of an ASD, which typically manifests as transient ST elevation in the inferior leads.[1,2,6,46] This reflects that when air embolism occurs affecting the coronary arteries, it will typically involve the right coronary artery due to the position of its origin in the right coronary cusp. The effects of air embolism are variable and range from chest discomfort to hemodynamic collapse. These consequences tend to resolve spontaneously over a period of minutes.[47]

Insuring the delivery sheath is appropriately de-aired is the most critical component in preventing air embolism. Given the shunt is predominantly left to right, one could anticipate most air emboli being directed through the right heart before being filtered by the lungs. Systemic embolization may also be avoided by using general anesthesia with mechanical ventilation, rather than heavy sedation with spontaneous breathing. The negative intrathoracic pressure generated by spontaneous respiration may precipitate right to left shunting, especially in a heavily sedated patient whose airway is partially obstructed.

Management of coronary artery air embolism involves the removal of air from the coronary vasculature and supportive management of the typically transient hemodynamic effects of air embolization. Optimal supportive therapy includes administration of 100% oxygen, parenteral analgesia, as well as inotropic and intra-aortic balloon pump counterpulsation support for hemodynamic instability. Insertion of a temporary pacing wire or DC cardioversion may be appropriate in cases of arrhythmia. In terms of methods of treating the underlying cause, injection of saline in the coronary vessel, aspiration, or the use of rheolytic therapy are described.[47,48]

Sudden death

Early in the experience of transcatheter device closure at least one episode of sudden death was reported. The mechanism in this case was unclear; however, as mentioned previously, the recognition of late device erosion and subsequent cardiac tamponade suggests that this may represent, at least in part, a potential etiology for sudden death after device implantation. In at least one patient who died suddenly, autopsy data failed to demonstrate hemopericardium, thus raising the possibility of an arrhythmic death.

Fortunately, sudden death remains a rare complication of this interventional technique. With the possibility of late device erosion now well recognized, physicians are less likely to oversize ASD devices, hopefully reducing the likelihood of future late deaths.

SUMMARY

Transcatheter closure of ASDs is safe, with satisfactory efficacy and long-term outcomes now reported. The need for adequate training and familiarity with these procedures is critical to provide optimum care and to prevent complications. In cases where complications do occur, experienced operators can provide prompt recognition and appropriate treatment. Judicious use of transcatheter closure, accompanied by meticulous technique and careful assessment, both before and after the procedure, is essential in optimizing delivery of this technology.

REFERENCES

1. Chan KC, Godman MJ, Walsh K et al. Transcatheter closure of atrial septal defect and interatrial communications with a new self expanding nitinol double disc device (Amplatzer septal occluder): multicentre UK experience. Heart 1999; 82(3): 300–6.
2. Fischer G, Stieh J, Uebing A et al. Experience with transcatheter closure of secundum atrial septal defects using the Amplatzer septal occluder: a single centre study in 236 consecutive patients. Heart 2003; 89(2): 199–204.
3. Butera G, Carminati M, Chessa M et al. Percutaneous versus surgical closure of secundum atrial septal defect: comparison of early results and complications. Am Heart J 2006; 151(1): 228–34.
4. Masura J, Gavora P, Formanek A, Hijazi ZM. Transcatheter closure of secundum atrial septal defects using the new self-centering Amplatzer septal occluder: initial human experience. Cathet Cardiovasc Diagn 1997; 42(4): 388–93.
5. Nugent AW, Britt A, Gauvreau K et al. Device closure rates of simple atrial septal defects optimized by the STARFlex device. J Am Coll Cardiol 2006; 48(3): 538–44.
6. Egred M, Andron M, Albouaini K et al. Percutaneous closure of patent foramen ovale and atrial septal defect: procedure outcome and medium-term follow-up. J Interven Cardiol 2007; 20(5): 395–401.
7. Jones TK, Latson LA, Zahn E et al. Results of the U.S. multicenter pivotal study of the HELEX septal occluder for percutaneous closure of secundum atrial septal defects. J Am Coll Cardiol 2007; 49(22): 2215–21.
8. Eerola A, Pihkala JI, Boldt T et al. Hemodynamic improvement is faster after percutaneous ASD closure than after surgery. Cathet Cardiovasc Interven 2007; 69(3): 432–41; discussion 442.
9. Spies C, Timmermanns I, Schrader R. Transcatheter closure of secundum atrial septal defects in adults with the Amplatzer septal occluder: intermediate and long-term results. Clin Res Cardiol 2007; 96(6): 340–6.
10. Patel A, Lopez K, Banerjee A et al. Transcatheter closure of atrial septal defects in adults > or = 40 years of age: immediate and follow-up results. J Interv Cardiol 2007; 20(1): 82–8.
11. Butera G, De Rosa G, Chessa M et al. Transcatheter closure of atrial septal defect in young children: results and follow-up. J Am Coll Cardiol 2003; 42(2): 241–5.
12. Kay JD, O'Laughlin MP, Ito K et al. Five-year clinical and echocardiographic evaluation of the Das AngelWings atrial septal occluder. Am Heart J 2004; 147(2): 361–8.
13. Koenig P, Cao QL, Heitschmidt M, Waight DJ, Hijazi ZM. Role of intracardiac echocardiographic guidance in transcatheter closure of atrial septal defects and patent foramen ovale using the Amplatzer device. J Interven Cardiol 2003; 16(1): 51–62.
14. Patel A, Cao QL, Koenig PR, Hijazi ZM. Intracardiac echocardiography to guide closure of atrial septal defects in children less than 15 kilograms. Cathet Cardiovasc Interven 2006; 68(2): 287–91.
15. Jux C, Bertram H, Wohlsein P, Bruegmann M, Paul T. Interventional atrial septal defect closure using a totally bioresorbable occluder matrix: development and preclinical evaluation of the BioSTAR device. J Am Coll Cardiol 2006; 48(1): 161–9.
16. Mullen MJ, Hildick-Smith D, De Giovanni JV et al. BioSTAR Evaluation STudy (BEST): a prospective, multicenter, phase I clinical trial to evaluate the feasibility, efficacy, and safety of the BioSTAR bioabsorbable septal repair implant for the closure of atrial-level shunts. Circulation 2006; 114(18): 1962–7.
17. Vogel M. Partial anomalous pulmonary venous connection and the scimitar syndrome. In: Gatzoulis MA, Webb GD, and Daubeney PEF, eds. Diagnosis and Management of Adult Congenital Heart Disease. London: Churchill Livingstone, 2004: 205–10.

18. Amin Z, Hijazi ZM, Bass JL et al. Erosion of Amplatzer septal occluder device after closure of secundum atrial septal defects: review of registry of complications and recommendations to minimize future risk. Cathet Cardiovasc Interven 2004; 63(4): 496–502.

19. Dehghani P, Collins N, Benson L, Horlick E. Sheath stabilizing technique for balloon sizing of large atrial septal defects response to article by Dr. Zahid Amin entitled 'Transcatheter closure of secundum atrial septal defects'. Cathet Cardiovasc Interven 2007; 70(1): 156–7; author reply 158–9.

20. Awad SM, Garay FF, Cao QL, Hijazi ZM. Multiple Amplatzer septal occluder devices for multiple atrial communications: immediate and long-term follow-up results. Cathet Cardiovasc Interven 2007; 70(2): 265–73.

21. Bonvini RF, Sigwart U, Verin V. Interatrial septum rupture during balloon measurement of a patent foramen ovale in a young patient presenting cryptogenic stroke. Cathet Cardiovasc Interven 2007; 69(2): 274–6.

22. Alsaileek AA, Omran A, Godman M, Najm HK. Echocardiographic visualization of laceration of atrial septum during balloon sizing of atrial septal defect. Eur J Echocardiogr 2007; 8(2): 155–7.

23. Cooke JC, Gelman JS, Harper RW. Cobrahead malformation of the Amplatzer septal occluder device: an avoidable complication of percutaneous ASD closure. Cathet Cardiovasc Interven 2001; 52(1): 83–5; discussion 86–7.

24. Meier B. Crowded atrial septum. Cathet Cardiovasc Interven 2007; 70(2): 274–5.

25. Chessa M, Carminati M, Butera G et al. Early and late complications associated with transcatheter occlusion of secundum atrial septal defect. J Am Coll Cardiol 2002; 39(6): 1061–5.

26. Post MC, Suttorp MJ, Jaarsma W, Plokker HW. Comparison of outcome and complications using different types of devices for percutaneous closure of a secundum atrial septal defect in adults: a single-center experience. Cathet Cardiovasc Interven 2006; 67(3): 438–43.

27. Preventza O, Sampath-Kumar S, Wasnick J, Gold JP. Late cardiac perforation following transcatheter atrial septal defect closure. Ann Thorac Surg 2004; 77(4): 1435–7.

28. Harper RW, Mottram PM, McGaw DJ. Closure of secundum atrial septal defects with the Amplatzer septal occluder device: techniques and problems. Cathet Cardiovasc Interven 2002; 57(4): 508–24.

29. Spies C, Boosfeld C, Schrader R. A modified Cook sheath for closure of a large secundum atrial septal defect. Cathet Cardiovasc Interven 2007; 70(2): 286–9.

30. Kannan BR, Francis E, Sivakumar K, Anil SR, Kumar RK. Transcatheter closure of very large (> or = 25 mm) atrial septal defects using the Amplatzer septal occluder. Cathet Cardiovasc Interven 2003; 59(4): 522–7.

31. Lopez K, Dalvi BV, Balzer D et al. Transcatheter closure of large secundum atrial septal defects using the 40 mm Amplatzer septal occluder: results of an international registry. Cathet Cardiovasc Interven 2005; 66(4): 580–4.

32. Levi DS, Moore JW. Embolization and retrieval of the Amplatzer septal occluder. Cathet Cardiovasc Interven 2004; 61(4): 543–7.

33. Mashman WE, King SB, Jacobs WC, Ballard WL. Two cases of late embolization of Amplatzer septal occluder devices to the pulmonary artery following closure of secundum atrial septal defects. Cathet Cardiovasc Interven 2005; 65(4): 588–92.

34. Mahadevan VS, Horlick EM, Benson LN, McLaughlin PR. Transcatheter closure of aortic sinus to left atrial fistula caused by erosion of Amplatzer septal occluder. Cathet Cardiovasc Interven 2006; 68(5): 749–53.

35. Divekar A, Gaamangwe T, Shaikh N, Raabe M, Ducas J. Cardiac perforation after device closure of atrial septal defects with the Amplatzer septal occluder. J Am Coll Cardiol 2005; 45(8): 1213–8.

36. Chun DS, Turrentine MW, Moustapha A, Hoyer MH. Development of aorta-to-right atrial fistula following closure of secundum atrial septal defect using the Amplatzer septal occluder. Cathet Cardiovasc Interven 2003; 58(2): 246–51.

37. Suda K, Raboisson MJ, Piette E, Dahdah NS, Miro J. Reversible atrioventricular block associated with closure of atrial septal defects using the Amplatzer device. J Am Coll Cardiol 2004; 43(9): 1677–82.

38. Du ZD, Hijazi ZM, Kleinman CS, Silverman NH, Larntz K. Comparison between transcatheter and surgical closure of secundum atrial septal defect in children and adults: results of a multicenter nonrandomized trial. J Am Coll Cardiol 2002; 39(11): 1836–44.

39. Hill SL, Berul CI, Patel HT et al. Early ECG abnormalities associated with transcatheter closure of atrial septal defects using the Amplatzer septal occluder. J Interven Card Electrophysiol 2000; 4(3): 469–74.

40. Hessling G, Hyca S, Brockmeier K, Ulmer HE. Cardiac dysrhythmias in pediatric patients before and 1 year after transcatheter closure of atrial septal defects using the amplatzer septal occluder. Pediatr Cardiol 2003; 24(3): 259–62.

41. Silversides CK, Siu SC, McLaughlin PR et al. Symptomatic atrial arrhythmias and transcatheter closure of atrial septal defects in adult patients. Heart 2004; 90(10): 1194–8.

42. Krumsdorf U, Ostermayer S, Billinger K et al. Incidence and clinical course of thrombus formation on atrial septal defect and patent foramen ovale closure devices in 1,000 consecutive patients. J Am Coll Cardiol 2004; 43(2): 302–9.

43. Braun MU, Fassbender D, Schoen SP et al. Transcatheter closure of patent foramen ovale in patients with cerebral ischemia. J Am Coll Cardiol 2002; 39(12): 2019–25.

44. Ellis SG, Bhatt D, Kapadia S et al. Correlates and outcomes of retroperitoneal hemorrhage complicating percutaneous coronary intervention. Cathet Cardiovasc Interven 2006; 67(4): 541–5.

45. Mahadevan VS, Jimeno SS, Benson LN, McLaughlin PR, Horlick EM. Preclosure of femoral venous access sites used for large sized sheath insertion with the Perclose™ device in adults undergoing cardiac intervention. Heart 2006.

46. Cardenas L, Panzer J, Boshoff D, Malekzadeh-Milani S, Ovaert C. Transcatheter closure of secundum atrial defect in small children. Cathet Cardiovasc Interven 2007; 69(3): 447–52.

47. Khan M, Schmidt DH, Bajwa T, Shalev Y. Coronary air embolism: incidence, severity, and suggested approaches to treatment. Cathet Cardiovasc Diagn 1995; 36(4): 313–18.

48. Dudar BM, Kim HE. Massive air embolus treated with rheolytic thrombectomy. J Invas Cardiol 2007; 19(7): E182–4.

25 Closure of patent foramen ovale with the Amplatzer PFO device

Jonathan Tobis and Tim Provias

A patent foramen ovale (PFO) is an evolutionary mechanism designed to allow blood oxygenated by the placenta to pass through the fetal right atrium and directly enter the left atrium. This blood bypasses the non-functional pulmonary circulation and delivers oxygenated blood directly to the systemic circulation. The opening is a dynamic passageway between the atria formed by the septum secundum superiorly and the septum primum inferiorly. With an infant's first breath, the left atrial pressure quickly rises over that of the right atrium and the flap of the septum primum is pressed against the septum secundum, sealing the foramen ovale. In most individuals the septa fuse during the first year of life, permanently closing the foramen and creating the fossa ovale.

In up to 25% of adults, however, the foramen ovale does not completely fuse and a valve-like opening between the atria persists. The anatomic presence of a PFO was described nearly two millennia ago by the Greek physician Galen, who studied cardiac anatomy in mammals.[1,2] In situations during which right atrial pressure transiently exceeds left, such as Valsalva maneuvers or even normal respiratory cycles, intermittent right-to-left shunting may occur. The clinical significance of this interatrial opening had long been considered trivial since the degree of hemodynamic shunting is generally minimal. In 1877, however, Julius Cohnheim postulated that the presence of a PFO could result in a paradoxical embolism.[3] A venous thrombosis that appears as an arterial embolus is considered 'paradoxical' because the thrombus would not be expected to be able to pass through the pulmonary circulation. By deductive reasoning, it is assumed that the venous embolus could not enter the arterial circulation unless there was an anomalous connection.

PFO, along with atrial septal aneurysm (ASA), has been implicated as a risk factor for stroke of undetermined etiology, or cryptogenic stroke. Up to 40% of ischemic strokes do not have a clear etiology and therefore are defined as cryptogenic.[4] The increased use of transesophageal echocardiography has demonstrated worm-like echogenic structures consistent with thrombus straddling the atrial septum through a PFO[5] (Figure 25.1). This evidence has strengthened the theory that

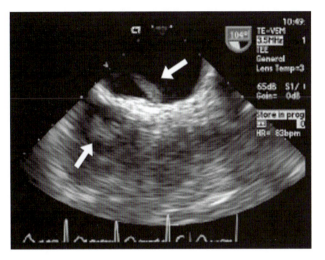

Figure 25.1 Evidence that thrombus can pass from the right atrium through a patent foramen ovale into the left atrium. This still frame from an echocardiogram shows a worm-like structure (arrow) straddling the interatrial septum. This structure is consistent with a venous thrombus cast of a peripheral vein that has lodged temporarily across a patent foramen ovale.

small venous emboli could pass from the venous circulation into the left atrium via a PFO and travel to the cerebral circulation, causing ischemia or infarction. Such paradoxical emboli may be responsible for a significant portion of cryptogenic strokes or transient ischemic attacks.

The diagnosis of cryptogenic stroke is made by exclusion of the common etiologies of stroke such as atherosclerosis of the cerebral or carotid arteries or the aortic arch, atrial fibrillation, or other potential intracardiac abnormalities that could result in thrombus such as mitral stenosis or left ventricular aneurysm or dilatation. Cryptogenic stroke is considered in younger individuals (less than 55 years old) who present with neurologic deficits and radiologic findings consistent with cerebral infarct and who do not have an obvious cause for the neurologic deficit. Patients should be screened for hypercoagulable states that could predispose them to developing venous blood clots. Pregnancy and the use of estrogen-containing contraceptive medications or hormone replacement therapy predispose women to venous thrombosis. Patients should also be screened for inherited or acquired thrombophilic conditions such as protein C or S deficiency, factor V Leiden, prothrombin mutation, and the antiphospholipid syndrome.

Observational studies have demonstrated that the prevalence of PFO in patients with cryptogenic stroke is higher than that of the general population. In one study of 60 patients with ischemic stroke who were under the age of 55, the prevalence of PFO was higher (40% vs 10%, $p < 0.001$) compared to the control group. Furthermore, the prevalence of PFO in patients with no identifiable cause of stroke was highest (54%) compared to those with no identifiable cause but at least one risk factor (40%) and those with an identifiable cause (21%, $p < 0.1$).[6] A second study of 146 patients similarly showed a higher prevalence of PFO (48% vs 4%, $p < 0.001$) in patients less than 55 years old with cryptogenic stroke compared to controls.[7] A meta-analysis by Overell et al. estimated that, in patients younger than 55 years, the odds ratio for stroke was 3.1 if a PFO was present, 6.1 if an ASA was identified, and 15.6 if both a PFO and ASA were present.[8] Various groups have also looked at the presence of PFO, ASA, or both as risk factors for recurrent stroke. In a study of 581 patients with cryptogenic stroke, the risk of recurrent stroke was 2.3% (95% CI 0.3 to 4.3%) in patients with PFO, 15.2% (95% CI 1.8 to 28.6%) in those with both PFO and ASA, and 4.2% (95% CI 1.8 to 6.6%) in individuals with neither abnormality.[9] These studies are all subject to the inaccuracy of diagnosing a PFO and must be interpreted with some caution.

Several studies have assessed the safety and efficacy of percutaneous closure of PFO for presumed cryptogenic stroke. Prior to the development of atrial septal occluder devices, patients with a documented PFO were treated with combinations of antiplatelet and anticoagulant medications. In rare cases, these patients underwent surgical closure. The incidence of recurrent stroke after surgical closure is not known as the number of cases is small. In one study, none of the 91 patients who underwent surgical closure of PFO had a recurrent stroke during a mean follow-up of 1.9 years. Eight patients had symptoms consistent with transient ischemic attack (TIA), but with no residual deficits.[10] There are no randomized controlled studies comparing these treatment options. However, in one non-randomized study, investigators compared medical therapy, consisting of aspirin (325 mg/day) and clopidogrel (75 mg/day), to device closure of PFO. They reported that over a 24-month follow-up period, the incidence of recurrent thromboembolic events per year was 14.7% in the medically treated group ($n = 44$), whereas none of the intervention group patients ($n = 48$) had a recurrence.[11]

Onorato et al. reported one of the largest series of transcatheter closures of PFO. This group performed 256 device closures for various indications, but primarily for ischemic stroke ($n = 101$) and TIA ($n = 144$). All but 8 of the devices were Amplatzer® PFO Occluders. Over a mean follow-up time of 19 months, there were no recurrent thromboembolic events.[12] Two more recent smaller studies of 55 and 40 patients similarly documented no recurrent thromboembolic events after PFO closure over mean follow-up times of 19 and 11 months, respectively.[13,14] Our group published a 5-year experience with PFO closure. In 131 (77% Amplatzer and 23% CardioSEAL) patients who underwent percutaneous closure of a PFO and were followed for a mean of 30 months, there were no recurrent TIAs, strokes, or peripheral thromboembolic events.[15] These observational studies must be interpreted with caution. It is impossible to clinically distinguish a TIA from a transient neurologic deficit associated with a complex migraine (especially without a headache), since both diagnoses will have transient neurologic features and a negative MRI. In the case of a TIA, lack of recurrent events after PFO closure supports the presumption that the device is preventing emboli to the brain. However, this assumption may not be correct. A similar mechanism may be responsible for reducing complex migraine symptoms after PFO closure. In these cases, the device may be preventing the right-to-left shunt of a chemical substance that triggers or potentiates symptoms. The fact that transient neurologic symptoms may not recur after PFO closure does not prove that the original episode was due to an embolic event (TIA) versus a chemical trigger (complex migraine). The inability to distinguish between these two diagnoses would argue against using TIA as an endpoint in clinical trial design to determine whether PFO closure prevents recurrent stroke.

Multiple devices have been developed for PFO closure. The most widely used are the Amplatzer® PFO Occluder (AGA Medical Corp, Plymouth, MN) and the CardioSEAL®/STARFlex® (NMT Medical, Boston, MA). The Amplatzer PFO Occluder has emerged as the preferred device in our group because of ease of use and low complication rates. The Amplatzer PFO Occluder is a self-expandable, double-disk device with a connecting waist made from a Nitinol wire mesh (0.004–0.0075 inch). Dacron patches are sewn within each disk and serve to occlude blood flow through the device. The occluder is available in three sizes (18 mm, 25 mm, and 35 mm), which describe the diameter of the larger right atrial disk. Animal studies have shown that complete endothelialization occurs by 3 months.[16]

There are variations in the technique for percutaneous closure with the Amplatzer PFO Occluder. The procedure can usually be done in an outpatient setting with conscious sedation; our preference is to use intravenous midazolam and fentanyl. Transvenous access is established via the right femoral vein, followed by placement of two 8 French vascular sheaths. One

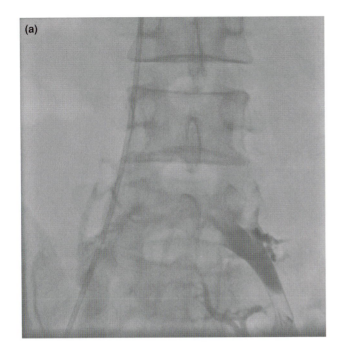

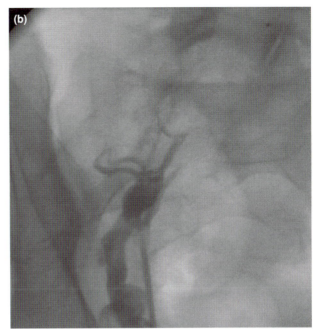

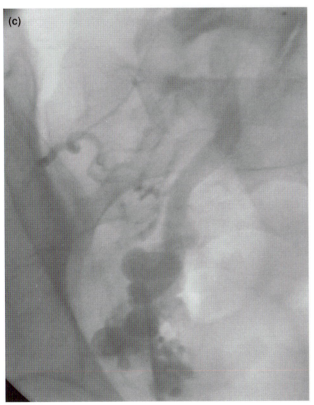

Figure 25.2 (a) An attempt was made to pass an intracardiac echocardiogram catheter from the left femoral vein. It was difficult to traverse the bifurcation into the inferior vena cava. The echo catheter was removed and an angiogram from the left femoral vein was performed. This picture shows residual hang-up of contrast in the left iliac vein, which is consistent with obstruction due to external compression of the left iliac vein between the right iliac artery and the spine. This phenomenon is known as the May-Thurner syndrome. (b) In this second patient, the guide wire would not pass through the right femoral vein. A venogram demonstrates obstruction of venous flow at the level of the iliac vein. (c) A later phase of the venogram reveals a tortuous collateral proceeding caudally and then reversing in a cephalad direction through an alternative vein.

sheath is used for the device delivery catheter, and the other sheath is used to insert an intracardiac echo (ICE) catheter. Although the ICE catheter can be placed from the left femoral vein, it is more difficult to maneuver the catheter in the right atrium from this position, and there is a slight risk of perforation of the femoral vein if the catheter is pushed against resistance. (Figure 25.2). An angiographic multipurpose catheter is used to localize the PFO under fluoroscopic guidance, and a soft guide wire with a J curve is placed through the foramen. The guide wire and catheter are positioned preferentially into the left superior pulmonary vein. The guide wire is then removed and replaced with a J curve Amplatz stiff exchange-length guide wire. We have switched from using an Amplatz super stiff exchange-length guide wire because we had a patient who developed pericardial tamponade from a left atrial puncture with this very stiff guide wire (Figure 25.3).

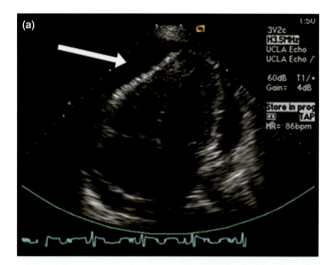

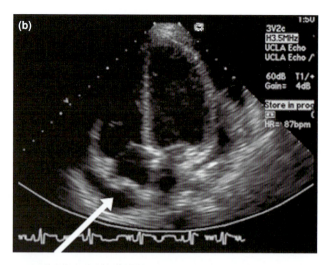

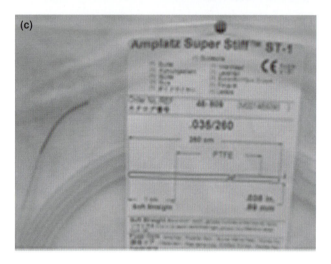

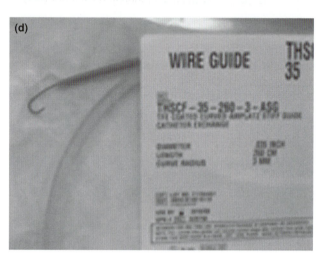

Figure 25.3   This 45-year-old man with cryptogenic stroke had an uneventful implantation of an Amplatzer PFO occluding device. However, 10 minutes after the procedure was over, the patient's blood pressure dropped to 75/40 mmHg and his pulse slowed to 50 beats/minute. A transthoracic echocardiogram demonstrated a pericardial effusion (a). In addition, there was evidence of tamponade physiology with indentation of the right atrial wall (arrow, b). In this patient, an Amplatzer Super Stiff exchange-length wire (c) had been used to pass the introducing catheter across the atrial septum into the left atrium. We believe that during manipulation of this wire, it perforated the left atrial free wall. We currently only use a J-tipped wire known as the Amplatz Stiff guiding wire (d). Although it is not as rigid, the strength of the Super Stiff guide wire is not necessary for support in passing an introducing catheter through the PFO.

The multipurpose catheter is removed and an 8–9 French guiding sheath is introduced over the guide wire and advanced under fluoroscopy into the right atrium. At this point the introducer is removed and the catheter is allowed to back bleed. This step is important to prevent air from being sucked into the catheter when it is within the left atrium. The catheter sheath is then advanced over the guide wire into the left atrium and the exchange-length wire is removed. The catheter is flushed and the back end is closed with a luer-lock syringe. The occluding device is then placed in a water bath and is loaded onto the delivery cable. While the device is still under water, the cable and device are retracted into a 6 inch loading catheter adapted with an O-ring to permit flushing

and prevent air from entering into the loading device. Meticulous care is necessary at this point to prevent any air from being introduced into the guiding catheter which could then embolize if released at the end of the catheter within the left atrium. If an air embolus occurs, it tends to travel through the left ventricle and passes along the superior aspect of the aortic root, thereby entering the superiorly positioned right coronary artery (since the patient is supine) (Figure 25.4).

The device within the loading tube is then attached to the main catheter and advanced within the sheath. The left atrial disk is advanced out of the catheter and expands to its original shape within the left atrium. The catheter and the left atrial disk are retracted as a

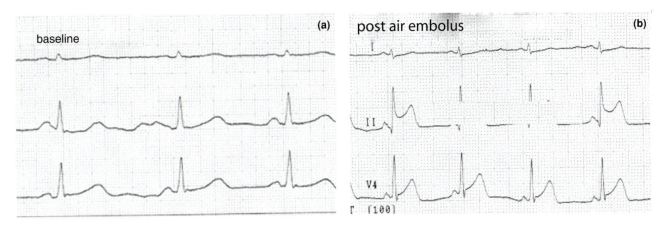

Figure 25.4 (a) Electrocardiogram at baseline shows normal sinus rhythm and normal morphology in a 21-year-old woman who was undergoing PFO closure. (b) Electrocardiogram following placement of a PFO occluding device. Although no air was visualized in the catheter, the ST segment elevation in the inferior leads occurred within minutes of passing the occluding device through the introducing catheter into the left atrium. With the patient in the supine position, air may have embolized from the left atrium to the aorta, and from there to the right coronary artery, the origin of which takes off anteriorly towards the chest wall.

unit until the left atrial disk abuts against the interatrial septum. This process is visualized both by fluoroscopy as well as ICE guidance. The right atrial disk is then deployed by withdrawing the sheath. The expanded right atrial disk is readvanced up against the septum. It is important to visualize that the pliable interatrial septum is clearly positioned between the right and left atrial disks. Placement of the device is confirmed by fluoroscopy and ICE.

The closure procedure is usually accomplished with echocardiographic guidance as well as fluoroscopy. In the past, the procedure was performed with transesophageal echocardiography (TEE); but more recently, studies have described the feasibility of ICE. TEE is an uncomfortable procedure for the patient, and, in some cases, may require general anesthesia with endotracheal intubation. Hijazi *et al.* first reported their experience with ICE compared to TEE in a study of 11 patients.[17] The study included patients with either secundum atrial septal defects (ASDs) or PFO, and in 6 cases, images were obtained sequentially, first with TEE and then ICE. The investigators used the 10 French ACUSON AcuNav™ ultrasound-tipped catheter (Siemens Medical Solutions USA, Inc, Malvern, PA). For adult patients, the ICE catheter was introduced via a separate 11 French sheath through the same femoral vein as the occluder device. The median diameters of the defects were 16.7 mm and 16.1 mm by TEE and ICE, respectively. The measurements correlated well with a coefficient of 0.97. In patients with ASD, the balloon-stretched diameters were also measured with a correlation coefficient of 0.98. In one case, a short inferior-posterior rim not visualized well by TEE was visible by ICE. The investigators also noted that

images of the upper left pulmonary vein and left atrium, or near field images on TEE due to their proximity to the esophagus, were clearer by ICE. Positioning of the wire, catheter, and device into the left atrium, as well as deployment of the left atrial disk, were visualized with greater clarity by ICE.

In a second study, Koenig *et al.* reported their experience with ICE-guided transcatheter closure of 111 patients with both secundum ASD (n = 82) and PFO (n = 29).[18] This study used the same 10 French ACUSON AcuNav™ catheter. This modality allowed for successful placement of the device in all patients, which resulted in immediate complete closure in all but 11 cases with trivial or small residual shunts. More recently, an 8 French version of the ICE catheter has become available which potentially decreases the risk of bleeding. In the United States, the FDA has approved this device to be resterilized up to 4 times, which significantly reduces the cost of the product.

There are various peri- and postprocedural complications associated with device closure of PFO. Twelve studies were reviewed between 2002 and 2007 for reports of specific complications and rates of occurrence. At the femoral venous puncture site, there is a risk of hematoma formation or other vascular injury. The risk of this complication is not unique to this closure procedure and is expected to be similar to other percutaneous, transvenous procedures. In most studies, this complication rate is reported to be between 2.0 and 4.7%.[12–15,19–26] Obese patients are at higher risk of hematoma formation because of the difficulty in isolating the femoral vein. For this reason, patients with a BMI greater than 35 are excluded from the PREMIUM trial of PFO closure in patients with severe migraine

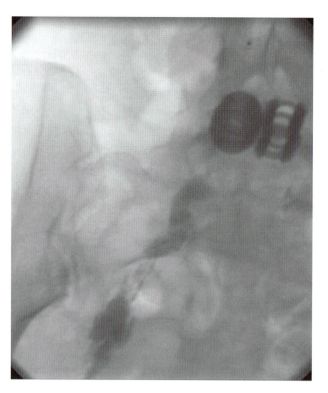

Figure 25.5 Perforation of the right iliac vein occurred in this 43-year-old woman who had a history of five abdominal operations. A J-tipped 0.038 inch guide wire met resistance in the iliac vein. A venogram revealed obstruction of the right iliac vein. The procedure was then performed from the left iliac vein without problems. An hour after the procedure, when the patient was back in the recovery area, her blood pressure dropped to 70/40 mmHg. An abdominal CT examination revealed extravasation of blood and a large hematoma. Surgical exploration demonstrated a lacerated right iliac vein that was extremely friable.

headaches. We have seen one patient who had a friable iliac vein secondary to multiple abdominal operations. Passage of a standard J wire through the right femoral vein resulted in a perforation of the iliac vein which was not recognized until one hour later when the patient became hypotensive (Figure 25.5).

Another complication is the development of transient arrhythmias, primarily atrial fibrillation, which can occur from catheter stimulation of the atrium during device implantation or within the first few months after the closure. All of the devices irritate the heart and induce inflammation and subsequent scar tissue formation. Patients who are allergic to nickel are more likely to develop an atrial arrhythmia (see below). Although approximately 20% of patients complain of some palpitations in the first 2 months following insertion of the device, paroxysmal atrial

tachycardia or atrial fibrillation is rare, occurring in 1–2% of patients.[12–15,19–26] A more serious complication is embolism of air into the left atrium causing occlusion of coronary or cerebral arterial blood flow. There are reports of transient ST segment elevations on electrocardiography and neurologic symptoms during or immediately after the procedure that have been attributed to air emboli.[27] The risk of ST segment elevation suggestive of coronary artery embolism ranges between 1.4 and 3.9%.[12–15,19–26] In all cases, the ischemic changes were temporary without long-term sequelae. TIA from presumed cerebral arterial embolism is even lower, between 0.3 and 0.7%, again with no residual neurologic deficits reported.[12–15,19–26]

There are also reports of pericardial effusion leading to cardiac tamponade occurring in 0.4 to 1.8% of cases.[12–15,19–26] Trepels *et al.* described a case of cardiac tamponade in a patient who became hypotensive 24 hours after device closure.[28] TTE confirmed a pericardial effusion with tamponade physiology and subsequent pericardiocentesis returned 600 ml of blood. The effusion reaccumulated with continued bleeding, and the patient was sent to surgery, where a small 2 mm erosion was found on the right atrial roof extending to the aortic root caused by the right atrial disk of the occluder. The true incidence of erosion with the Amplatzer PFO device is unknown. According to the manufacturer and the FDA MAUDE database (www.accessdata.fda.gov), there have been 5 reported cases of erosion with the PFO device out of approximately 40 000 implants (0.0125%). Erosion with the PFO device should be distinguished from that of the Amplatzer ASD device. Studies suggest that erosion is more likely to occur when oversized ASD devices are used. Since the most frequently used Amplatzer PFO devices are either 25 or 35 mm, size does not appear to be a major determinant for erosion with this device (Figure 25.6).

The procedural success rate for deployment of the Amplatzer PFO Occluder is reported to be 100%.[12–15,19–26] Most studies describe some residual shunt after closure that is detected immediately post-deployment. The degree of shunting decreases during a 1- to 6-month follow-up period with TEE. Measurement of the shunt depends on the sensitivity of the technique that is used. For example, transcranial Doppler imaging produces the largest shunt estimates, followed by TEE and then transthoracic echocardiography. The presence of a minor residual shunt is reported to be between 6 and 47%. Braun *et al.* performed a more detailed analysis of residual shunting and compared rates between the Amplatzer and CardioSEAL devices. In 69 patients receiving the Amplatzer PFO Occluder, 40% had small to moderate residual shunts and 1% had a large shunt. Among those patients who received the CardioSEAL, 36% were found to have small to moderate shunting, and 3% had

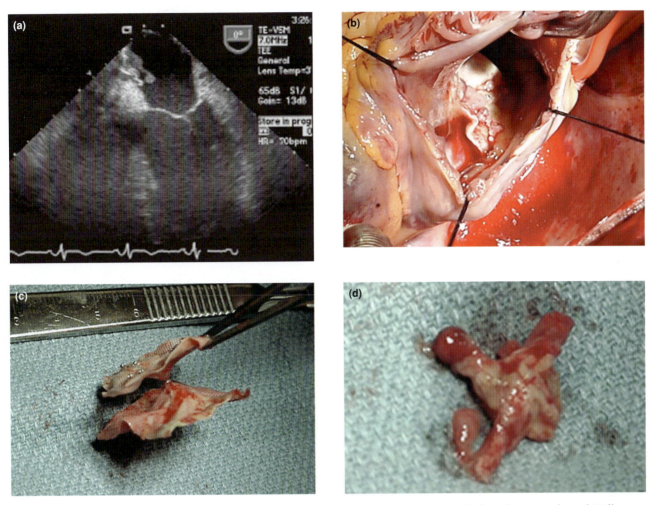

Figure 25.6 This 32-year-old man with cryptogenic stroke had a CardioSEAL PFO occluding device implanted. Follow-up transesophageal echocardiogram at 4 weeks revealed a large echogenic mobile structure on the right and left atrial sides of the device. The patient was initially treated with anticoagulation, but when the follow-up echocardiogram at 6 weeks still revealed mobile fronds consistent with thrombus in the left atrium (a), we elected to remove the device surgically. The opened left atrium demonstrated the CardioSEAL device with a pedunculated mass on the left atrial side (b). (c) The removed CardioSEAL device. The mass of tissue (d) was a pedunculated mobile combination of organizing thrombus and fibrous tissue.

large shunts. In this study, only 1 patient who received the CardioSEAL had a recurrent TIA without long-term deficits.[19] Therefore, the clinical significance of a residual shunt is unclear, with inadequate data to draw a conclusion about the incidence of clinically significant shunts and recurrent thromboembolic events.

Although complete endothelialization of the PFO devices tends to occur within 3 months, there are reports of thrombus formation on the device postimplantation. In one study of 593 patients who received one of four devices – Amplatzer PFO Occluder, CardioSEAL, StarFLEX, and PFO-Star – the rates of thrombus formation were 0%, 7.1%, 5.7%, and 6.6%, respectively. The difference between the Amplatzer device and the other three was statistically significant.[29] In this study, postprocedural atrial fibrillation and the presence of an atrial septal aneurysm were predictors for thrombus formation. Two of the patients required

surgical removal of thrombus and device, and one had thrombus alone evacuated.

Recurrent thromboembolic events may be a complication of patent foramen ovale closure and depend on the type of device that was implanted. In addition, a distinction must be drawn between thrombus formation on the device, specifically on the left atrial disk which may embolize, and residual shunt with continued risk for paradoxical embolism. In our series of 200 cases, we have not seen thrombus formation on an Amplatzer PFO or ASD device, but have found a 22% incidence of thrombus on the CardioSEAL.[15] One of our patients required surgical removal of the CardioSEAL device secondary to the formation of a large mobile thrombus (Figure 25.6). The fibrothrombotic material on the left atrial side was polypoid and extremely sessile. The incidence of dislodgement of these types of thrombus with possible embolic

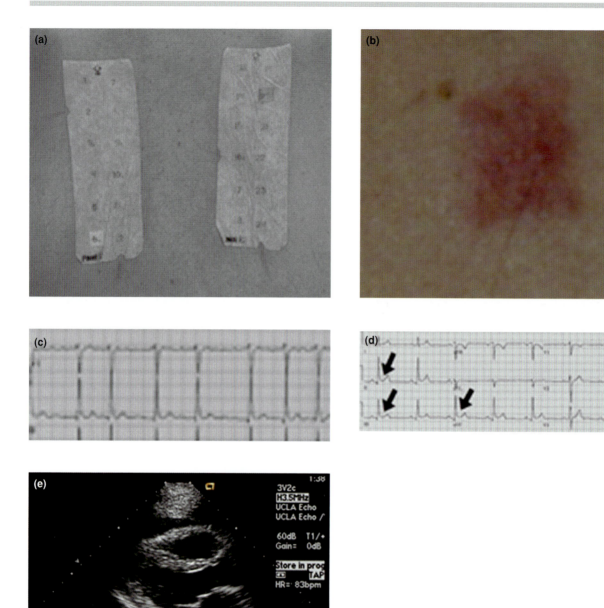

Figure 25.7   A 38-year-old man with a history of migraine headaches with aura developed right-sided visual loss and paraphasic speech. He was found to have a small ischemic stroke in the territory of the left middle cerebral artery. A work-up revealed antibodies to cardiolipin and the presence of a PFO. His PFO was closed using the Amplatzer PFO Occluder as part of the RESPECT registry. Two weeks after the procedure he developed episodes of chest pain that were pleuritic and positional in nature, with tingling down his left arm. He also began to have more frequent migraine headaches with visual auras. A TEE revealed a small pericardial effusion. Allergy patch testing (a) showed a 2+ reaction to nickel, suggesting a type IV hypersensitivity reaction (b). He was treated with steroids with significant improvement. Three weeks later he had recurrence of chest pain associated with atrial fibrillation (c) and diffuse ST segment changes consistent with pericarditis (d). The echocardiogram showed an increase in the size of the pericardial effusion, but there was no evidence of tamponade (e). The effusion was not tapped. He was treated with another course of oral steroids (60 mg prednisone/day tapered to 10 mg/day over one week) and the symptoms resolved. He continued to have intermittent migraines with visual aura and occasional chest discomfort for one year, but the symptoms eventually resolved.

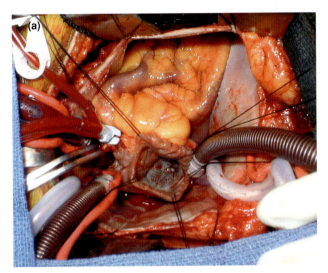
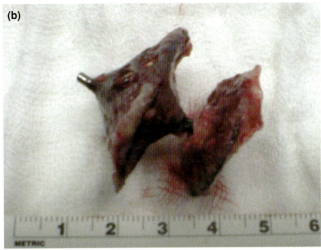

Figure 25.8   Open-heart surgery (a) in a 32-year-old man who complained of severe chest pain, which was intermittent over 4 months following implantation of an Amplatzer PFO occluding device. The device was placed secondary to a cryptogenic stroke. Despite medical therapy with steroids and analgesics, the pain continued and he was referred to surgery for device removal. The explanted Amplatzer device (b) demonstrated dense fibrous tissue covering both the left and right atrial sides. From the surgical observations, there was no obvious cause of the severe chest pain.

sequelae is unknown, and, in fact, the thrombus material may resorb and eventually adhere to the device as scar tissue. We have not observed any secondary strokes or peripheral embolic events in our patients who have primarily received the Amplatzer and Cribriform Occluders over a mean follow-up period of 30 months and up to 6 years.[15] On the other hand, according to a report of PFO occlusion in 237 patients where the CardioSEAL was the predominant device used (86% CardioSEAL vs 14% Amplatzer), the incidence of recurrent stroke was 3.4% during a mean follow-up of 1.6 years.[30]

Dislocation or embolization of ASD and PFO closure devices has been reported. The rate of this complication is less than 1% among all devices.[12–15,19–26] There is one report of an embolized ASD device that required surgical removal, but no similar cases with PFO occluders.[24] Embolization of PFO devices, and specifically the Amplatzer PFO Occluder, is extremely rare with only anecdotal reports. Braun *et al.* described two cases of embolization of the PFO-Star into the left atrium and into the systemic circulation as far as the descending aorta. In both cases, the devices were successfully retrieved with snare tools.[20] In a case involving the Amplatzer PFO Occluder, there was partial retraction of the right atrial disk of the device into the PFO channel, a complication which was attributed to a particularly long channel.[19]

PFO closure in some patients leads to new onset of migraine headaches or exacerbation of pre-existing symptoms usually associated with visual aura.[31] This effect appears to be paradoxical in light of multiple reports of the benefit of PFO closure in reducing migraine headache symptoms.[32,33] We have associated this flare-up in migraine headaches with patients who have a hypersensitivity reaction to nickel. All of the Amplatzer devices, including the PFO Occluder, are composed of Nitinol, an alloy containing 55% nickel and 45% titanium. In an analysis of 37 patients receiving closure devices with documented nickel allergy testing, the incidence of chest discomfort or new or worsening migraine headaches with aura was 60% among patients with a nickel allergy, compared with 11% in those who tested negative for the allergy ($p = 0.005$).[34] One potential hypothesis for the new onset or exacerbation of migraine headaches is that a local inflammatory response to the Amplatzer device leads to platelet aggregation and thrombus formation with embolization to the brain. Support for this theory comes from the fact that institution of clopidogrel therapy improves the symptoms. However, thrombus on an Amplatzer device has not been documented in any of these cases. We believe that an allergy to nickel leads to an exaggerated inflammatory response, and that inflammatory factors themselves, such as chemokines, travel to the cerebral circulation and trigger the migraine symptoms. We have also seen the induction of migraine headaches in two patients who were not allergic to nickel, but had the largest size ASD device (38 mm) implanted. In addition to the 9 patients in our series, we have received reports from 10 other physicians around the world who have described similar findings. These physicians also note significant improvement in their patients' symptoms with treatment using clopidogrel or steroids.

In addition to exacerbation of migraine headaches, about 20% of the patients complain of chest discomfort. Usually this sensation is mild and intermittent, and only lasts for a few weeks. Depending on the severity of these complaints, patients may respond to non-steroidal anti-inflammatory agents, but most patients choose not to take any medication. However, in the patients with nickel allergy, the pain can be more severe with evidence of pericardial irritation either by EKG changes showing concave-up ST elevation or new onset of pericardial effusion. (Figure 25.7) The symptoms respond to treatment with oral steroids.

In the 150 patients in our series of Amplatzer device implantation, we have had one patient who had such severe chest discomfort that he requested to have open-heart surgery to remove the device (Figure 25.8). This individual had unusual anatomy and required a transseptal puncture to position the Amplatzer device. The initial puncture created a small dissection plane within the septum, but a second puncture was successful and the device was implanted. It is unclear if the excessive discomfort was due to the trauma created by the transseptal puncture or if it was from a reaction to the Amplatzer device alone. He was not allergic to nickel and there was no evidence of pericarditis. The pain did not respond to steroid therapy. After 3 months without abatement of his symptoms, he elected to have the device surgically removed.

The Amplatzer PFO Occluder is remarkable because it is a percutaneously placed device that is easily implanted and effectively seals the foramen ovale. In addition, it is usually very well tolerated by the patients. However, as with any interventional procedure, there are potential complications that are described in this chapter. It is our hope that by presenting this information, operators will gain from past experience and reduce the incidence of these complications.

REFERENCES

1. Shah S, Shindler D. Patent foramen ovale. Echoes from the past and questions for the future. N J Med 2002; 99(6): 25–6.
2. Galen. De usu partium L. Nicolaus. De usu partium corporis humani, magna cura ad exemplaris Graeci veriritatem [sic] castigatum, universo hominum generi apprime necessarium. 1528, Parisiis,: Ex officina Simonis Colinaei. [32], 484.
3. Cohnheim J, Vorlesungen über allgemeine Pathologie: ein Handbuch für Aerzte und Studirende. Berlin: Hirschwald, 1877.
4. Homma S et al. Effect of medical treatment in stroke patients with patent foramen ovale: patent foramen ovale in Cryptogenic Stroke Study. Circulation 2002; 105(22): 2625–31.
5. Kessel-Schaefer A et al. Migrating thrombus trapped in a patent foramen ovale. Circulation 2001; 103(14): 1928.
6. Lechat P et al. Prevalence of patent foramen ovale in patients with stroke. N Engl J Med 1988; 318(18): 1148–52.
7. Di Tullio M et al. Patent foramen ovale as a risk factor for cryptogenic stroke. Ann Intern Med 1992; 117(6): 461–5.
8. Overell JR, Bone I, Lees KR. Interatrial septal abnormalities and stroke: a meta-analysis of case-control studies. Neurology 2000; 55(8): 1172–9.
9. Mas JL et al. Recurrent cerebrovascular events associated with patent foramen ovale, atrial septal aneurysm, or both. N Engl J Med 2001; 345(24): 1740–6.
10. Dearani JA et al. Surgical patent foramen ovale closure for prevention of paradoxical embolism-related cerebrovascular ischemic events. Circulation 1999; 100(19 Suppl): II171–5.
11. Thanopoulos BV et al. Transcatheter closure versus medical therapy of patent foramen ovale and cryptogenic stroke. Cathet Cardiovasc Interven 2006; 68(5): 741–6.
12. Onorato E et al. Patent foramen ovale with paradoxical embolism: mid-term results of transcatheter closure in 256 patients. J Interven Cardiol 2003; 16(1): 43–50.
13. Chatterjee T et al. Interventional closure with Amplatzer PFO occluder of patent foramen ovale in patients with paradoxical cerebral embolism. J Interven Cardiol 2005; 18(3): 173–9.
14. Bijl JM et al. Percutaneous closure of patent foramen ovale. Intern Med J 2005; 35(12): 706–10.
15. Slavin L et al. Five-year experience with percutaneous closure of patent foramen ovale. Am J Cardiol 2007; 99(9): 1316–20.
16. Han YM et al. New self-expanding patent foramen ovale occlusion device. Cathet Cardiovasc Interven 1999; 47(3): 370–6.
17. Hijazi Z et al. Transcatheter closure of atrial septal defects and patent foramen ovale under intracardiac echocardiographic guidance: feasibility and comparison with transesophageal echocardiography. Cathet Cardiovasc Interven 2001; 52(2): 194–9.
18. Koenig P et al. Role of intracardiac echocardiographic guidance in transcatheter closure of atrial septal defects and patent foramen ovale using the Amplatzer device. J Interven Cardiol 2003; 16(1): 51–62.
19. Braun M et al. Transcatheter closure of patent foramen ovale (PFO) in patients with paradoxical embolism. Periprocedural safety and mid-term follow-up results of three different device occluder systems. Eur Heart J 2004; 25(5): 424–30.
20. Braun MU et al. Transcatheter closure of patent foramen ovale in patients with cerebral ischemia. J Am Coll Cardiol 2002; 39(12): 2019–25.
21. Hong TE et al. Transcatheter closure of patent foramen ovale associated with paradoxical embolism using the amplatzer PFO occluder: initial and intermediate-term results of the U.S. multicenter clinical trial. Cathet Cardiovasc Interven 2003; 60(4): 524–8.
22. Khositseth A et al. Transcatheter Amplatzer device closure of atrial septal defect and patent foramen ovale in patients with presumed paradoxical embolism. Mayo Clin Proc 2004; 79(1): 35–41.
23. Post MC, Van Deyk K, Budts W. Percutaneous closure of a patent foramen ovale: single-centre experience using different types of devices and mid-term outcome. Acta Cardiol 2005; 60(5): 515–19.
24. Purcell IF, Brecker SJ, Ward DE. Closure of defects of the atrial septum in adults using the Amplatzer device: 100 consecutive patients in a single center. Clin Cardiol 2004; 27(9): 509–13.
25. Schwerzmann M et al. Percutaneous closure of patent foramen ovale: impact of device design on safety and efficacy. Heart 2004; 90(2): 186–90.
26. Varma C et al. Clinical outcomes of patent foramen ovale closure for paradoxical emboli without echocardiographic guidance. Cathet Cardiovasc Interven 2004; 62(4): 519–25.

27. Schwerzmann M, Salehian O. Hazards of percutaneous PFO closure. Eur J Echocardiogr 2005; 6(6): 393–5.

28. Trepels T et al. Cardiac perforation following transcatheter PFO closure. Cathet Cardiovasc Interven 2003; 58(1): 111–13.

29. Krumsdorf U et al. Incidence and clinical course of thrombus formation on atrial septal defect and patient foramen ovale closure devices in 1,000 consecutive patients. J Am Coll Cardiol 2004; 43(2): 302–9.

30. Harms V et al. Outcomes after transcatheter closure of patent foramen ovale in patients with paradoxical embolism. Am J Cardiol 2007; 99(9): 1312–15.

31. Rodes-Cabau J et al. Migraine with aura related to the percutaneous closure of an atrial septal defect. Cathet Cardiovasc Interven 2003; 60(4): 540–2.

32. Azarbal B et al. Association of interatrial shunts and migraine headaches: impact of transcatheter closure. J Am Coll Cardiol 2005; 45(4): 489–92.

33. Morandi E et al. Transcatheter closure of patent foramen ovale: a new migraine treatment? J Interven Cardiol 2003; 16(1): 39–42.

34. Wertman B et al. Adverse events associated with nickel allergy in patients undergoing percutaneous atrial septal defect or patent foramen ovale closure. J Am Coll Cardiol 2006; 47(6): 1226–7.

26 Complications of the CardioSEAL Occluder (NMT Medical)

Mark Reisman

In Europe, CardioSEAL was awarded the CE mark in September 1997 and is now commercially available. The CE mark signifies that the product has been designed, tested, and manufactured in a manner which demonstrates safe use in humans. In the US, the CardioSEAL device is only approved for ventricular septal defects, but is used in an off-label fashion for patent foramen ovale.

DEVICE DESCRIPTION

The CardioSEAL is a third generation device (Figure 26.1) consisting of a double umbrella which is a combination of two squares of knitted polyester frabric and a metal frame MP35n alloy, which incorporates two tandem coil hinges in each rib of metal that goes across the fabric. Each square patch is 45° rotated relative to the opposing counterpart.

Using spring coils in the framework, the CardioSEAL implant can be collapsed into a delivery sheath of 10 French. With one umbrella positioned on each side of the defect, the spring coil design promotes apposition to the right and left sides of the septum. Once in position the CardioSEAL is released from the delivery system.

PROCEDURE

Imaging

The deployment of the CardioSEAL device is a catheter-based procedure and is done in a cardiac catheterization laboratory. The cath lab for this procedure should be maintained with similar precautions placed when implanting a permanent prosthesis. Transesophageal (TEE) or intracardiac (ICE) echocardiography should be performed to interrogate several aspects of the structural anatomy, specifically the septum primum for presence or absence of an atrial septal aneurysm (ASA), the length of the tunnel, and the thickness of the septum secundum. Imaging is helpful in determining the presence of an Eustachian valve or Chiari network, and thus alerting the physician of the potential for entanglement in these structures. Imaging

has also been helpful to detect the presence of clot in the patent foramen ovale (PFO) tunnel, or occasionally the presence of clot on the device or the guide wire.

PFO Balloon sizing

We use both fluoroscopy and ICE to balloon size of the PFO (Figure 26.2). The general rule is that the device should be twice as large as the maximal balloon diameter. Several caveats should be considered when doing the balloon sizing technique. (1) The inflation should be at very low pressure so as to not increase the opening of the PFO iatrogenically. (2) The balloon shape should be interrogated to appreciate the inflow from the right side, the tunnel length and uniformity of compliance, and the left-sided exit of the PFO. (3) A bubble study should be performed with the balloon inflated to ascertain that there is no transmission of bubbles, with concomitant transcranial Doppler, thus providing information on whether a secondary atrial level or pulmonary arteriovenous shunt is present.

Access and device delivery

We generally initiate the procedure with 9 French (for balloon sizing) and 11 French (for the ICE catheter), both in the right femoral vein. Once the ICE is in position we then use a multipurpose diagnostic catheter and a 0.032 inch J-wire to cross the left atrium and optimally place the wire into the left upper pulmonary vein. One positioned, we exchange the J-wire for an extra-support Amplatz guide wire, and then deliver the sizing balloon. The PFO is sized and the device selected. Once the device is prepped we then place the 10 French Mullins sheath and carefully evacuate air from the catheter. It is important to get blood flow back from the catheter to assure that the catheter is not up against any cardiac structures. The selected device is than advanced to the tip of the sheath, the left side is opened, the sheath device system withdrawn to the intra-atrial septum, then, with slight pullback pressure, the right side of the device is

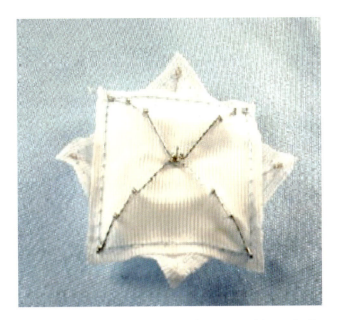

Figure 26.1 The CardioSEAL device. Double umbrella device composed of 2 square sheets of polyester fabric each attached to four nitinol springs.

deployed. If the device is superiorly straddling the primum, the device is released and the delivery catheter removed. With release the appearance should be that of a chromosome.

COMPLICATIONS OF THE CardioSEAL DEVICE

The next sections discuss the array of suboptimal outcomes that can occur with PFO devices, with specific attention to CardioSEAL. Some may not have significant clinical relevance, but help in understanding the limitations and challenges of the device.

Thrombosis

Thrombosis is one of the major concerns of any implantable device. There have been reports of both left- and right-sided thrombosis on the device. One patient, a 48-year-old female who suffered a stroke 2 months after implantation with a CardioSEAL device had two large pedunculated thrombi on the left atrial side of the device, despite postimplantation aspirin therapy.[1]

A second report found microthrombi formed more frequently on the CardioSEAL device (22%) than on the Amplatzer device (0%) 1 month after implantation ($p = 0.02$).[2] This was also consistent with another study that found higher rates of thrombi on the CardioSEAL device (Figure 26.4).

Nonetheless, thrombus does occur and the management of such complications can be quite challenging. In one case of a right-sided thrombosis at our centre, the patient was treated with Coumadin (warfarin). The clot resolved after one month. We elected to continue the Coumadin for 6 months. The initial diagnosis was picked up on routine 1-month thransthoracic echocardiography (TTE). Thrombosis on the left side creates a greater clinical danger to the patient. Although no evidence-based recommendation can be made, options of thrombolysis, open heart surgery, and oral anticoagulation remain part of the therapeutic algorithm.

At present our recommendation for postimplant therapy is chronic ASA and three months of Plavix (clopidogrel). The latter is predicated on the TTE and TCD evidence of an complete closure. If at one year

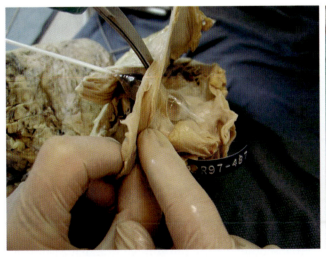
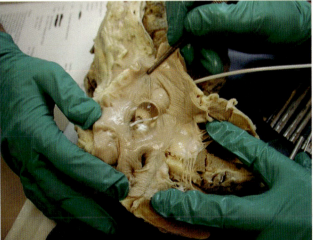

Figure 26.2 Balloon sizing in cadaveric heart.

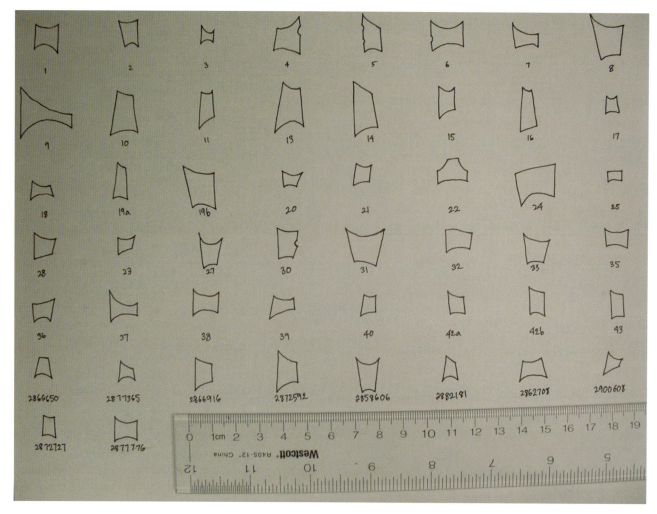

Figure 26.3 These shapes represent casts from human cadaveric hearts of the intra-atrial tunnel. Note the significant variation of length and width.

the patient continues to have a significant residual leak we perform TEE to assess the device.

We have also seen clot on the device during the procedure (Figure 26.5). This particular case was most probably due to stasis of blood in the delivery catheter and that ultimately was captured on the CardioSEAL device. Management of this was by gently withdrawing the device back, and not attempting to pull it into the delivery sheath until the device was low in the inferior vena cava (IVC).

Impact of anatomy and CardioSEAL positioning

After the CardioSEAL device has been opened on the right side of the intra-atrial septum, it remains on the delivery system until the operator decides to release it. Since delivery is from the IVC the device is generally being 'pulled' inferiorly and posteriorly. This will often make it difficult to ascertain how the device will lie on the secundum once released. The tunnel (the overlap between the septum primum and the septum secundum) compliance can be rigid and other times very elastic and thus floppy, with the extreme being an atrial septal aneurysm. The ubiquitous length and width of the tunnel adds to the challenges of discerning how the device will finally be positioned (Figure 26.3). Specifically: (1) juxtaposition on the septum, i.e. how flat the device sits on the septum; (2) whether an arm will be flaired either due to the central pin moving high onto the limbus or due to a thick secundum; and (3) whether the release will impact the left side of the device. The primum is less impacted on release, except with a large ASA, where the device may move excessively in its inferior portion, or with a very thin primum, where there is excessive space between the device and the tissue, setting up a situation for flow to easily traverse and maintain patency of the right to left shunt.

Finally, another challenge of the 'folding devices' is that, with Valsalva or excessive motion of the intra-atrial septum, we see the arms go from flat against the septum to the geometry of a 'V.' This is most probably secondary to the central pin moving inferiorly into the

Device	TEE Due (n)		TEE Performed (%)		Thrombus (%, n)	
	n	6 months	4 weeks	6 months	4 weeks	6 months
Rashkind	1	1	100%	100%	0%	0%
Buttoned Device	52	52	67%	69%	0%	0%
ASDOS	42	42	66%	83%	3.6% (n=1)	0%
Angel Wings	30	30	0%	97%	0%	3.3% (n=1)
CardioSEAL	27	27	52%	93%	7.1% (n=1)*	0%
StarFLEX	142	111	74%	70%	5.7% (n=6)*	0%
Amplatzer	418	375	78%	70%	0%	0.3% (n=1)
PFO-Star	127	127	60%	66%	6.6% (n=5)*	1.5% (n=1)
Helex	161	138	76%	80%	0.8% (n=1)	0%

* Significant difference between the Amplatzer-PFO against the CardioSEAL, StarFLEX, and PFO-Star

Figure 26.4   Septal Occlusion Devices: Thrombus Formation.

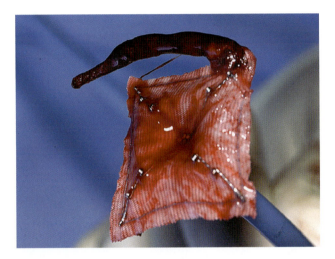

Figure 26.5   Thrombus on the CardioSEAL device. This was most probably caused by stasis in the delivery sheath and subsequent advancement of the device reulted in it adhering to the CardioSEAL.

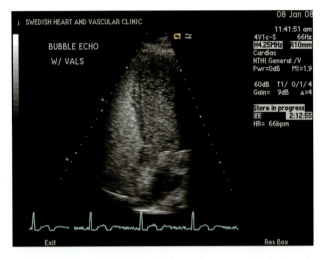

Figure 26.6   This patient had no shunt at rest, but with valsalva the patient has a significant shunt as demonstrated on this bubble study.

tunnel and slightly collapsing the device. This may cause a situation of no residual shunt at rest and a large shunt with Valsalva (Figure 26.6).

Primary placement malaposition

As described above, the majority of primary malpositions can be adjudicated at the time of release of the device, the caveat being that prior to release it may not look ideal, but on release the device lies down very flat and snug along the intra-atrial wall (Figure 26.7). The types of primary malpostioning that we see are (1) arm extended out and not lying on the septum (Figure 26.8); (2) the device not well opposed to the septal wall, either on the right or left side (Figure 26.9); (3) the central pin deep into the tunnel, thus trapping part

of the device and not allowing for full expansion of the arms – typically this is seen on the left.

This primary placement malposition may affect healing of the device, completeness of closure, or risk for recurrent events. If this is noted then it is worthwhile to retract the device and remove it from the body. Device retrieval is possible with the CardioSEAL device. We routinely place a 12 French sheath over our 10 French Mullins sheath if recapture of the larger devices is necessary. Once the right side has been released and the device retrieved, then device should not be reused and a new one should be placed. In our experience, we have not been able to relate primary malaposition to recurrent clinical events. In fact, when looking at residual shunt from our data set, we have not been able to correlate the presence of persistent right to left shunt with the recurrence of stroke or death (Figure 26.10).

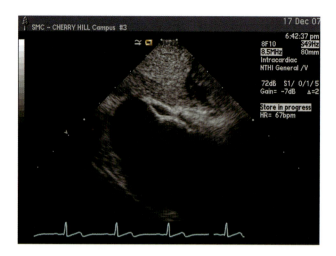

Figure 26.7   As a reference a well deployed CardioSEAL device demonstrating no shunt. Immediately post procedure by Intracardiac echo.

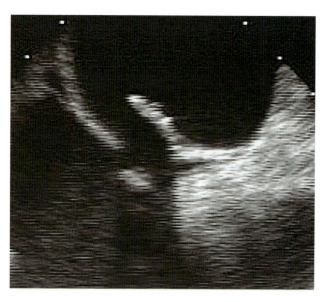

Figure 26.8   As a reference a well deployed CardioSEAL device demonstrating no shunt. Immediately post procedure by Intracardiac echo.

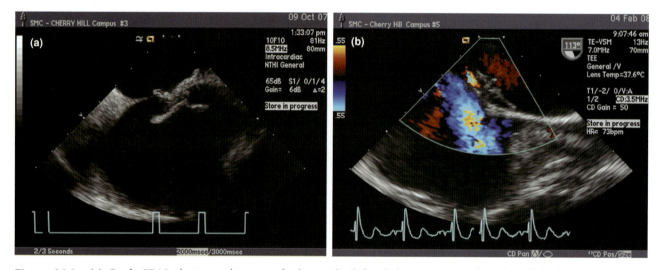

Figure 26.9   (a) CardioSEAL device at the time of release. The left sided arms are significantly off the left atrial septum. (b); The patient had a four month f/u TEE do to persistent shunt which demonstrated flow under the left arms of the device and a significant residual shunt.

	Patients with large residual RLS N=19	Patients without large residual RLS N=150	P value
Recurrent Stroke	1 (5.3%)	5 (3.3%)	0.52
All Cause Death	1 (5.3%)	2 (1.4%)	0.30
Surgical Device Explantation	1 (5.3%)	1 (0.7%)	0.21

Fuller CJ, Jesurum JT, Spencer MP, Reisman M et al. International Stroke Conference 2006.

Figure 26.10   Large residual RLS after PFO Closure does NOT mean more adverse outcomes.

One final comment is in regard to device selection. The recommendation is for the balloon diameter to be doubled for selection of the appropriate device. In many cases the balloon diameter, when doubled, is between two sizes and both may be acceptable to use. We generally will use the larger device in the presence of a thick secundum or in the presence of a significant ASA. Also, in some cases with a very floppy primum and a very short tunnel, i.e. borderline atrial septal defect, we may choose a larger device to reduce the possibility for embolization. It is our impression that, with the relatively rigid CardioSEAL device once deployed, the tunnel overlap makes it unlikely the device can completely fold and sublux into the tunnel.

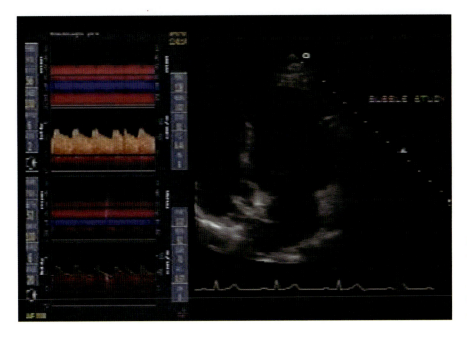

Figure 26.11 Malapposition of a CardioSEAL device resulting in a significant bidirectional shunt. The device was ultimately explanted (see Figure 11). Alongside the TTE image is the Transcranial doppler signal.

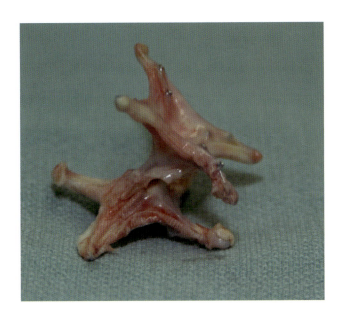

Figure 26.12 An explanted CardioSEAL device, removed after the patient developed significant dyspnea on exertion. TTE demonstrated a large right to left shunt.

Embolization

Although methodical reporting is limited with this device, it is our impression that postdeployment embolization is very rare. The highest risk for embolization arises if the device is not correctly attached to the delivery system at the time of implantation. The operator should check that the locking mechanism is appropriately positioned, and 'tug' the CardioSEAL to assure the security of the device.

In the event that a device embolizes it is important to have snares and retrieval baskets available in the cath lab, and some degree of experience with these devices.

Infection

Once again the true incidence of infection is probably not known, but we believe that it is very infrequent. We pretreat our patients with antibiotics and maintain rigorous catheterization laboratory policies and procedures for an implantable device.

Arrthyhmia

The incidence of atrial arrhythmias is unknown, but in our experience is about 15% and transient. We have had a few patients with persistent atrial fibrillation whom we needed to treat with Coumadin. In these patients it is often a question of whether the atrial fibrillation was the antecedent event that caused the transient ischemic attack/stroke prior to the procedure. This is the reason it is always sound judgement to perform a TEE prior to these procedures, and also in the older population specifically to consider Holter or event monitors prior to the procedure.

Secondary device malposition

With the CardioSEAL device, retraction of the arms has occurred over time as the device healed (Figures 26.11

and 26.12). This is generally associated with the device having the appearance of a 'V.' In our single case this event was associated with a bidirectional shunt and symptoms of dyspnea. The device was ultimately explanted.

SUMMARY

Overall, the CardioSEAL device has been associated less with complications such as embolization and erosion, but more with suboptimal positioning on the septum and residual leaks. The double umbrella devices continue to undergo rapid evolution, with better centering systems and bioabsorbable components currently available in Europe, or being evaluated in randomized clinical trials.

REFERENCES

1. Schuchlenz HW et al. J Thorac Cardiovasc Surg 2005; 130: 591–2.
2. Anzai H et al. Am J Cardiol 2004; 93: 426–31.
3. Krumsdorf et al., JACC, 2004; 43(2): 302–9.

27 Device closure of patent foramen ovale with the St Jude's Premere device

Robert J Sommer

INTRODUCTION

The technique of transcatheter patent foramen ovale (PFO) closure, using double occluder type devices, has been well described in the literature,[1–5] and in earlier chapters in this book. While the implantation of such a device is generally quite safe, there have been a number of late, device-related complications which continue to cause concern, including device thrombosis,[6] atrial arrhythmia,[7] device erosion,[8–11] and anatomic/device distortion with residual shunting in a patient with a long, non-compliant PFO tunnel.[12,13] The St Jude's Premere PFO Closure system, a modified double occluder, was designed to minimize these specific risks. Early clinical results are available.[14,15]

DEVICE DESIGN

The St Jude's Premere PFO Closure system (Figure 27.1), like its counterparts, is a self-expanding, dual-anchor, occlusion device. The right and left atrial anchors are constructed of Nitinol, with only the right anchor entirely enveloped by a knitted polyester fabric. A flexible polyester braided tether, running through the center of the device, allows the anchors to be locked together after delivery. The final distance separating the two anchors is adjustable. A snare-type release mechanism, as well as the braided tether, allows for device retrieval at any point of the implantation procedure. The device is designed specifically for PFO closure. It is not indicated for atrial septal defects (ASDs), or a multiply fenestrated atrial septum.

Left atrial occluder surface area

The left atrial anchor is left free of the fabric covering that characterizes most double occluder systems. This modification reduces the surface area of the left atrial anchor, compared with that of the right atrial anchor, by over 95%. Since the thrombogenicity of the left atrial occluder is in part related to the amount of surface exposed to left atrial blood, the reduction of the left atrium (LA) surface area is intended to minimize the risk of device thrombus formation, and hence the systemic thromboembolism.

With less atrial tissue in direct contact with the device, the irritant/inflammatory effects of the implant should also be reduced, perhaps minimizing the risk of the atrial arrhythmia seen with other devices, in the first few weeks following implantation.[7]

Variable anchor separation

The most unique feature of the Premere design is its ability to adjust to variations in the PFO anatomy. All other double occluder devices are designed so that, upon deployment, the left and right atrial occluders will assume a position abutting one another, separated by a short, fixed distance. This is a vestige of their original design as closure devices for ASDs where there is no distance between the right atrium (RA) and the LA surfaces.

The embryologic formation of the atrial septum[16] involves the overlapping and partial fusion of the thin septum primum to the left of the more rigid septum secundum. Because the two septal portions are not fully adherent to one another, the thinner septum primum acts as a flap-valve, allowing one-way, right-to-left shunting during fetal life when RA pressure exceeds LA pressure. Postnatally, LA pressure rises, shutting the flap-valve, and the two septal portions are intended to fuse completely, eliminating the fetal pathway.

When fusion is incomplete, the resulting PFO anatomy is extremely variable. The persistent tracks, or 'tunnels,' from the RA to the LA vary widely in both width and in length from patient to patient. Any device intended to rest securely on the RA and LA septal surface must traverse the length of the tunnel. Typically, with the compliant nature of septum primum tissue, a short tunnel length, and the typical wide 'mouth' on the LA surface, the occluder pulled back against the LA septal surface will distort septum primum, collapse the tunnel, and allow the two occluders to rest immediately adjacent to one another, as in an ASD. However, when the tissue of septum primum is more rigid, the tunnel is longer, and/or the hinge points of the LA septal attachments are closely spaced, the tunnel may not collapse as easily. Because of the

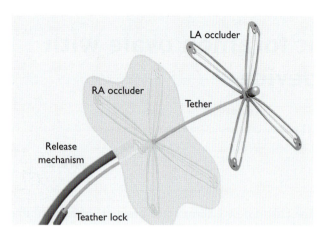

Figure 27.1   The right and left atrial Nitinol anchors of the Premere device are independent of one another. Only the right atrial (RA) occluder is covered by the knitted polyester. A flexible polyester braided tether, running through the center of the device, allows the anchors to be locked together after delivery. A snare-type release mechanism and the braided tether allow for device retrieval at any point of the implant, up to cutting the tether.

fixed, short separation between the occluders, the RA occluder of most devices may deploy within the tunnel of the PFO, not on the RA septal surface. This may lead to an unstable device position, may damage septal or surrounding tissue, or may effectively stent open the PFO leading to increased shunting. If the device is retracted further into the tunnel, the LA occluder will begin to evert, again with potential adverse effects.

In contrast, the connecting tether of the Premere system provides the mechanism for adjustable occluder separation, allowing the device to span even the longest tunnel lengths, with both occluders flat against the septal surface with no anatomic distortion. It is anticipated that this will lead to better closure rates in long tunnel defects, and less risk of tissue injury.

TECHNIQUE OF PFO CLOSURE WITH THE PREMERE DEVICE

Choice of echocardiography

The first consideration in closing a PFO is choosing which echocardiographic modality is to be used to guide the implant, and to assess outcome at the conclusion of the procedure. While some authors have reported PFO closure without echocardiography,[17] the goal of the procedure is the elimination of the right-to-left shunt, not simply the implantation of a device. Additional defects in the septum, and/or the presence of pulmonary arteriovenous malformations, will not be detectable without echocardiography and bubble contrast injection. Transesophageal (TEE) and intracardiac echocardiography (ICE) are both excellent options for this procedure.

TEE has several advantages compared with ICE. TEE imaging allows a far greater number of angles with which to view the septum, the PFO, and the implanted device. It has the advantage of being done by another physician. This minimizes distractions for the implanting physician, and may provide him or her with valuable additional input. Since TEE images are routine in clinical use, these images may also be more immediately helpful to the new device implanter. However, TEE requires deeper sedation or general anesthesia, as it is unpleasant for the patient, and airway compromise, methemoglobinemia, and esophageal injury are possible complications.[18,19]

ICE imaging's single greatest advantage is the ability of the operator to obtain the images him- or herself. It requires no additional sedation, no additional personnel, and makes use of conscious sedation practical for the implantation procedure. Imaging of the septum may equal that of TEE, but depends to a large extent on the experience and the patience of the operator. A second venous access is required for the ICE catheter, and may be placed from the same femoral vein as the device delivery catheter, from the opposite femoral vein, or from a superior approach if need be. Tortuous venous pathways, and branch points, may complicate passing the catheter from the insertion site to the right atrium. Care must be taken to avoid injuring or perforating a side branch as the echo catheter has no end hole and cannot be passed over a wire. We prefer to use the same femoral vein as the device delivery sheath, so we may use the other catheter as a guide for advancing the echo catheter. In difficult cases, we will use a 25–30 cm venous sheath, introduced over a J-wire, to bypass the tortuous veins proximal to the inferior vena cava.

For the Premere PFO system, PFO tunnel length less than 5 mm or the presence of a markedly aneurysmal septum primum (> 20 mm septal excursion), with a wide separation between septum primum and septum secundum, are poor prognostic predictors for success with this device, and should have been ruled out prior to the procedure.

Venous access and crossing the PFO

As with other PFO and closure techniques, the access of choice is the femoral vein, as the inferior vena cava's entry into the RA is aligned embryologically with the flap-valve of the PFO. A second venous access is obtained if ICE imaging is being used. After access is obtained, heparin is administered to maintain an activated clotting time (ACT) of > 250 seconds (~50 units/kg). From the femoral vein, a multipurpose or similarly curved catheter can be used to cross the PFO. This can be accomplished with or without a floppy guide wire. Echocardiography can be very helpful in guiding the catheter into the defect, particularly when the RA is dilated, or when diaphragmatic elevation

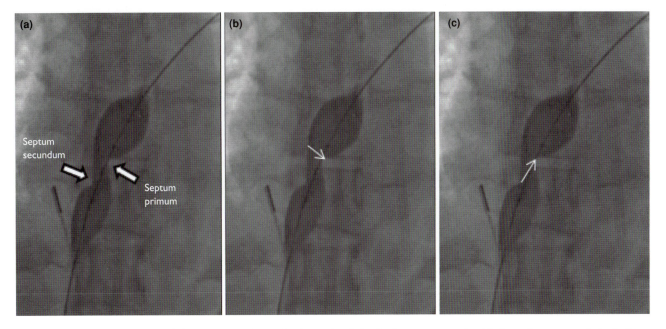

Figure 27.2   Balloon sizing of the PFO reveals much about the defect's characteristics. In (a) the indentations of the balloon are offset, consistent with a long PFO tunnel. The indentations on the balloon demarcate septum secundum (entrance to the tunnel) and septum primum (exit from the tunnel). (b) This figure demonstrates a line drawn perpendicular to the wire course from the superior indentation, defining the 'stretched diameter' of the PFO. (c) A line drawn connecting the two indentations defines the tunnel length.

changes the usual fluoroscopic landmarks. Once across the septum, the catheter should be directed to the left upper pulmonary vein, which enters the back of the atrium over the spine, as seen from a straight antero-posterior (AP) projection. This catheter course provides the straightest path for later delivery of the transseptal sheath. A stiff 0.035 inch guide wire, ideally one with a short, floppy J-tip, is then advanced through the catheter to the pulmonary vein. Injury to the pulmonary vein is possible with excessive force and a stiff, straight-tipped wire. Care must also be taken to insure that the wire is in the pulmonary vein and not the left atrial appendage which sits immediately anterior to the pulmonary vein. This thin-walled structure is particularly susceptible to wire-related injury.

Balloon sizing the PFO and device size selection

Once an acceptable wire position is obtained, balloon sizing is recommended, as the 'stretched' diameter of the defect will determine appropriate device implant size. A low-pressure, compliant sizing balloon is advanced over the wire to straddle the defect, and is inflated to pressures of less than 1 atmosphere. Both the distal and proximal balloon will inflate, leaving a 'waist' or indentation in the balloon. The size and shape of this indentation on the balloon tell the operator much about the characteristics of the PFO, including PFO opening size, tunnel length, and tunnel

compliance (Figure 27.2). The Premere device is currently available in 20 and 25 mm sizes (measured from one edge of the occluder frame to the other). Stretched diameters of greater than 18 mm preclude use of the Premere device. A 30 mm device, for larger defects, is soon to be released by the manufacturer. From early studies of the device in unselected populations,[14] the data suggest that the smaller the device, the larger the risk of residual shunt. This observation is believed to be related to the fact that the Premere has only one occlusive surface. Therefore, having an adequately sized RA occluder becomes that much more critical. Choice of device size seems to be more important than with other devices. Some European operators are using the largest device for all but the smallest PFOs.

In addition to the defect diameter, balloon sizing provides information about the non-reducible length of the PFO tunnel (Figure 27.2), and may be used at a later stage of the procedure as a guide to the optimal separation of the two occluders.

Premere device implantation

Once sizing is completed, the balloon is removed, leaving the stiff wire in the pulmonary vein. The long delivery sheath and dilator are both flushed well with heparinized saline using a 20 cc syringe. The dilator is loaded into the long blue sheath, and the sheath/dilator is advanced over the guide wire to the pulmonary vein. The sheath is advanced over the dilator into the vein, and the wire and dilator are removed. The sheath must then be carefully debubbled again. Debubbling of the sheath is probably the most important step in the procedure, as air embolization is one of the most common and potentially dangerous complications of the PFO closure procedure (see below).

The white device delivery catheter and its loader are then flushed carefully. While flushing continuously, the loading tube is advanced into the hub of the blue delivery sheath, and the device is transferred into the sheath by advancing the white catheter 10–20 cm through the loading tube. The loader can then be withdrawn to the hub of the delivery catheter. Under fluoroscopic guidance, the device is advanced to the end (but not out) of the blue sheath in the pulmonary vein. The sheath and delivery catheter are then withdrawn slowly together, until the tip is free in the left atrium.

The left atrial anchor is then deployed under fluoroscopic guidance by advancing the white delivery catheter. The radio-opaque tips of the anchor will emerge together from the sheath, and will then expand away from each other as the anchor opens. It is critical to stop advancing the white catheter immediately at this point, so that the right atrial anchor is not deployed inadvertently. Once the LA anchor is opened, the operator must take hold of the tether at the back of the delivery catheter. This tether is connected directly to the LA anchor. Slight tension should be applied to the tether, until the opened LA anchor is withdrawn against the mouth of the sheath in the LA. Tension is maintained as both tether and the blue sheath are withdrawn together under fluoroscopic guidance. The anchor will soon change its orientation as it comes into contact with the left side of the septum (Figure 27.3a). The operator should be able to feel the change in tension on the tether as this occurs.

The tether is then grounded on the table, and the white delivery catheter and blue sheath are withdrawn, over the tether, as a unit, back through the PFO to the mid RA. While maintaining tension on the tether with the right hand, and fixing the blue delivery catheter with the left, the white delivery catheter is advanced, delivering the RA occluder. When opened, the occluder is advanced until it is seated gently against the RA septal surface (Figure 27.3b). Too much forward pressure can push the RA occluder into the PFO tunnel, everting the anchor arms. Separation of the occluders should be approximately equal to the tunnel length as defined by balloon sizing.

When the device position is confirmed by fluoroscopy and by echocardiography, the two occluders are locked together. Maintaining tension on the tether, the lock mechanism is advanced over the tether by depressing and pushing forward on the 'lock advance' button on the handle of the white delivery system, until it is in contact with the hub of the RA anchor (Figure 27.3c). The lock moves in only one direction

over the tether; it cannot be retracted. It is important not to overtighten the lock (see below). Once the lock is in place, the 'implant release' button is depressed and pushed forward, releasing a snare mechanism at the RA anchor hub. The implantion is now completed.

Traction on the tether, at this point, allows the operator to test the device stability. The tether is released, and the white delivery catheter withdrawn from the blue sheath. The cutter is threaded onto the tether and advanced into the blue sheath, using the tether as a rail. Under fluoroscopic guidance, the cutter is advanced until the distal tip is adjacent to the lock device. It is critical that the cutter is not advanced too far on the tether, or it will push the lock forward, and may overtighten the anchors. The tether is cut by rotating the wheel on the cutter handle clockwise. The cutter will 'jump' away from the implanted device as the tether is cut. The cutter wheel is then rotated two turns back counterclockwise, and the cutter and tether are withdrawn from the sheath. Follow-up fluoroscopic, echocardiographic, and bubble contrast studies can be performed to confirm proper implant position (Figure 27.3d). All catheters and sheaths are then removed from the body.

POTENTIAL COMPLICATIONS OF THE PFO CLOSURE PROCEDURE

Potential complications of the Premere implantation procedure include all of the general risks of cardiac catheterization, the general risks of a PFO closure procedure using any device, and the risks related to the unique design and deployment of the Premere device.

General catheterization risks

Anesthesia/sedation risks depend to a large extent on what type of echocardiography is being used. For TEE imaging, a much deeper anesthetic technique will be required, which increases the risks of hypoventilation, apnea, and airway obstruction. Injuries to femoral vessels and surrounding structures are possible, including hematoma, AV fistula formation, and pseudoaneurysm formation. The additional access for a second venous sheath (for ICE imaging) increases these risks somewhat. There are risks related to topical agents including allergic/hypersensitivity reactions to tape, drapes, and cleansers. Reactions may occur to intravenous antibiotics given for prophylaxis. Thrombus formation on the device or on the catheters, during the procedure, is possible, and an adequate ACT should be maintained throughout the procedure. Injectable contrast materials may cause allergic reactions, but are not required for a PFO closure, and can be avoided in hypersensitive patients. Each of these risks is discussed in earlier chapters, and will not be addressed further here.

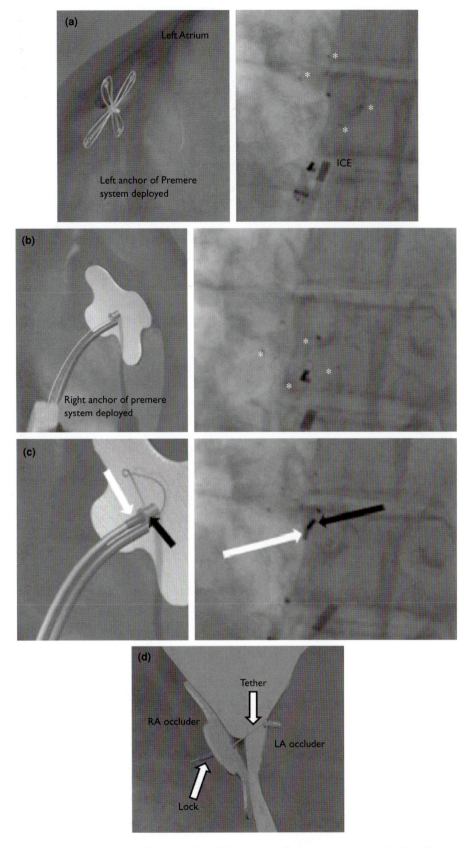

Figure 27.3   Steps of implantation. (a) Left: LA anchor delivered, pulled against septum. Right: Fluoroscopy with asterisks marking the corners of the LA anchor. ICE, echo catheter. (b) Left: RA anchor pushed against septal surface. Right: Fluoroscopy; the LA anchor is in position and asterisks mark the corners of the RA anchor. (c) Cartoon: lock delivered and snare released. Fluoroscopy: the lock device (white arrow) has been advanced over the tether to contact the hub of the RA anchor (black arrow). (d) Final deployed device position. The LA and RA occluders are flush against the septal surfaces, connected by the tether, with the lock mechanism maintaining the appropriate tether length and separation.

General risks of PFO closure

As outlined in prior chapters, all PFO closures require large venous sheaths which reach the left atrium, and the implantation of a foreign body. Proper heparinization (ACT > 250 seconds) will preclude the formation of thrombus, either on the advancing device or on the indwelling wires and catheters. Thrombus in the LA can have dire consequences, including stroke, myocardial infarction, or embolization to another critical structure. Device implantation can be complicated by device malposition and immediate embolization is a complication attributable almost entirely to operator error/inexperience. These issues can be avoided with proper technique and with careful use of both echocardiographic and fluoroscopic images. Atrial perforations/erosions with pericardial effusions have been reported with other devices,[8–11] and are a potential risk of the Premere or any other device. Infection of an implanted device has been reported,[20] with the largest risk the introduction of mouth bacteria into the bloodstream, with dental work, in the few months after the implant (prior to device endothelialization).

Atrial arrhythmia

Manipulation of the catheters and wires in the atria may induce atrial arrhythmia. Frequent premature atrial contractions are seen commonly, as are short runs of atrial tachycardia. The repositioning of catheters, including the ICE catheter, may be needed. In our experience, atrial fibrillation may be induced in about 1% of cases by this atrial ectopy. This is particularly common in the older patient populations, who presumably are more prone to atrial fibrillation. In a series of > 450 patients receiving the CardioSEAL device, 16 (~4%) developed atrial fibrillation in the first 4 weeks after implantation. All but one was greater than 55 years of age.[7] Similarly, a small percentage of patients developed atrial fibrillation in the early European studies with the Premere device.[14]

Migraine headache postimplant

Some patients will develop true migraine headache symptoms with visual aura following implantation of a PFO device.[21,22] This has been seen primarily in patients with a previous history of migraines, though the symptoms may rarely appear de novo. The etiology/mechanism of this complication is unknown, but has been seen in a number of PFO and ASD closure devices. In most patients, it is not related to residual shunting, though increased flow from a poorly positioned device may also trigger such symptoms. It has been speculated that this may be a platelet-mediated phenomenon, as clopidogrel seems to relieve the postimplant migraine symptoms.[23] The syndrome of chest discomfort, palpitations, and headaches may

represent a form of nickel sensitivity, and in our experience seems to resolve in nearly all cases over several months, in the time frame usually associated with device endothelialization.

Avoiding air embolization

With large sheaths in the left atrium, the risk of air embolization should not be underestimated. Small bubbles may be flushed from the sheath, may be pushed out of the sheath by the device, or may be trapped within the collapsed device itself. With the patient in a supine position, the right coronary ostium arises almost directly anteriorly from the aortic root, and thus is the most likely place that an air bubble may become lodged. Patients will present acutely with chest discomfort, shortness of breath, anxiety, and diaphoresis and may become bradycardic and hypotensive, as the ST segments rise and the QRS widens on the surface ECG. The operator should be prepared for this complication, and should be prepared to administer oxygen, atropine, and inotropic and mechanical support, including temporary pacing and placement of an intra-aortic balloon pump.

Transient ST segment changes occur during these procedures in approximately 1% of our cases, despite meticulous care taken to evacuate all air from the system. The following steps should be used to minimize this frequently avoidable complication:

1. Flush all sheaths and dilators well before introduction into the body.
2. Upon reaching the LA with the delivery sheath, it is acceptable to debubble the sheath by opening the side port on the sheath when the patient is intubated and being managed with a positive pressure ventilator. Positive airway pressure increases intrathoracic pressure relative to the outside air pressure, and helps flush the air out of the catheter system passively. However, a patient who is sedated and breathing spontaneously may develop a degree of airway obstruction. Breathing against a closed glottis will create significant negative intrathoracic pressure, which has the potential to suck air rapidly into the open sheath, and into the left heart. With a spontaneously breathing patient, we prefer to keep the system closed as much as possible, and use gentle suction with a large syringe to debubble the sheath.
3. Debubble the sheath, if possible, in the pulmonary vein. The advantage of placing the sheath tip in the pulmonary vein, rather than in the LA, is that, within the lumen of the vein, there will be free blood flow. If the sheath is placed instead in the left atrium, the sheath tip may contact the posterior wall and a vacuum is produced (with cardiac

motion and suction on the sheath), drawing air into the sheath through the back-stop valve.

4. Because the volume of the sheath will be between 15 and 20 cc, a full 20 cc of blood should be removed, to ensure that no air remains. The hub and side arm of the sheath should be tapped vigorously, as blood is being withdrawn, to free up any trapped bubbles. Similarly, the sheath must be flushed with an adequate amount of heparinized saline to insure that no undiluted blood remains in the sheath.

5. While debubbling, pay attention to the hubs and connections of the delivery catheters and sheaths, where air is most likely to collect.

6. Before introducing the collapsed device into the sheath, flush the device forcefully, preferably underwater, to remove any air that might accompany the device into the delivery sheath.

7. After advancing the device into the sheath, remove any introducers from the hub of the delivery sheath that may allow the introduction of air into the closed system.

Potential problems unique to the Premere PFO system

Unlike any of the current double umbrella devices, the Premere PFO Closure system requires delivery of two separate anchors and has additional steps required to lock the two anchors to one another. There are a number of problems which are predictable, given these unique steps.

Lock-related issues

As discussed above, overtightening of the lock can evert the RA occluder into the tunnel of the PFO, and diminish its effective coverage of the defect. Most operators, early in their experience, are likely to overtighten the locking device, fearing that the device might otherwise be unstable. Similarly, the lock can be inadvertently advanced with the cutter device, distorting the RA occluder.

It is generally preferable to have the lock initially too loose rather than too tight. If, after release of the snare, by echocardiography, the device appears to be moving, or is unstable in the septum, the cutter can be used to advance/tighten the lock slightly, prior to cutting the tether.

Echocardiography remains the optimal way to assess the tightness of the lock, as it is deployed. The RA anchor should remain flat against the septal surface throughout deployment. The lock should be advanced just to the hub of the RA anchor. No space should be left between the lock and the anchor hub. If, however, with tightening of the lock, the edges of the RA anchor lift off the septal surface, the occlusive covering on the RA surface will be compromised. The lock is too tight and the device should probably be removed and replaced.

Cutter failure

Rarely, operators have described failure of the cutter device. In this unusual situation, a new device can be opened and the cutter from the new package can be used. If this is unsuccessful, the basket retrieval device can be used to retrieve the device (as below).

Device retrieval

If, during the procedure, the device is in a suboptimal position, the operator may wish to redeploy or remove the device from the patient. The Premere device is unlike some other double occluder devices, which retract easily into the delivery sheath and can be immediately redeployed.

If only the LA anchor has been deployed and needs to be repositioned (i.e. pulled through the defect to the RA), traction on the tether will easily recollapse the anchor into the delivery sheath. If the delivery sheath remains on the LA side of the septum, the anchor can be immediately redeployed.

If both anchors are deployed, one on each side of the septum (prior to locking them together), and the operator feels that the device is inappropriately positioned, traction on the tether will collapse the RA anchor back into the sheath. The sheath can then be advanced over the tether, to the LA, and the LA anchor can be retracted into the sheath. The delivery catheter and device can then be removed from the blue sheath by replacing the introducer through the back-stop valve of the blue sheath.

If both anchors are inadvertently deployed on the same side of the septum, or if the device needs to be retrieved after locking the two anchors together, the Premere device comes with a proprietary retrieval basket to facilitate the safe removal of the device (Figure 27.4). If attempts are made to remove locked anchors or unlocked anchors on the same side of the septum, the anchors may become entangled with one another, and not collapse fully into the sheath.

The white delivery catheter is withdrawn over the tether, and removed from the blue sheath. The retrieval basket is threaded onto the tether (in similar fashion to the cutter). Grounding the tether allows the basket to slide over the tether, through the sheath, to the site of the device. If the anchors are both in the LA, the sheath and basket are advanced over the tether to the LA. The basket is opened in the LA (Figure 27.4a). Traction on the tether and manipulation of the basket will draw the two anchors fully into the mouth of the retrieval basket (Figure 27.4b). Maintaining traction on the tether, and while grounding the blue sheath, the tether and basket are pulled back into the

(a)

(b)

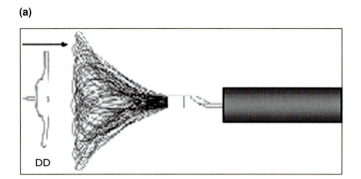

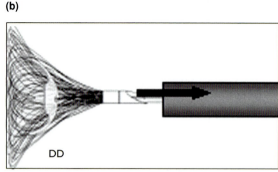

Figure 27.4 Basket retrieval device: (a) The Nitinol retrieval basket is delivered over the tether, and is opened proximal to the deployed device (DD) for retrieval. (b) The device is pulled fully into the wire mesh of the retrieval basket, which is then retracted into the sheath, eliminating the risks of the device edges damaging the sheath or surrounding vascular structures.

sheath. If the anchors are both in the RA, the basket is delivered similarly to the RA. If the device is locked, and straddling the septum, traction on the tether will pull the LA anchor through the PFO to the RA, and retrieval is performed for both anchors in the RA. Replacement of the introducer through the back-stop valve of the blue sheath will allow removal of the basket containing the device, with simultaneous traction on the basket and the tether. If the basket device is used, there is a good chance that the tip of the delivery sheath will be damaged, and should probably be replaced prior to the next attempt to close the PFO.

CONCLUSIONS

The Premere PFO Closure system is a relatively new entrant into the field of percutaneous PFO closure. As a result, long-term outcomes and late complications remain poorly defined. Initial short- and medium-term follow-up indicates that, in terms of closure and complication rates, the Premere is comparable to many of the better established double occluder devices. However, the unique features of the device, particularly its ability to adapt to long PFO tunnel anatomy, have made it an attractive alternative to the better established devices with fixed separation of the two occluders. In many large European laboratories, where a number of PFO devices are commercially available, the Premere system has become the option of choice for long tunnels.

REFERENCES

1. Schräder R. Indication and techniques of transcatheter closure of patent foramen ovale. J Interven Cardiol 2003; 16: 543–51.
2. Martín F, Sánchez PL, Doherty E et al. Percutaneous transcatheter closure of patent foramen ovale in patients with paradoxical embolism. Circulation 2002; 106: 1121–6.
3. Wahl A, Krumsdorf U, Meier B et al. Transcatheter treatment of atrial septal aneurysm associated with patent foramen ovale for prevention of recurrent paradoxical embolism in high-risk patients. J Am Coll Cardiol 2005; 45: 377–80.
4. Schuchlenz HW, Weihs W, Berghold A, Lechner A, Schmidt R. Secondary prevention after cryptogenic cerebrovascular events in patients with patent foramen ovale. Int J Cardiol 2005; 101: 77–82.
5. Windecker S, Wahl A, Nedeltchev K et al. Comparison of medical treatment with percutaneous closure of patent foramen ovale in patients with cryptogenic stroke. J Am Coll Cardiol 2004; 44: 750–8.
6. Krumsdorf U, Ostermayer S, Billinger K et al. Incidence and clinical course of thrombus formation on atrial septal defect and patent foramen ovale closure devices in 1,000 consecutive patients. J Am Coll Cardiol 2004; 43: 302–9.
7. Kiblawi FM, Sommer RJ, Levchuck SG. Transcatheter closure of patent foramen ovale in older adults. Cathet Cardiovasc Interven 2006; 68: 136–42.
8. Cecconi M, Quarti A, Bianchini F et al. Late cardiac perforation after transcatheter closure of patent foramen ovale. Ann Thorac Surg 2006; 81: e29–30.
9. Palma G, Rosapepe F, Vicchio M et al. Late perforation of right atrium and aortic root after percutaneous closure of patent foramen ovale. J Thorac Cardiovasc Surg 2007; 134: 1054–5.
10. Trepels T, Zeplin H, Sievert H et al. Cardiac perforation following transcatheter PFO closure. Cathet Cardiovasc Interven 2003; 58: 111–13.
11. Christen T, Mach F, Didier D et al. Late cardiac tamponade after percutaneous closure of a patent foramen ovale. Eur J Echocardiogr 2005; 6: 465–9.
12. Zajarias A, Thanigaraj S, Lasala J, Perez J. Predictors and clinical outcomes of residual shunt in patients undergoing percutaneous transcatheter closure of patent foramen ovale. J Invas Cardiol 2006; 18: 533–7.
13. Harms V, Reisman M, Fuller CJ et al. Outcomes after transcatheter closure of patent foramen ovale in patients with paradoxical embolism. Am J Cardiol 2007; 99: 1312–15.
14. Büscheck F, Sievert H, Kleber F et al. Patent foramen ovale using the Premere device: the results of the CLOSEUP trial. J Interven Cardiol 2006; 19: 328–33.
15. Rigatelli G, Cardaioli P, Braggion G et al. Resolution of migraine by transcatheter patent foramen ovale closure with Premere Occlusion System in a preliminary series of patients with previous cerebral ischemia. Cathet Cardiovasc Interven 2007; 70: 429–33.
16. Moore KL, Persaud TVN. The Developing Human: Clinically Oriented Embryology, 7th edn. Philadelphia: Saunders Books, 2003.

17. Surmely JF, Meier B. Percutaneous closure of the patent fora-men ovale. Minerva Cardioangiol 2007; 55: 681–91.

18. BheemReddy S, Messineo F, Roychoudhury D. Methemo-globinemia following transesophageal echocardiography: a case report and review. Echocardiography 2006; 23: 319–21.

19. Min JK, Spencer KT, Furlong KT et al. Clinical features of complications from transesophageal echocardiography: a single-center case series of 10,000 consecutive examinations. J Am Soc Echocardiogr 2005; 18: 925–9.

20. Goldstein JA, Beardslee MA, Xu H, Sundt TM, Lasala JM. Infective endocarditis resulting from CardioSEAL closure of a patent fora-men ovale. Cathet Cardiovasc Interven 2002; 55: 217–20.

21. Fernández-Mayoralas DM, Fernández-Jaén A, Muñoz-Jareño N et al. Migraine symptoms related to the percutaneous closure of an ostium secundum atrial septal defect: report of four paediatric cases and review of the literature. Cephalalgia 2007; 27: 550–6.

22. Riederer F, Kaya M, Christina P, Harald G, Peter W. Migraine with aura related to closure of atrial septal defects. Headache 2005; 45: 953–6.

23. Wilmshurst PT, Nightingale S, Walsh KP, Morrison WL. Clopidogrel reduces migraine with aura after transcatheter clo-sure of persistent foramen ovale and atrial septal defects. Heart 2005; 91: 1173–5.

28 Device closure of patent foramen ovale with the Cardia Intrasept device

Massimo Chessa, Gianfranco Butera, and Mario Carminati

Following the introduction of the Cardia PFO Occluder (Cardia, Inc Burnsville, MN) in 1998, it has been systematically modified without changing the general concept of the device, which consists of a double umbrella design with Ivalon sails mounted on Nitinol wires. The sails (0.5 mm thick) are attached to the struts with polypropylene sutures. The free end of each of the stiff Nitinol 'arms' is blunted with a smooth metal tip, in order to prevent their digging into the tissues. The last generation (IV) of the device is called Intrasept (Figure 28.1). The peculiarity is the dual articulating sails with a titanium center post and struts with 19 individual strands of Nitinol that are supposed to maximize fatigue resistance, reducing the risk of wire fracture. The device is available in 20, 25, 30, and 35 mm sizes. The size represents the maximum diameter of the umbrella when measured from tip to tip of an arm.

The Cardia device comes as a Cardia PFO kit, which includes a delivery cable and a 5 French bioptome. Each jaw of the bioptome has a tiny notch which creates a small hole when they are closed. In addition to the hole in the jaws, there is a very secure locking screw mechanism at the proximal end of the delivery cable. The legs of the Cardia devices are flexible from the center, but the individual legs do not bend or flex at any point. This characteristic makes them less conforming to a constraining tunnel; the titanium pivoting center post of the IV generation is supposed to help in this case.

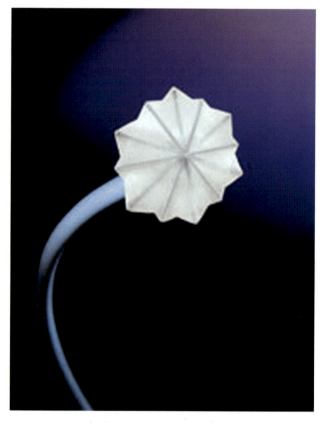

Figure 28.1   The last generation (IV) of the Intrasept device.

COMPLICATIONS

The best way to deal with misadventures in the implantation of the device is to avoid and prevent them.

Groin complications may result from arterial injury, premature ambulation, excessive anticoagulation, or a combination of these, as reported for other devices.[1] Strict attention to anatomic landmarks and allowing for sufficient bed rest after sheath removal should prevent nearly all such complications.

Peri-interventional complications (within 24 hours) occur in 2–4% of cases.[2–4] ST segment elevation appears more frequently in the inferior leads, presumably due to air embolism through the transseptal sheath during device delivery. The ECG changes are usually transient. Most complications were observed using the first-device generations because of the original cumbersome underwater introduction system, which may have produced embolization of small air bubbles. The introduction system was subsequently changed to a more practicable and safer high-pressure flushing-loading system. We suggest that the dilator is retrieved gently to prevent vacuum in the sheath, and well controlled for spontaneous backflow of blood via the sheath side port. This practice may reduce the risk of air embolism. Supraventricular extra beats, atrial tachycardia, and/or atrial fibrillation have been described as transient complications in the peri-interventional period.

The risk of device embolization is far less during patent foramen ovale (PFO) occlusion, assuming that the proper device is used, correct techniques are utilized, and that all of the equipment functions properly. Poor and/or unusual position or setting of the device on the septum can happen. The arms of the device are very flexible and allow the easy withdrawal of the

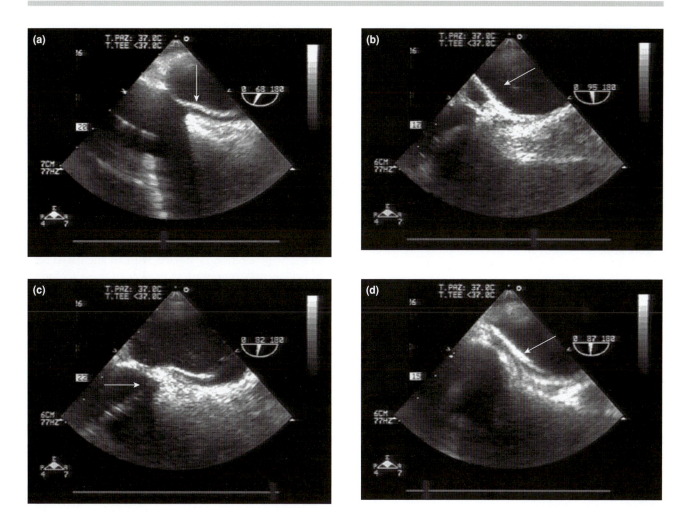

Figure 28.2   (a) The lung tunnel PFO (arrow). (b) The malpositioned device through the PFO (arrow). (c) The transseptal needle pushing the septum primum part of the PFO (arrow). (d) The well positioned implanted device passing through the little hall created with the transseptal puncture (arrow).

device back into the delivery sheath before the device is released, even after both disks have been deployed and without destroying the device. However, if the device is withdrawn back into the sheath after deployment of the proximal umbrella, the right atrial disk is averted within the long sheath. In that case the short introducing sheath (8 French) must be reintroduced into the proximal end of the long sheath and the device withdrawn from the long sheath back into the short sheath, in order to withdraw it through the valve of the long delivery sheath. Once out of the long sheath, the device is delivered from the short sheath and released from the delivery cable. The loading procedure must than be repeated, starting from the beginning, with the new device.

In the case of device embolization the device may be snared either by a simple snare or by using a basket. It is helpful to advance a 0.018 inch guide wire through the 10 French sheath to avoid losing the access during retrieval. For retrieval of the device a 14 French long sheath is necessary.

In order to prevent device malposition/embolization when attaching the closure device to the delivery system (bioptome) ensure it is firmly secured by tugging on the device, and also by confirming that the locking mechanism is fully blocked. Malposition of the device may be the result of the presence of a lung tunnel (Figure 28.2); in this case we can suggest to avoid to pass the PFO, encasing both sides of the atrial septum with a device passed through a created new hall using a transeptal puncture (Figure 28.3).[5] Thrombus formation has been reported on the surface of all the interatrial closure devices, with an occurrence rate of 3–27%.[6–8] Device-adherent thrombus formation has been detected both at the center of the left atrial disc and attached to the expanded Nitinol arms in generation I and II devices.[2] Hence, placement of all Nitinol parts medial to the Ivalon sails, oriented towards the interatrial septum, a design change implemented in the generation III device, may have led to the remarkable reduction in thrombus formation compared with the previous generations.

In order to minimize the risk, it is important to maintain the activated clotting time (ACT) > 200 seconds at the time of device deployment. The use of postprocedural prothrombotic (protamine) therapy should be avoided. The implementation of dual

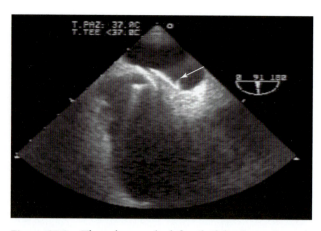

Figure 28.3 Thrombus on the left sail of the device (arrow).

antiplatelet therapy with ASA and clopidogrel for the first 4 weeks postprocedure may help, but there are no randomized studies to support this protocol.

If thrombus is detected before release of the device, it must be taken into account during device withdrawals, as there is a risk of thrombus embolization. If the thrombus is detected at the end of the procedure, after the device has been released, the patient must be put immediately on oral anticoagulation initially with intravenous heparin, and later with warfarin. Repetitive transesophageal echocardiographic (TEE) examinations must be done in order to monitor the thrombus evolution. The device may also be removed surgically, but this is very unusual.

FOLLOW-UP

It is recommended that TEE is performed at 6 months after device implantation, although late thrombotic problems are rare. The rapidity of endocardial coverage of the device is not known; animal studies and examination of devices removed at different time periods after implantation have shown that coating with fibrinogen occurs within the first few hours, and that endocardialization is complete in 4–6 months at the latest.

Arm fractures have been described, but most of them occurred in generation I and II devices, and just a few in generation III;[2] this complication has not been reported for the generation IV device.

The follow-up of all patients must include a detailed 12-lead ECG at rest and a 24-hour Holter test – and ECG if patient complains of palpitations. Supraventricular

tachycardia has been observed,[2] and atrial fibrillation is also possible. As with any occurrence of this arrhythmia, correcting it within the first 24–36 hours after onset is simple, whereas treatment beyond this time frame may necessitate at least 2–3 months of anticoagulation associated with antiarrhythmic drugs.

Pericardial effusion has been detected in few cases;[4] it can be related to the procedure or to device-related cardiac perforation. Perforation seems to be associated with device malposition,[9] which may cause perforation of the aortic wall and a left-to-right shunt between the aortic root and the right atrium. Use of the appropriate size device is important. Thus, devices must fit as well as possible into the individual anatomic structures. The generation IV device, with an angulated central bridge, may represent an answer to these technical problems.

Endocarditis is a potential complication with the device. Careful screening of the patients for infection before the implant, the use of strict sterile techniques, and antibiotic prophylaxis during the implant procedure, avoiding any elective interventions during the 6 months immediately following the implant, should be sufficient to avoid this complication.

REFERENCES

1. Kramer P. Percutaneous closure of PFO with the CardioSEAL/STARFLex occluder in Percutaneous Interventions for Congenital Heart Disease. Informa Health Care 2007; UK Ltd.
2. Braun MU, Fassbender D, Schoen SP et al. Transcatheter closure of patent foramen ovale in patients with cerebral ischemia. J Am Coll Cardiol 2002; 39: 2019–25.
3. Braun MU, Gliech V, Boscheri A et al. Transcatheter closure of PFO in patients with paradoxical embolism. Eur Heart J 2004; 25(5): 424–30.
4. Spies C, Strasheim R, Timmermanns I et al. PFO closure in patients with cryptogenic thrombo-embolic events using the Cardia PFO occluder. Eur Heart J 2006; 27: 365–71.
5. Ruiz CE, Alboliras ET, Pophal, SG. The puncture technique: a new method for transcatheter closure of patent foramen ovale. Cathet Cardiovasc Interven 2001; (53): 369–72.
6. Meier B, Lock JE. Contemporary management of patent foramen ovale. Circulation 2003; 107: 5–9.
7. Jux C, Bertram H. Thrombus formation on intracardiac devices: a complex issue. J Am Coll Cardiol 2004; 44: 1712–13.
8. Meier B. Closure of patent foramen ovale: technique, pitfalls, complications, and follow-up. Heart 2005; 91: 444–8.
9. Lange SA, Schoen SP, Braun MU et al. Perforation of aortic root as secondary complication after implantation of patent foramen ovale occlusion device in a 31-year-old woman. J Interven Cardiol 2006; 19: 166–9.

29 Complications of coarctation stenting in the adult patient

Roy P Venzon and Ziyad M Hijazi

Coarctation of the aorta is a congenital narrowing of the descending thoracic aorta distal to the origin of the left subclavian artery and in the region of the ductus arteriosus. It is a relatively common disorder and accounts for 7% of cases of all known congenital heart disease.[1] The severity of the disease can vary from mild stenosis to complete interruption of the aorta (acquired atresia). Patients who present in adulthood are typically found to be hypertensive and have discrepant pulses between the upper and lower extremities. If left untreated, significant coarctation results in serious morbidity and has a mortality rate of 50% by the age of 32 years, and 92% by the age of 60 years.[2] Because of this, therapy is generally recommended when a pressure gradient of at least 20 mmHg exists between the upper and lower extremities.[3]

Surgical repair was originally the only treatment option available for coarctation of the aorta. However, surgical therapy is associated with potential complications, including paraplegia due to perioperative spinal cord ischemia, recurrent or residual coarctation, aneurysmal formation, and even death.[4] With recent advances in transcatheter interventional techniques, percutaneous therapy has emerged as an alternative treatment for coarctation of the aorta. In particular, the use of angioplasty and stenting has been shown to be effective in the management of aortic coarctation in the adult population.[5-8] The percutaneous approach is less invasive than surgery, and obviates the potential surgical complications mentioned previously. As such, it is currently recommended that stent placement be the treatment of choice for native and recurrent coarctation of the aorta in adult-sized adolescents and adult patients.[3] However, as with any new modality, complications unique to stent implantation have been noted, and great care should be taken to avoid these.

TECHNIQUE

The use of angioplasty and stenting in the treatment of coarctation of the aorta requires the utilization of proper technique by the operator as well as the availability of a wide selection of balloons, stents, wires, and catheters in order to be successful.[3,6,9]

The procedure is ideally performed under general anesthesia. Femoral arterial access is obtained and the coarctation is crossed in a retrograde fashion using an appropriate diagnostic catheter and wire. Hemodynamic evaluation is done to assess the pressure gradient across the coarctation. Aortography is then performed to allow for assessment of the diameter and length of the coarctation, the diameter of the aorta proximal and distal to the stenosis, and the relationship of the narrowed segment to the left subclavian artery and other branches of the aorta. Based on these measurements, balloon and stent sizes are chosen.

After the above diagnostic evaluation is done, a stiff wire with a soft tip is passed retrograde across the coarctation with the aid of an appropriate catheter. The soft tip of the wire is positioned either in the ascending aorta or the left subclavian artery. When stenting the coarctation, it is preferable to position the guide wire in the ascending aorta. This is important so that, if the isthmus is short, the tip of the balloon is not inside the subclavian artery. Inflation of a large balloon inside the subclavian artery may result in damage to this vessel. Further, if the guide wire is in the subclavian artery during stent expansion, the proximal part of the stent may lie unapposed to the wall of the arch, preventing future access to the ascending aorta. A long delivery sheath is then advanced over the wire beyond the lesion. The chosen stent is manually crimped onto the balloon and pushed into the sheath until it reaches the level of the lesion. At this point, the balloon–stent assembly is kept in place while the delivery sheath is withdrawn to uncover the stent. Contrast injection via the side arm of the delivery sheath is performed to confirm proper positioning of the stent in relation to the coarctation. In addition, a catheter from either the brachial artery or via a transseptal approach to the aortic arch may also be used for angiographic monitoring during stent positioning. Once proper positioning is confirmed, the balloon is inflated to deploy the stent. Additional balloon dilatations are performed as needed.

Following stent implantation, repeat hemodynamic evaluation is performed to assess for residual gradient. Repeat aortography is also done to document the final angiographic result and to look for any potential complication.

EQUIPMENT NEEDED

Stents

A wide variety of stents should be available in the cardiac catheterization laboratory when performing coarctation stenting. The stent should be long enough to cover the narrowed segment and the segment of the aorta immediately above and below the coarctation. Furthermore, the stent must have enough radial strength to prevent recoil of the coarctation after it is deployed.

Frequently used stents include the Palmaz XL 10 series stents (Johnson & Johnson Interventional Systems, Warren, NJ), the Palmaz Genesis XD stents (Johnson & Johnson Interventional Systems, Warren, NJ), the IntraStent LD Max stents (ev3, Plymouth, MN), and the covered and bare Cheatham–Platinum stents (NuMED, Inc, Hopkinton, NY). The Palmaz XL stents can expand to a minimum diameter of 10 mm and a maximum diameter of 25 to 28 mm, and come in lengths of 31, 40, and 50 mm. However, they have the disadvantage of significant shortening when fully expanded, as well as having sharp edges. The Palmaz Genesis XD stents have minimal shortening when deployed, but cannot be expanded beyond 18 to 20 mm in diameter. The IntraStent LD Max stents can be expanded to a diameter of 24 to 26 mm, and are available in lengths of 16, 26, and 36 mm with minimal shortening when fully expanded. Finally, the Cheatham–Platinum stents are manufactured as either bare or covered stents. However, they are not readily available in the US.

In addition to the above stents, one should have in the hospital various stent grafts to deploy in cases of dissection of the aorta. Our vascular surgical colleagues have the AneuRx stent graft system (Medtronic Corporation, Santa Rosa, CA) readily available for them and we have used it in one case of dissection with a very good result.

Balloons

Balloons in various lengths and diameters should be available in the cardiac catheterization laboratory when performing coarctation stenting. The balloon used to deploy the stent needs to be slightly longer than the chosen stent, but not by more than 1 cm. The diameter of the balloon should approximate the diameter of the aortic segment above the coarctation.[10] In severe cases, it is recommended that the balloon diameter should not be more than 3.5 times the diameter of the narrowed segment.[11]

The most commonly used balloons include the Z-Med II balloon (NuMED, Inc, Hopkinton, NY) and the Balloon-in-Balloon (BiB) catheter (NuMED, Inc, Hopkinton, NY). The Z-Med II balloon is a high-pressure balloon that is available up to a diameter of 20 mm. The BiB catheter, as the name implies, features a balloon inside a balloon. During stent deployment, inflation of the inner balloon stabilizes the stent on the balloon and allows exact positioning of the stent while minimizing the risk of stripping it off. Once proper placement is achieved, the outer balloon is inflated to deploy the stent. The BiB catheter is available in diameters of 8 to 24 mm. Other less commonly used balloons include the Cordis balloons (Warren, NJ).

Wires

Wires that are stiff, but with a soft tip, are preferred in coarctation stenting. Stiff wires positioned in either the ascending aorta or left subclavian artery are needed to provide an adequate rail for advancing the stent–balloon assembly to the lesion. Frequently used wires include the 260 cm 0.35 inch Rosen wire (Cook, Inc, Bloomington, IN) or the Amplatz Super-Stiff wire (Cook Inc, Bloomington, IN).

Sheaths

Manually crimped stents require delivery via long sheaths in order to minimize the risk of stripping the stent off the balloon while advancing the stent–balloon assembly. With a stent hand crimped on the balloon, the sheath has to be 1 to 2 French sizes greater than what would have been required by the balloon alone. Straight RB-Mullins design sheaths (Cook, Inc, Bloomington, IN) or similar sheaths are preferred.

COMPLICATIONS

Aortic coarctation stenting can be a technically challenging procedure. Even with the use of proper technique and appropriate equipment, complications can still occur. The multi-institutional Congenital Cardiovascular Interventional Study Consortium (CCISC) evaluated 565 aortic coarctation stenting procedures. In their report, procedural complications occurred in 14.3% of cases.[12] However, it was also noted that the frequency of complications has decreased in recent years, partly due to improvement in balloon and stent design as well as operator experience. Complications are generally classified as aortic wall complications, technical complications, and peripheral vascular complications.

Aortic wall complications

Aortic wall complications include intimal tears, dissection, rupture, and aneurysm formation. In the CCISC study, aortic wall complications were noted in 3.9% of the procedures.[12]

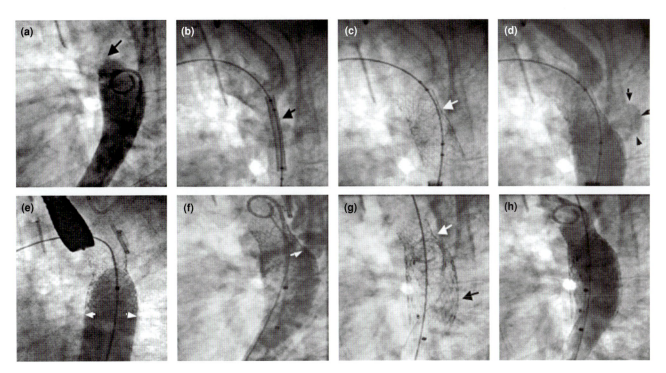

Figure 29.1   Cine angiographic images in the lateral projection in a 26-year-old female patient who underwent coarctation of the aorta stenting. (A) Angiogram in the descending thoracic aorta demonstrating the presence of severe coarctation of the aorta (arrow). (B) Cine image during positioning of a 36 mm long Intrastent Max-LD covered with PFTE (arrow) at the area of coarctation. The stent is mounted on a 16 mm BiB balloon catheter. (C) Cine image after expansion of the stent (arrow). (D) Angiogram via the side arm of the delivery sheath prior to removal of the BiB balloon demonstrating extravasation of contrast outside the vessel (arrows). (E) Cine image during expansion of the distal part of the stent (arrows) using a 20 mm balloon to fully appose the stent to the distal wall of the aorta to prevent extravasation of contrast. (F) Repeat angiogram still demonstrates extravasation of contrast (arrow). (G) Cine image after the deployment of a 3.375 cm long, 22 mm diameter stent graft (AneurRx) partially overlapping the first stent (arrows). (H) Final angiogram demonstrates good result with no extravasation of contrast.

Intimal tears are defined as filling defects within the vessel lumen without any evidence of extravasation outside the vessel lumen. A dissection involves extravasation of contrast outside the vessel lumen (Figure 29.1). These events are most likely due to overdilatation during balloon angioplasty, as well as vessel trauma caused by wire and sheath maneuvering across the coarctation. If possible, prestent angioplasty should be avoided in order to minimize vessel injury. In addition, care should be used when crossing the coarctation with wires or sheaths. Primary stenting minimizes the risk of developing intimal tears or dissections. However, these can still occur in the proximal or distal margins of the stent. If hemodynamically significant dissections are noted at the stent margins, deployment of additional stents may be necessary to tack the dissection against the vessel wall. We prefer to use a stent graft or a covered stent to tack the dissection (Figure 29.1).

Aortic rupture is a potentially catastrophic complication following balloon angioplasty or stenting of aortic coarctation.[13–16] It is frequently caused by the use of oversized balloons or very high pressure inflations. It is imperative that the size of the balloon should not exceed the diameter of the aorta proximal and distal to the coarctation. In more severe cases, it is suggested that the balloon diameter to coarctation diameter ratio should not exceed 3.5:1.[11] In these cases, the achievement of hemodynamic improvement, rather than a perfect angiographic outcome, should be the goal. One can always bring the patient back for redilatation later on, while this is not always possible if catastrophic aortic rupture occurs. In addition to proper balloon sizing, the use of covered stents has also been recommended as a primary therapeutic tool in order to minimize the risk of aortic rupture.[17] The previously mentioned Cheatham–Platinum stents are available as covered stents. Alternatively, hand sewing stretched polytetrafluoroethylene or similar material onto a stent can be done. If aortic rupture does occur, it invariably leads to hemodynamic compromise that requires prompt intervention. The deployment of a covered stent has been used to successfully treat aortic rupture.[18] The availability of premounted balloon dilatable covered stents or self-expanding stent grafts in the cardiac catheterization laboratory is imperative if aortic rupture is to be treated percutaneously in a timely manner.[5,18] Emergent surgical repair may be necessary, and it is always prudent to arrange for surgical back-up prior to performing coarctation stenting.

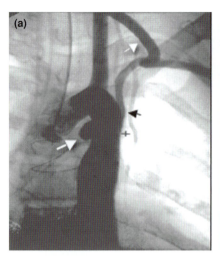
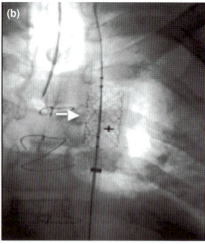
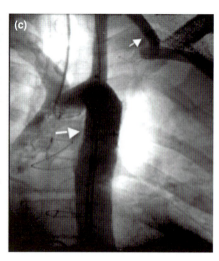

Figure 29.2 Cine angiographic images in the frontal projection. (A) Angiogram in the arch demonstrates the saccular aneurysm (white large arrow) and the left subclavian artery (black arrow) arising opposite to the aneurysm. Note, there is a graft from the left carotid artery to the left subclavian artery (white small arrow). (B) Cine fluoroscopy demonstrating the Genesis covered stent (arrow) deployed at the site of aneurysm. (C) Final angiogram demonstrating total exclusion of the aneurysm (white large arrow) and the left subclavian artery filling from the graft (white small arrow) arising from the left carotid artery (Courtesy of the Journal of Invasive Cardiology: Holzer R, Concilio K, Hijazi ZM. Self-fabricated covered stent to exclude an aortic aneurysm after balloon angioplasty for post-surgical recoarctation. J Invas Cardiol 2005; 17: 177–9.)

Aneurysm formation is defined as an expansion of the aortic wall by greater than 10% compared to the adjoining native lumen that was not present prior to intervention.[12] It may occur around the time of the procedure, or be noted during a follow-up imaging study. As with aortic dissection and rupture, overaggressive balloon dilatation that leads to significant vessel injury and weakening of the aortic wall is the likely cause of aneurysm formation.[6] Proper balloon sizing is needed to avoid this complication. If a small aneurysm is found, this can generally be followed conservatively. However, if the aneurysm is large or is rapidly expanding, it will need to be treated with a covered stent (Figure 29.2) or surgical repair.

Technical complications

Technical complications include stent migration, balloon rupture, and overlap of the stent with a brachiocephalic vessel. In the CCISC study, stent migration occurred in 5.0% and balloon rupture occurred in 2.3% of aortic coarctation stenting procedures.[12]

Stent migration is the most frequent technical complication that occurs with coarctation stenting and is often caused by balloon oversizing, balloon undersizing, or balloon rupture. The use of a balloon that is larger than the segment of the aorta proximal to the coarctation can cause the balloon–stent assembly to slip down during inflation and lead to deployment of the stent distal to the coarctation. On the other hand, undersizing the balloon may result into poor apposition of the stent with the walls of the aorta, and lead to distal migration of the stent as

the balloon is withdrawn. These underscore the need for accurate measurement of the segments of the aorta and proper balloon sizing. Measures that lower stroke volume, such as rapid cardiac pacing or administration of adenosine, may also be used to minimize movement of the balloon–stent assembly during deployment.[19] This allows for more precise stent placement and lowers the risk of stent migration. If stent migration does occur, attempts to retrieve the stent via the delivery sheath should be made. If this cannot be safely done, the stent should be deployed in a segment of the aorta that has no significant side branches.

Balloon rupture during initial stent deployment is the second most common technical complication. Issues associated with balloon rupture include embolization of balloon fragments with subsequent need for surgical removal, and stent migration due to incomplete expansion of the stent.[3] Balloon rupture is primarily linked to the use of Palmaz 8 series stents (Johnson & Johnson Interventional Systems, Warren, NJ), which have sharp edges. With advancement in balloon technology and the availability of stents that have rounded edges, the occurrence of balloon rupture has decreased. The use of balloons that are much longer than the stent also predisposes to balloon rupture by causing an exaggerated dumbbell shape during inflation. It is important that the balloon used should not be more than 1 cm longer than the stent to minimize this risk.

Stent placement over the origin of one or more brachiocephalic vessels should be avoided, although this is not always possible. Careful examination of the arch aortogram and other imaging studies should be done to determine the exact relationship of the coarctation to the arch vessels. If the origin of the left subclavian artery is in close proximity to the coarctation, then placing a stent across its origin is unavoidable. Fortunately, this has not been demonstrated to have any harmful sequelae.[3] For obvious reasons, covered stents should not be used in these situations.

Peripheral vascular complications

Peripheral vascular complications include cerebrovascular accidents and access vessel complications. In the CCISC study, cerebrovascular accidents occurred in 0.7% and access vessel complications occurred in 2.3% of aortic coarctation stenting procedures.[12]

Neurologic events such as cerebrovascular accidents happen very infrequently, and when they do occur, they most often occur in association with other complications, such as balloon rupture, stent migration, and aortic dissection.[3,12] Adequate heparinization is a standard part of coarctation stenting. However, measures taken to avoid the associated complications mentioned above likely have as much of an impact on decreasing the occurrence of neurologic complications.

Access site complications include bleeding complications and acute vessel closure.[3,12] The use of large-sized sheaths during coarctation stenting places these patients at a relatively higher risk of access site bleeding. Care should be taken to ensure that the vessel is punctured at the common femoral artery level. In these cases, manual compression of the access site usually provides adequate hemostasis. However, puncture above the inguinal ligament renders manual compression less effective and may lead to hematoma formation or retroperitoneal bleeding. The use of micropuncture technique may be used to confirm puncture of the artery at the common femoral level prior to placing a large bore sheath. Transcatheter vessel closure devices may also be employed, especially when larger bore sheaths are used.

Acute vessel closure involving the femoral artery may also occur. Patients with coarctation of the aorta frequently have smaller caliber vessels in the lower extremities. This, in conjunction with the use of large sheaths, puts them at risk of developing acute femoral artery closure. Patients should be monitored closely after the procedure, and particular attention should be paid to peripheral pulses. In patients who do develop acute closure of the femoral artery, heparinization and thrombolytic therapy should be initiated. If distal pulses fail to return despite these measures, surgical intervention may be necessary.

CONCLUSION

In conclusion, angioplasty and stenting for aortic coarctation in adults is a highly demanding procedure that requires the use of meticulous technique on the part of the operator and the availability of proper equipment in the cardiac catheterization laboratory in order to be successful. The operator needs to be aware of the possible complications associated with this procedure in order to be able to prevent them from happening, or to be able to treat them when they do occur.

REFERENCES

1. Fyler DC, Buckley LP, Hellenbrand WE, Cohn HE. Report of the New England Regional Infant Cardiac Program. Pediatrics 1980; 65(Suppl): 376–60.
2. Campbell M. Natural history of coarctation of the aorta. Br Heart J 1970; 32: 633–40.
3. Golden AB, Hellenbrand WE. Coarctation of the aorta: stenting in children and adults. Cathet Cardiovasc Interven 2007; 69: 289–99.
4. Gibbs JL. Treatment options for coarctation of the aorta. Heart 2000; 84: 11–13.
5. Mahadevan VS, Vondermuhll IF, Mullen MJ. Endovascular aortic coarctation stenting in adolescents and adults: angiographic and hemodynamic outcomes. Cathet Cardiovasc Interven 2006; 67: 268–75.
6. Piechaud JF. Stent implantation for coarctation in adults. J Interven Cardiol 2003; 16: 413–18.
7. Shah L, Hijazi ZM, Sandhu S, Joseph A, Cao QL. Use of endovascular stents for the treatment of coarctation of the aorta in children and adults: immediate and midterm results. J Invas Cardiol 2005; 11: 614–18.
8. Harrison DA, McLaughlin PR, Lazzam C, Connelly M, Benson LN. Endovascular stents in the management of coarctation of the aorta in the adolescent and adult: one year follow up. Heart 2001; 85: 561–6.
9. Cheatham, JP. Stenting of coarctation of the aorta. Cathet Cardiovasc Interven 2001; 54: 112–25.
10. Pedra CA, Fontes VF, Esteves CA et al. Stenting vs balloon angioplasty for discrete unoperated coarctation of the aorta in adolescents and adults. Cathet Cardiovasc Interven 2005; 64: 495–506.
11. Forbes TJ, Moore P, Pedra CA et al. Intermediate follow-up following intravascular stenting for treatment of coarctation of the aorta. Cathet Cardiovasc Interven 2007; 70: 569–77.
12. Forbes TJ, Garekar S, Amin Z et al. Procedural results and acute complications in stenting native and recurrent coarctation of the aorta in patients over 4 years of age: a multi-institutional study. Cathet Cardiovasc Interven 2007; 70: 276–85.
13. Varma C, Benson LN, Butany J, McLaughlin PR. Aortic dissection after stent dilatation for coarctation of the aorta: a case report and literature review. Cathet Cardiovasc Interven 2003; 59: 528–35.
14. Korkola SJ, Tchervenkov CI, Shum-Tim D, Roy N. Aortic rupture after stenting of a native coarctation in an adult. Ann Thorac Surg 2002; 74: 936.
15. Kulick DL, Kotlewski A, Hurvitz RJ et al. Aortic rupture following percutaneous catheter balloon coarctoplasty in an adult. Am Heart J 1990; 119: 190–3.
16. Balaji S, Oommen R, Rees PG. Fatal aortic rupture during balloon dilatation for recoarctation. Br Heart J 1991; 65: 100–1.
17. Hijazi ZM. Catheter intervention for adult aortic coarctation: be very careful! Cathet Cardiovasc Interven 2003; 59: 536–7.
18. Tan JL, Mullen M. Emergency stent graft deployment for acute aortic rupture following primary stenting for aortic coarctation. Cathet Cardiovasc Interven 2005; 65: 306–9.
19. Daehnert I, Rotzsch C, Wiener M, Schneider P. Rapid right ventricular pacing is an alternative to adenosine in catheter interventional procedures for congenital heart disease. Heart 2004; 90: 1047–50.

30 Complications of alcohol septal ablation

Karen M Smith

HYPERTROPHIC CARDIOMYOPATHY

Hypertrophic cardiomyopathy (HCM) is the most commonly occurring genetic cardiovascular disease with a prevalence in the general population estimated to be 0.2%[1,2] It is caused by mutations in any one of 10 genes encoding cardiac sarcomeric proteins with structural, regulatory, or contractile functions.[3–5] Phenotypic expression is influenced not only by genetic mutation, but also by modifier genes and environmental factors, and may result in substantial molecular, anatomic, pathophysiologic, and clinical heterogeneity.[3,5] Patients may have global hypertrophy, apical hypertrophy, mid cavity obliteration, and/or basal septal hypertrophy. Diastolic dysfunction, myocardial ischemia, and obstruction to late blood flow out of the left ventricle appear to be pathophysiologic features which are responsible for reduced exercise capacity, functional limitations, and other symptoms.[3–7] Twenty-five percent of patients with HCM have evidence of obstruction of the left ventricular outflow tract (LVOT).[3,8] As stated in the American College of Cardiology/European Society of Cardiology Clinical Expert Consensus Document on Hypertrophic Cardiomyopathy:[5]

> It is important to distinguish between obstructive and nonobstructive forms of HCM, based on presence or absence of a LV outflow gradient at rest and/or with provocation since management is tailored to the hemodynamic state. Outflow gradients are responsible for a loud apical systolic ejection murmur associated with a constellation of unique clinical signs, hypertrophy of the basal portion of ventricular septum and small outflow tract, and an enlarged and elongated mitral valve in many patients. Obstruction may either be subaortic or mid-cavity in location. Subaortic obstruction is caused by systolic anterior motion (SAM) of the mitral valve leaflets and mid-systolic contact with the ventricular septum. This mechanical impedance to outflow occurs in the presence of high velocity ejection in which a variable proportion of the forward blood flow may be ejected early in systole. Systolic anterior motion is probably attributable to a drag effect or possibly a Venturi phenomenon and is responsible not only for subaortic obstruction, but also the concomitant mitral regurgitation (usually mild-to-moderate in degree) due to incomplete

> leaflet apposition, which is typically directed posteriorly into the left atrium. When the mitral regurgitation jet is directed centrally or anteriorly into the left atrium or if multiple jets are present, independent abnormalities intrinsic to the mitral valve should be suspected (e.g. myxomatous degeneration, mitral leaflet fibrosis, or anomalous papillary muscle insertion). Occasionally (perhaps in 5% of cases), gradients and impeded outflow are caused predominately by muscular apposition in the mid-cavity region – usually in the absence of mitral-septal contact – involving anomalous direct insertion of anterolateral papillary muscle into the anterior mitral leaflet, or excessive mid-ventricular or papillary muscle hypertrophy and malalignment.

> There is general agreement that a subaortic gradient > 30 mm Hg and associated elevations in intra-cavitary LV pressure reflect impedance to outflow that is of pathophysiologic and prognostic importance. Obstruction is a strong, independent predictor of disease progression to death (relative risk vs. nonobstructed patients, 2.0), to severe symptoms (NYHA class III or IV), and to death due to heart failure and stroke (relative risk vs. nonobstructed patients, 4.4). However, the likelihood of severe symptoms and death from outflow tract obstruction was not greater when the gradient was > 30 mm Hg.

> Clinical consequences of chronic outflow gradients are believed to be mediated by the resultant increase in LV wall stress, ischemia and eventual cell death and fibrosis. Therefore, outflow obstruction justifies intervention to reduce subaortic gradients in severely symptomatic patients refractory to medical management. The obstruction is characteristically dynamic as the magnitude of an outflow gradient may vary spontaneously or with physiologic alterations (e.g. drugs, heavy meal or ingestion of alcohol).

> Patients may be divided into hemodynamic subgroups by peak instantaneous gradient with continuous wave Doppler: **Obstructive** – ≥ 30 mm Hg (2.7 m/s by Doppler) with basal (resting) conditions, **Latent (provocable) obstructive** – < 30 mm Hg under basal conditions and ≥ 20 mm Hg with provocation, and **Nonobstructive** – < 30 mm Hg under both basal and provocable conditions. LV outflow gradients are measured noninvasively with

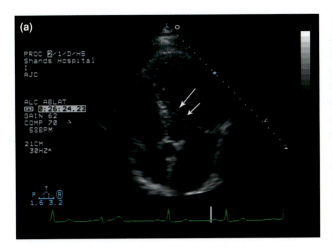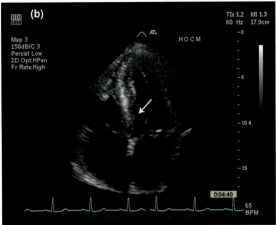

Figure 30.1   (A) Apical four-chamber view of a patient with hypertrophic cardiomyopathy prior to ASA. ASH (large arrow) and SAM (small arrow) were present and the LVOT Doppler flow velocity was 3.4 m/s, reflecting a resting pressure gradient of 45.2 mmHg. (B) Apical four-chamber view of the same patient 3 months following ASA showing regression in basal septal thickness. SAM and LVOT gradient were no longer present.

continuous wave Doppler echocardiography, generally obviating need for serial cardiac catheterizations except when CAD or other associated anomalies such as valvular disease are suspected.

A variety of interventions have been used to elicit gradients (i.e. amyl nitrite inhalation, Valsalva maneuver, post-premature ventricular contraction response, isoproterenol or dobutamine infusion, standing posture, and physiologic exercise), however, rigorous standardization for these maneuvers has been lacking, and many are non-physiologic. To define latent pressure gradients during and/or immediately following exercise for management decisions, exercise testing with Doppler echocardiography is the most physiologic and preferred provocative maneuver since symptoms often occur with exertion.[5]

THERAPEUTIC OPTIONS

Alcohol septal ablation (ASA) is a percutaneous procedure originally introduced to treat HCM instead of surgical septal myectomy/myotomy. While the surgical approach yielded somewhat better results in terms of improved exercise parameters in uncontrolled trials, both approaches were similarly effective at reducing obstruction and subjective exercise limitation in appropriately selected patients.[9] But the ease of use, safety, and possibility of repeat ablations have resulted in an increased use of the percutaneous approach. These qualities have also prompted earlier referral of patients in the course of disease, particularly for those who do not tolerate large doses of β-blockers and calcium channel blockers (Figure 30.1).

SELECTION OF PATIENTS

While there may be some minor variations, most interventionalists use the following as criteria to select candidates for alcohol septal ablation:[5,10–16]

1. Symptoms despite medical therapy (NYHA class III/IV), or intolerant of medical therapy.
2. Asymmetric septal hypertrophy (ASH) with septal thickness ≥ 13 mm and/or a septal-to-posterior wall ratio of 1.3.
3. Systolic anterior motion of the mitral valve (SAM).
4. Left ventricular outflow tract obstruction (due to ASH and SAM) demonstrated by resting gradient ≥ 30 mm Hg and/or provocable gradient ≥ 50 mm Hg. Provocation may be accomplished with Valsalva maneuver, inhalation of amyl nitrite, postPVC beat, but is most reliably and physiologically evaluated with exercise.
5. Possibly late systolic closure of the aortic valve.
6. Acceptable coronary artery anatomy.
7. Absence of concomitant cardiac disease that requires surgical correction.
8. Patients with increased surgical risk due to comorbid conditions.

PROCEDURE TECHNIQUE

The objective of ASA is to safely administer 100% ethanol into the muscular interventricular septum producing LVOT obstruction and contributing to systolic anterior motion of the mitral valve. This is accomplished by injection of alcohol through the central lumen of an over-the-wire balloon catheter into the septal perforator branches of the left anterior descending coronary artery which supply the septal myocardium in the region of obstruction. Therefore, ASA uses techniques and methodology similar or identical to the performance of percutaneous coronary interventional (PCI) procedures such as balloon angioplasty. Most operators perform the procedure under fluoroscopic guidance in the cardiac catheterization laboratory as well as live echocardiographic monitoring.[10–13,16–18]

Preparation

The patient is prepared for the procedure in a similar manner to diagnostic cardiac catheterization and coronary interventional procedures. Appropriate informed consent is obtained. The procedure is performed under typical sterile technique in the cardiac catheterization laboratory. Due to the potential for the development of complete heart block (CHB), if the patient does not have a permanent pacemaker or implantable cardioverter defibrillator (ICD), then a temporary pacemaker is placed percutaneously via central vein access and appropriate function is confirmed.[5,10,12]

Diagnostic cardiac catheterization

If the patient has not previously had a diagnostic cardiac catheterization, it is performed at this time.[5,10,12] It is particularly important to evaluate for communication of septal perforator arteries between the left anterior descending (LAD) and posterior descending (PDA) coronary arteries. It is also important to identify and quantify the severity of coronary artery disease (CAD) or any coronary anomalies that may be present. The number, distribution, size, and anatomy of the septal perforator arteries supplying the interventricular septum should be carefully identified. Most septal perforators which supply the interventricular septum in the area of the LVOT originate from the proximal portion of the LAD. However, septal perforators supplying this area have also been noted to originate from ramus intermedius, circumflex or obtuse marginal branches, the proximal right coronary artery (RCA), and PDA.[5,10,12] During angiography it is important to note which septal perforators may supply the area of obstruction. This is later confirmed under echocardiographic guidance.[5,10,17,18] It is also important to note the size and the angle from which septal branches originate from the LAD, as it may be important in gaining access to the arteries with a guide wire as well as in selection of balloon size (Figure 30.2).

Concomitant CAD

It may be desirable to treat obstructive coronary artery lesions at the time of angiography, and return to the

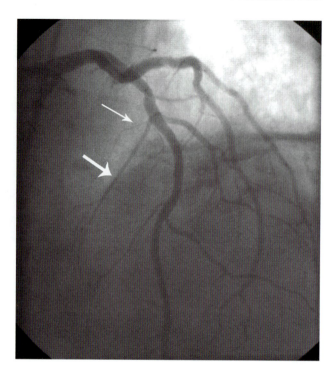

Figure 30.2 AP cranial view angiogram demonstrating the septal perforator (large arrow) and its origin from the proximal LAD (small arrow).

cath lab at a later date for the performance of the ASA procedure. However, percutaneous treatment of coronary lesions in the same procedure as the ASA has been described and can be safely accomplished.[19]

Measuring the gradient

A catheter is placed in the left ventricle for monitoring of the gradient between the left ventricle and aorta throughout the procedure.[5,10,12] A guiding catheter is placed via (usually) femoral arterial access with the tip in the ostium of the left main coronary artery (LMCA). It is important to use a coaxial guiding catheter and avoid pressure of the catheter against the wall of the left main coronary artery in order to avoid potential dissections.[12] The pressure gradient is measured between the left ventricular and guiding catheters. Sometimes, if the patient is sedated, if the blood pressure is low, or due to the dynamic nature of hypertrophic cardiomyopathy, a resting gradient is not observed in the cath lab, although a significant gradient has been documented on many occasions. In this case, the gradient may be provoked by postPVC beat, Valsalva, or inhalation of amyl nitrite. Rarely, the gradient will not be seen under resting or even provocable conditions in the cath lab. If the gradient has previously been definitively documented, I will proceed with the ASA procedure even under these circumstances.

Wires and balloon catheters

The septal perforator coronary artery estimated to supply the area of asymmetric septal hypertrophy and obstruction is wired with a 0.014 inch × 300 cm angioplasty guide wire.[5,10,11] Generally a medium-weight, floppy-tipped, all-purpose guide wire is most effective, such as a Balance Middle Weight™ (Guidant Corporation, Santa Clara, CA), Traverse® (Guidant), or Asahi Prowater™ (Abbott Vascular Devices, Redwood City, CA). Often septal perforators are angulated and considerable steering and finesse are required to wire the vessel.

An over-the-wire balloon catheter is advanced over the guide wire into the septal perforator artery.[5,10,11] It is important to choose an appropriately sized balloon (1.0 or 1.1 ratio to the perforator diameter). Oversized balloons may result in vessel dissection and undersized balloons may result in incomplete occlusion. When this procedure was first developed, only balloons of 15 mm in length were available. The shorter balloons available today are easier to track into septal perforator vessels and allow more precise placement fully within the septal perforator without projecting into the LAD.[5,10,11] Most frequently I employ a 1.5, 2.0, or 2.5 mm (diameter) by 9 mm (length) Maverick™ (Boston Scientific Corporation, Natick, Massachusetts) over-the-wire angioplasty dilation catheter. The balloon is advanced into the proximal portion of the septal perforator so that it is located entirely within the perforator branch and does not project backwards into the LAD, which may result in alcohol tracking retrograde along the sides of the inflated balloon and into the parent coronary artery.[5,10,11]

In general, the balloon should be inflated to a nominal or moderate inflation pressure, but should completely occlude the septal artery. Angiography should be performed with injection of radiographic contrast through the guiding catheter into the LAD (or parent) coronary artery, and should demonstrate no flow of contrast around the balloon into the septal artery. Radiographic contrast is injected through the central lumen of the balloon catheter into the septal artery under cine angiography. This should demonstrate no reflux of contrast retrograde around the balloon catheter into the parent coronary artery. Likewise, communication with other septal perforator arteries, the RCA, the distal LAD, or other vessels or structures should be noted. Simultaneous echocardiography should be performed. Radiographic contrast often enhances the area of the septum supplied by the septal perforator on echocardiography. This will confirm that the septal perforator supplies the area of the interventricular septum desirable for alcohol injection. Sometimes, radiographic contrast is not visible on echocardiography.[10,11]

If radiographic contrast tracks retrograde around the balloon, then adjustments should be made. Possibilities include choosing a larger balloon size, inflating the balloon to a higher pressure, or repositioning the balloon, usually more distally in the septal perforator. Under no circumstances should alcohol be injected if there is

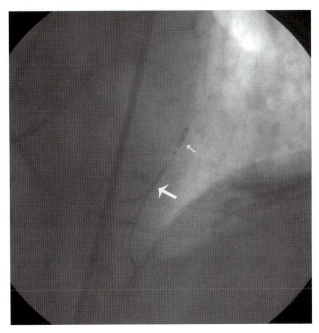

Figure 30.3 AP cranial view angiogram of injection of radiographic contrast through the central lumen of the balloon catheter. Contrast fills the septal artery (large arrow)and does not track retrograde around the inflated balloon (small arrow).

evidence of contrast leak around the balloon or communication with other cardiac structures[10,11] (Figure 30.3).

Myocardial contrast echocardiography

Most operators use myocardial contrast echocardiography (MCE) to confirm appropriate balloon placement in the arterial supply to the interventricular septum.[5,10–12,16–18] Between 1 and 2 cc of an echo contrast agent such as Definity® (Bristol Myers Squibb, North Billerica, MA) is administered by injection through the central lumen of the balloon catheter and visualized under echocardiography. The area of the septum supplied by the septal perforator will be enhanced by the echo contrast agent. If the contrasted area correlates with the area of Doppler flow acceleration and coaptation between the septum and SAM, then this is the appropriate septal perforator into which to inject alcohol. Assessment in multiple views should be performed to rule out echo contrast enhancement of other areas of the myocardium, indicating septal artery communication with other important structures, such as the right ventricular moderator band, right side of the ventricular septum, inferior walls, apex, papillary muscles, and other cardiac structures[10,11,13,20,21] (Figure 30.4).

In postmarketing use, 4 patients who received Definity® Injectable Suspension experienced fatal cardiac arrests during or within 30 minutes of administration. The US Food and Drug Administration (FDA) issued a Healthcare Provider Advisory alert in October 2007

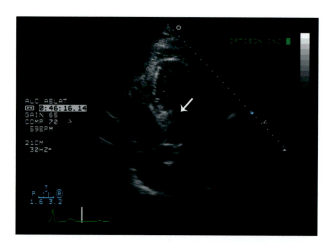

Figure 30.4 Apical four-chamber view. Injection of echo-cardiographic contrast through the central lumen of the balloon catheter into the septal artery enhances the area of the interventricular septum (arrow) causing LVOT obstruction.

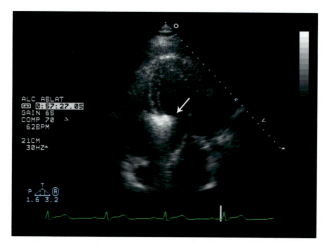

Figure 30.5 Apical four-chamber view of the same patient following injection of alcohol through the central lumen of the balloon catheter into the septal artery. Note the 'bright' or enhanced area of the septum (arrow).

advising that patients be assessed for conditions that preclude Definity administration and monitoring patients for 30 minutes following administration.[22] We continue to use Definity in accordance with these recommendations.

Some operators advocate the use of agitated saline instead of echocardiographic contrast for visualization of the interventricular septum. I have found this to be unreliable for optimal visualization. Others report injecting no contrast whatsoever, but using decrease of the pressure gradient which occurs due to occlusion of the septal perforator with balloon inflation as evidence of balloon location in the appropriate septal artery.[14,23] While this appears to be effective, it does not provide visual evidence of communication of the septal artery with other areas of the heart which could be injured by alcohol injection.

Injection of echo contrast agents into a septal perforator artery frequently produces rapid opacification of the left ventricular cavity. This generally occurs within 2–3 heartbeats. On two occasions I have observed the instantaneous appearance of echo contrast in the LV cavity by a jet from the area of the septum. Because this may represent direct communication between the septal artery and left ventricle, and could potentially jeopardize LV endocardial tissue, I did not inject alcohol.[24]

Alcohol administration

After the balloon is appropriately placed in the septal perforator artery, the balloon is demonstrated to completely occlude the septal perforator, and the area supplied by the septal perforator has been confirmed to be the obstructing area, then 98–100% dehydrated alcohol (American Regent, Inc, Shirley, New York) is injected through the central lumen of the balloon catheter into the septal perforator artery.[5,10–18,25] Continuous echocardiographic visualization will show enhancement of the interventricular septum when alcohol perfuses the myocardium. Echo visualization of other areas of the heart such as the distal septum, left ventricular apex, anterior wall, papillary muscles, and inferior walls should be frequently monitored for enhancement and hypokinesia which is evidence of alcohol penetration into undesirable areas of the heart. If this should occur, the procedure should be immediately terminated (Figure 30.5).

The volume of alcohol to be injected , the rate of injection, and the number of septal perforator arteries to be injected are issues of considerable discussion, vary somewhat among operators, and appear to require some amount of judgment and experience. In general, 1–3 cc absolute alcohol are injected into the area of the interventricular septum which contributes to LVOT obstruction. In some patients this involves injection of one large septal perforator, and in other patients this may involve injection of two or more smaller arteries or branches.

Fernandez *et al.*, under the direction of Prinicipal Investigator Dr William H Spencer III, who first performed this procedure in the United States, reported the average amount of alcohol injected as 3.5 ± 1.5 cc and the average number of septal perforators injected as 1.5 ± 0.6 after 5 years of experience performing the procedure in 130 patients.[12] Ten-year data (619 patients) indicate a slight decrease in these averages to 2.6 ± 1.0 cc of alcohol and 1.3 ± 0.5 septal arteries injected.[26] In our experience of about 106 patients we have injected a mean of 2.3 ± 0.6 cc of alcohol and the average number of septal perforators injected was 1.3 ± 0.6. Injection of higher volumes of alcohol has been reported to result in a higher occurrence of complete heart block and may needlessly injure adjacent cardiac structures.[5,10,21,23,27–29]

While it might seem reasonable to believe the injection of substantially less alcohol may result in a less effective procedure, this is not necessarily the case. Veselka et al. found that, while higher doses of alcohol correlated with higher peak CK-MB, there was no correlation between peak CK and LVOT gradient in the follow-up period.[28] Nagueh et al. found only moderate correlation between MCE septal area and reduction in LVOT gradient. Larger areas of infarction did correlate with larger reductions in outflow gradient. But precision appears to be more important: when alcohol injection was directed to the main area of the septum causing obstruction, patients had small defects with a large reduction in gradient. Therefore, 'targeted delivery of ethanol is of great potential importance in view of the detrimental effects of large infarctions on left ventricular function and the subsequent risks of ventricular arrhythmias and complete heart block'.[18]

Rate of alcohol delivery varies among operators. Holmes et al. reported typically injecting 1–1.5 ml of alcohol over approximately 10 minutes, depending on the size of the septal perforator artery and the volume of septum to be ablated.[10] We inject at a rate of approximately 1 cc over 5 minutes. Faster rates of injection may result in higher instances of complete heart block and the need for permanent pacemaker implantation[10–12,24,26] and perhaps less effective procedures. Slower rates of injection are likely unnecessary. However, one study in piglets found significant differences in myocardial infarct size with different amounts of alcohol injected, but no apparent differences in infarct size with different speeds of alcohol injection.[30,31]

The number of septal perforating arteries injected with alcohol varies somewhat between operators, and is influenced by septal anatomy, but most reports indicate an average number between 1.0 and 2.0.[5,10,12,26] The number of septal branches injected is associated with larger infarcts and may correlate with total area of the septal myocardial injury.[18,29] It is likely that focused delivery to the area of obstruction, whether accomplished by injection of one artery or more, is the important issue.

Following injection of the desired amount of alcohol, the balloon is left in place for another 2–10 minutes and the alcohol is allowed to dwell or disperse.[5,10,11,18,32] This may lessen the incidence of alcohol spill into the parent coronary artery when the balloon is deflated and may allow more time for the alcohol to produce the desired effect.

Many operators flush saline through the central lumen of the balloon before it is deflated to clear the balloon lumen of alcohol, so as to reduce the risk of alcohol spilling out of the catheter as it is withdrawn into the parent coronary artery.[10,18] However, this is not my usual practice, because I feel it may potentially dilute the alcohol injected into the septal myocardium. Without reinsertion of the guide wire, a 3 cc luer-lock syringe is placed on the central lumen of the balloon catheter and the contents are aspirated as the balloon is deflated and withdrawn through the guiding catheter. In order to avoid alcohol contamination with any other equipment the balloon catheter is discarded immediately. In order to avoid the potential for mistakenly injecting the alcohol into unwanted areas or through other equipment, we do not open the alcohol until we are ready to inject it through the central lumen of the balloon catheter. We use a 3 cc luer-lock syringe, carefully note the initial amount of alcohol in the syringe, and inject approximately 1.0 to 1.5 cc of alcohol per septal perforator depending on the size of the artery and area of the vascular bed perfused by the vessel.

Postinjection angiography, echocardiography, and evaluation of gradient

It is extremely important to monitor coronary blood flow intermittently throughout the injection of alcohol. With any evidence of impaired blood flow into any of the coronary arteries, the procedure should be terminated immediately because this most likely indicates alcohol 'spill' or injection into an unwanted area. Because alcohol produces myocardial cell death, it is unlikely that any vasodilators will improve slow-flow or no-reflow into the coronary arterial system. It is important to continue to monitor the entire myocardium with echo throughout the procedure, being vigilant for enhancement or hypokinesis which could indicate alcohol in unwanted areas.

Angiography should be performed following the procedure to rule out evidence of impairment of coronary blood flow, coronary artery dissection, disruption of atherosclerotic plaques, and other complications. The septal perforator which has been injected with alcohol usually appears occluded following the procedure.

Echocardiography should be performed immediately afterwards to confirm normal wall motion in all other areas and to evaluate LVOT gradient.

Most operators use immediate postinjection reduction of the LV gradient to assess efficacy of the procedure and guide their judgment on the amount of alcohol to administer.[10,18] Holmes et al. reported criteria as follows: 'If the resting gradient is more than 30 mm Hg, the goal is to decrease it to less than 10 mm Hg. If the resting gradient is less than 30 mm Hg at baseline, but there is a significant provokable gradient, the goal is to decrease that provokable gradient by more than 50%'.[10] I have found that if a resting and/or provocable gradient is present at the beginning of the procedure, this is quite useful in determining efficacy of the procedure. However, in some cases, due to the dynamic nature of hypertrophic cardiomyopathy, and possibly due to sedation in some patients, resting or provocable gradient is not present during the procedure although it has been reliably documented previously. In-lab reduction in gradient and postprocedure CK elevation have been shown to correlate with procedural efficacy.[33] (Figures 30.6 and 30.7).

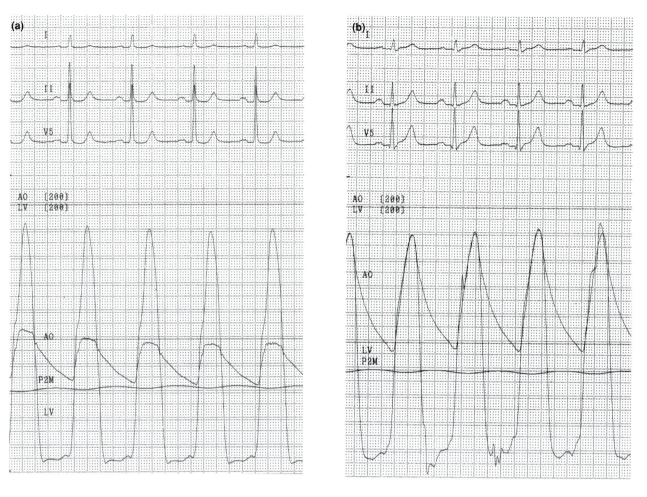

Figure 30.6 Hemodynamic tracings of simultaneous left ventricular and arterial pressure waveforms before (A) and immediately after (B) injection of alcohol indicating reduction of the pressure gradient from 60 to 0 mmHg.

Pain

Injection of the alcohol into the myocardium typically produces chest pain in most patients. Frequently it is moderately intense for 1 to 2 minutes and then gradually subsides. Therefore, I generally sedate patients prior to alcohol injection until they are asleep but still arousable. If patients experience severe, prolonged, or escalating chest pain, and particularly if it is not very responsive to medications, an alcohol 'spill' or communication into another myocardial area is likely. If the patient experiences this type of pain, particularly if accompanied by significant ST elevation, a vigilant search for problems with coronary blood flow and occurrence of remote myocardial injury should be immediately undertaken.

Follow-up echocardiography

Because the myocardium becomes non-contractile when injected with alcohol, the left ventricular pressure gradient frequently resolves in the catheterization laboratory. However, probably due to inflammation and edema of the LVOT myocardium, gradients are often seen the following day and do not correlate with ultimate results of the procedure. Therefore, it is recommended that echocardiography not be performed in the days immediately following alcohol ablation other than to assess for complications. I generally do not perform echocardiographic evaluation until 3 months postprocedure.

COMPLICATIONS

Because the alcohol septal ablation procedure involves techniques identical to those used in diagnostic cardiac catheterization, PCI, and placing of temporary pacing wires, complications encountered with those procedures may occur with ASA. These include vascular access site complications such as infection, bleeding (local, retroperitoneal, rectus abdominus, etc.), hematoma, vascular injury (dissection, perforation, thrombosis, embolization, acute closure), arteriovenous fistula, and pseudoaneurysm.

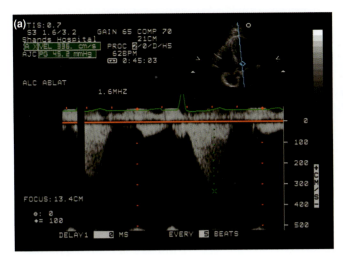
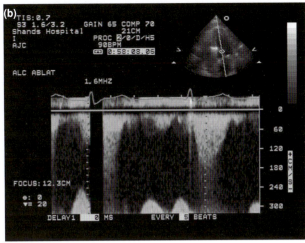

Figure 30.7   Apical four-chamber Doppler waveform before (A) and immediately after (B) injection of alcohol demonstrating reduction in LVOT flow velocity from 3.4 to 1.8 m/s (normal).

Cardiac or central vascular complications may include coronary artery dissection, perforation, occlusion/acute closure, thrombosis, distal embolization, occlusion of branch vessels, myocardial infarction, and transient ischemia attack (TIA) or stroke. Other complications include contrast nephropathy/renal failure, cholesterol embolization syndrome, hypoventilation, allergic or anaphylactoid reaction/anaphylaxis, arrhythmia, need for emergency surgery, need for blood transfusion, postprocedure pulmonary embolism, and death. Complications associated with placing temporary pacing wires may include bleeding, vessel or cardiac perforation, pericardial effusion/cardiac tamponade, pneumothorax/chest tube, air embolus, arrhythmias, and impairment of visualization of cardiac structures. Detailed discussions of these complications are outlined elsewhere relative to these procedures.[34–36] Table 30.1 outlines the complications associated with ASA.

Inability to perform procedure/no alcohol administered

Occasionally it is not safe or possible to administer alcohol. Reasons for this include poor access to septal arteries, anatomic barriers, collateral blood flow into other vessels or cardiac structures, or other procedural complications. Singh *et al.* evaluated the anatomic characteristics of the septal perforating arteries in 10 autopsy hearts and found substantial variability in size and distribution.[35] Patients may have one large branching septal perforator; multiple moderately sized branches that originate individually from the LAD; multiple tiny branches; first and second septals originating from a common ostium or second septal branch originating from the first; anomalous origins from coronary arteries other than the LAD; as well as significant variation in length, diameter, branching patterns, systolic compression, communication with other vessels, etc. Septal

arteries have been identified which supply the inferior wall, right side of the septum, moderator band, papillary muscles, and right ventricular free wall.[5,10,12,18,25,37] In addition, the area producing obstruction may not be supplied by the first septal artery, but by the second, or third, or a branch of one artery, or a combination. Large septals may also communicate with septal branches originating from the PDA, or may give rise to collaterals to the apical, inferior, or posterior walls[10,12,25,29,37] (Figure 30.8).

Inability to access septal arteries

1. Septal perforator branches may arise from the LAD or from other vessels such as the ramus intermedius, circumflex, proximal RCA, or PDA.[10] Often it is possible to gain access to these branches, map them with MCE to ensure that they supply the area of LVOT obstruction, and successfully inject alcohol. However, these vessels may be located too distally to allow successful navigation of devices, may be too tortuous, or may not reliably supply the involved interventricular septum. We encountered one patient in whom the proximal LAD was extremely tortuous and affected the ability to wire the septal artery. We placed a stiff guide wire in the LAD which straightened the tortuous segment and resulted in successful access to the septal perforator with a separate wire (Figure 30.9).

2. Sometimes septal perforator branches are too small to allow successful balloon inflation of even the smallest balloon. To do so may risk vessel dissection or perforation. In addition, the vessel may supply such a small territory that injection of an adequate amount of alcohol would be unlikely. Often, however, injection of multiple, small septal perforators may allow administration of enough alcohol in a confluent manner to be effective in reducing LVOT obstruction.

Table 30.1 Complications of alcohol septal ablation.

- Inability to perform procedure/no alcohol administered
  - Inability to gain access to septal artery with guide wire or balloon catheter
  - Septal artery communicates with other cardiac structures
  - Other procedural complications
- Incomplete procedure and/or inadequate result
- Coronary artery dissection
- Alcohol spill into parent coronary artery
- Alcohol penetration into undesirable locations
- Ventricular arrhythmias
- Conduction abnormalities
  - CHB requiring placement of permanent dual chamber pacemaker
  - Others
- Persistent symptoms despite successful procedure
- Risk of sudden cardiac death/need for ICD
- Long-term effects unknown
- Ventricular septal defect
- Death

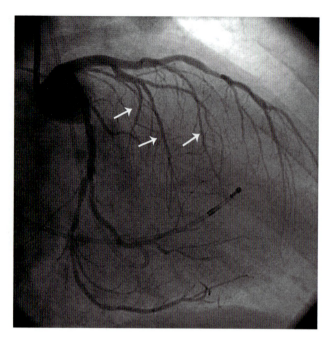

Figure 30.8 RAO caudal view angiogram demonstrating large septal artery with three branches.

3. Septal perforator branches may have very angulated origins from the LAD, making it extremely difficult to steer guide wires successfully into the vessel or to advance a balloon. Sometimes it is possible to steer the tip of the guide wire into the origin of the septal perforator, but attempts to advance the wire result in prolapse down the LAD. Devising various bends on the tip of the wire may enhance access into the vessel and steerability down the artery. I find that a Judkins left bend with a primary and secondary curve is often helpful, with the primary bend approximately 1 mm from the tip of the wire and the secondary bend approximately 3 mm from the tip of the wire. Sometimes a long, gentle, smooth curve is beneficial. Attempting different types of wires may also enhance success. For example, using a guide wire which is flexible or has a hydrophilic coating, such as a Whisper™ (Abbott Vascular) wire may allow access to the vessel. However, depending on the angulations and the size of the vessel, it may be difficult to advance the balloon catheter over such a wire. In this instance, the use of a Transit™ infusion catheter (Cordis Neurovascular, Inc, Miami Lakes, FL), which has no balloon or other device at the tip, may be used to exchange the initial wire for a more substantial wire that will allow tracking of the balloon into the vessel. At times, I have found that the use of a stiff-tipped wire such as a Cross-it® wire (Guidant) will hold a bend on the end of the wire more reliably and permanently and allow tracking of the wire into the septal perforator. This type of wire should be used with vigilance and finesse to avoid vessel dissection and perforation.

In addition, an angulated origin of the septal perforator from the LAD may inhibit advancement of the balloon catheter down the septal perforator despite initial access with the guide wire. In this case, use of a heavier wire, or a gentle curve on the wire, may enhance balloon advancement. Also, using the lowest profile balloon available may enhance tracking, but adequate sizing of the balloon within the septal perforator and complete occlusion of the vessel before alcohol injection is imperative. Use of a 'buddy' wire has not reliably enhanced success, but may be tried. Another trick which may enhance balloon advancement is to advance the guide wire as far down the septal perforator as deemed safe.[10] Working on a more substantial area of the guide wire several centimeters proximal to the tip may be of benefit.

Inability to adequately maintain a stable position of the inflated balloon within the septal perforator due to backward movement caused by systolic myocardial compression of the septal artery has been described.[38]

Septal artery communicates with other cardiac structures

Occasionally the selected septal perforator artery communicates with other cardiac structures into which it would be unsafe to inject ethanol. For example, septal perforator branches which originate from the LAD may communicate with other septal perforators located more distally along the LAD or with septal perforators from the PDA. Injection of alcohol in this situation may result in alcohol traversing the communicating vessels and entering the anterior, apical, or inferior myocardium.[29] Inferior myocardial infarction resulting from communications of septal branches of the LAD with septal branches from the PDA has been described.[12,37] Injection of angiographic contrast through the balloon lumen into the septal perforator should demonstrate

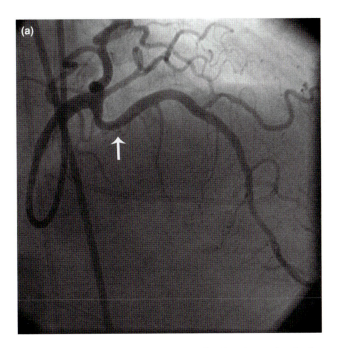 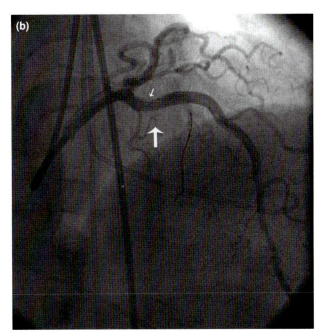

Figure 30.9 (A) Tortuous proximal LAD (arrow) which prevented adequate manipulation of the guide wire to access the septal perforator (RAO cranial view). (B) A stiff guide wire was directed through the tortuous segment into the distal LAD. This straightened the proximal segment (large arrow) (note wire bias, small arrow) enabling successful navigation of a second wire into the septal branch.

such communication, and, if present, alcohol should not be injected. Septal perforator branches supplying a papillary muscle have also been observed. Due to the potential for papillary muscle rupture and resultant mitral regurgitation it is not recommended that alcohol be injected in this situation. Not infrequently, the right side of the interventricular septum and/or the moderator band will enhance with MCE. Most operators choose not to inject alcohol in this situation.

Other complications

Occasionally, there is inability to perform the alcohol ablation procedure due to encountering another complication. The operator should be vigilant throughout the procedure regarding respiratory and hemodynamic compromise, electrocardiographic changes, blood flow in the coronary arteries, evidence of dissection, perforation, acute closure, disruption of atherosclerotic plaque, loss of branches, alcohol spill down the coronary artery, as well as vascular access and other complications of percutaneous cardiac procedures. At times these complications may be immediately correctable and the alcohol ablation procedure may be completed. At other times, the procedure should be postponed until the patient can be stabilized, or cancelled altogether.

Incomplete procedure and/or inadequate result

Another complication of the ASA procedure is incomplete procedure or inadequate result. Either the operator is unable to inject the desirable amount of

alcohol, or the patient has persistent gradient and/or symptoms in the follow-up period, or both.

Inability to inject the desired amount of alcohol may result from encountering a complication either before alcohol is given or during the administration of alcohol, resulting in early termination of alcohol injection. Examples of this include alcohol spill down the coronary artery, significant arrhythmias, hemodynamic instability, etc. Complications should be addressed immediately and the alcohol injection postponed until the patient is stabilized, or abandoned altogether.

Sometimes the vessel is so small that only a small amount of alcohol can be injected safely because of the small territory supplied by the vessel. If other branches are not easily accessible, then the myocardial injury induced may not be adequate to provide regression of septal thickness to relieve obstruction and symptoms.

It may not be possible to access the desired number of septal perforators in order to accomplish complete injection of the territory contributing to LVOT obstruction. In this case, there may be a small area of akinesis and thinning of the septum, but the area may be inadequate to provide total relief of gradient and/or symptoms.

Sometimes the septal perforator arteries bifurcate shortly after the origin from the LAD and it is impossible to place a balloon proximal to the bifurcation without the balloon projecting into the LAD. In this case, it is usually possible to advance the balloon and inject alcohol into each branch separately, but occasionally only one branch is accessible. This may result in incomplete resolution of obstruction. In cases of an incomplete or inadequate procedure, many patients are candidates for repeat procedures or myectomy[12,39] (Figure 30.10).

Coronary artery dissection

Coronary artery dissection is one of the more common complications of ASA.[12] It is important to differentiate coronary artery dissection from other causes of impaired flow such as vasospasm and alcohol spill in order to provide appropriate treatment.[41] In the case of alcohol spill, branch vessels are equally affected and flow is not affected by vasodilators. The use of guiding catheters which point upward toward the superior wall of the LMCA may cause dissection. It is therefore recommended that soft-tipped catheters are used, that catheters are seated in the ostium of the left main artery in a coaxial manner, and that vigilance regarding catheter position is maintained throughout the procedure.[12] As with other intracoronary procedures, dissection may also be caused by the manipulation of guide wires and other devices within the artery or by disruption of atherosclerotic plaques.[12,39] The use of soft- or floppy-tipped guide wires is recommended.

I have encountered dissection associated with coronary atherosclerotic plaques on two occasions. In one case it was noted that the patient had diffuse, non-obstructive CAD, and guide wire manipulation near the origin of the septal branch resulted in disruption of a plaque and acute closure of the LAD and a large diagonal branch. Guide wire access to both branches was established and bifurcation stenting was performed with excellent angiographic result and restoration of TIMI 3 flow into the vessel. The alcohol septal ablation procedure was successfully performed 6 months later (Figure 30.11).

In the second situation, it was noted that the patient had an atherosclerotic plaque near the origin of the intended septal artery. It was felt that this plaque could potentially be disrupted by guide wire maneuvers and therefore a guide wire was placed across this lesion into the distal LAD in order to preserve access into the distal vessel. Following ASA there was a hazy appearance to the plaque which indicated that it had been disrupted, so the LAD was stented, 'jailing' the involved septal perforator. Although we could have treated the plaque in the LAD prior to the procedure, it was felt that we might jeopardize our access to the septal artery, so we elected to perform the alcohol ablation first and stent the LAD at the end of the procedure.

We have encountered coronary dissection in a third setting. In this case it appeared that the septal perforator originated from the proximal aspect of the ramus intermedius artery. We accessed the septal and performed multiple balloon inflations and repositioning in the proximal portion of this artery as we attempted to confirm balloon sizing, appropriate occlusion of the vessel, and map the septal territory echocardiographically. This produced a dissection in the proximal portion of the artery which propagated retrograde into the left main coronary artery. In this situation the dissection was not treatable by stenting because the left main, LAD, ramus intermedius, and circumflex arteries were all affected by the dissection.

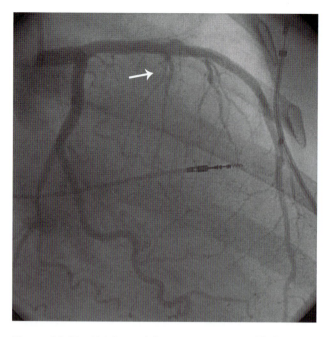

Figure 30.10 RAO caudal view angiogram of bifurcating first septal perforator (arrow). The proximal segment was too short to allow balloon positioning between the LAD and the bifurcation, so each branch was selectively engaged and injected with alcohol.

The patient underwent successful emergency bypass grafting and myectomy. In order to avoid this situation, it is recommended that an appropriately sized balloon is inflated to a low or nominal inflation pressure and not overexpanded in the coronary artery. The balloon should be located entirely within the septal perforator artery and not partially in the LAD. The balloon should be inflated, the positioned confirmed, and the balloon remain inflated, even if it takes several minutes to accomplish appropriate mapping before alcohol is injected. It appears that multiple balloon inflations and repositioning in the artery may contribute to the possibility of dissection (Figure 30.12).

Alcohol spill down the left anterior descending coronary artery

One of the most devastating complications of ASA is alcohol 'spill' down the LAD. Alcohol spill down the parent artery may occur when the balloon does not completely occlude the septal artery. This may be due to the fact that the balloon is undersized, underinflated, or located proximally in the septal perforator so it projects into the parent coronary artery. This allows for potential retrograde flow of alcohol along the inflated balloon and down the coronary artery. Injection through the central lumen of the balloon catheter may displace the balloon backward, dislodging it and allowing retrograde flow around the balloon into the parent coronary artery. Therefore it is imperative that the

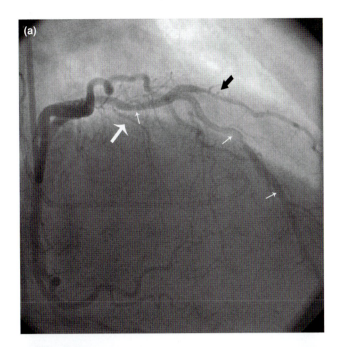

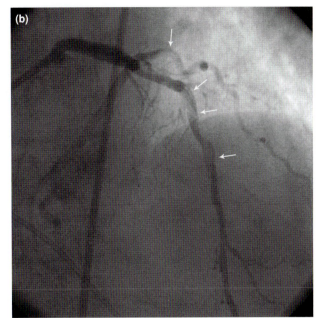

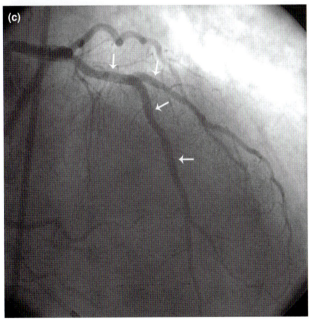

Figure 30.11 (A) RAO cranial view angiogram of septal perforator (large arrow) originating proximal to the LAD in the vicinity of the LAD/diagonal bifurcation. There is diffuse non-obstructive disease throughout the LAD (small arrows) and obstructive disease in the diagonal (black arrow). The septal perforator has an ostial stenosis. Guide wire manipulation near the septal perforator resulted in dissection of the proximal LAD which propagated down the LAD and into the diagonal. (B) AP cranial view demonstrating dissection (arrows) of the LAD and diagonal vessels secondary to efforts to maneuver a guide wire into the septal artery. (C) The same vessels after stenting (arrows). The ASA procedure was successfully performed 6 months later (AP cranial view).

balloon be appropriately sized, appropriately inflated, and location confirmed within the septal artery. Injection through the central lumen of the balloon should be gentle, and dislodgment of the balloon ruled out angiographically following every injection. It is recommended that frequent injections through the guiding catheter be performed throughout the alcohol ablation procedure to confirm normal flow in the parent coronary arterial system. If there is any impairment of flow, the alcohol injection should be immediately terminated.

We have experienced alcohol spill on three occasions. On two occasions there was minor impairment of flow in the LAD. The procedures were terminated and intracoronary vasodilators such as adenosine and nitroprusside were administered; but it is not clear whether or not they provided any benefit. In two cases

the most distal aspect of the LAD became and remained occluded, with TIMI 3 flow in the rest of the vessel. There was a focal area of apical hypokinesia that did not resolve in the months following the procedure.

In the third incidence, alcohol spill down the coronary artery resulted in complete closure of the LAD and a large diagonal branch. This was complicated by hemodynamic compromise, ventricular tachycardia, and was unresponsive to all efforts to 'open' the artery. Intracoronary ultrasound was performed to rule out dissection or thrombus and showed a completely normal appearing lumen. Administration of heparin, abciximab, and intracoronary vasodilators did not improve flow whatsoever. The patient survived hospitalization and was discharged. Echocardiogram several weeks later showed anterior and apical akinesis and apical ventricular septal defect

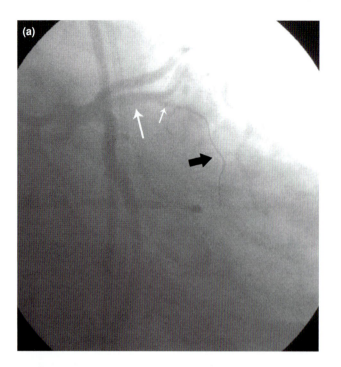

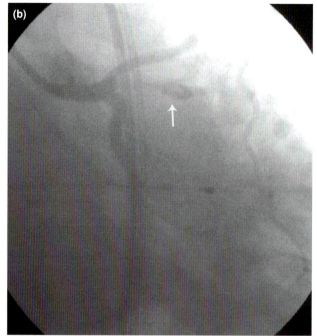

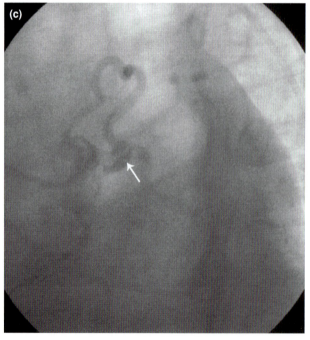

Figure 30.12 (A) RAO caudal view angiogram of possible septal artery originating from ramus intermedius (large arrow) branch with balloon (small arrow) and guide wire in place (black arrow). (B) RAO caudal angiogram showing dissection of septal perforator (arrow) originating from ramus intermedius artery due to multiple manipulations of the balloon catheter during mapping to determine if the vessel supplied the area of obstruction. (C) LAO caudal view. Retrograde propagation of the dissection into the LMCA (arrow) affecting the origins of the circumflex, LAD, and ramus intermedius coronary arteries.

(VSD). The patient underwent repair of the VSD and grafting of the LAD. She moved to a different state and was lost to follow-up. Obviously alcohol spill down the coronary artery is a devastating complication. The operator should be vigilant for any impairment of flow or contractility throughout the procedure and abort the procedure immediately if this occurs (Figure 30.13).

Alcohol penetration into undesirable locations

Alcohol may penetrate into undesirable locations remote from the targeted septal area by several mechanisms.

Septal anatomy is complex and variable, so exquisite attention to mapping with MCE is imperative to reduce the chances of this complication. Septal arteries may supply the right side of the septum or right ventricular free wall; the moderator band; papillary muscles; the distal septum; and other walls of the left ventricle directly. These areas should be detectable with MCE and should be injected with great care and trepidation or not at all. We have successfully injected septal arteries that supply the right side of the septum and/or the moderator band with no adverse consequences and efficacious results if enhancement was mild, but many operators avoid alcohol injection in this situation due to the potential for right ventricular infarction.[10]

Long or branching septal perforators may supply a large area of the septum even if they originate from the proximal LAD. Injection of alcohol in this situation may produce a larger injury than needed. Also, it appears that alcohol administration focused on the area of obstruction may provide an effective result with a lower incidence of complete heart block. Therefore, it is probably worthwhile to try to determine if injecting only one or two branches, or some smaller portion of a large, branching septal perforator would focus the injury on the desired area. Long, complex septal arteries may supply the distal septum, apex, or communicate with other septal arteries. We have observed several situations where injection of one septal perforator with radiographic contrast demonstrated flow into another septal perforator and subsequently into the LAD.

Septal arteries may also have complex collateral networks and may communicate with vessels that supply the apex, anterior, inferior, or posterior left ventricular walls.[29,38] These should be visible with MCE, but vigilance throughout the procedure for other evidence of remote injury is important. Intense or escalating chest pain, or pain that is not very responsive to medications, ST segment elevation on ECG, ventricular arrhythmias, hypokinesis of remote areas visible on echo, and enhancement of remote myocardial areas by the contrast or alcohol visible on echo, are all important signs of remote injury and should be investigated thoroughly.

We encountered a situation of alcohol penetration into the inferior wall likely through a septal perforator connection to the PDA which was not evident on preprocedure angiography. The patient experienced chest pain and significant ST elevation in the inferior leads during the procedure. Echocardiography did not reveal any enhancement of the inferior, apical, or posterior myocardium by the alcohol or hypokinesia of these areas. The patient had two episodes of ventricular tachycardia/ventricular fibrillation which were terminated with defibrillation and did not recur with pacing at 90 beats per minute and administration of intravenous amiodarone. Angiography revealed occlusion of the distal PDA and left ventriculography showed diaphragmatic hypokinesia. Apparently this area was not completely visualized with echocardiography. The patient recovered clinically and had no further arrhythmias, no evidence of heart failure, and reported improvement in symptoms related to HCM.

Ventricular arrhythmias and conduction abnormalities

Ventricular premature beats will frequently be encountered when accessing the septal perforator coronary arteries and injecting alcohol. These are usually transient and do not require treatment. Episodes of non-sustained ventricular tachycardia (NSVT) may also be seen.[10,40]

Patients should be monitored for at least 72 hours postprocedure.[10]

At least three cases of sustained ventricular tachycardia (VT) following alcohol ablation have been reported.[41–43] One patient experienced VT with syncope on postprocedure day 8. He was treated with transient intravenous amiodarone and subsequently underwent electrophysiology (EP) evaluation, which showed normal sinus and AV node function and sustained monomorphic ventricular tachycardia (SMVT) which appeared to originate from the basal septum. A dual chamber implantable cardioverter debrillator (ICD) was placed and he was maintained on β-blocker therapy. Approximately 3 weeks later he experienced SMVT which was appropriately terminated with ICD discharge. The authors pointed out that 'NSVT occurs in 20% of patients [with HCM] and is a predictor of sudden death in adults, whereas SMVT occurs only rarely. In contrast, scar-related VT is well-described post MI, which is why concern has been raised that this may be a complication of ASA'.[41] As only one case of VT was reported among 325 ASA patients in two studies, it appears to be a rare occurrence.[43,44] The low incidence following ASA as compared with MI may be due to the more focused, smaller, well defined scar created with the ASA procedure.[41] The reported cases occurred within 3 weeks of alcohol ablation, the significance of which is not clear. It appears that the incidence of VT does not increase in the follow-up period after ASA up to 10 years.[26]

On two occasions, we encountered VT/fibrillation immediately following the procedure, and both were associated with evidence of alcohol penetration into remote areas. Both cases were successfully treated with overdrive pacing and administration of anti-arrhythmic agents, and did not recur.

Conduction abnormalities can occur as a consequence of the ASA procedure due to the fact that the first septal perforator generally supplies the septum in the vicinity of the ventricular conduction axis.[45] Right bundle branch block (RBBB) is the most frequently occurring conduction abnormality, which may occur in up to 80% of patients.[10,46,47] Patients with a left bundle branch block (LBBB) prior to the alcohol ablation procedure are at higher risk, perhaps 50–68%, for developing CHB during or following the procedure.[10, 46–49] The incidence of CHB requiring permanent dual chamber pacemaker implantation has been reported to be 0–40%, with higher rates occurring early in the experience with the procedure.[5,10,12,48–50] Faber et al. reported the development of CHB in 13 of their initial 25 patients (52%), 5 (20%) of whom required permanent DDD pacemaker implantation.[51] In their one-year follow-up data, Lakkis et al. reported the following data on their first 50 patients, 12 of whom already had permanent pacemakers in place at the time of ASA: 11 (~30%) developed CHB and required pacer placement; 20 patients developed new RBBB; 14 patients developed RBBB and left anterior fascicular

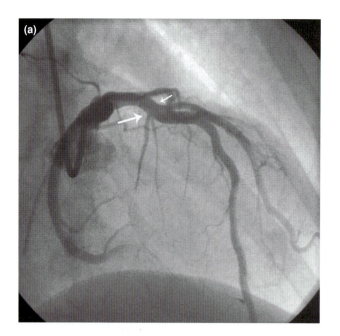

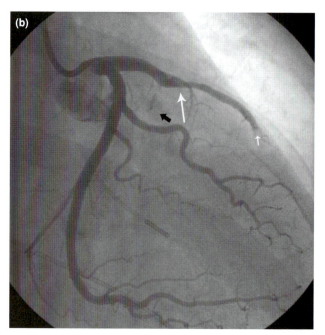

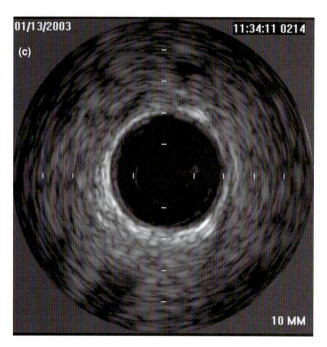

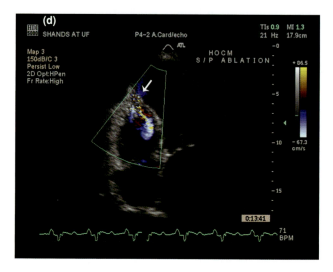

Figure 30.13 (A) RAO cranial view angiogram of septal perforator originating from the LAD (large arrow) in the area of LAD/diagonal bifurcation (small arrow). (B) Occlusion of the LAD (large arrow) and diagonal (small arrow) vessels due to alcohol spill. Flow into the vessels was not restored. Balloon inflated in the septal perforator is also shown (black arrow). (C) Intracoronary ultrasound cross-sectional view of LAD with normal-appearing lumen. (D) Apical four-chamber view with color Doppler demonstrating VSD (arrow) due to large anteroapical-septal infarction 3 months after ASA.

block; and 6 patients developed LBBB.[40] Five-year data from the same investigators on 130 patients revealed a 9% pacer rate in the last 80 patients for an overall rate of 13%.[12] Data on the first 50 patients at Medical University of South Carolina indicate a permanent pacer rate of 6.7%.[52] The decrease in the incidence of CHB and the need for permanent pacemaker implantation is probably the result of the learning curve felt to be present with the procedure; increasing

experience and available data; injection of less alcohol with smaller area of myocardial injury; more focused administration of alcohol into the septal area of obstruction; and possibly slower rates of injection.[12]

CHB may occur at the time of the procedure or in the first several days thereafter. Occurrence beyond 2–3 days postprocedure is very rare, but has been reported.[10,48,53,54] It is also of note that in many patients who develop CHB, the ventricular escape rhythm is very slow, often in the range of 30 beats per minute, and frequently results in syncope.[53,55] CHB is often transient and may not require placement of a permanent pacemaker. Observation of the patient in the hospital for 3–4 days postprocedure is recommended, especially if the patient has experienced transient CHB during the immediate postprocedural period.[5,10,12,53]

Predictors of CHB following ASA include baseline LBBB, advanced age, volume of alcohol injected, and perhaps fast rate of injection.[10,56] Surgical myectomy-myotomy is associated with the development of LBBB rather than RBBB and has a rate of CHB requiring permanent DDD pacemaker implantation of ~10%.[55,56]

Because the ASA procedure produces acute myocardial injury in the region of the basal interventricular septum with resultant permanent injury and scar formation (infarction), ECG changes typical of septal infarction are common. In addition to the frequent development of RBBB, ECG changes include ST elevation in septal leads which may be persistent for days or weeks; tendency for the QRS axis to rotate leftward; and loss of R-wave or the development of Q-waves in lead V1. QTc may be prolonged, but generally returns to baseline by 3 months.[46,57]

Persistent symptoms

Despite a completely successful and effective procedure with complete resolution of the left ventricular outflow gradient, thinning of the septum, and resolution of systolic anterior motion of the mitral valve, some patients remain somewhat symptomatic and continue to require medications. This is likely due to diastolic dysfunction due to hypertrophic cardiomyopathy affecting all of the myocardium, not just the left ventricular outflow area. However, we have seen that in the majority of patients with a successful procedure, symptoms and requirements for medication are diminished, and some patients may discontinue their medications altogether and remain completely free of symptoms.[12] There is a spectrum of anatomic and clinical responsiveness to the ASA procedure, which probably correlates with the heterogeneity demonstrated by HCM, as well as variance in degree of myocardial injury and healing.

Risk of sudden cardiac death/need for ICD

It appears that while the ASA procedure may alleviate obstruction to left ventricular outflow and symptoms, it may not modify the risk of sudden cardiac death in patients with hypertrophic cardiomyopathy. Some physicians believe that it may contribute to the risk of sudden cardiac death, but this notion is not accepted by all cardiologists.[12,26] In our series of over 100 patients who have undergone ASA we have had no occurrence of sudden cardiac death in the follow-up period.

Long-term effects unknown

The alcohol ablation procedure was initially performed in Europe and reported in 1995, and in the US in 1998.[58,59] Five-year data on 130 patients indicate that the procedure effectively reduces symptoms and LVOT gradient 'which is usually permanent.'[12] Procedural mortality is < 2%. The rate of repeat procedures was 17%, but this reflected early experience. As procedural experience and technology increase the rate of repeat procedures is expected to be lower.[12] There is no evidence that the ablated tissue is regenerated. Publication of 10-year data is pending.[26]

Ventricular septal defect

Although ASA creates a permanent injury in the area of the membranous intraventricular septum, the occurrence of VSD is virtually unheard of, most likely due to the fact that the septum is significantly hypertrophied. I located one case report of a VSD discovered 5 weeks postASA in an 82-year-old female. 2.5 cc of alcohol had been injected 'slowly' into a 'large septal perforator,' and she had had no in-hospital complications. Echocardiographic measurement of the septal diameter preprocedure was 18 mm. The VSD was successfully closed percutaneously with a 20 mm Amplatzer postMI VSD occluding device (AGA Medical, Golden Valley, MN).

We encountered the occurrence of an apical VSD following alcohol spill into the LAD (see above).

Death

The most devastating complication of the ASA procedure is death. This may occur due to a variety of complications including alcohol spill down the parent coronary artery with large infarction, untreated CHB, and others. We have had two procedure-related deaths in our series of patients, one from pulmonary embolism which occurred on postprocedure day 3 while the patient was in the CCU and on subcutaneous heparin; and one with cardiac arrest at home on postprocedure day 4 due to development of CHB. No pacemaker was placed due to the patient's prior directives and the family's wishes and the patient expired.

In their 5-year postprocedure data on 130 patients who had procedures between 1996 and 2002, Fernandez et al. reported 10 deaths in the entire cohort. There were 3 cardiac deaths. Only two of these appear to be related to the procedure. One death was due to LAD dissection complicated by ventricular fibrillation. The patient died during emergency cardiac surgery. The other procedural death was due to an inferior and right ventricular myocardial infarction and cardiogenic shock 10 days after the procedure. The third was sudden cardiac death in the follow-up period. These data suggest a cardiac mortality rate of 2.3%.[12] It is possible that, with experience and the evolution of the procedure, current mortality is lower. Evaluation of data on more patients would be valuable in determining if this is the case.

CONCLUSION

ASA has proven to be an effective procedure which has provided benefit to selected patients with immediate and sustained improvement in LVOT gradient and symptoms. The procedure should be performed by an experienced interventional cardiologist and echocardiologist in a cardiac catheterization laboratory which has immediate access to anesthesia and respiratory therapy services; cardiothoracic surgical services experienced in myectomy-myotomy and complex cases; an intensive care unit; and dual chamber pacing.[1] It should be performed with meticulous attention to detail, and with patience, vigilance, finesse, courage, and great care.

Acknowledgments

I am indebted to Dr William H Spencer III for his mentorship, advice, and discussion of his experience with this procedure. Thanks to Dr Carl J Pepine and Dr C Richard Conti for their review of this manuscript and for suggesting improvements. I am grateful to Mrs Evette Hutchinson, Ms Ivy Strawder, and Mrs Lisa Hamilton for their assistance in preparation of this manuscript. Finally, I offer my thanks and appreciation to the editors of this book for inviting my participation.

ABBREVIATIONS FOR FIGURES

ASA	alcohol septal ablation
ASH	asymmetric septal hypertrophy
SAM	systolic anterior motion of the mitral valve
LVOT	left ventricular outflow tract
m/sec	meters per second
mm Hg	millimeters of mercury
RAO	right anterior oblique
LAO	left anterior oblique
AP	anteroposterior
LAD	left anterior descending coronary artery
LMCA	left main coronary artery
VSD	ventricular septal defect

REFERENCES

1. King SB III, Aversano T, Ballard WL et al. ACCF/AHA/SCAI 2007 update of the clinical competence statement on cardiac interventional procedures: a report of the American College of Cardiology Foundation/American Heart Association/American College of Physicians Task Force on Clinical Competence and Training (Writing Committee to Update the 1998 Clinical Competence Statement on Recommendations for the Assessment and Maintenance of Proficiency in Coronary Interventional Procedures). J Am Coll Cardiol 2007; 50: 82–108.

2. Maron BJ, Gardin JM, Flack JM et al. Prevalence of hypertrophic cardiomyopathy in a general population of young adults. Echocardiographic analysis of 4111 subjects in the CARDIA Study. Coronary Artery Risk Development in (Young) Adults. Circulation 1995; 92: 785–9.

3. Watkins H. Multiple disease genes cause hypertrophic cardiomyopathy. Br Heart J 1994; 72: S4–9.

4. Ruzyllo W, Chojnowska L, Demkow M et al. Left ventricular outflow tract gradient decrease with non-surgical myocardial reduction improves exercise capacity in patients with hypertrophic obstructive cardiomyopathy. Eur Heart J 2000; 21: 770–7.

5. Maron BJ, McKenna WJ, Danielson GK et al. ACC/ESC clinical expert consensus document on hypertrophic cardiomyopathy: a report of the American College of Cardiology Task Force on Clinical Expert Consensus Documents and the European Society of Cardiology Committee for Practice Guidelines (Committee to Develop an Expert Consensus Document on Hypertrophic Cardiomyopathy). J Am Coll Cardiol 2003; 42: 1687–1713.

6. Maron BJ, Bonow RO, Cannon RO, Leon MB, Epstein SE. Hypertrophic cardiomyopathy: interrelation of clinical manifestations, pathophysiology and therapy. N Engl J Med 1987; 316: 780–9.

7. Grigg LE, Wigle ED, Williams WG, Daniel LB, Rakowski H. Transesophageal Doppler echocardiography in obstructive cardiomyopathy: clarification of pathophysiology and importance of intraoperative decision making. J Am Coll Cardiol 1992; 20: 42–52.

8. Henry WL, Clark CE, Griffith JM, Epstein SE. Mechanism of left ventricular outflow obstruction in patients with obstructive asymmetric septal hypertrophy (idiopathic hypertrophic subaortic stenosis). Am J Cardiol 1975; 35: 337–45.

9. Firoozi S, Elliott PM, Sharma S et al. Septal myotomy-myectomy and transcoronary septal alcohol ablation in hypertrophic obstructive cardiomyopathy. A comparison of clinical, hemodynamic and exercise outcomes. Eur Heart J 2002; 23: 1617–24.

10. Holmes DR, Valeti US, Nishimura RA. Alcohol septal ablation for hypertrophic cardiomyopathy: indications and technique. Cathet Cardiovasc Interven 2005; 66: 375–89.

11. Lakkis NM, Nagueh SF, Kleiman NS et al. Echocardiography-guided ethanol septal reduction for hypertrophic obstructive cardiomyopathy. Circulation 1998; 98: 1750–5.

12. Fernandez VL, Nagueh SF, Franklin J et al. A prospective follow-up of alcohol septal ablation for symptomatic hypertrophic obstructive cardiomyopathy – The Baylor Experience (1996–2002). Clin Cardiol 2005; 28: 124–30.

13. Knight CJ. Alcohol septal ablation for obstructive hypertrophic cardiomyopathy. Heart 2006; 92: 1339–44.

14. Gietzen FH, Leuner CJ, Raute-Kreinsen U et al. Acute and long-term results after transcoronary ablation of septal hypertrophy (TASH). Eur Heart J 1999; 20; 1342–54.

15. Gietzen FH, Leuner CJ, Obergassel L, Strunk-Mueller C, Kuhn H. Role of transcoronary ablation of septal hypertrophy in patients with hypertrophic cardiomyopathy, New York Heart Association Functional Class III or IV, and outflow obstruction only under provocable conditions. Circulation 2002; 106: 454–9.

16. Faber L, Seggewiss H, Welge D et al. Echo-guided percutaneous septal ablation of symptomatic hypertrophic obstructive cardiomyopathy: 7 years of experience. Eur J Echocardiogr 2004; 5: 347–55.

17. Faber L, Seggewiss H, Gleichmann U. Percutaneous transluminal septal myocardial ablation in hypertrophic obstructive cardiomyopathy. Results with respect to intraprocedural myocardial contrast echocardiography. Circulation 1998; 98: 2415–21.

18. Nagueh SF, Lakkis N, He ZX et al. Role of myocardial contrast echocardiography during nonsurgical septal reduction therapy for hypertrophic obstructive cardiomyopathy. J Am Coll Cardiol 1998; 32: 225–9.

19. Seggewiss H, Faber L, Meyners W et al. Simultaneous percutaneous treatment in hypertrophic obstructive cardiomyopathy and coronary artery disease. Cathet Cardiovasc Diagn 1998; 44: 65–9.

20. Alfonso F, Isla LP, Seggewiss H. Images in cardiology. Contrast echocardiography during alcohol septal ablation: friend or foe? Heart 2005; 91 e18.

21. Faber L, Seggewiss H, Ziemssen P, Gleichmann U. Intraprocedural myocardial contrast echocardiography as a routine procedure in percutaneous transluminal septal myocardial ablation: detection of threatening myocardial necrosis distant from the septal target area.Cathet Cardiovasc Interven 1999; 47: 462–6.

22. Dear Healthcare Provider Letter http://www.definityimaging .com/pdf/T6Doo35DefinityDear HCPlette.V4.10.11.pdf.

23. Bockstegers P, Steinbigler P, Molnar A et al. Pressure-guided nonsurgical myocardial reduction induced by small septal infarctions in hypertrophic obstructive cardiomyopathy. J Am Coll Cardiol 2001; 38: 846–53.

24. Elliot PM, Brecker SJ, McKenna WJ. Left ventricular opacification during selective intracoronary injection of echocardiographic contrast in patients with hypertrophic cardiomyopathy. Heart 2000; 83: e7.

25. Singh M, Edwards WD, Holmes Dr, Tajik AJ, Nishimura RA. Anatomy of the first septal perforating artery: a study with implications for ablation therapy for hypertrophic cardiomyopathy. Mayo Clin Proc 2001; 76: 799–802.

26. Fernandes V, Nielsen C, Nagueh S et al. A prospective follow up of alcohol septal ablation for symptomatic hypertrophic obstructive cardiomyopathy the ten year Baylor and MUSC experience. Accepted for publication by J Am Coll Cardiol, International.

27. Chang SM, Lakkis NM, Franklin J, Spencer WH, Nagueh SF. Predictors of outcome after alcohol septal ablation therapy in patients with hypertrophic obstructive cardiomyopathy. Circulation 2004; 109: 824–7.

28. Veselka J, Procházková Š, Duchonová R et al. Alcohol septal ablation for hypertrophic obstructive cardiomyopathy: lower alcohol dose reduces size of infarction and has comparable hemodynamic and clinical outcome. Cathet Cardiovasc Interven 2004; 63: 231–5.

29. Parham WA, Kern MJ. Apical infarct via septal collateralization complicating transluminal alcohol septal ablation for hypertrophic cardiomyopathy. Cathet Cardiovasc Interven 2003; 60: 208–11.

30. Li ZQ, Cheng TO, Liu L et al. Experimental study of relationship between intracoronary alcohol injection and the size of the resultant myocardial infarct. Int J Cardiol 2003; 91: 93–6.

31. Cheng TO. Percutaneous transluminal septal myocardial ablation for hypertrophic obstructive cardiomyopathy: how much alcohol should be injected? Cathet Cardiovasc Interven 2005; 65: 313–14.

32. Seggewiss H. Percutaneous transluminal septal myocardial ablation: a new treatment for hypertrophic obstructive cardiomyopathy. Eur Heart J 2000; 21: 704–7.

33. Chang SM, Lakkis NM, Fanklin J, Spencer WH III, Nagueh SF. Predictors of outcome after alcohol ablation therapy in patients with hypertrophic obstructive cardiomyopathy. Circulation 2004; 109: 824–7.

34. Butman SM. Complications of Percutaneous Coronary Interventions. New York: Springer Science and Business Media, Inc, 2005.

35. Kerensky RA. Complications of Cardiac Catheterization and Strategies to Reduce Risks. Baltimore: Williams and Wilkins, 1998.

36. Baim DS, Simon DI. Complications and the Optimal Use of Adjunctive Pharmacology. Philadelphia: Lippincott Williams and Wilkins, 2006.

37. Chowdary S, Galiwango P, Woo A, Schwartz L. Inferior infarction following alcohol septal ablation: a consequent of 'Collateral Damage'? Cathet Cardiovasc Interven 2007; 69: 236–42.

38. Dudek D, Gil R, Dimitrow PP et al. Balloon positioning difficulties during nonsurgical septal reduction therapy in a patient with hypertrophic obstructive cardiomyopathy. Cathet Cardiovasc Interven 2000; 49: 314–17.

39. Nagueh S, Buergler JM, Quinones MA, Spencer WH, Lawrie GM. Outcome of surgical myectomy after unsuccessful alcohol septal ablation for the treatment of patients with hypertrophic obstructive cardiomyopathy. J Am Coll Cardiol 2007; 50: 795–8.

40. Lakkis NM, Nagueh SF, Dunn JK, Killip D, Spencer WM III. Nonsurgical septal reduction therapy for hypertrophic obstructive cardiomyopathy: one-year follow-up. J Am Coll Cardiol 2000; 36: 852–5.

41. Ziaee A, Lim M, Stewart R, Kern MJ. Coronary artery occlusion after transluminal alcohol septal ablation: differentiating dissection, spasm and alcohol-induced no reflow. Cathet Cardiovasc Interven 2005; 64: 204–8.

41. Simon RDB, Crawford FA, Spencer WH III, Gold MR. Sustained ventricular tachycardia following alcohol septal ablation for hypertrophic obstructive cardiomyopathy. PACE 2005; 28: 1354–6.

42. Boltwood CM, Chien W, Ports T. Ventricular tachycardia complicating alcohol septal ablation. N Engl J Med 2004; 351:1914–15.

43. McGegor JB, Rahman A, Rosario S et al. Monomorphic ventricular tachycardia: a late complication of percutaneous alcohol septal ablation for hypertrophic cardiomyopathy. Am J Med Sci 2004; 328: 185–8.

44. Crawford FA III, Killip D, Franklin J et al. Implantable cardioverter-defrillators for primary prevention of sudden cardiac death in patients with hypertrophic obstructive cardiomyopathy after alcohol septal ablation. Circulation 2004; 108: 386–7.

45. Sigwart U, Gibson D, Henein M et al. Clinical significance of obstruction of the first major septal branch. Circulation 1998; 98: 377–8.

46. Runquist LH, Nielson DC, Killip D, Gazes PC, Spencer WH III. Electrocardiographic changes after alcohol septal ablation therapy for obstructive cardiomyopathy. Am J Cardiol 2002; 990: 1020–2.

47. Henein MY, O'Sullivan CA, Ramzy IS, Sigwart U, Gibson DG. Electromechanical left ventricular behavior after nonsurgical septal reduction in patients with hypertrophic obstructive cardiomyopathy. J Am Coll Cardiol 1999; 34: 1117–22.

48. Chang SM, Hagueh SF, Spencer WH III, Lakkis NM. Complete heart block: determinants and clinical impact in patients with hypertrophic obstructive cardiomyopathy undergoing non-surgical septal reduction therapy. J Am Coll Cardiol 2003; 42: 296–300.

49. Faber L, Seggewiss H, Welge D et al. Predicting the risk of atrioventricular conduction lesions after percutaneous septal ablation for obstructive hypertrophic cardiomyopathy. Z Kardiol 2003; 92: 39–47.

50. Knight CJ. Five years of percutaneous transluminal septal myocardial ablation. Heart 2000; 83: 255–6.

51. Faber L, Meissner A, Ziemssen P, Seggewiss H. Percutaneous transluminal septal myocardial ablation for hypertrophic obstructive cardiomyopathy: long term follow up of the first series of 25 patients. Heart 2000; 83: 326–31.

52. Nielsen CD, Killip D, Spencer WH III. Nonsurgical septal reduction therapy for hypertrophic obstructive cardiomyopathy: short-term results in 50 consecutive procedures. Clin Cardiol 2003; 26: 275–9.

53. Kern MJ, Holmes DG, Simpson C, Bitar SR, Hassan R. Delayed occurrence of complete heart block without warning after alcohol septal ablation for hypertrophic obstructive cardiomyopathy. Cathet Cardiovasc Interven 2002; 56: 503–7.

54. Faber L, Seggewiss H, Fassbender D et al. Identification of patients requiring ddd-pacemaker after percutaneous transluminal septal myocardial ablation in hypertrophic obstructive cardiomyopathy. J Am Coll Cardiol 1998; 1011–28.

55. Valettas N, Rho R, Besai J et al. Alcohol septal ablation complicated by complete heart block and permanent pacemaker failure. Cathet Cardiovasc Interven 2003; 58: 189–93.

56. Lawrenz T, Lieder F, Bartelsmeier M et al. Predictors of complete heart block after transcoronary ablation of septal hypertrophy. Results of a prospective electrophysiological investigation in 172 patients with hypertrophic obstructive cardiomyopathy. J Am Coll Cardiol 2007; 49: 2356–63.

56. Heric B, Lytle BW, Miller DP et al. Surgical management of hypertrophic obstructive cardiomyopathy. Early and late results. J Thorac Cardiovasc Surg 1995; 110: 195–208.

57. Kazmierczak J, Kornacewicz-Jach Z, Kisly M, Gil R, Wojtarowicz A. Electrocardiographic changes after alcohol septal ablation in hypertrophic obstructive cardiomyopathy. Heart 1998; 80: 257–62.

58. Sigwart U. Non-surgical myocardial reduction for hypertrophic obstructive cardiomyopathy. Lancet 1995; 346: 211–14.

59. Lakkis N, Nagueh S, Kleiman N et al. Echocardiographic-guided ethanol septal reduction for hypertrophic obstructive cardiomyopathy. Circulation 1998; 98: 1750–5.

61. Aroney CN, Goh TH, Hourigan LA, Dyer W. Ventricular septal rupture following nonsurgical septal reduction for hypertrophic cardiomyopathy: treatment with percutaneous closure. Cathet Cardiovasc Interven 2004; 61: 411–14.

31 Complications related to percutaneous transluminal aortic valvuloplasty and their management

Yoshihito Sakata

Percutaneous transluminal aortic valvuloplasty (PTAV) is indicated for the patients with symptomatic severe aortic stenosis, who are contraindicated or very high risk for surgical valve replacement due to extremely advanced age, concomitant illness, and poor general condition.[1,2] As the candidate patients tend to be physically debilitated and hemodynamically labile, a variety of adverse events can be anticipated during these procedures. In order to avoid potential PTAV-related complications, it is critically important to perform a thorough evaluation of the baseline cardiac condition, to prepare for any potential adverse events in advance, and to pay meticulous care to details of technique based on a detailed understanding of the nature of this procedure.

APPROACHES TO PTAV: ANTEGRADE VS RETROGRADE TECHNIQUES

There are two different approaches in PTAV to reach the aortic valve – the retrograde approach by arterial access through the aorta, and the antegrade approach by venous and transseptal access, in which the balloon is advanced over a wire loop traversing the heart from right to left.[3,4] Each approach has its merits and disadvantages. The retrograde approach is more straightforward to perform, technically being similar to regular cardiac catheterization. Its downside includes the limited size of arterial catheters and sheaths, and frequent arterial complications as a consequence of the 12–14 French sheaths used. The antegrade approach is less traumatic on the arteries and allows introduction of the larger sized devices using venous access. When we discuss complications related to PTAV, some of them are more approach-specific, while others are commonly seen in any percutaneous aortic valve intervention.

BRADYARRHYTHMIAS

The assessment of baseline EKG prior to the procedure is important. The mechanical stress on any cardiac structure can cause a transient increase of vasovagal activity,

causing bradycardia with or without hypotension.[5] Inflation of the balloon catheter across the aortic valve by any approach can also disturb the electrical conduction system by direct trauma, causing intraventricular conduction defect or bundle branch block. In particular, the patients with an underlying defect of the conduction system such as pre-existing left or right bundle branch block or atrioventricular (AV) block are more susceptible to developing advanced atrioventricular block and severe bradycardia with hemodynamic compromise, and temporary pacemaker placement supporting the procedure is mandatory for this high-risk group. In the majority of cases, this is a transient disorder with recovery within 48 hours, rarely requiring permanent pacemaker implantation (Figure 31.1). In the antegrade approach, mechanical trauma by the intraventricular wire loop can cause transient conduction disturbances. An advance consideration is to discontinue any medication which exerts a negative chronotropic effect, such as β-receptor antagonists and antiarrhythmic agents.

TACHYARRHYTHIMAS

Ventricular arrhythmias are routinely provoked during wire or balloon manipulation and are a ubiquitous part of every PTAV procedure. In both the antegrade and retrograde approaches, the extra-stiff guide wire used to deliver the balloon provokes serious ventricular arrhythimas. These may result in ventricular tachycardia or even fibrillation, accompanying significant hemodynamic compromise (Figure 31.2). Gentle wire manipulation is crucial, avoiding mechanical stress on the left ventricle. One might consider administering antiarrhythmic agents such as lidocaine beforehand to minimize ventricular arrhythimas.

PROCEDURE-RELATED STRUCTURAL INJURIES

During the procedure, both careful observation of patients' symptoms and monitoring of hemodynamics are crucial.[6] Any clinical symptom in the middle of the

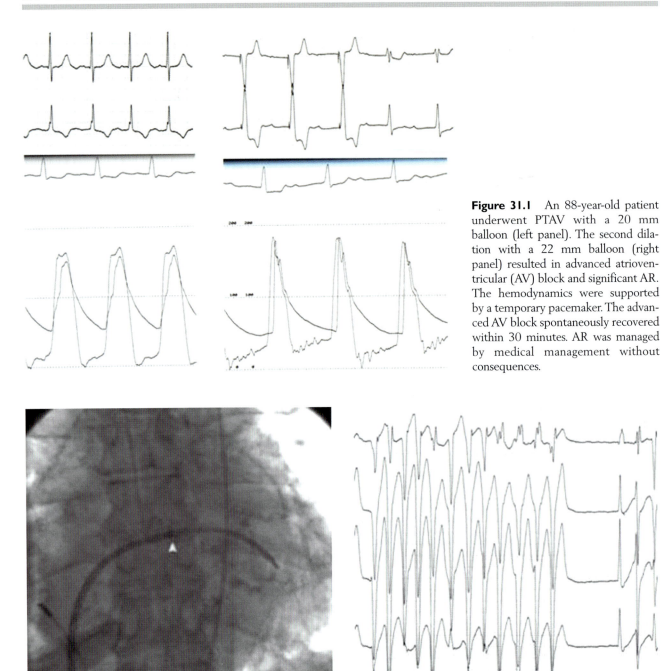

Figure 31.1 An 88-year-old patient underwent PTAV with a 20 mm balloon (left panel). The second dilation with a 22 mm balloon (right panel) resulted in advanced atrioventricular (AV) block and significant AR. The hemodynamics were supported by a temporary pacemaker. The advanced AV block spontaneously recovered within 30 minutes. AR was managed by medical management without consequences.

Figure 31.2 The intraventricular loop is formed in the apex of the left ventricle for antegrade PTAV. Manipulation of the catheter while creating a turn in the LV apex prior to wire placement caused ventricular tachycardia (VT) and transient hypotension. Transient catheter-related VT is always part of these procedures and must be minimized to avoid creating prolonged hypotension and myocardial ischemia.

procedure, such as local pain, dypsnea, discomfort, mental status change, or gastrointestinal symptom could be the initial hint of major intracardiac trauma or other complication. Particularly when it accompanies a change in vital signs such as hypotension, vascular or cardiac perforation with active bleeding or cardiac tamponade needs to be ruled out (Figure 31.3). The heart rate may be accelerated with aggravation of vascular volume loss and increased sympathetic activity, or it may exhibit bradycardia due to vasovagal reaction associated with injury.

VASCULAR COMPLICATIONS RELATED TO ACCESS (RETROGRADE APPROACH WITH ARTERIAL ACCESS)

As the vascular access is performed on frail patients of advanced age, whose arteries are significantly atherosclerosed, there is always a risk of inadvertent trauma of a vessel, resulting in hematoma formation, retroperitoneal bleeding, vascular perforation, dissection, or atheroembolization. For the introduction of

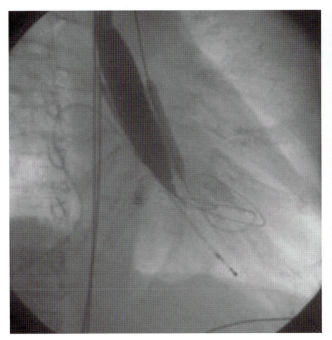
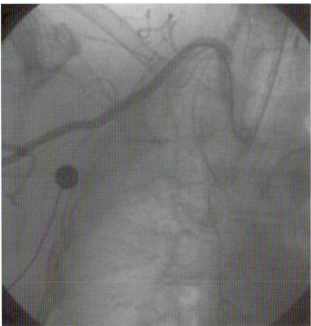

Figure 31.3   In order to gain appropriate dilation, the double-balloon technique was utilized for a 90-year-old female case with critical aortic stenosis. One PTAV balloon was approached from the right brachial artery. Subsequent to successful PTAV, the patient became agitated and diaphoretic, and her blood pressure dropped acutely from 130/70 to 70/40. The right subclavian angiogram demonstrated contrast dye leak from a branch of the right subclavian artery (arrow). The PTAV balloon was kept inflated in the right subclavian artery. Repeated occlusions by the balloon inflation for a limited time provided complete hemostasis without compromising the blood flow to her right arm. It is speculated that the guide wire perforated the branch.

the balloon catheter, a 9–12 French sheath is required for the retrograde arterial approach, and 14 French sheath for the transvenous antegrade approach. The manipulation of the large bore sheath or catheter can lead to major hemorrhage, formation of superficial hematoma, and pseudoaneurysm, occasionally requiring surgical repair or blood product transfusion.[7,8] These major vascular complications are associated with increased mortality and morbidity, and the treatment of the arteriotomy site is critical. Prolonged manual compression of the groin due to difficult hemostasis could potentially cause venous thrombosis and consequent pulmonary embolism in the patient who is immobile with low cardiac output. It is critically important to obtain the puncture in the appropriate location of the common femoral artery. A low puncture in the superficial or deep femoral branches has a higher risk of hematoma, and a higher puncture above the inguinal ligament could cause retroperitoneal bleeding. The use of preprocedural fluoroscopy to identify the anatomy is helpful. As the iliac and femoral arteries of these severely diseased patients are typically heavily calcified and tortuous (Figure 31.4), the placement of a long sheath is recommended in order to minimize vascular trauma.

As soon as a vascular complication is suspected, an angiogram or CT scan needs to be performed in order to confirm the diagnosis and its location. Occasionally

the compression of intrabladder contrast medium or deviation of the pyelo-urethra system may indicate acute retroperitoneal hemorrhage. Reversal of heparin anticoagulation with intravenous protamine is essential. Administration of one or two doses of 10–15 mg of protamine at a time is often adequate to reduce the activated clotting time to less than 200 seconds. Blood products such as packed red blood cells and FFP should be prepared, and the vascular surgical team should be called. For temporary occlusion, the PTAV balloon could be inflated at the site of perforation (Figure 31.3). If indicated, stent graft or coil embolization of the culprit artery may be considered.

In contrast, the transvenous antegrade approach is much less traumatic on the vascular system, making it the most useful method in avoiding vascular or atheroembolic complications deriving from injuries of arteries and the aorta.[3,4] Vascular surgery for femoral arterial complications is required in as many as 5% of patients. This has been dramatically reduced by applying suture closure in association with the retrograde or antegrade approach. The preclosure of 14 French venous puncture with sutures provides complete hemostasis with good success. Significant hematoma occurs in up to 10% of the patients treated by manual compression, and transfusion rates in some series are as high as 20%. The need for transfusion is almost completely eliminated in our practice using suture closure.[9–11]

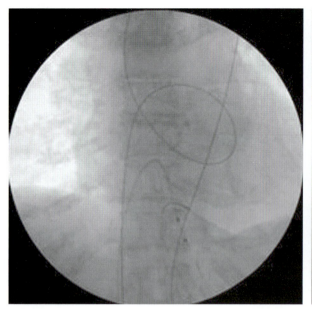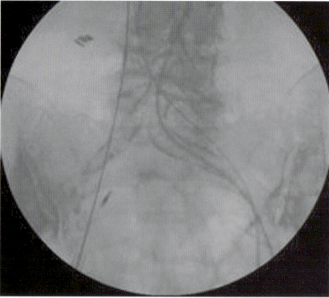

Figure 31.4   Wire placement for antegrade PTAV is demonstrated. There is a notably calcified and torturous iliac artery, and the patient has significantly high risk for vascular trauma or difficulty in advancing a large caliber device through the arterial system. The Inoue balloon catheter was advanced from the femoral venous access up to the aortic valve in the antegrade approach. In this approach, the potential for damage to the arteries and aorta is minimal, essentially making vascular-related complications negligiable.

COMPLICATIONS INVOLVING THE AORTA (RETROGRADE APPROACH USING THE FEMORAL ARTERIAL AND AORTIC SYSTEM)

With the manipulation of the catheter through a severely diseased aorta with atherosclerosis, plaque atheroembolization or cholesterol embolization could occur, causing ischemic symptoms involving the lower extremities or abdominal organs.[12] Cerebrovascular ischemia and infarct is one of the most debilitating potential complications. The aortic arch with atheroma is the source of iatrogenic atheroembolization. The friable or mobile atheroma in the aortic arch and ascending aorta may be scraped by the passage of wires or the balloon, with detached plaque showered into the cerebrovascular circulation. Furthermore, manipulation of a diseased aortic valve can cause atheroembolizaion or embolization of calcific debris from the leaflets, and this is more easily triggered by the retrograde approach, as leaflet calcification tends to be localized on the aortic side rather than on the left ventricular side of the aortic valve.

Any deterioration of mental status during or after PTAV could be a hint of low cerebral perfusion. Maintenance of appropriate anticoagulation during the procedure, avoidance of hypotension, and freedom from oversedation are all essential.

Preoperative evaluation of the aortic arch by transesophageal echocardiography (TEE), contrast-enhanced CT, or MRI in order to identify and localize the friable atheroma is helpful, so that mechanical stress on those structures by wire and catheter should be best avoided.

TEE has been the most commonly employed tool in our practice, since it is also used to exclude left atrium (LA) and left ventricle (LV) clot in patients with atrial fibrillation or a dilated LV, respectively.

CARDIAC PERFORATION AND TAMPONADE

Cardiac tamponade due to catheter or wire perforation has been reported in about 1% of PTAV cases. In the transarterial retrograde approach, the stiff wire placed in the LV is pushed against the apex of the left ventricle in order to support the advancement of the catheter. Although the distal end of the stiff wire is curved, it could apply excessive mechanical force, particularly when the aggressive advancement of the balloon is attempted due to difficulty in crossing the stenotic valve. Avoidance of excessive stress during the wire manipulation or advancement of the balloon is important. Futhermore, the balloon tip may traumatize the LV apex during balloon inflation. In the transvenous antegrade approach, cardiac perforation predominantly occurs in association with transseptal puncture. With the development of perforation, the patient may experience discomfort accompanying vasovagal response. Subsequent hemodynamic change is diverse, depending on the location, presence of pericardial adhesion (postpericardiotomy), and the size of the perforation. The development of tamponade may be a slow process with oozing, requiring several hours until there is accumulation of

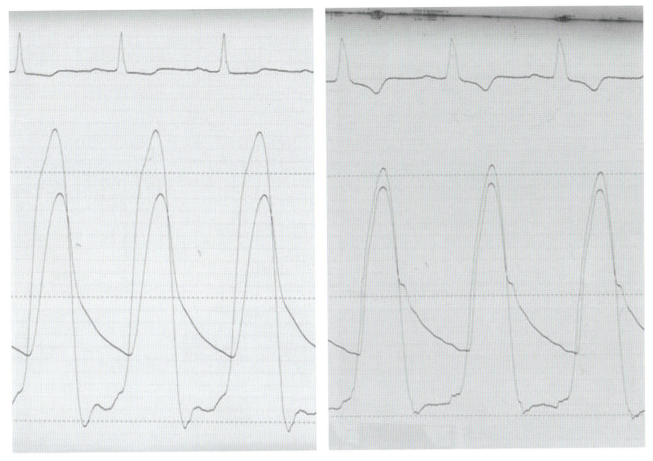

Figure 31.5   The presence of concomitant severe AR occasionally makes a case a contraindication for PTAV. Utilization of the Inoue balloon with antegrade aortic valve crossing enables the efficient and less mechanical trauma of a heavily calcified valve. This case is an 88-year-old with severe AS and concomitant severe AR, as illustrated by the wide aortic pressure difference. The controlled dilation successfully treated the AS, while not aggravating the AR. It is noted on the EKG trace that PTAV caused a transient intraventricular conduction defect.

enough effusion for tamponade, or in some cases frank bleeding with rapid hemodynamic compromise.

Whenever development of cardiac perforation is suspected, the procedure needs to be discontinued and intracardiac pressures followed with close echocardiographic observation. The catheter or wire causing the perforation is kept in place, as its removal could lead to fatal tamponade. If perforation is by puncture of the transseptal access needle alone, simply the reversal of anticoagulation may be enough. If insertion of the 8 French transseptal sheath or dilator creates the perforation, the instruments need to be left in place, and the surgical team must be called. Performance of pericardiocentesis is a requisite skill for these procedures.

VALVULAR OR LEAFLET DAMAGE RESULTING IN AR

As the mechanism of PTAV is based on the creation of microfractures of ostified valve in its mid segment, not commisurectomy, and some degree of dilation of the aortic valve ring, the procedure is essentially a form of therapeutic trauma of the valve. Therefore, if its effect is excessive, unfavorable valvular damage or avulsion could occur. Clinically significant aggravation of AR or development of new AR could occur in both the antegrade and retrograde approaches, however its incidence and degree are dependent on the technique utilized (Figure 31.5). The retrograde advancement of the wire or balloon causes distortion of the aortic valve, a less favorable balloon orientation, and more traumatic dilation, as compared to the antegrade approach. It is recommended to dilate the valve in a stepwise fashion from the small-sized to the larger-sized balloon or adding the balloon (double or triple balloon technique) to minimize the risk of undesirable valvular damage. Use of the Inoue balloon in the antegrade transvenous approach provides a favorable mechanical profile in dilating a heavily calcified aortic stenosis, with more secure positioning of the balloon.

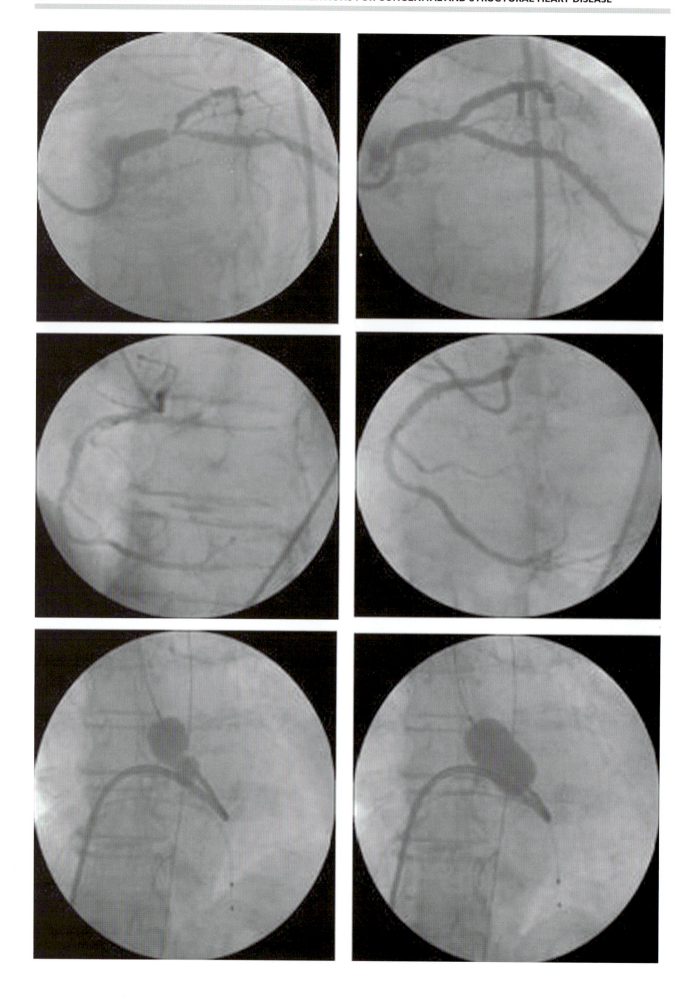

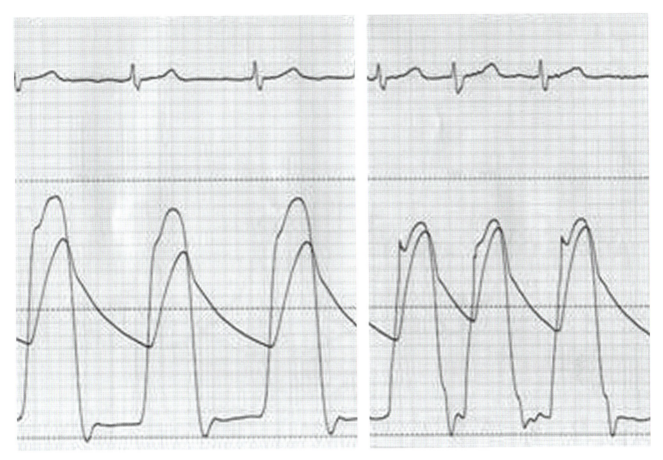

Figure 31.6   This illustrates the case of an 86-year-old patient who had critical calcific aortic stenosis (AS) and concomitant severe coronary artery stenosis involving the left main trunk, left anterior descending (LAD) artery, and right coronary artery (RCA). Due to the patient's poor general condition and refusal of surgery, transcatheter treatment was performed. In order to avoid myocardial insult both by ischemia and mechanical stress due to AS, the treatment was electively performed in the stepwise fashion. On the first day, the left coronary system was treated by PCI with left main stent implantation using the modified T technique and LAD stenting. On the second day, the RCA lesion was stented. Approximately a week later, AS was successfully treated by antegrade PTAV with a 26 mm Inoue balloon dilation, as demonstrated in the hemodynamic trace (AVA dilated from 0.7 to 1.2 cm^2).

LV FAILURE AND LOW CARDIAC OUTPUT ASSOCIATED WITH PTAV

Rarely, a progressive low-output state has been encountered after valvuloplasty, sometimes ending in death. Several technical factors can cause this disastrous syndrome. Each balloon inflation causes a transient but substantial stress on the LV. Outflow obstruction is acutely worsened and chamber dilation occurs. Ventricular pressure generation decreases, with elevation of intracardiac pressure and impairment of coronary perfusion. Arrhythmias further depress cardiac output and coronary perfusion.

Efficient balloon inflation with stable positioning, coupled with rapid deflation and withdrawal of the balloon from the valve, helps to avoid prolonged ouflow obstruction and minimizes hemodynamic compromise. Use of the Inoue balloon in the antegrade transvenous approach is most beneficial for this purpose. A rest period between inflations of several minutes is often useful. If the patient has severely compromised baseline LV systolic dysfunction or low cardiac output (<2.5 l/min), use of positive inotropic agents and/or LV support devices could be useful as a hemodynamic support.

As there is left ventricular hypertrophy and underlying subendomyocardial ischemia associated with pressure overload in aortic stenosis, concomitant epicardial coronary artery obstruction could cause significant myocardial ischemia. With additional hemodynamic stress by PTAV, myocardial ischemia is aggravated and this leads to further myocardial dysfunction or arrhythmia. Therefore it is important to perform percutaneous coronary intervention (PCI) of epicardial coronary artery disease prior to PTAV when large ischemic territories are present. In order to minimize both ischemic and mechanical stress on the myocardium, it is desirable to perform PCI and PTAV separately, allowing sufficient time for myocardial function to recover from each individual insult (Figure 31.6). In many cases separate sessions are not feasible, and a decision must be made regarding which lesion to treat first. In most cases, symptoms can be attributed to either the valve or the coronary lesion, and the more clinically important problem should be treated first.

COMPLICATIONS SPECIFIC TO THE TRANSVENOUS ANTEGRADE APPROACH

In the transvenous antegrade approach, there are several procedural steps which can potentially cause cardiovascular trauma. Where the iliac vein crosses over atherosclerotic iliac artery is the point where advancement of the transseptal needle may encounter significant resistance. The use of a 14 French long sheath is recommended prior to insertion of the 8 French Mullins sheath, to straighten the path of the Mullins sheath and eliminate friction where the iliac vein or inferior vena cava crosses the iliac artery. The stylet should be inserted through the inner lumen of the transseptal needle to facilitate its passage. As transseptal puncture is the critical step of this procedure, the related complications such as cardiac perforation with tamponade, and air or thromboembolization, need to be avoided. The use of intracardiac echocardiography (ICE) should be considered if any difficult is encountered, and this will greatly improve the safety profile.

In the antegrade approach, the wire is passed from the right to left atrium, across the mitral valve, looped in the LV, and then passed into the descending aorta. The wire can mechanically distort the mitral and aortic valves, keeping them propped open, and causing significant MR and AR.

In cases where the wire loop causes excessive mechanical stress on the mitral valve, mitral valve damage ensues, potentially resulting in permanent, critical MR and hemodynamic compromise. Furthermore, in the antegrade approach, when the wire travels through subvalvular structures, balloon inflation can cause significant subvalvular damage such as rupture of chordae, resulting in severe MR. When removing the wire at the completion of the procedure, it is important to advance a 5 or 6 French catheter, such as a pigtail or multipurpose one, over the wire to cover it and reduce friction as the wire is removed, and thus avoid the cutting effect of the wire on the mitral valve apparatus.

Another potential source of cardiac damage in the antegrade approach is the formation of an iatrogenic atrial septal defect (ASD). Transseptal tearing created by the wire and the catheter is usually small and is closed within 6 months of the procedure. However, when a clinically significant ASD results, repair may be necessary. This can be accomplished with septal closure devices in most cases.

In conclusion, PTAV is an underutilized palliative procedure, in part because complications can be severe and difficult to manage. Most patients have 1–2 years of relief of symptoms after these procedures.[13,14] Careful attention to procedural technique and a high index of suspicion for the occurrence of complications can lead to early treatment of problems before they are catastrophic. Hopefully this will allow more of these elderly, high-risk patients to derive the considerable relief of symptoms associated with PTAV.

REFERENCES

1. Feldman T. Balloon aortic valvuloplasty appropriate for elderly patients. J Interven Cardiol 2006; 19: 276–9.
2. Hara H, Pedersen WR, Ladich E et al. Percutaneous balloon aortic valvuloplasty revisited: time for a renaissance. Circulation 2007; 115: e334–8.
3. Eisenhauer AC, Hadjipetrou P, Piemonte TC. Balloon aortic valvuloplasty revisited: the role of the Inoue balloon and transseptal antegrade approach. Cathet Cardiovasc Interven 2000; 50: 484–91.
4. Sakata Y, Syed Z, Salinger M, Feldman T. Percutaneous balloon aortic valvuloplasty: antegrade transseptal vs. conventional retrograde transarterial approach. Cathet Cardiovasc Interven 2005; 64: 314–21.
5. Carlson MD, Palacios I, Thomas JD et al. Cardiac conduction abnormalities during percutaneous balloon mitral or aortic valvotomy. Circulation 1989; 79: 1197–203.
6. Isner JM. Acute catastrophic complications of balloon aortic valvuloplasty. The mansfield scientific aortic valvuloplasty registry investigators. J Am Coll Cardiology 1991; 17: 1346–444.
7. Letac B, Cribier A, Koning R, Lefebvre E. Aortic stenosis in elderly patients aged 80 or older. Treatment by percutaneous balloon valvuloplasty in a series of 92 cases. Ciruculation 1989; 80: 1514–20.
8. Lewin RF, Dorros G, King JF, Mathiak L. Percutaneous transluminal aortic valvuloplasty: acute outcome and follow-up of 125 patients. J Am Coll Cardiol 1989; 14: 1210–17.
9. Feldman T. Percutaneous suture closure for management of large French size arterial and venous puncture. J Interven Cardiol 2000; 13: 237–42.
10. Mylonas I, Sakata Y, Salinger M, Sanborn T, Feldman T. The use of percutaneous suture-mediated closure for the management of 14 French venous access. J Invas Cardiol 2006; 18: 299–302.
11. Solomon LW, Fusman B, Jolly N et al. Percutaneous suture closure for management of large French size arterial puncture in aortic valvuloplasty. J Invas Cardiol 2001; 13: 592–6.
12. Safian RD, Berman AD, Diver DR et al. Balloon aortic valvuloplasty in 170 consecutive patients. N Engl J Med 1988; 319: 125–30.
13. Sherman W, Hershman R, Lazzam C et al. Balloon aortic valvuloplasty in adult aortic stenosis: determinants of clinical outcome. Ann Intern Med 1989; 110: 421–5.
14. Agarwal A, Kini AS, Attanti S et al. Results of repeat balloon valvuloplasty for treatment of aortic stenosis in patients aged 59 to 104 years. Am J Cardiol 2005; 95(1): 43–7.

32 Percutaneous mitral commissurotomy

Alec Vahanian, Dominique Himbert, Eric Brochet, and Bernard Iung

INTRODUCTION

Percutaneous mitral commissurotomy (PMC) has been in use in the treatment of mitral stenosis since 1984.[1] The good immediate and mid term results obtained during the last 20 years have led to its wide spread dissemination. It has now virtually replaced surgical commissurotomy and is a complement of mitral valve replacement.[2]

The several thousand procedures performed in patients with different clinical conditions and valve anatomy have allowed us to accurately assess the risk involved.[3–12] Generally speaking, the occurrence of complications can be patient-related due to their clinical and anatomic condition or operator-related, since the importance of training in this procedure has been demonstrated by the comparison of early and late experience in the same groups and of large-volume center reports and multicenter studies, including centers with variable experience (Table 32.1).

COMPLICATIONS

Hemopericardium

Hemopericardium may be related to transseptal catheterization or to left ventricular perforation by the guide wires or the balloons. Its incidence varies from 0.5% to 12%. Hemopericardium usually has immediate clinical consequences resulting in tamponade and should always be suspected when hypotension occurs during PMC. Hemopericardium related to the transseptal puncture mostly occurs when the operator is less experienced.[3,7,10] Unfavorable patient characteristics such as severe atrial enlargement or severe thoracic deformity also increase risk. Furthermore, the occurrence of hemopericardium may be technique dependent. The double-balloon technique and its variant the multitrack technique[12] or the metallic commissurotome[9] carry a higher risk than the Inoue technique, which is now almost the only technique worldwide where the risk of left ventricular perforation is virtually eliminated.[11]

If hemopericardium is suspected, echocardiography should be performed urgently before deterioration occurs (Figure 32.1). This stresses the importance of immediate availability of echocardiography when performing PMC.

Hemopericardium requires immediate pericardiocentesis, ideally performed under echocardiographic guidance after reversal of anticoagulation. If this is successful, PMC can be reattempted and the patient should be closely monitored. In most cases, hemopericardium due to transseptal catheterization can be managed by pericardiocentesis, especially when it results from only an incorrect puncture by the transseptal needle. This underlines the fact that the transseptal catheter should only be advanced over the needle when fluoroscopy and pressure monitoring have confirmed a satisfactory positioning of the needle.

The prevention of this complication firstly includes proper training in transseptal catheterization. PMC clearly should be restricted to teams that have extensive experience with transseptal catheterization and are able to perform an adequate number of procedures.[13] The interventionists must also be able to perform emergency pericardiocentesis.

Echographic monitoring using either the transesophageal or intracardiac approach can be helpful for transseptal catheterization.[14] In experienced teams, echocardiographic guidance is restricted to cases with known difficulties, such as severe thoracic deformity, or where unexpected difficulties occur.

PMC should not be performed in patients with bleeding disorders, in particular those with too high anticoagulation. Transseptal catheterization should not be performed if the INR is >1.2, in particular in patients who have not had a previous cardiac operation, i.e. pericardial opening. In patients receiving intravenous heparin, it should be discontinued 4 hours before the procedure and can be restarted 2 hours after.[15,16] Vitamin K should not be given before the procedure in patients who are at high risk for left atrial thrombosis, and PMC should be delayed until a satisfactory level of coagulability is reached. To further increase safety, the absence of hemopericardium could be verified using echocardiography before administering heparin after the transseptal puncture.

Embolism

Embolism may be due to a thrombus that was pre-existing, mostly in the left atrial appendage (Figure 32.2), or it may have developed during the procedure due to air leaking from the balloon or, very rarely, to calcium.

Table 32.1   Severe complications of percutaneous mitral commissurotomy.

Study	Number	Mortality (%)	Hemopericardium (%)	Embolism (%)	Severe mitral regurgitation (%)
Ben Farhat et al.[4]	463	0.4	0.7	2	4.6
Chen et al.[5]	4832	0.12	0.8	0.5	1.4
Iung et al.[7]	2773	0.4	0.2	0.4	4.1
NHLBI.[6]	738	3	4	3	3
Stefanadis et al.[8]	893	0.3	0	0	3.1
Tuzcu et al.[3]	311	1.7	NA	–	8.7 (>2+ increase)

NA, not available; NHLBI, National Heart, Lung, and Blood Institute.

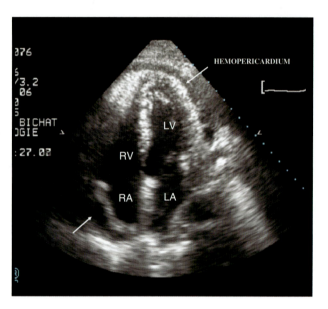

Figure 32.1   Hemopericardium after PMC shown by transthoracic echocardiography. Apical four-chamber view.

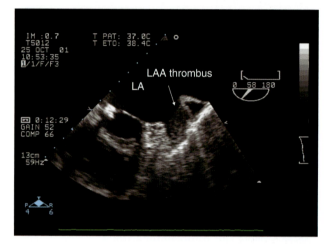

Figure 32.2   Transesophageal echocardiography showing a large thrombus in the left atrial appendage (arrow). LA, left atrium; LAA, Left atrial appendage.

Embolism is encountered in 0.5 to 5% of cases. Cerebral embolism usually results in a stroke. Coronary embolism leads to transient ST segment elevation in inferior leads, which is well tolerated when it is due to microbubbles of air that can occur when using the Inoue balloon and will resolve spontaneously. If it is due to embolization of a large quantity of air, such as when the balloons rupture with the double-balloon technique, it may lead to vagal reaction and hypotension.

The treatment of cerebral embolism should be in collaboration with a stroke center. Cerebral imaging should be performed on an emergency basis to rule out hemorrhage, then intra-arterial fibrinolytic therapy should be administered early in the absence of contraindication. In the case of persistent ST segment elevation, coronary angiography should be performed. If a coronary occlusion is present, coronary angioplasty can be performed, while thrombo-aspiration could be an appealing alternative.

Although the incidence of embolism is low, its potential consequences are severe and all possible precautions

should be taken to prevent it. Thus, transesophageal echocardiography (TEE) should be performed a few days prior to intervention to rule out the presence of such thrombi. PMC is contraindicated in patients with a thrombus floating in the left atrial cavity or located on the atrial septum. No consensus has been reached regarding patients with thrombosis in the left atrial appendage.[15–18] The indications for PMC are limited to patients with contraindications to surgery or those without urgent need for intervention when oral anticoagulation can be given for at least 2 and up to 6 months,[17] and a new TEE examination shows the disappearance of the thrombus.[15,16] During this period the level of oral anticoagulation should be increased (INR 3–3.5). Aspirin can be added in patients at low bleeding risk.

During PMC, heparin should be given as a bolus at a dose of around 3 to 5000 IU after the transseptal catheterization. In addition the duration of the procedure should be kept to a minimum.

The occurrence of air embolism may be decreased by careful venting of the Inoue balloon and repeated inflations in saline to flush out the last bubbles of air before use.

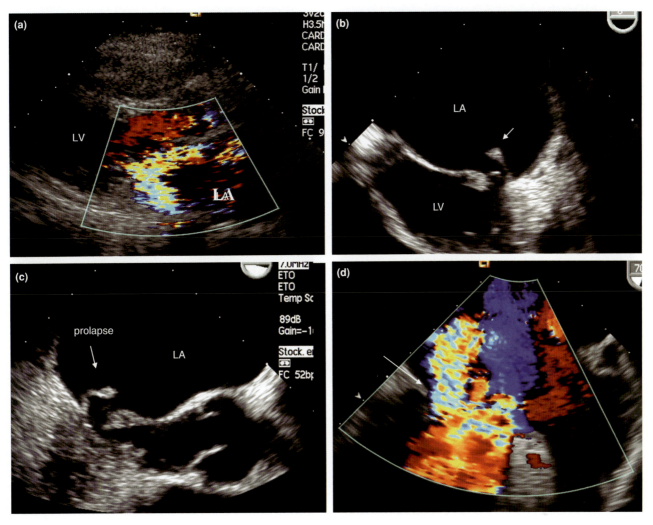

Figure 32.3 Severe mitral regurgitation (MR) occurring during PMC. (A) Transthoracic parasternal long axis view; diffracted color Doppler jet of MR. (B–D) Transesophageal echocardiography; prolapse of posterior leaflet with severe eccentric mitral regurgitant jet (arrow).

Severe mitral regurgitation

Severe mitral regurgitation is rare but represents an ever-present risk.[19–23] Surgical findings[19,22,23] have shown that it is most often related to non-commissural leaflet tearing, which could be associated with chordal rupture (Figure 32.3). In these cases, one or both commissures are often too tightly fused to be split. Severe mitral regurgitation may also be due to excessive commissural splitting or, in very rare cases, rupture of a papillary muscle. The majority of cases of severe mitral regurgitation occur in patients with unfavorable anatomy.

The frequency of severe mitral regurgitation ranges from 2 to 19%.[3–12] As mitral regurgitation is usually initially well tolerated, surgery can be performed on a scheduled basis. The precise timing of intervention should be based on functional tolerance and surgical risk. Subsequent surgical treatment is usually necessary because the prognosis of patients with severe mitral regurgitation after PMC, or surgical commissurotomy, is usually poor, with secondary objective deterioration and a lack of symptom alleviation. In most cases, valve replacement is required because of the severity of the underlying valve disease. Conservative surgery has been successfully performed in cases of less severe valve deformity.[22]

At the present stage, the occurrence of severe mitral regurgitation remains largely unpredictable for a given patient[7] and its development depends more on the distribution of morphologic changes than on their severity. Scores that take into account the uneven distribution of anatomic deformities of the leaflets or commissural area have been developed.[24] Preliminary results for their use are promising but disputed.[25]

The available data suggest, but do not prove, that the stepwise Inoue technique, combined with echocardiographic monitoring, is likely to decrease the incidence of severe regurgitation, even if it does not eliminate it.

The balloon should be properly sized and the procedure should be stopped if the degree of regurgitation increases. The following criteria have been proposed for the desired endpoint of the procedure: (1) mitral valve area of more than 1 cm^2/m^2 of the body surface area; (2) complete opening of at least one commissure; or (3) appearance or increment of regurgitation of more than ¼, especially if the regurgitation is located in a commissural area and if its mechanism is leaflet tear or chordal rupture.[11] The strategy should be tailored to the individual circumstances, taking into account clinical factors, such as the risk and availability of surgery, together with anatomic factors and the cumulative data of periprocedural monitoring. For example, balloon size, increments of size, and expected final valve area are smaller in elderly patients and in the presence of tight mitral stenosis, extensive valve and subvalvular disease, and nodular commissural calcification. The same holds to be true for pregnant patients in whom the goal of the procedure should be to allow for delivery and where emergency surgery could have dramatic consequences for the fetus.

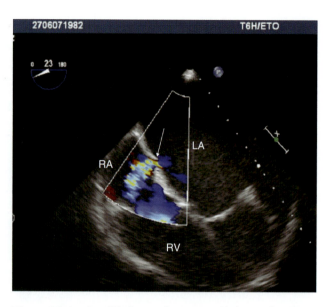

Figure 32.4 Small left to right interatrial shunt after PMC assessed by transesophageal echocardiography (arrow). LA, left atrium; RA, right atrium; RV, right ventricle.

RESCUE SURGERY

Although urgent surgery (within 24 hours) is seldom needed for complications (<1%), it may be required for massive hemopericardium resulting from left ventricular perforation intractable to treatment by pericardiocentesis. According to circumstances, this could be drainage of the pericardial effusion alone or also include valve surgery. Less frequently, severe mitral regurgitation, leading to hemodynamic collapse or refractory pulmonary edema, may necessitate emergency surgery with the support o f an intra-aortic balloon pump en route to the operating room. The exact arrangement for surgical back-up varies from institution to institution, according to the severity of the condition being treated and the experience of the cardiologic and surgical teams.

MORTALITY

The main causes of death are massive hemopericardium or the poor condition of the patient. The latter condition is often a factor in end stage patients, such as an elderly patient where PMC is attempted as a palliative procedure,[26] or in emergency cases performed in patients in pulmonary edema or, very occasionally, in cardiogenic shock.[27,28] The fatality rate ranges from 0 to 3%. The decrease in fatality is related to the experience of the team in PMC, the availability of rescue surgery, and also the selection of the patients. In respect of this latter factor, it is probably better to withhold PMC in elderly patients in shock where the outcome is particularly poor and the efficacy of PMC very limited.

INTER-ATRIAL SHUNTS

The clinical importance of this complication was largely overemphasized in the early days of PMC. These shunts are usually small and without consequence, since most of them will disappear on follow-up after successful PMC because of a reduced interatrial pressure gradient. The persistence of shunts is related to their magnitude (diameter of the defect > 0.5 cm or Qp/Qs ratio > 1.5) or to unsatisfactory relief of the valve obstruction. In rare circumstances, right to left shunts may occur in patients with severe pulmonary hypertension when PMC is not successful and leads to hypoxemia.

The frequency of interatrial shunts varies from 10 to 90%, depending on the technique used for detection[4–12,29] (Figure 32.4).

Surgery has very seldom been necessary because of interatrial shunting. On the other hand, if surgery is needed for unsuccessful PMC or restenosis, the interatrial septum should be looked at and septal tears sutured at the time of surgery. No cases of percutaneous closure of such defects have been reported to our knowledge, and such a procedure is unlikely to be successful because the interatrial shunts are not due to defects similar to patent foramen ovale or congenital atrial septal defects, but to longitudinal tears.

The use of the Inoue technique has significantly decreased the incidence of this complication in comparison with other techniques. To further decrease the magnitude of the problem it is necessary to fully slenderize the Inoue balloon before withdrawal and also to pull the guide wire so that only the soft part protrudes from the balloon during withdrawal across the interatrial septum in order to avoid the 'cutting effect' which may occur if the stiff part of the guide wire is out of the tip of the balloon during the maneuver.

OTHER COMPLICATIONS

Atrial fibrillation rarely occurs during the procedure. When it does, it is usually transient and resolves within a few hours under medical treatment. In rare cases where it persists, it requires electric counter shock a few days after.

The incidence of transient, *complete heart block* is rare (<1%) and exceptionally requires implantation of a permanent pacemaker.

Vascular complications are the exception when using the antegrade or transvenous approach, but were more frequently seen with the retrograde approach, which is now almost abandoned. In teams experienced in transseptal catheterization, left heart catheterization may be avoided to simplify the procedure and further reduce the incidence of vascular complication as well as shorten the duration of hospital stay.[30]

Endocarditis is extremely rare and does not justify prophylaxis before the procedure. The risk is higher when balloons are reused, which occurs in many centers in developing countries. The same holds to be true for transmissible infections such as hepatitis or aids.

With regard to *specific risks of PMC during pregnancy*,[31,32] concerns were initially raised regarding the fetal tolerance of the procedure and the potential risk related to radiation, since the procedure is monitored using fluoroscopy. The use of cardiac fetal monitoring during the procedure showed that PMC during pregnancy was not associated with signs of fetal distress. Semiquantitative radiation dose assessment showed that the radiation dose remains at very low levels and this is unlikely to have any consequence on the short- as well as long-term outcome of the fetus. The alternative of performing the procedure uniquely under TEE has been proposed in short series. However, this was associated with a high complication rate, including tamponade. This approach is, therefore, not recommended.

In particular during pregnancy, PMC should be performed by experienced operators. This is an important condition to keep the risk of complications as low as possible and to shorten the duration of the procedure and fluoroscopy time. The use of the Inoue balloon is particularly attractive in this setting. The abdomen of the patient should be covered using a lead apron during the procedure. The monitoring of valve opening relies on echocardiographic examination, thereby avoiding the use of cardiac catheterization and angiography to decrease radiation and avoid hypothyroidy due to dye injections.

Maternal complications could be partly related to the fact that PMC may be performed as an emergency procedure in critically ill patients. Thromboembolic complications are rare but may be favored by hypercoagulability, which is present during pregnancy. Consequences of traumatic mitral regurgitation can be particularly harmful in pregnant patients because severe, acute, mitral regurgitation is poorly tolerated given the increase in blood volume and cardiac output. Urgent valvular surgery could be needed in such cases, with the inherent risk for the fetus. If the tolerance is good it is preferable to wait for the fetus to be viable and perform Cesarean section quickly before cardiac surgery.

CONCLUSION

After over 20 years of extensive clinical evaluation, PMC appears to be an effective procedure that carries a small but definite risk.[33,34] Overall, the considerable simplification resulting from use of the Inoue balloon could lead to a false sense of security and must not overshadow the importance of training. Due to the low prevalence of mitral stenosis in developed countries, maintenance of experience will be difficult. It seems appropriate to concentrate the performance of the procedure among experienced centers to improve the management of the interventional procedure by decreasing the risk and improving the selection of patients by means of clinical evaluation and echocardiographic assessment.

REFERENCES

1. Inoue K, Owaki T, Nakamura T et al. Clinical application of transvenous mitral commissurotomy by a new balloon catheter. J Thorac Cardiovasc Surg 1984; 87: 394–402.
2. Iung B, Baron G, Butchart EG et al. A prospective survey of patients with valvular heart disease in Europe: the Euro Heart Survey on valvular heart disease. Eur Heart J 2003; 13: 1231–43.
3. Tuzcu EM, Block PC, Palacios IF et al. Comparison of early versus late experience with percutaneous mitral balloon valvuloplasty. J Am Coll Cardiol 1991; 17: 1121–4.
4. Ben Farhat M, Betbout F, Gamra H et al. Results of percutaneous double-balloon mitral commissurotomy in one medical center in Tunisia. Am J Cardiol 1995; 76: 1266–70.
5. Chen CR, Cheng TO. Percutaneous balloon mitral valvuloplasty by the Inoue technique: a multicenter study of 4832 patients in China. Am Heart J 1995; 129: 1197–1202.
6. The National Heart, Lung, and Blood Institute Balloon Valvuloplasty Registry. Complications and mortality of percutaneous balloon mitral commissurotomy. Circulation 1992; 85: 2014–24.
7. Iung B, Nicoud-Houel A, Fondard O et al. Temporal trends in percutaneous mitral commissurotomy over a 15-year period. Eur Heart J 2004; 25: 702–8.
8. Stefanadis CI, Stratos CG, Lambrou SG et al. Accomplishments and perspectives with retrograde nontransseptal balloon mitral valvuloplasty. J Interven Cardiol 2000; 13: 269–80.
9. Cribier A, Eltchaninoff H, Carlot R. Percutaneous mechanical mitral commissurotomy with the metallic valvotome: detailed technical aspect and overview of the results of the multicenter registry 882 patients. J Interven Cardiol 2000; 13: 255–62.

10. Harrison KJ, Wilson JS, Hearne SE et al. Complications related to percutaneous transvenous mitral commissurotomy. Cathet Cardiovasc Diagn 1994; 2: 52–60.

11. Vahanian A, Cormier B, Iung B. Percutaneous transvenous mitral commissurotomy using the Inoue balloon: international experience. Cathet Cardiovasc Diagn 1994; 2: 8–15.

12. Bonhoeffer P, Hausse A, Yonga G. Technique and results of percutaneous mitral valvuloplasty with the multi-track system. J Interven Cardiol 2000: 13: 263–9.

13. King SB 3rd, Aversano T, Ballard WL et al American College of Cardiology Foundation; American Heart Association; American College of Physicians Task Force on Clinical Competence and Training (writing Committee to Update the 1998 Clinical Competence Statement on Recommendations for the Assessment and Maintenance of Proficiency in Coronary Interventional Procedures). ACCF/AHA/SCAI 2007 update of the clinical competence statement on cardiac interventional procedures: a report of the American College of Cardiology Foundation/American Heart Association/American College of Physicians Task Force on Clinical Competence and Training (writing Committee to Update the 1998 Clinical Competence Statement on Recommendations for the Assessment and Maintenance of Proficiency in Coronary Interventional Procedures). J Am Coll Cardiol 2007; 50: 82–108.

14. Green NE, Hansgen AR, Carroll JD. Initial clinical experience with intracardiac echocardiography in guiding balloon mitral valvuloplasty: technique, safety, utility, and limitations. Cathet Cardiovasc Interven 2004; 63: 385–94.

15. Bonow RO, Carabello BA, Chatterjee K et al. ACC/AHA 2006 Guidelines for the Management of Patients With Valvular Heart Disease. A Report of the American College of Cardiology/American Heart Association Task Force on Practice Guidelines. J Am Coll Cardiol 2006; 48: e1–148.

16. Vahanian A, Baumgartner H, Bax J et al. Task Force on the Management of Valvular Heart Disease of the European Society of Cardiology; ESC Committee for Practice Guidelines. Guidelines on the management of valvular heart disease: The Task Force on the Management of Valvular Heart Disease of the European Society of Cardiology. Eur Heart J 2007; 28: 230–68.

17. Silaruks S, Thinkhamrop B, Kiatchoosakun S, Wongvipaporn C, Tatsanavivat P. Resolution of left atrial thrombus after 6 months of anticoagulation in candidates for percutaneous transvenous mitral commissurotomy. Ann Intern Med 2004; 140: 101–5.

18. Chen WJ, Chen MF, Liau CS et al. Safety of percutaneous transvenous balloon mitral commissurotomy in patients with mitral stenosis and thrombus in the left atrial appendage. Am J Cardiol 1992; 70: 117–19.

19. Herrmann HC, Lima JAC, Feldman T et al. Mechanisms and outcome of severe mitral regurgitation after Inoue balloon valvuloplasty. J Am Coll Cardiol 1993; 27: 783–9.

20. Hernandez R, Macaya C, Benuelos C et al. Predictors, mechanisms, and outcome of severe mitral regurgitation complicating percutaneous mitral valvotomy with the Inoue balloon. Am J Cardiol 1993; 70: 1169–74.

21. Choudhary SK, Talwar S, Venugopal P. Severe mitral regurgitation after percutaneous transmitral commissurotomy: underestimated subvalvular disease. J Thorac Cardiovasc Surg 2006; 131: 927.

22 Acar C, Jebara VA, Grare PH et al. Traumatic mitral insufficiency following percutaneous mitral dilation: anatomic lesions and surgical implications. Eur J Cardiothorac Surg 1992; 6: 660–4.

23. Varma PK, Theodore S, Neema PK et al. Emergency surgery after percutaneous transmitral commissurotomy: operative versus echocardiographic findings, mechanisms of complications, and outcomes. J Thorac Cardiovasc Surg 2005; 130: 772–6.

24. Padial LR, Abascal VM, Moreno PR et al. Echocardiography can predict the development of severe mitral regurgitation after percutaneous mitral valvuloplasty by the Inoue technique. Am J Cardiol 1999; 83: 1210–13.

25. Mezilis ME, Salame MY, Oakly DG. Predicting mitral regurgitation following percutaneous mitral valvotomy with the Inoue balloon: comparison of two echocardiographic scoring systems. Clin Cardiol 1999; 22: 453–58.

26. Shaw TRD, Sutaria N, Prendergost B. Clinical and hemodynamic profiles of young, middle aged and elderly patients with mitral stenosis undergoing mitral balloon valvotomy. Heart 2003; 89: 1430–6.

27. Vahanian A, Iung B, Nallet O. Percutaneous valvuloplasty in cardiogenic shock. In: Hasdai D, Berger P, Battler A, Holmes D, eds. Cardiogenic Shock: Diagnosis and Treatment. New Jersey: Humana Press Inc, 2002; 181–93.

28. Goldman J, Slade A, Clague J. Cardiogenic shock to mitral stenosis treated by balloon mitral valvuloplasty. Cathet Cardiovasc Diagn 1998; 43: 195–7.

29. Cequier A, Bonan R, Dyrda I et al. Atrial shunting after percutaneous mitral valvuloplasty. Circulation 1990; 81: 1190–7.

30. Gupta S, Schiele F, Xu C et al. Simplified percutaneous mitral valvuloplasty with the Inoue balloon. Eur Heart J 1998; 19: 610–6.

31. Presbitero P, Prever SB, Brusca A. Interventional cardiology in pregnancy. Eur Heart J 1996; 17: 182–8.

32. Weiss BM. Managing severe mitral valve stenosis in pregnant patients – percutaneous balloon valvuloplasty, not surgery, is the treatment of choice. J Cardiothorac Vasc Anesth 2005; 19: 277–8.

33. Feldman T. Core curriculum for interventional cardiology: percutaneous valvuloplasty. Cathet Cardiovasc Interven 2003; 60: 48–56.

34. Vahanian A, Palacios IF. Percutaneous approaches to valvular disease. Circulation 2004; 109: 1572–9.

33 Balloon pericardial window

Andrew O Maree, Hani Jneid, and Igor F Palacios

BACKGROUND

Percutaneous transcatheter aspiration of fluid from the pericardium or pericardiocentesis is performed for both diagnostic and therapeutic purposes. It is indicated as a diagnostic procedure to establish the etiology of a pericardial effusion. Therapeutic pericardiocentesis is most commonly performed emergently to relieve cardiac tamponade and thereby prevent progression to pulseless electrical activity and cardiac arrest. Diagnostic information is also gained in this setting through analysis of the pericardial fluid and evaluation of the pericardial pressure. When pericardial hemodynamic assessment is performed with concomitant right heart catheterization, processes such as effusive-constrictive pericarditis can be confirmed or ruled-out.[1]

In most cases of pericardial effusion, once-off pericardiocentesis will confirm the etiology and correct hemodynamic impairment. Postprocedure, an indwelling catheter is usually left in place to facilitate near complete drainage of the pericardium. However, patients in whom pericardial fluid continues to accumulate are at significant risk of recurrent tamponade.

Percutaneous balloon pericardiotomy (balloon pericardial window) is performed in follow-on from pericardiocentesis, primarily to prevent recurrent pericardial effusion and the possibility of tamponade.[2,3] As such, it provides a less invasive alternative to the surgical creation of a pericardial window.

Cardiac surgery has replaced malignancy as the leading cause of pericardial effusion requiring percutaneous drainage.[4] However, patients with malignant pericardial effusion or uremic pericardial disease are most at risk of fluid reaccumulation. Pericardial disease is the most common indication for cardiology consultation among hospitalized patients with cancer.[5] Effusions related to malignancy or radiotherapy are five times more likely to require repeat pericardiocentesis when compared to those with non-malignancy-related effusions. Malignant effusions are most commonly associated with lung and breast cancer. Balloon pericardiotomy in this population is highly successful, with approximately 88% freedom from recurrence at 4 months.[5]

Large idiopathic chronic pericardial effusions, though frequently well tolerated, may progress unexpectedly to severe tamponade. Catheter drainage of such effusions is associated with lower recurrence rates than conservative treatment, and thus pre-emptive treatment may be warranted.[4] Any patient with recurrent tamponade should also be considered a candidate for a more definitive percutaneous or surgical pericardial procedure. Options include pericardiocentesis followed by instillation of sclerosant, or alternatively, percutaneous or surgical creation of a pericardial window.[6]

PROCEDURAL TECHNIQUE

Pericardiocentesis

The percutaneous balloon pericardial window technique was pioneered at Massachusetts General Hospital, initially as a procedure to treat patients with malignant pericardial effusion who were poor surgical candidates.[2] The technique was developed to follow on from standard pericardiocentesis via the subxiphoid approach. Although now performed in a variety of settings (non-invasive laboratory, intensive care units with bedside echocardiographic guidance) pericardiocentesis preceding percutaneous balloon pericardiotomy should be performed in the cardiac catheterization laboratory. Initial pericardiocentesis is carried out in standard fashion using the Seldinger technique. The skin and subcutaneous tissue are infiltrated with local anesthesia (2% lidocaine) 1 cm below and to the left of the xiphocostal junction. The pericardial needle is connected to an ECG lead and inserted, directing it towards the left shoulder (under fluoroscopic or echocardiographic guidance). The needle passes through the diaphragm (a discrete pop may be felt) and advanced into the pericardial space. ST-segment elevation on the ECG tracing indicates contact with the epicardium. On entry into the pericardial space a guide wire is inserted via the needle into the pericardial sac. The needle is then removed, the track dilated, and a percutaneous catheter (usually pigtail) or sheath is then inserted into the pericardial space. An opening pericardial pressure should be recorded and fluid samples collected for analysis (biochemical, cytologic, bacteriologic, and immunologic). In the setting of pericardial tamponade, fluid is aspirated until hemodynamic and clinical improvement occurs.

Percutaneous balloon pericardiotomy (balloon pericardial window)

A percutaneous pericardial window can be created safely with minimal discomfort under conscious sedation with local anesthesia. A small amount of iodinated contrast (5–10 ml) is introduced under fluoroscopy via the indwelling pericardial catheter or sheath to define the pericardial space (Figure 33.1A). A preshaped stiff guide wire (0.038 inch) with a broad curve on the tip is advanced through the indwelling catheter until it loops in the pericardial sac and the catheter is removed. The skin and subcutaneous tissue are predilated with a 10 French dilator prior to insertion of the balloon dilating catheter (typically 20 mm diameter × 3 cm long) over the wire. Biplane fluoroscopy is the optimal imaging modality, with one plane in the left lateral projection. The balloon is positioned such that its mid portion straddles the parietal pericardium, taking care to insure that the proximal end is inserted beyond the skin and subcutaneous tissue (Figure 33.1B). The balloon is then inflated until both sides of the waist caused by the pericardial sac are obliterated (Figure 33.1C). Two to three inflations may be required. The balloon dilation catheter is then exchanged for an indwelling (pigtail) catheter which is left in place to insure complete clearance of the effusion.

In vitro evaluation of the technique demonstrates that the balloon disrupts collagen and elastic fibers at the edge of the pericardiotomy site, resulting in localized tearing of the parietal pericardium. In most cases this results in communication between the pericardial and pleural cavity. Rarely, communication with the abdominal cavity occurs.[7]

Double-balloon technique

Modification of the single-balloon technique involves simultaneous use of two balloon catheters to create the window.[8,9] In this technique, two 0.035 inch J-tipped wires are introduced via a 7 French sheath. The point of separation of the two wires in the pericardial space helps to determine the border of the parietal pericardium. Two sheaths are then inserted over the wires and two balloon catheters (8–12 mm × 2 cm and 8–12 mm × 4 cm, depending on body habitus) inserted via the sheaths. The balloons are inflated simultaneously until the waists are gone. The larger balloon is then fixed and the smaller one advanced and withdrawn through the defect in the pericardium to establish the window further.

Postprocedure, patients can be monitored in a general medical ward. The pericardial catheter should be aspirated at 6 to 8 hourly intervals and flushed with sterile heparinized saline until pericardial drainage volumes are less than < 50–75 ml in 24 hours. A chest X-ray should be performed to determine if a pleural effusion has developed from the draining pericardial fluid. Some advocate antibiotic coverage while the catheter is in place (usually first-generation cephalosporin for empirical coverage of gram-positive bacteria).

HOW TO STAY OUT OF TROUBLE

Although a relatively simple procedure, there are several pitfalls that need to be avoided when performing percutaneous balloon pericardiotomy. It is noteworthy that major complications accompany 1.3–1.6% of cases of pericardiocentesis and all contraindications to pericardiocentesis extend to balloon pericardiotomy.[10] Firstly, the pericardial effusion should be of sufficient size, non-loculated, and causally associated with the process that you intend to correct to make percutaneous drainage a reasonable approach. Drainage of more than 1 l of pericardial fluid at a time may be associated with right ventricular dilatation and therefore fluid replacement may be required in these cases.[11]

Patients with bleeding diatheses, thrombocytopenia (platelet count < 50 000/mm³), or on anticoagulant therapy are at significant risk of hemorrhage associated with pericardiocentesis. This risk is significantly greater with balloon pericardiotomy where trauma to pericardial vessels requiring surgical intervention is a recognized complication.[3]

Pericardial effusions frequently accompany aortic dissection (17–45%).[12] Pericardial tamponade complicating aortic dissection occurs most commonly with De-Bakey type II (18–45%) and less frequently type I (17–33%) or type III dissections (6%). These patients are at considerable risk of further hemorrhage and extension of the dissection if treated percutaneously (increases dp/dt (pressure over time)) and therefore should be managed with open surgical repair.[13] The pericardium is highly innervated and mechanical disruption is associated with considerable discomfort, therefore care should be taken to administer adequate analgesia and sedation in advance. Patients with reduced pulmonary reserve should be assessed carefully prior to consideration for percutaneous balloon pericardiotomy. Development of a left pleural effusion within 24 to 48 hours is common and thoracentesis is frequently required (approximately 16% of cases).[3] Thus patients postpneumonectomy or those with a coexistent pleural effusion may tolerate the procedure poorly, and risks and benefits should be weighed carefully in advance. When performing balloon pericardiotomy, particular care must be taken to insure that the proximal portion of the balloon catheter is clear of the skin and subcutaneous tissue prior to inflation to avoid pericardiocutaneous fistula formation. The best way to achieve this is by performing the procedure using biplane fluoroscopy, with one plane in the left lateral position and confirming balloon position in both planes prior to inflation.[14]

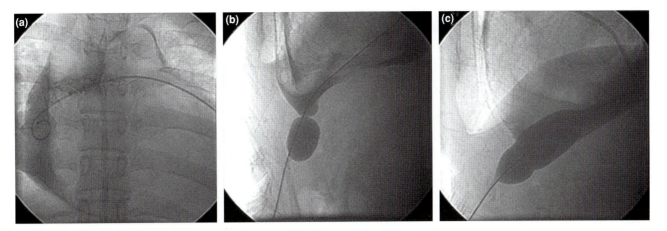

Figure 33.1 (A) Cinematographic image of the heart in an anteroposterior projection depicting a pigtail catheter in the pericardial sac through which contrast has been introduced to demonstrate the pericardial effusion. (B) Cinematographic image of the heart in a lateral projection illustrating inflation of a balloon against the parietal pericardium resulting in generation of a waist in the balloon. (C) Cinematographic image of the heart in a lateral projection demonstrating further inflation of the balloon with obliteration of the waist.

It is noteworthy that one-third of patients with large malignant pericardial effusions who undergo pericardiotomy will have a fever post procedure.[9]

COMPLICATIONS

Complications associated with pericardiocentesis via the left xiphocostal route also apply to percutaneous balloon pericardiotomy. These include puncture of the right atrium or right ventricle and laceration of the heart or a coronary vessel with either the needle or guide wire. Hemopericardium, arrhythmia, and air embolism may result.[6] The guide wire used during percutaneous balloon pericardiotomy is considerably stiffer than the regular pericardiocentesis wire, therefore great care should be taken to shape the tip with a broad curve prior to insertion under fluoroscopic guidance. Acute decompression of pericardial tamponade may also result in pulmonary edema.[11] Pneumothorax, puncture of the peritoneal cavity, and laceration to abdominal viscera have also been reported.

Thirteen percent of patients who undergo percutaneous balloon pericardiotomy suffer minor complications.[3] Many patients develop a left pleural effusion, although this usually resolves spontaneously. A persistent clinically significant pleural effusional is of more concern. To minimize risk from pericardial effusion it is prudent to remove as much of the fluid as possible during pericardiocentesis prior to creating a pericardial window.

Palacios et al. reported the first human experience of percutaneous balloon pericardiotomy in 8 patients with malignant pericardial effusion and tamponade.[2] The technique was successful in all patients, with no recurrence of pericardial effusion after a mean follow-up of 6 months. Mean time to development of a new

or significantly increased pleural effusion was 2.9 days. A subsequent 16-center registry enrolled 130 patients between 1987 and 1994. Eight patients developed recurrent pericardial effusions (mean time to recurrence 54 days). Seven of these patients underwent a surgical window procedure (4 developed recurrent effusions). Fifteen percent of patients with pre-existing pleural effusions required thoracocentesis or chest tube placement, compared to 9% of patients without pre-existing pleural effusions. Three patients developed persistent pericardial bleeding postpericardiotomy that required surgical intervention.[3]

We have encountered balloon rupture at our institution on two occasions. On the first occasion, while the ruptured balloon catheter was being withdrawn, a balloon fragment separated and remained in the pericardium. Thoracotomy was required to remove the residual fragment. On a different occasion, balloon rupture occurred again (Figure 33.2). During catheter withdrawal the distal portion of the balloon separated and remained free within the pericardial effusion (Figure 33.2B). Access to the pericardium was maintained with a J-wire and a sheath was inserted. Via the sheath, a snare was used to secure and remove the fragment from the pericardium, avoiding the need for surgical intervention (Figure 33.2C).

Management

Bleeding complications should be treated with reversal of anticoagulation and transfusion of blood products where appropriate. Pericardiocentesis via the indwelling catheter may also be necessary. Ultimately, surgical intervention may be required if bleeding from pericardial vessels persists. Accumulation of a large pleural

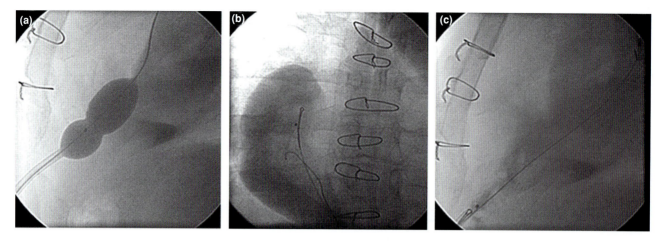

Figure 33.2 (A) Cinematographic image of the heart in a left lateral projection depicting inflation of the pericardiotomy balloon with a waist on either side. (B) Cinematographic image of the heart in an anteroposterior projection. The detached distal portion of the balloon is seen within the pericardium. A J-wire is left in place securing pericardial access while a snare is used to secure the balloon fragment. (C) Cinematographic image of the heart in a lateral projection depicts the balloon fragment within the loop of the snare being withdrawn towards a sheath at the apex of the heart.

effusion may require thoracentesis. In many cases this can be anticipated and will usually occur 2 to 3 days postprocedure. Reaccumulation of the pericardial effusion may necessitate surgical intervention. Thoracoscopic surgical techniques are associated with lower morbidity than the earlier open procedure.[15]

Puncture of the right atrium or ventricle, or laceration of the heart or a coronary vessel, may require emergent surgical correction and surgical assessment should be requested early. Echocardiography should also be performed and, depending on the extent of the cardiac injury, pericardiocentesis may be appropriate. Hemodynamic instability should be treated with volume expansion, blood transfusion, and inotropes.

Balloon rupture may occur, particularly when the parietal pericardium is resistant, necessitating high balloon inflation pressures (Figure 33.2). If rupture does occur, balloon fragmentation during removal is a possibility and should be anticipated. In this setting, continued pericardial access is essential. The J-wire should be kept in place and the balloon catheter exchanged for a large sheath to facilitate snare retrieval of the balloon fragment.

REFERENCES

1. Maree AO, Jneid H, Palacios IF. Percutaneous balloon pericardiotomy for patients with pericardial effusion and tamponade. In: Mukherjee D, Cho L, Moliterno DJ, eds. 900 Questions: An Interventional Cardiology Board Review. Philadelphia, PA: Lippincott Williams & Wilkins, 2006.
2. Palacios IF, Tuzcu EM, Ziskind AA, Younger J, Block PC. Percutaneous balloon pericardial window for patients with malignant pericardial effusion and tamponade. Cathet Cardiovasc Diagn 1991; 22(4): 244–9.
3. Ziskind AA, Pearce AC, Lemmon CC et al. Percutaneous balloon pericardiotomy for the treatment of cardiac tamponade

and large pericardial effusions: description of technique and report of the first 50 cases. J Am Coll Cardiol 1993; 21(1): 1–5.
4. Tsang TS, Enriquez-Sarano M, Freeman WK et al. Consecutive 1127 therapeutic echocardiographically guided pericardiocenteses: clinical profile, practice patterns, and outcomes spanning 21 years. Mayo Clin Proc 2002; 77(5): 429–36.
5. Gornik HL, Gerhard-Herman M, Beckman JA. Abnormal cytology predicts poor prognosis in cancer patients with pericardial effusion. J Clin Oncol 2005; 23(22): 5211–16.
6. Jneid H, Maree AO, Palacios IF. Pericardial tamponade: clinical presentation, diagnosis and catheter-based therapies. In: Parrillo JE, Dellinger RP, eds. Critical Care Medicine: Principles of Diagnosis & Management in the Adult, 3rd edn: St Louis, MO: Elsevier, 2007.
7. Chow LT, Chow WH. Mechanism of pericardial window creation by balloon pericardiotomy. Am J Cardiol 1993; 72(17): 1321–2.
8. Iaffaldano RA, Jones P, Lewis BE et al. Percutaneous balloon pericardiotomy: a double-balloon technique. Cathet Cardiovasc Diagn 1995; 36(1): 79–81.
9. Wang HJ, Hsu KL, Chiang FT et al. Technical and prognostic outcomes of double-balloon pericardiotomy for large malignancy-related pericardial effusions. Chest 2002; 122(3): 893–9.
10. Maisch B, Seferovic PM, Ristic AD et al. Guidelines on the diagnosis and management of pericardial diseases executive summary; The Task Force on the Diagnosis and Management of Pericardial Diseases of the European Society of Cardiology. Eur Heart J 2004; 25(7): 587–610.
11. Armstrong WF, Feigenbaum H, Dillon JC. Acute right ventricular dilation and echocardiographic volume overload following pericardiocentesis for relief of cardiac tamponade. Am Heart J 1984; 107(6): 1266–70.
12. Erbel R. Diseases of the thoracic aorta. Heart 2001; 86(2): 227–34.
13. Erbel R, Alfonso F, Boileau C et al. Diagnosis and management of aortic dissection. Eur Heart J 2001; 22(18): 1642–81.
14. Ziskind AA, Palacios IF. Percutaneous balloon pericardiotomy for patients with pericardial effusions and tamponade. In: Topol EJ, ed. Textbook of Interventional Cardiology, 3rd edn. Philadelphia: WB Saunders, 1999: 869–77.
15. Ozuner G, Davidson PG, Isenberg JS, McGinn JT Jr. Creation of a pericardial window using thoracoscopic techniques. Surg Gynecol Obstet 1992; 175(1): 69–71.

34 Left atrial appendage occlusion

Yves L Bayard, Stefan H Ostermayer, and Horst Sievert

INTRODUCTION

In patients with non-rheumatic atrial fibrillation, more than 90% of all thrombi are isolated to or originate in the left atrial appendage.[1] Percutaneous left atrial appendage occlusion has been performed since 2001 to prevent thromboembolism in patients who are suboptimal candidates for long-term anticoagulation treatment. Three devices have been used for left atrial appendage occlusion by catheter technique: the PLAATO™ system (ev3, Inc, Plymouth, MN), the WATCHMAN® left atrial appendage system (Atritech, Inc, Plymouth, MN), and the Amplatzer® Septal Occluder (AGA Medical Corporation, Golden Valley, MN). So far, left atrial appendage closure has been performed in more than 1000 patients, predominantly within international multicenter studies.

To avoid complications during interventional left atrial appendage occlusion, one has to be aware of the particular features of the different devices as well as the anatomic characteristics of the left atrial appendage. Operator-related complications tend to occur more often in centers that start their left atrial appendage occlusion experience.

HOW TO AVOID GENERAL COMPLICATIONS DURING LEFT ATRIAL APPENDAGE OCCLUSION

Preparations prior to the procedure

The left atrial appendage ranges from 20 to 45 mm in length and 15 to 35 mm in orifice diameter.[2] Prior to left atrial appendage occlusion, the individual left atrial appendage anatomy should be assessed using transesophageal echocardiography (TEE) and left atrial thrombi must be exluded. When using the WATCHMAN or the PLAATO device, the left atrial appendage orifice diameter should not extend 29 mm in order to achieve a minimal residual device compression of 10% with the largest device available (33 mm and 32 mm, respectively). If the orifice diameter is larger, the device will not be stable after implantation. When using the Amplatzer Septal Occluder, it is beneficial to have an appendage with a 'neck,' a narrowing distally to the orifice. In this case, the device may be implanted in a stable position with one disk in the left atrial appendage and one disk covering its orifice (Bernhard Meier refers to this as the 'pacifier position'[3]). In more than two-thirds of the population, the left atrial appendage consists of two or more lobes originating from one common orifice.[2] If only one lobe can be occluded, complete occlusion of the left atrial appendage cannot be achieved and the procedure should not be performed.

All patients should be screened for possible thrombi in the left atrial appendage. As for preprocedure medication, patients should be on aspirin 300 mg per day and clopidogrel 75 mg per day.

HOW TO AVOID PROCEDURAL COMPLICATIONS

General procedural complications such as vascular access complications (see Chapter 4), arrhythmias, air or thrombus embolization, and pericardial tamponade due to transseptal puncture (see Chapter 6) requiring pericardiocentesis have been described elsewhere.

Percutaneous appendage occlusion can be performed either under general or local anesthesia. In our experience, general anesthesia is usually not required. It is sufficient to administer 0.5–1 mg per kg propofol, even if the procedure is performed under TEE guidance.

Although left atrial appendage closure may be performed by experienced operators under fluoroscopy only, we recommend TEE guidance. It is useful for safe transseptal puncture, sizing of the left atrial appendage, and device positioning.

After venous groin access, transseptal puncture is performed using standard techniques. Septal puncture should be performed in the fossa ovalis. Thus, the WATCHMAN delivery sheath – we prefer the double curve sheath – points directly to the left atrial appendage. It is also possible to use a patent foramen ovale (PFO) or an atrial septal defect (ASD) to access the left atrium.

After successful puncture verified by pressure monitoring, 10 000 units of heparin are administered in order to keep the activated clotting time above 250 seconds. For the first dye injection into the appendage ('appendogram') we suggest a 4 French angulated pigtail catheter. It allows for deep and safe positioning of the catheter and reduces the risk of perforation of the very thin left atrial appendage wall.

Bleeding complications due to perforation of the left atrial appendage or during transseptal puncture are the most common complications in left atrial appendage occlusion. They are mainly observed in centers who are beginning their learning curve with left atrial appendage occlusion, and are seen less frequently as experience increases. TEE guidance can be very helpful to assure a safe transseptal puncture site. After needle crossing, pressure monitoring is useful to confirm left atrium (LA) position before the transseptal sheath is advanced. End-hole catheters should be avoided when approaching the left atrial appendage. Instead, a pigtail catheter should be routinely used for safe and deep insertion into the left atrial appendage. In addition, only J-tip guide wires are used for catheter exchange.

Standard management comprehends administration of protamin and/or pericardiocentesis. If the device is already positioned in the left atrial appendage, the procedure should be completed if possible.

Thrombus formation was occasionally noted with the PLAATO procedure when heparin was not given immediately after successful transseptal puncture. The thrombi were located between the tip of the sheath and the surface of the occluder. Adequate heparin administration and timing is crucial. Immediately after transseptal puncture, 10 000 units of heparin should be administered in order to keep the activated clotting time above 250 seconds.

If a thrombus is detected while the device is still within the transseptal sheath, we recommend removing the device from the sheath and attempting aspiration of the thrombus. In doing so, it can be helpful to slightly advance the sheath towards the thrombus to allow for aspiration. In case that the thrombus is located between the sheath and the surface of the unfolded occluder, we recommend not recollapsing the device before the thrombus has been removed. If these attempts fail, thrombolysis should be considered.

To choose the appropriate size of the device, several fluoroscopic and TEE measurements of the left atrial appendage should be taken. According to our experience, the most helpful projections are right anterior oblique (RAO), RAO cranial, and RAO caudal. Besides the orifice diameter, the length and shape of the appendage can influence device selection as well. In the case of a wide, but short appendage, a smaller device could potentially be introduced deeper into the appendage than a larger device size as it is recommended by the manufacturer according to the proximal opening diameter. However, compression of the device of at least 8% must be achieved before it can be released!

Prior to the release from the delivery catheter, the device position should be assessed with a stability test. The implanted device must not change its configuration and position within the left atrial appendage when the delivery catheter is carefully pushed and pulled. The device should move only together with the left atrial appendage. Additionally, when using the WATCHMAN device, a residual compression of at least 8% is necessary to guarantee a stable position of the occluder.

DEVICE-RELATED COMPLICATIONS AND MANAGEMENT

PLAATO device

Percutaneous left atrial appendage closure was introduced into clinical practice in 2001 using the PLAATO system.[4] The results of the PLAATO Feasibility Study published in July 2005 showed the feasibility and safety of this procedure.[5] Despite good clinical results, the ev3 company discontinued the production of the PLAATO device in December 2005 for financial reasons.

Pericardial effusion (2.5%) or *tamponade* (2.5%) due to perforation of the left atrial appendage or complications during transseptal puncture were the most common complications noted with the PLAATO device. It is helpful to use TEE guidance for transseptal puncture and guidance of the transseptal sheath. The initial visualization of the left atrial appendage ('appendogram') should be performed with a 4 French pigtail catheter to prevent perforation of the appendage wall. In almost all cases, pericardiocentesis performed in the catheterization laboratory was effective to handle these complications.

Embolization of the PLAATO occluder is a possible, but rare, complication that occurred only in patients in whom the release criteria were not fully met (residual device compression of at least 10%). The devices ended up in the aorta and were retrieved in the catheterization laboratory. Due to the device's hooks, it is important to snare the distal hub of the device in order to allow retrieval into the sheath. A second snare introduced either from the same or contralateral femoral artery side may be useful to center the device during its retrieval into the arterial introducer sheath.

Thrombus formation on the occluder during the healing process is a rare complication that may be detected by TEE during early follow-up. In our experience, these thrombi were firmly attached to the device surface and not of a mobile or floating character. Continuous administration of aspirin and clopidogrel or low-molecular-weight heparin alone were effective in resolving these thrombi.

WATCHMAN device

Compared with the PLAATO occluder, the WATCHMAN device is much softer. It is covered with a polyester filter membrane on its atrial facing side only. Device sizes range from 21 to 33 mm. At present, it is the only device available that is specifically designed for the left atrial appendage. In 2007, Sick and colleagues published the final results of a feasibility study with this device with promising results.[6] Although it is CE approved in Europe, it is currently only available within the Protect AF study (WATCHMAN Left Atrial Appendage System for Embolic PROTECTion in Patients With Atrial Fibrillation), comparing left atrial appendage occlusion with long-term warfarin intake in patients with non-rheumatic atrial fibrillation.

If repositioning of the device within the left atrial appendage is necessary, the device can be retrieved leaving the sheath in place.

Embolization of the WATCHMAN occured twice in the first generation of the device. After modification of the barbs around the device body, no more embolizations occured in the WATCHMAN feasibility study. Similar to the PLAATO device, a residual compression of at least 10% after implantation is the most important criterion to guarantee a stable position of the device within the left atrial appendage. In case of an embolization, the device may be snared and removed via a large sheath. Special attention is required to avoid injury caused by the fixation barbs surrounding the device.

Thrombus formation on the device was the most common complication in the feasibility study of the WATCHMAN device. Warfarin administration for 6 months was effective to resolve these thrombi in all patients.

Pericardial effusion (2.5%) occured twice as a complication of transseptal puncture, and once as a result of a vigorous 'tug test' when evaluating the device stability within the left atrail appendage. Continous TEE observation of the procedure might help to avoid these complications.

Amplatzer device

In contrast to the WATCHMAN or the PLAATO device, Amplatzer ASD and PFO occluders were not specifically designed to fit the left atrial appendage. However, Amplatzer occluders offer a number of favorable characteristics such as easy handling, a smaller, possibly less thombogenic introducer sheath (8 French vs 12 French with the WATCHMAN and PLAATO systems) and the fact that they may adapt to a large diversity of left atrial appendage shapes because of their flexibility. The initial experience of using Amplatzer septal devices for left atrial appendage closure was described by Meier and colleagues in 2003.[3]

Implanting both device disks in the left atrial appendage is advantageous, as less foreign material is exposed to the blood stream. However, residual flow into the left atrial appendage is more frequent with this implantation method. An alternative placement method has been described by Bernhard Meier as the 'pacifier position'[3]: the left atrial disk is expanded into the left atrial appendage body, the central connection part is bridging the neck of the left atrial appendage and the right atrial disk is covering its orifice.

Amplatzer occluders do not have hooks to stabilize their position, therefore the risk of perforation and pericardial bleeding may be lower than with the PLAATO and WATCHMAN devices. The downside of the missing hooks is obvious: early device embolizations are the most common complications when using Amplatzer occluders for left atrial appendage occlusion. Amplatzer occluders can be snared at the right atrial hub and can be removed through a sheath.

COMPLICATIONS AFTER LEFT ATRIAL APPENDAGE OCCLUSION AND MANAGEMENT

To detect postprocedural complications, patients should be followed with chest X-ray, transthoracic echocardiogram, and clinical examination before hospital discharge, and at 1- and 6-month follow-up. Furthermore, we recommend TEE after 1 and 6 months to assess for implant position, LAA occlusion, and exclusion of thrombus formation on the device.

Postprocedure, we suggest clopidogrel (75 mg) and an endocarditis prophylaxis for the first 6 months. Aspirin (300 mg) should be prescribed on a continuing basis.

SUMMARY

In experienced hands, left atrial appendage occlusion by the catheter technique can be safely performed with all devices decribed. WATCHMAN and PLAATO are devices specifically designed for left atrial appendage occlusion. In these devices, bleeding complications caused by transseptal puncture or perforation of the left atrial appendage wall are the most common complications. Careful catheter and sheath manipulation in the left atrium under TEE guidance is essential. Device embolization of the WATCHMAN and PLAATO device is a rare complication that can be avoided by assuring a residual compression of at least 10% after expansion within the left atrial appendage. Amplatzer Septal Occluders are easy to handle and can be used for left atrial appendage occlusion in selected patients. However, with the Amplatzer device shapes currently available, embolization occurs more frequently than with the other occluders.

REFERENCES

1. Blackshear JL, Odell JA. Appendage obliteration to reduce stroke in cardiac surgical patients with atrial fibrillation. Ann Thorac Surg 1996; 61: 755–9.
2. Veinot JP, Harrity PJ, Gentile F et al. Anatomy of the normal left atrial appendage. Circulation 1997; 96: 3112–15.
3. Meier B, Palacios I, Windecker S et al. Transcatheter left atrial appendage occlusion with Amplatzer devices to obviate anticoagulation in patients with atrial fibrillation. Cathet Cardiovasc Interven 2003; 60(3): 417–22.
4. Sievert H, Lesh MD, Trepels T et al. Percutaneous left atrial appendage transcatheter occlusion to prevent stroke in high-risk patients with atrial fibrillation – early clinical experience. Circulation 2002; 105: 1887–9.
5. Ostermayer SH, Reisman M, Kramer PH et al. Percutaneous left atrial appendage transcatheter occlusion (PLAATO system) to prevent stroke in high-risk patients with non-rheumatic atrial fibrillation: results from the international multicenter feasibility trials. J Am Coll Cardiol 2005; 46(1): 9–14.
6. Sick PB, Schuler G, Hauptmann KE et al. Initial worldwide experience with the WATCHMAN left atrial appendage system for stroke prevention in atrial fibrillation. J Am Coll Cardiol 2007; 49(13): 1490–5.

35 Complications of percutaneous aortic valve replacement

Jean-Bernard Masson and John G Webb

INTRODUCTION

Conventional aortic valve replacement (AVR) can be performed in good surgical candidates with an expectation of an excellent outcome. However, surgery in patients with comorbidities may be associated with significant morbidity and mortality. In some such patients percutaneous AVR may offer durable benefit while avoiding many of the problems associated with sternotomy, aortotomy, and cardiopulmonary bypass.[1–3] However, a percutaneous procedure is associated with its own unique risks. Knowledge of the potential complications of percutaneous AVR is necessary both in the selection of appropriate candidates and in optimizing outcomes for this new therapeutic alternative.

Percutaneous AVR is generally performed utilizing a retrograde approach from the femoral artery. Two types of valves have seen extensive use: a balloon-expandable valve (Cribier Edwards™ or more recently the Edwards SAPIEN™ valve, Edwards Lifesciences, Inc) and a self-expanding valve (CoreValve™, CoreValve, Inc). While there are many differences between these valves and procedures there are even more commonalities, particularly in terms of the potential risks (Table 35.1). An understanding of the nature of these potential complications, their avoidance, and mitigation is the subject of this chapter.

COMPLICATIONS

Access-related complications

The large profile of current devices is a major concern with respect to arterial access. First-generation valves and delivery systems were high profile, as large as 24 French in diameter. A sheath with a lumen appropriate for such a device would typically have an outer diameter of 9 mm, larger than many femoral arteries. Typically, patients with femoral arteries larger than this, or even slightly smaller but still elastic, can accommodate sheaths of this size. However, patients with smaller, stenotic, calcified, or tortuous arteries are at considerable risk of vascular injury. The femoral and iliac arteries and, more rarely, the aorta can suffer damage from wires, dilators, and sheath manipulation, ranging from non-flow-limiting dissection to occlusion or perforation.

Perhaps the most important lesson learned in the early experience is that the risk of vascular injury can be greatly reduced by careful screening. We routinely perform detailed abdominal aortography with opacification of both iliac and femoral arteries utilizing a marker catheter to allow accurate calibration and vessel measurement. CT angiography is often useful, particularly in patients with borderline arterial access. Patients with marginal arterial access are best avoided if complications are to be avoided.

We attempt to assure large sheath placement in an area of the common femoral artery relatively free of atheroma and away from the femoral bifurcation. At the time of abdominal aortography it is helpful to image the common femoral artery to the level of the femoral bifurcation. Most commonly, this will confirm the ideal puncture site overlies the upper portion of the bony femoral head, although this may vary. Following puncture we perform femoral angiography through the sheath to assure there is no retroperitoneal leak from a high puncture and that the puncture site is suitable for placement of a large sheath or percutaneous closure if planned.

Arterial perforation during sheath placement or aggressive manipulation of large catheters within the aorta may result in dissection or perforation. Should unexpected hypotension be encountered this possibility should be promptly considered. Angiography may be necessary. Arterial occlusion using a very compliant occlusion balloon may be invaluable in rapidly controling bleeding (Figure 35.1). In the high-risk patients with comorbidities who are currently being considered for percutaneous AVR, dissection or perforation of the aorta is likely to be fatal unless non-surgical management is feasible (Figure 35.2). However, ilio-femoral complications can generally be managed successfully. Perforations can be treated with a covered stent or open surgical repair (Figure 35.3). Dissections can most often be managed conservatively, although, if extensive, stenting may be necessary.

Removal of a large sheath which is relatively occlusive within an artery is associated with a unique concern. If a sheath is allowed to remain in contact with

Table 35.1   Equipment for management of complications during percutaneous AVR.

Equipment	Example	Comments and usage
Wires	Meier™ 0.035 inch exchange (Boston Scientific)	Stiff wire to facilitate difficult sheath insertion
	Hydrophilic angled tip 0.035 inch GlideWire™ (Terumo)	Steerable wire to facilitate contralateral or tortuous access
Occlusion balloon*		For aortic, iliac, or femoral perforation, or hemostasis during sheath removal
	CODA™ (Cook, Inc)	Compliant, suitable for 6 to 30 mm vessels
Cross-over catheter	e.g. Internal Mammary, Cobra catheters	Facilitate contralateral iliac angiography
Cross-over sheath	Balkin™ sheath (Cook, Inc)	Facilitate contralateral iliac access and stent placement
Covered stents*	Fluency™ (Bard, Inc)	Ilio-femoral perforation; self-expanding 7–10 mm × 40–60 mm
Uncovered stent	Zilver™ (Cook, Inc)	Ilio-femoral dissection
Aortic stent	CP™ covered stent (Numed, Inc)	Aortic dissection, perforation, reversed aortic valve
Cardiopulmonary support*		Temporary hemodynamic support in the presence of reduced cardiac ouput
	IABP	Pre- or postprocedural only
	Impella™ (Abiomed)	Post-procedural only
	Femoral femoral bypass	Pre-, intra- or postprocedural
	TandemHeart™ (Cardiac Assist Technologies)	Pre-, intra-, or postprocedural

*Strongly recommended.

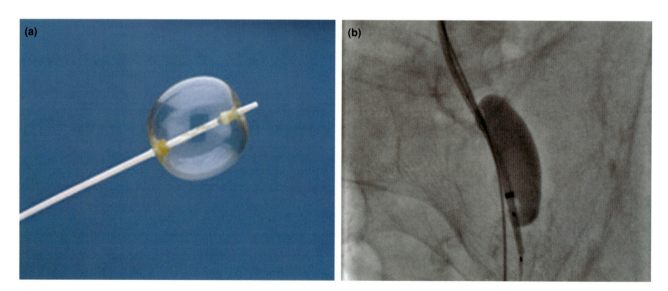

Figure 35.1   Occlusion balloon. (A) Example of a very compliant occlusion balloon (Cook, Inc). (B) The occlusion balloon can be inflated in the aorta or iliac artery to assist in management of perforation or vascular closure.

the artery wall too long adhesion can occur. Forceful withdrawal of the sheath can lead to avulsion and possibly perforation of the artery wall (Figure 35.4). To avoid the risk of sheath–artery adhesion it is important to minimize the duration an occlusive, oversized sheath remains in place.

Because the sheath is often occlusive, arterial injury may not be evident until after removal. Postprocedural

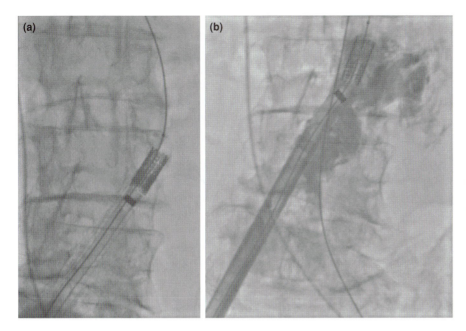

Figure 35.2 Aortic perforation. (A) The sheath can be seen to be directed towards the wall of the aorta. (B) Forceful, but unsuccessful, attempts to pass the prosthetic valve through the native valve resulted in the sheath sliding in and out and aortic injury. Sudden hypotension was followed by angiographic documentation of perforation.

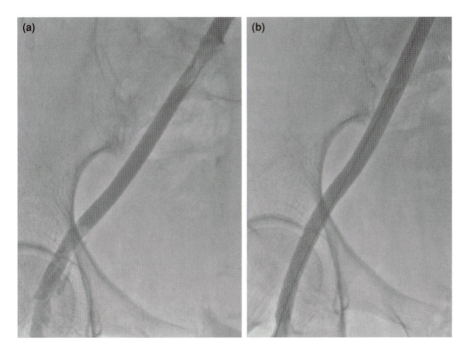

Figure 35.3 Vascular injury. (A) Hypotension and inguinal swelling developed following sheath removal and surgical closure of the arteriotomy site. Angiography showed retroperitoneal extravasation just above the femoral head as well as femoral and iliac dissection. (B) The perforation was effectively sealed with a covered self-expanding stent.

hypotension may be the first sign of ilio-femoral perforation or retroperitoneal bleed. We routinely perform an ilio-femoral angiogram through a sheath in the contralateral femoral artery following removal of a large sheath so as to identify vascular injury before it is clinically evident.

Stroke

Stroke is a major concern with conventional aortic valve surgery. In the first-in-man transarterial balloon-expandable valve experience, the incidence of clinical stroke was 4%.[2] In the subsequent 145 patients included in the REVIVE II and REVIVAL II trials, the incidence of neurologic events was 5.5% (unpublished data). Utilizing the CoreValve™ device in 86 patients an incidence of 10% was reported.[3]

Unique to a percutaneous transarterial procedure is the risk of mobilizing friable atheroma as wires and catheters are passed through the aortic arch. As percutaneous valve delivery systems evolve, a major design goal is to reduce the potential for aortic injury. Early bulky, stiff catheters with uncovered stents are being replaced with progressively lower profile systems with atraumatic tapered tips and smoother surfaces to reduce the potential for aortic injury.

There are multiple potential causes for perprocedural stroke. Hypotension might result in cerebral

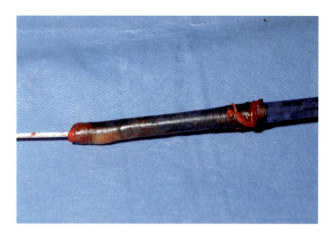

Figure 35.4 Artery on a stick. Resistance to sheath withdrawal was encountered with subsequent avulsion of the adherent iliac artery. An occlusion balloon (white catheter) placed in the aorta provided good vascular control, allowing controlled vascular repair.

hypoperfusion, particularly in the presence of pre-existing cerebrovascular disease. On occasion we have observed thrombus on a guide wire by echocardiography. This can best be avoided by adequate anticoagulation and reducing procedural duration. Premedication with aspirin and/or clopidogrel and administration of heparin to maintain an activated clotting time above 250 seconds has been our standard regimen. Although dissection (Figure 35.5) and occlusion of arch vessels might result in stroke,[4] this risk appears low.

Prior surgical experience suggested that calcified debris from the native valve itself is a major concern. However, in the case of valve implantation, unlike surgery, the cellular layer covering this relatively amorphous, friable calcified atheroma is not incised and remains largely intact.[5] Although embolization of calcified or atheromatous material from the valve likely does occur (Figure 35.6), this appears to be less of a clinical concern than might be anticipated.

Malposition

Improper positioning of a prosthetic valve (i.e. somewhere other than within the aortic annulus) may occur. Implications may be relatively benign or potentially life-threatening.

A valve that is implanted too low within the ventricle below the level of the annulus could be associated with residual aortic stenosis, paravalvular insufficiency, ventricular arrhythmias, or mitral regurgitation. If positioned within the outflow tract, a second overlapping prosthesis may restore valvular function. If unstable within the left ventricular cavity, surgery may be the only option.

Failure to cross the native valve with the prosthesis and inability to pull it back within the sheath has been seen. In this case, deployment of the prosthesis in the aorta may have to be considered. Ideally, aortography

is utilized to select an appropriate sized segment of the aorta free of side branch. As long as the valve remains oriented in the flow direction, hemodynamic consequences are negligible. Potential concerns relate to distension of the aorta and the possibility of dissection or occlusion of side branch by the sealing cuff, but up to this point complications have not been reported.

Implanting a valve too high in the aorta can result in embolization, paravalvular regurgitation, or coronary obstruction. Embolization is likely to be well tolerated as long as the valve remains oriented in the direction of flow. Should the prosthesis be allowed to rotate freely, aortic obstruction is likely and implanting a large diameter stent within the prosthesis or emergency surgical removal may be necessary. The preferable mode of management is to maintain guide wire position through the prosthesis to prevent the valve from rotating. The balloon catheter should be readvanced into the prosthesis and inflated just enough to allow the prosthesis to be withdrawn to a safe location within the arch or descending aorta, where it can be further expanded and secured (Figures 35.7 and 35.8).

In our first-in-man experience, successful implantation was achieved in 76% in the first 25 patients, compared with 96% in the next 25 patients.[2] Pooled data from the subsequent REVIVE II and REVIVAL II trial using the balloon-expandable Edwards–Cribier valve showed an implant success rate of 89.5% (unpublished data). Implant success rate in the initial experience with the self-expandable Core Valve™ in 86 patients was 88%.[3] Currently, success rates with both devices exceed 95 percent.

Coronary occlusion

Coronary occlusion might theoretically occur due to embolization of thrombus, atheroma, or calcific valve material. Initial concerns that percutaneous prostheses would directly occlude the coronary ostium have not been borne out with current prostheses. The open cells of current balloon-expandable Edwards valves may on occasion extend to the level of the coronary ostium, whereas the aortic component of the self-expanding CoreValve device routinely extends over the coronary ostia without apparent ill effect. Moreover, because of the shape of the Valsalva sinuses, blood can flow around the prosthesis and into the coronaries.

Theoretically, a stent strut in front of a coronary ostium may displace ostial atheroma or interfere with coronary cannulation. The potential for a bulky and calcified native valve leaflet to be displaced over the coronary ostia appears real. We reported left main occlusion (Figure 35.9) with pathologic confirmation.[2] Subsequently, left main occlusion with hemodynamic collapse and successful reperfusion with angioplasty or off-pump aortocoronary bypass has been observed. The risk of left main obstruction has been somewhere around 1%, however it appears likely that a better

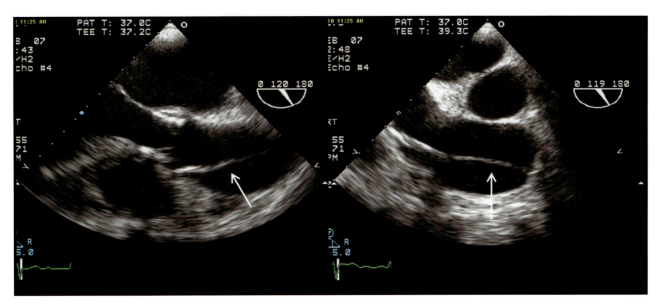

Figure 35.5   Type A aortic dissection. TEE images with evidence of type A aortic dissection. Left panel: parasternal long axis of the aortic valve and ascending aorta. Right panel: long axis view of the aortic arch. This patient was asymptomatic and remains well one year later.

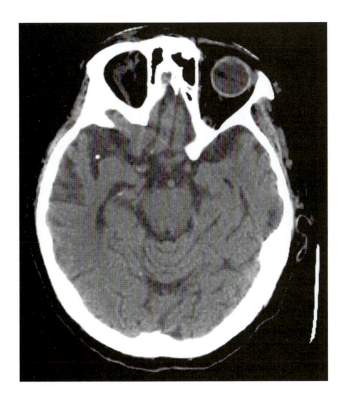

Figure 35.6   Calcified debris embolization. A calcific embolus and hypodensity are visible in the right temporal lobe. Clinical features of stroke were evident.

understanding along with echocardiographic and angiographic screening will reduce this risk.

Arrhythmia

New onset atrial fibrillation may occur and is often poorly tolerated in this setting. Early cardioversion may

be desirable. Similarly, ventricular fibrillation may occur, particularly in the presence of ventricular catheter-induced ectopy, ischemia, burst pacing (Figure 35.10), adrenergic stimulation, or medications. We routinely apply defibrillator pads to facilitate prompt defibrillation when necessary.

Complete heart block has been reported to be as high as 6.4% after surgical AVR.[6] Among our first 77 patients receiving a balloon-expandable transcatheter aortic valve, 6% have developed new and sustained atrioventricular block requiring pacemaker implantation.[7] The most plausible explanation seems to be pressure effect and ischemia on the conducting tissues. The left bundle branch may be more subject to this complication due to its proximity to the aortic annulus, hence a higher risk of complete heart block among patients with pre-existing right bundle branch block.

Cardiac perforation

Cardiac tamponade may occur as a complication of pacemaker placement or left ventricular perforation. Unexplained hypotension should prompt echocardiographic evaluation for this treatable complication. Tamponade has been observed in incidence ranging from 2[2] to 7%[3] in feasibility studies, attributed to the use of a stiff, traumatic ventricular guide wire.[3] Manual shaping of the guide wire to form a less traumatic pigtail curve can reduce the incidence of left ventricle perforation.

Rupture of the aortic annulus is a rare complication of aortic balloon valvuloplasty and has been seen with percutaneous AVR. Oversizing and postdilating to reduce paravalvular leaks is ultimately limited by this potential complication. The risk of annular rupture

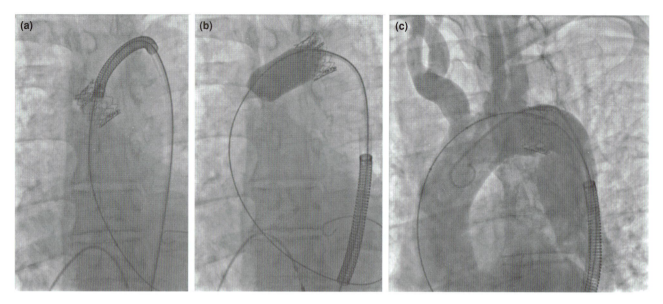

Figure 35.7 Valve malposition and embolization. The valve was positioned too aortic prior to balloon inflation and burst pacing was terminated too early. (A) The expanded stent is free-floating in the ascending aorta. (B) The partially inflated balloon is used to pull back the valve into a secure location. (C) The valve was overexpanded within the aortic arch in an area free of side branches and has not caused problems at follow-up of over 2 years.

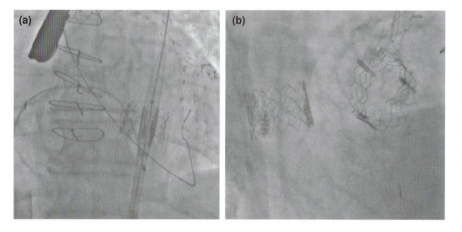

Figure 35.8 Successful valve implantation following malposition. An unsuccessfully deployed valve was redeployed in the abdominal aorta. A second valve was easily advanced through the malpositioned valve (A) and placed in the correct position. The patient remains well at 6-month follow-up. (B) Follow-up fluoroscopy in the RAO cranial angulation.

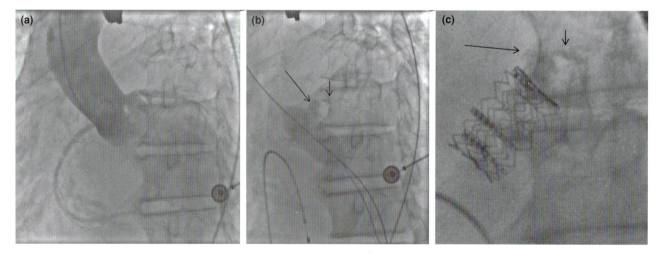

Figure 35.9 Coronary occlusion caused by displacement of a bulky leaflet. (A) Diagnostic aortic angiogram showing a bulky and calcified left coronary leaflet. (B) During balloon valvuloplasty, the calcified left coronary leaflet (long arrow) comes in contact with left main coronary artery calcification (short arrow). (C) After valve implantation, the left coronary leaflet and left main artery calcifications remain in contact. This patient died of LV failure and left coronary obstruction was observed at necropsy.

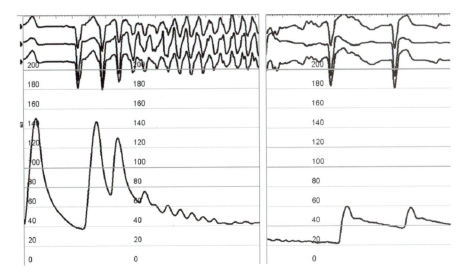

Figure 35.10 Induction of ventricular fibrillation. Rapid pacing degenerated into ventricular fibrillation. On the right panel, normal sinus rhythm was restored after external defibrillation.

may be greater with a more calcified, less compliant aortic annulus, and with more aggressive dilation. In the current global balloon-expandable valve experience, the risk of annular rupture has been <0.5% despite routine oversizing.

Cardiogenic shock

Patients with severe aortic stenosis are not tolerant to myocardial ischemia and hypotension, particularly in the presence of coronary disease, left ventricular dysfunction, or hypertropy. Hypotension of any cause may precipitate ischemia in a ventricle with little reserve. A reduction in blood pressure is common during valve implantation as a consequence of vasodilator anesthetic agents, vagal stimulation, burst pacing, arrhythmias, blood loss, and transient occlusion of the aortic valve during balloon valvuloplasty or deployment of the prosthesis. Additional causes of ischemia include tachycardia and excess inotropic stimulation. Ischemia may lead to a potentially irreversible spiral of progressive hypotension, ischemia, myocardial dysfunction, and cardiogenic shock.

Chronotropic agents such as dopamine, dobutamine, or epinephrine administered to maintain cardiac output may exacerbate ischemia and result in paradoxic deterioration. We favor liberal use of vasoconstrictor agents, such as phenylephrine or norepinephrine, and volume to maintain coronary perfusion pressure. Most important is to maintain a judicious procedural pace to allow for a stable procedure and avoidance of unnecessary stress. Unexpected hypotension should prompt consideration and exclusion of treatable cause (e.g. bleeding, tamponade, arrhythmia). If hypotension is unresponsive, mechanical cardiopulmonary support may be life-saving and allow recovery of left ventricular function.

Acute renal failure

Renal dysfunction is common in aortic stenosis patients. Procedural stresses include transient hypotension, contrast, and atheroembolism. Diagnostic angiography is ideally performed at a separate setting and contrast exposure minimized at the time of valve implantation. Although transient worsening of renal function may occur, we have more often observed a prompt improvement in renal function as a consequence of improved renal perfusion with relief of aortic stenosis.

Acute valve failure

Obviously a percutaneous valve placed completely above or below a stenotic native valve may not function as hoped. Percutaneous valves are at risk of failure due to manufacturing defects, damage during storage, crimping, compression or deployment, or by under- or overexpansion. Valves can be implanted with reversed orientation due to human error. Should this occur immediate implantation of a second valve within the reversed valve may be necessary. In general, currently available valves function well and have proven reliable when implanted correctly.

Paravalvular insufficiency

In our experience, at least a trace of paravalvular insufficiency is commonly present if carefully looked for with transesophageal imaging. However, with careful positioning of the sealing cuff within the native annulus and implantation of an oversized prosthesis, paravalvular insufficiency is rarely severe. When severe paravalvular insufficiency is observed, the cause is typically undersizing or suboptimal positioning of the sealing cuff. The initial indicator of severe paravalvular insufficiency may be

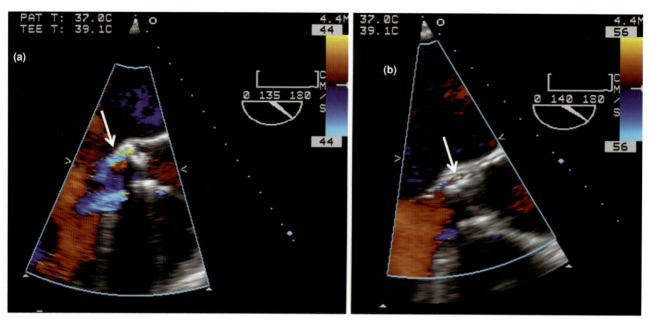

Figure 35.11 Paravalvular regurgitation. (A) TEE long axis view of the aortic valve after implantation with evidence of significant posterior paravalvular regurgitation. (B) After balloon redilation, the paravalvular leak is graded mild.

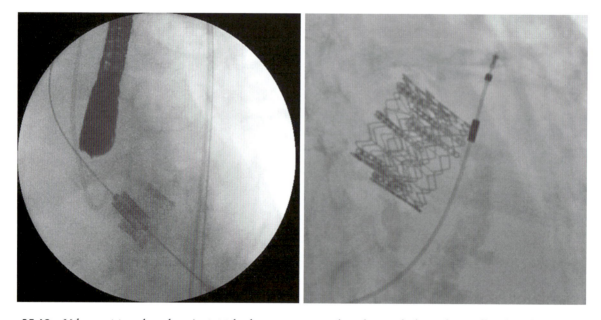

Figure 35.12 Valve positioned too low. An initial valve was positioned too low with the sealing cuff within the left ventricular outflow tract. Poor sealing resulted in paravalvular insufficiency. A second valve implanted slightly higher resulted in effective sealing and good valve function.

an inappropriate fall in diastolic pressure with fluoroscopic, angiographic, and echocardiographic evidence of suboptimal positioning and insufficiency.

Mild to moderate, and even moderately severe aortic regurgitation, may be well tolerated when aortic stenosis is relieved, and conservative management is most often appropriate. However, very severe paravalvular regurgitation may result in persistent heart failure or shock. When underexpansion of the prosthesis is present, redilation may be effective [8] (Figure 35.11). If the initial prosthesis is implanted too high or too low within the annulus, a second prosthesis partially overlapping the first valve may allow sufficient extension of the sealing cuff to reduce insufficiency (Figure 35.12). Anecdotal attempts at placing occlusive plugs have been unsuccessful. Conventional surgery may still be an option in the occasional patient.

Late valve failure

The initial long-term follow-up data after percutaneous valve implantation data are encouraging, but limited.[2,9] We have not observed hemolysis, despite prospective evaluation.[10] Valve thrombosis and infection may occur but, to date, have not been reported. Structural valve failure has not been reported to date. Nevertheless, failure of transcatheter bioprostheses is to be expected with time. Testing of current valves suggests failure will more often occur due to leaflet calcification and stenosis than due to leaflet tears. As new experimental stent designs are introduced, valve durability will be an ongoing concern.

SUMMARY

Percutaneous implantation of aortic valves is associated with the potential for significant benefit, but also significant risk. Better understanding of sources of risk and the management of complications will allow optimal patient outcomes.

REFERENCES

1. Webb JG, Chandavimol M, Thompson CR et al. Percutaneous aortic valve implantation retrograde from the femoral artery. Circulation 2006; 113(6): 842–50.

2. Webb JG, Pasupati S, Humphries K et al. Percutaneous transarterial aortic valve replacement in selected high-risk patients with aortic stenosis. Circulation 2007; 116(7): 755–63.

3. Grube E, Schuler G, Buellesfeld L et al. Percutaneous aortic valve replacement for severe aortic stenosis in high-risk patients using the second- and current third-generation self-expanding CoreValve prosthesis: device success and 30-day clinical outcome. J Am Coll Cardiol 2007; 50(1): 69–76.

4. Berry C, Cartier R, Bonan R. Fatal ischemic stroke related to non permissive peripheral artery access for percutaneous aortic valve replacement. Cathet Cardiovasc Interven 2007; 69: 56–63.

5. Cribier A, Eltchaninoff H, Tron C, Bauer F, Gerber L. Percutaneous implantation of aortic valve prosthesis in patients with calcific aortic stenosis: technical advances, clinical results and future strategies. J Interven Cardiol 2006; 19: S87–S96.

6. El-Khally Z, Thibault B, Staniloae C et al. Prognostic significance of newly acquired bundle branch block after aortic valve replacement. Am J Cardiol 2004; 94(8): 1008–11.

7. Sinhal A, Pasupati S, Humphries K et al. Atrioventricular block after transcatheter aortic valve. J Am Coll Cardiol Interv, in press.

8. Pasupati S, Chandimavol M, Nercolini D et al. Balloon-expandable aortic valve insertion: implications of re-dilatation. [abstract] Can J Cardiol, 2006; 22 (Suppl SD): 88.

9. Cribier A, Eltchaninoff H, Tron C et al. Treatment of calcific aortic stenosis with the percutaneous heart valve: mid-term follow-up from the initial feasibility studies: the French experience. J Am Coll Cardiol 2006; 47(6): 1214–23.

10. Murphy CJ, Pasupati S, Webb JG [abstract]. Hemolysis after transcatheter balloon-expandable aortic valve insertion. Can J Cardiol 2007; 23: 260C.

36 Transseptal catheterization in adults

Amr Bannan and Howard C Herrmann

INTRODUCTION

Prior to the introduction of transseptal left heart catheterization, left atrial and left ventricular pressures were measured via transbronchial, transthoracic, and direct percutaneous approaches. Transseptal left heart catheterization was introduced independently by Ross et al.[1] and Cope[2] in 1959. The procedure was later modified by Brockenbrough et al.[3] and Mullins.[4] Although transseptal catheterization gained enormous popularity in the 1960s, the development of the flotation pulmonary catheter in 1970[5] and retrograde catheterization of the left ventricle led to a significant decline in the utilization of this technique. With the introduction of percutaneous balloon mitral valvuloplasty, antegrade percutaneous aortic valvuloplasty, percutaneous repair of atrial septal defects, mitral valve repair, and electrophysiologic ablation procedures, there has been renewed interest in transseptal catheterization.

INDICATIONS

In order to avoid complications related to transseptal catheterization, one must first appreciate the appropriate indications. Transseptal catheterization may be performed both for diagnostic and therapeutic indications (Table 36.1). Diagnostic transseptal catheterization is performed when direct measurement of left atrial pressure is needed. In mitral stenosis with severe pulmonary hypertension, for example, a pulmonary capillary wedge pressure may be unobtainable or inaccurate, and there is a slightly higher incidence of pulmonary artery perforation with balloon flotation in the pulmonary arteries. Other indications include situations in which retrograde crossing of the aortic valve is difficult or potentially deleterious, such as the presence of severe aortic stenosis, a mechanical aortic prosthesis, or aortic valve endocarditis. The hemodynamic assessment of hypertrophic obstructive cardiomyopathy is also aided by transseptal catheterization.

Transseptal catheterization is increasingly performed for a number of interventional procedures such as percutaneous mitral valvuloplasty, antegrade percutaneous aortic valvuloplasty, percutaneous edge-to-edge mitral valve repair, percutaneous heart valve implantation, transseptal PFO closure, and left atrial appendage ablation.

A number of electrophysiologic procedures also require a transseptal approach. These include ablation of left-sided accessory pathways, pulmonary vein ablation for paroxysmal atrial fibrillation, and ablation of left atrial and left ventricular arrhythmias.

SEPTAL ANATOMY

The plane of the atrial septum runs from 1 o'clock to 7 o'clock (as viewed from the feet with the patient lying supine). The fossa ovalis is posterior and caudal to the aortic root and anterior to the free wall of the right atrium. The fossa ovalis is approximately 2 cm in diameter and is bounded superiorly by a ridge (the limbus).

This anatomy can be distorted by aortic or mitral valvular disease. In aortic stenosis, the plane of the septum becomes more vertical and the fossa may be located slightly anteriorly. In mitral stenosis, the intreratrial septum becomes flatter and more horizontal and the fossa ovalis itself tends to lie lower.

It is important to understand the fossa anatomy when trying to enter the left atrium in a specific location. For example, if one turns the transseptal needle clockwise in order to puncture more posteriorly, the needle will move inferiorly as well. These trade-offs for an exact puncture location may have important implications in some procedures.

THE PROCEDURE

The physician performing the procedure must be fully familiar with the transseptal apparatus.[6,7] Typically, this consists of a Mullins introducer (composed of a 59 cm sheath and a 67 cm dilator) and the Brockenbrough needle and stylet (79 cm). Other sheath and needle combinations may be preferred by some operators. The flange of the needle has an arrow that points to the position of the curved needle tip. Before use, the operator must be sure that the needle proximal to the tip is straight and that the arrow of the flange is perfectly aligned with the distal curve.

Right femoral venous access is obtained percutaneously and a 0.032 inch J-wire is advanced until it is positioned at the level of the junction of the superior vena cava and right innominate vein. Under fluoroscopic guidance, the Mullins sheath and dilator are

Table 36.1 Indications for transseptal catheterization.

Diagnosis of mitral gradients

- Unreliable capillary wedge pressure
- Mechanical aortic valve prosthesis

Diagnosis of aortic gradients

- Severe aortic stenosis when valve cannot be traversed
- Hypertrophic obstructive cardiomyopathy

Interventional procedures: structural and valvular heart disease

- Percutaneous mitral balloon valvuloplasty
- Percutaneous edge-to-edge mitral valve repair
- Antegrade aortic balloon valvuloplasty
- Percutaneous heart valve implantation
- Transseptal patent foramen ovale closure
- Left atrial appendage ablation

Electrophysiologic studies: ablation

- Left-sided accessory pathways
- Pulmonary vein ablation for paroxysmal atrial fibrillation
- Left atrial tachycardias
- Atypical left atrial flutters
- Left ventricular tachycardia

advanced over the guide wire into the superior vena cava. The sheath must never be advanced without the guide wire as the stiff dilator can readily perforate the inferior vena cava, superior vena cava, or the right atrium. Once the Mullins sheath is properly placed, the guide wire is removed. The Brockenbrough needle is then inserted into the Mullins sheath such that the needle tip lies within the dilator. When the needle tip lies just within the dilator, there is an approximately 1.5–2 cm distance between the dilator hub and the needle flange. This measurement (approximately 2 finger widths) should be noted in order to avoid inadvertent needle exposure beyond the dilator. When advancing the needle within the dilator, it must rotate freely and not be forcibly turned to avoid damage to the needle tip. With the needle in position, the stylet is removed and the needle is flushed and connected to pressure. Some operators remove the stylet before inserting the needle into the sheath. In another variation, the operator may use the dilator without a sheath to improve tactile feedback. Femoral arterial access may also be obtained percutaneously and a 5 French pigtail catheter advanced into the right coronary sinus to aid in identifying the aorta during transseptal puncture and for hemodynamic monitoring.

Prior to proceeding with the transseptal puncture, proper orientation of the assembly is crucial. The side arm of the sheath and flange of the needle should always have the same orientation. The entire system is rotated clockwise until the needle flange arrow and sheath side arm are positioned at 4 o'clock (with the patient's forehead being 12 o'clock and occiput 6 o'clock). This directs the assembly to the left and slightly posterior.

The assembly is then carefully withdrawn in a straight path, during which it will encounter three sequential bumps (leftward movements of the needle). These leftward movements occur at the superior vena cava/right atrium junction, as the needle moves over the ascending aorta and, finally, as it passes over the limbus and into the fossa ovalis.

At this point, fluoroscopy in the left anterior oblique (LAO) projection should demonstrate the needle pointing posteriorly towards the spine and lateral fluoroscopy should demonstrate the needle being inferior and posterior to the aorta (which can be marked by a pigtail catheter placed in the right coronary sinus). Accurate positioning can also be confirmed using a variety of echocardiographic techniques, as will be discussed later.

Once a satisfactory position is attained, the system is advanced (needle within the dilator) until further movement is limited and a damped right atrial pressure is observed. In approximately 10% of patients, the foramen ovale is patent and the apparatus enters the left atrium without needle puncture. In the remainder the needle is advanced into the left atrium under fluoroscopic and pressure monitoring.

Successful entry into the left atrium appears as a subtle but observed sudden leftward movement into the left atrium accompanied by an occasional palpable pop. Left atrial position is confirmed by a left atrial pressure tracing. If there continues to be doubt about position, contrast should be injected through the needle, which should flow freely in the left atrium. If there is staining of the interatrial septum, the needle should be advanced further. If there is aortic or pericardial staining, or the appearance of a pericardial or aortic waveform, the needle should be withdrawn and the patient evaluated for the potential complications of inadvertent needle puncture. If the left atrium cannot be entered, the entire system must be withdrawn to the inferior vena cava/right atrial junction, the needle removed, the J-wire reinserted and advanced into the superior vena cava, and the entire process repeated.

Once the needle tip is within the left atrium, the assembly is held together with the right hand and the unit advanced with the left hand near the groin for about 1 cm under fluoroscopic and hemodynamic monitoring until the tip of the dilator is in the left atrium. If dampening of the left atrial pressure waveform occurs, reorient the assembly more anteriorly (3 o'clock). The needle is then withdrawn out of the sheath and the guide wire reinserted and advanced into the left atrium, forming an exaggerated loop. The dilator and sheath are then advanced over the guide wire, followed by removal of the dilator and wire. The sheath is then flushed prior to connecting to pressure. At this point, systemic anticoagulation with heparin is instituted.

Table 36.2 Complications of transseptal catheterization.

Cardiac perforation

- Incidence: ~1%
- Consequences: hemopericardium, cardiac tamponade, death
- Minimized by strict adherence to technique, echocardiographic and hemodynamic guidance, experience
- Echocardiography can reduce the risk and allows early identification of effusion

Systemic embolization

- Incidence: < 1%
- Consequences: stroke most common but may also lead to limb, coronary, renal, and splanchnic ischemia
- Minimized by strict adherence to technique, especially flushing, and by anticoagulation

Inferior vena cava perforation

- Incidence: rare
- Consequences: retroperitoneal hemorrhage
- This is usually due to not allowing the needle to turn freely as it is inserted or forceful insertion despite resistance in tortuous Iliac vessels

Cardiac arrhythmias

- Incidence: common, including atrial tachycardias, heart block, bundle branch block
- Consequences: usually benign

COMPLICATIONS

In part, the decline in the frequency of transseptal catheterizations can be attributed to the concern over the potential complications (Table 36.2). Cardiac perforation is the most feared complication of transseptal catheterization. Cardiac perforation occurs with advancement of the large dilator into the pericardial sac, and not usually with inadvertent needle puncture alone. In one large series from a large volume academic center[6] there were 2 aortic and 13 atrial perforations in 1279 procedures resulting in cardiac tamponade, an incidence of 1.2%. The 13 patients who suffered atrial perforation survived. The only death in that series was secondary to aortic perforation, leading to an overall mortality rate of 0.08%. This describes the experience of a high-volume academic center, and the complication rates are likely to be higher in lower-volume centers.

Inadvertent pericardial puncture does not always result in tamponade. In one series, pericardial puncture occurred in 3 of 217 patients, and none resulted in tamponade.[8] Several series have noted that at operation following uneventful transseptal catheterization, blood-stained pericardium is not infrequently present, implying unnoticed atrial puncture during the procedure.[3,9,10] Cardiac tamponade occurs less frequently

in patients with prior cardiac surgery because of the obliteration of the pericardial space by adhesions.

Perforation of the IVC, resulting in a retroperitoneal bleed, may also occur. This is usually due to not allowing the needle to turn freely as it is inserted, or forceful insertion despite resistance in tortuous Iliac vessels. Systemic embolization (air or thrombus) is another potential complication of transseptal catheterization. Cerebral emboli are most frequently reported, but emboli to coronary, splanchnic, renal, and femoral arteries have also occurred. The incidence of an embolic event was reported to be 0.08% in the series of 1279 procedures described above.[6] Less serious complications include atrial arrhythmias, heart block, bundle branch block, and complications related to vascular access.

IMAGING MODALITIES FOR TRANSSEPTAL CATHETERIZATION

Fluoroscopy

Traditionally, fluoroscopy has been the imaging modality utilized during transseptal catheterization (Figure 36.1). Anteroposterior fluoroscopy allows accurate positioning of the transseptal puncture apparatus against the fossa ovalis in the interatrial septum in the vertical plane, defining the superior and inferior borders of the interatrial septum. However, it does not define the posterior border of the interatrial septum, leading to an increased risk of posterior puncture and left atrial perforation when only this single view is utilized.

A higher success rate has been reported using modified single-plane fluoroscopy.[11] A right anterior oblique (RAO) view (40–50°) provides an en face view of the interatrial septum and defines the inferior, posterior, and superior borders of the right atrium, decreasing the risk of atrial perforation. A pigtail catheter in the aorta demarcates its posterior wall and the level of the aortic valve. The recommended puncture in this projection lies midway between the posterior borders of the right atrium and the aorta, and 1–3 cm below the aortic valve.

Biplane fluoroscopy in the anteroposterior and lateral projections is a preferred modality. It allows accurate puncture site determination in both the vertical dimension and anteroposterior dimension simultaneously. In the anteroposterior view, proper positioning of the needle is at the mid portion of the right atrial silhouette. In the lateral view, it lies posterior and inferior to the aortic valve plane, demarcated by the pigtail catheter, with the needle pointing posteriorly (towards the spine).

However, there are limitations to utilizing fluoroscopy as the sole imaging modality. As mentioned previously, several series have noted that, at operation following transseptal catheterization, blood-stained

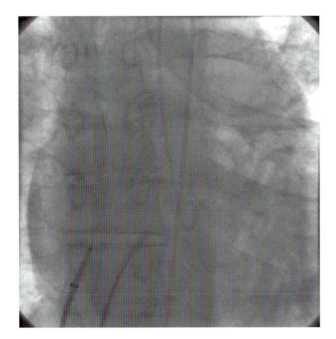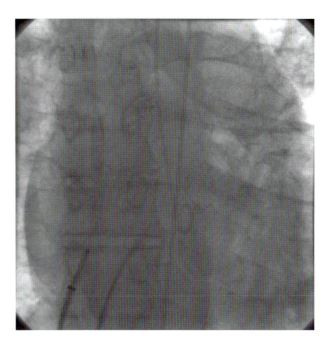

Figure 36.1 Biplane fluoroscopy demonstrating the location of optimal needle puncture. On the left is a posterior-anterior projection demonstrating the location of the dilator (with the needle not exposed beyond the tip) relative to the spine and a pigtail catheter in the right coronary sinus just prior to puncture. On the right is a 45° left anterior oblique projection confirming posterior needle orientation (toward the spine). Both views also show an 8 French AcuNav ICE catheter in the right atrium.

pericardial fluid is not infrequently present, indicating that atrial puncture occurs more frequently than is recognized clinically.[3,9,10] This may go unrecognized if there is perforation of the right atrial posterior wall followed by re-entry into the left atrium (the so-called stitching phenomenon).

Complications of transseptal catheterization are more common in certain disease states with distorted septal anatomy. The fossa ovalis is usually concave with respect to the right atrium, allowing easy identification on pull back from the superior vena cava (SVC) into the proper position as it jumps into the fossa ovalis. In patients with chronic elevation of left atrial pressure (as in mitral stenosis, for example), the fossa ovalis tends to bulge into the right atrium. This makes identification of the fossa ovalis more difficult. In addition, because of the bulge, the septal plane becomes parallel to the direction of the catheter and needle and puncture can result in septal dissection. These factors tend to result in a more caudal puncture, risking right atrial free wall perforation.

Puncture of atrial septal aneurysms poses another challenge. These are difficult to identify fluoroscopically. The placement of large-bore catheters and devices with repeated traction may cause extensive tearing of a thin aneurysmal septum.

Kyphoscoliosis and aortic root dilatation have also been considered relative contraindications to transseptal catheterization in the past as they distort normal intrathoracic anatomy and the relationships of cardiac structures to one another. Lipomatous hypertrophy of the interatrial septum may also make transseptal puncture more difficult due to increased septal thickness. Recently, a radiofrequency catheter has been introduced as a replacement for the sharp needle puncture and may have a specific utility in thick or lipomatous septa.[12] Because of the aforementioned situations and the necessity of precision of the transseptal puncture site required for specific therapeutic interventions, there is new interest in complimentary imaging modalities.

Transthoracic and transesophageal echocardiography

There are several reasons to consider adjunctive echocardiographic imaging during transseptal catheterization. First, it improves the overall safety of the procedure by confirming the needle location where it deforms or 'tents' the septum prior to actual puncture. In addition, it allows for improved precision with regard to the exact position of the septum, a feature of increasing importance for complex interventions. In the event of perforation or other patient symptoms such as chest pain, or hemodynamic alterations related to perforation, such as a vagal reaction, the presence of an echocardiographic probe can allow earlier identification of a complication or provide reassurance to its absence. Finally, the use of echocardiographic imaging for the transseptal puncture allows it to be already in place to be used as needed for other portions of the procedure, including assessment of mitral regurgitation, device placement, etc.

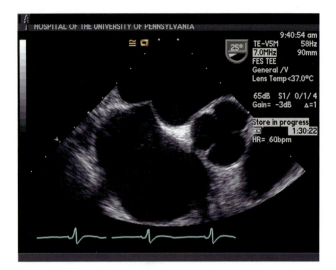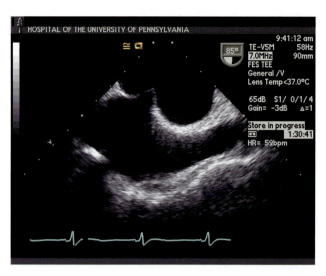

Figure 36.2 Tenting of the interatrial septum at the fossa ovalis by the needle as visualized just before puncture on transesophageal echocardiography in a patient with mitral stenosis. Note the bowing of the septum downward towards the right atrium due to the patient's elevated left atrial pressure (left atrium at the top nearer to the transducer). On the left is an anterior-posterior view with the aortic valve visible that allows the puncture to be as anterior (close to the valve) or posterior (away) as desired. On the right is a bicaval view (superior vena cava to the right) that allows for fine-tuning of the cranial vs caudal needle location.

The usefulness of two-dimensional transthoracic echocardiography (TTE) in guiding transseptal puncture has been reported.[13] Two-dimensional echocardiography allows delineation and spatial resolution of the aorta and interatrial septum. The interatrial septum is clearly demonstrated in the short-axis and four-chamber views, and clearly separated from the ascending aorta. The transseptal needle and catheter can be visualized by echocardiography while the needle tip is manipulated into the fossa ovalis, avoiding puncture of the aortic root. However, TTE is often limited by imaging windows and the fact that the patient must remain supine during the catheterization procedure. This may result in suboptimal visualization of the interatrial septum. Furthermore, it interferes with fluoroscopic imaging and exposes the echocardiographer to radiation. The need to preserve a sterile field is another limitation to the use of transthoracic echocardiography.

Transesophageal echocardiography (TEE) provides superior visualization of the interatrial septum and its usefulness has also been documented.[14] A small risk exists, however, for esophageal injury and lung aspiration. The need for heavy sedation or general anesthesia adds discomfort and stress for the patient. A final limitation of TEE is the requirement of an additional operator.

TEE can be useful for fine-tuning the septal puncture location. For instance, in the percutaneous edge-to-edge clip repair technique for mitral regurgitation, it is essential to have adequate height above the valve (assessed in a four-chamber view) as well as a superior and posterior puncture site in order to align the clip delivery system with the mitral valve line of leaflet coaptation. This is done using both the bicaval short-axis mid-esophageal view (for superior-inferior positioning) and the anteroposterior view (Figure 36.2). Recently, we have begun to use real-time live three-dimensional TEE imaging during this procedure. This technique allows for unprecedented appreciation of not only the septal puncture site, but also the tract and direction of entry into the left atrium (see Figure 36.3).

Intracardiac echocardiography

Intracardiac echocardiographic (ICE) guidance for transseptal catheterization offers several advantages.[15–18] In one case series, the utility of ICE in patients with a distorted anatomy of the fossa ovalis was examined.[16] Accurate localization of the fossa ovalis allowed successful, uncomplicated puncture in 12 patients with giant left atria and in 1 patient with kyphoscoliosis. Furthermore, in 2 patients with atrial septal aneurysms, avoiding puncture at these thin-walled areas was possible. Thus, it is clear that ICE not only allows superior visualization of the fossa ovalis as compared with TTE and TEE, but it also allows precise localization in those patients with distorted anatomy, a population which is at risk for increased complications and comprises the majority of patients who undergo transseptal catheterization for most interventional procedures.

In addition to superior imaging, patient comfort is also enhanced with ICE. Apart from the additional venous access required, there is no need for additional sedation or endotracheal intubation. Last, adequate imaging for many procedures can be obtained by the interventionalist eliminating the requirement for another operator or echocardiographer.

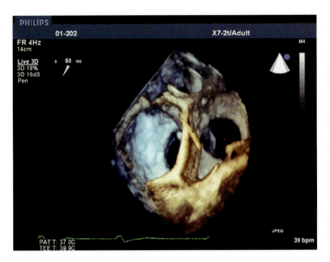

Figure 36.3 Three-dimensional transesophageal echocardiographic image of the interatrial septum just after needle puncture in a patient with severe mitral regurgitation and a massively enlarged left atrium undergoing percutaneous mitral valve repair. Note the posterior to anterior path of the sheath and needle from the right atrium (to the right of the figure) through the septum and the potential for the needle to continue through the left atrial wall if not reoriented.

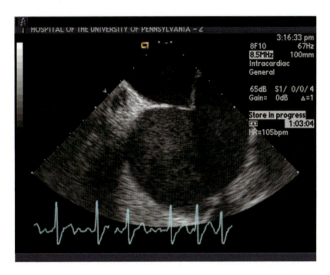

Figure 36.4 Intracardiac echocardiographic image with an 8 French AcuNav catheter in a patient with mitral stenosis undergoing percutaneous balloon valvuloplasty. The right atrium is on top (closer to the transducer) with tenting into the enlarged left atrium.

In our laboratory, all of our transseptal catheterizations are performed under ICE guidance. This involves insertion of an 8 French sheath, usually in the left femoral vein, to introduce the 8 French AcuNav ICE catheter (Bioscience-Webster Inc.). This is a steerable catheter with both color flow and spectral Doppler capabilities and excellent resolution. The ICE catheter is then advanced into the right atrium, where posterior and rightward angulation allows imaging of the interatrial septum, providing visualization of the transseptal apparatus as it traces the interatrial septum and enters the left atrium (Figure 36.4).

Although this catheter is the current 'gold standard' for ICE imaging, it adds significant additional cost to the procedure (approximately $2000). Costs can be reduced by using a resterilization process. The rotational ULTRAICE catheter (Boston Scientific Corp) is less expensive, but gives a smaller field of view and lacks color flow and Doppler capability. Nonetheless, it provides adequate imaging for transseptal puncture. Recently, a new planar ICE catheter with full color flow and Doppler has become available (EP Med Systems), although this catheter can only be flexed in one plane, potentially limiting its steerability as compared to the ACUNAV catheter, which can be manipulated in two planes.

MANAGEMENT OF COMPLICATIONS ASSOCIATED WITH TRANSSEPTAL CATHETERIZATION

Complications of transseptal catheterization are uncommon when performed by experienced operators.

Although most complications of transseptal catheterization are managed as they would be in the setting of retrograde left heart catheterization or right heart catheterization, the management of cardiac perforation in this setting requires further discussion. Tamponade occurs due to inadvertent puncture of the aorta or right atrial free wall, and less often the left atrium or pulmonary artery. Certainty about the site of needle puncture is of the utmost importance in preventing this complication. Adequate positioning of the needle prior to puncture can be evaluated using several modalities. On biplane fluoroscopy, the needle should be approximately at the mid portion of the right atrial silhouette in the anteroposterior view and inferior and posterior to the aortic root (demarcated by the pigtail catheter). TEE and ICE allow the accurate identification of the fossa ovalis in almost all patients, including those with altered anatomy, where fluoroscopy alone may be insufficient.

Puncture of adjacent cardiac structures is not always associated with catastrophic complications. As long as the patient is not anticoagulated and perforation is limited to the 21-gauge tip of the Brockenbrough needle, this is usually a benign event. However, if the 8 French catheter itself is advanced into the aorta or the pericardium, fatal complications may occur. This underscores the need for the operator to monitor closely the location of the transseptal catheterization apparatus. In general, if inadvertent needle perforation into the pericardium is suspected, it is best to withdraw the needle, terminate the procedure, and observe the patient for at least 24 hours before reattempting transseptal puncture and anticoagulation.

Following septal puncture, left atrial entry may be confirmed via several modalities. The pressure waveform should clearly demonstrate a left atrial waveform. A damped pressure waveform may indicate entry into the pericardium or incomplete septal penetration. An injection of a small amount of contrast through the needle may be helpful in this situation. Pericardial staining would indicate free right atrial perforation, whereas staining of the interatrial septum would indicate incomplete penetration. On the other hand, the appearance of an arterial waveform indicates aortic puncture. Aortic staining with contrast is another sign of aortic puncture. The transseptal puncture apparatus should never be advanced in the absence of a left atrial waveform. Oxygen saturation of blood aspirated from the needle may also aid in identifying the location of the needle.

In our laboratory, we routinely withdraw the needle after the tip of the dilator is across the septum and reinsert the 0.032 inch guide wire. The wire is curved in the left atrium before advancing the Mullins sheath, to protect against left atrial perforation by the tip of the dilator as it is advanced. This is particularly important when resistance is encountered, as the sheath meets septal resistance due to the 'shoulder' between the dilator and sheath. In this setting, further rotation and advancement can cause the dilator and sheath to jump into the left atrium and the wire helps protect the free wall from the dilator tip.

If needle puncture of the right atrial free wall or aorta occurs, the tip of the needle must be removed and the patient monitored for cardiac tamponade (although rare with needle-only puncture). Monitoring of right atrial pressures and systemic aortic pressure should be performed before a second attempt. An echocardiogram should also be obtained to ensure that there is no accumulation of blood in the pericardium.

A second attempt at transseptal puncture may be performed if there is no hemodynamic evidence of cardiac tamponade and if the procedure is performed for diagnostic purposes. If, however, transseptal catheterization is performed for interventional purposes, the procedure may be better postponed for another day in order to avoid the need for systemic anticoagulation.

CONCLUSIONS

Transseptal catheterization is an important diagnostic tool and of increasing importance for a number of therapeutic interventions. Avoiding complications, particularly perforation and cardiac tamponade, requires an understanding of the normal anatomy, distorted anatomy associated with various disease states, technical considerations, and the strengths and limitations of various imaging modalities. Echocardiography, and particularly ICE, has become an indispensible adjunct to transseptal catheterization in our laboratory due to its ability to optimize puncture location and minimize complications. With the combination of fluoroscopic imaging, hemodynamic monitoring, and echocardiography, complications of transseptal catheterization can be minimized, and rapidly recognized and treated if they occur.

REFERENCES

1. Ross J Jr, Braunwald E, Morrow AG. Transseptal left atrial puncture: new technique for the measurement of left atrial pressure in man. Am J Cardiol 1959; 3: 653–5.
2. Cope C. Technique for transseptal catheterization of the left atrium: preliminary report. J Thorac Surg 1959; 37: 482–6.
3. Brockenbrough EC, Braunwald E, Ross J Jr. Transseptal left heart catheterization: a review of 450 studies and description of an improved technique. Circulation 1962; 25: 15–21.
4. Mullins CE. Transseptal left heart catheterization: experience with a new technique in 520 pediatric and adult patients. Pediatr Cardiol 1983; 4: 239–46.
5. Swan HJ, Ganz W, Forrester J et al. Catheterization of the heart in man with use of a flow-directed balloon-tipped catheter. N Engl J Med 1970; 283: 447–51.
6. Roelke M, Smith AJ, Palacios IF. The technique and safety of transseptal catheterization: The Massachusetts General Hospital experience with 1,279 procedures. Cathet Cardiovasc Diagn 1994; 32: 332–9.
7. Baim DS. Percutaneous approach, including transseptal and apical puncture. In: Baim DS, ed. Cardiac Catheterization, Angiography and Intervention. Boston, MA: Williams and Wilkins, 2006. 7th edition: 79–132.
8. Ali Khan MA, Mulins CE, Bash SE et al. Transseptal left heart catheterization in infants, children, and young adults. Cathet Cardiovasc Diagn 1989; 17: 198–201.
9. Adrouny AZ, Sutherland DW, Griswold HE et al. Complications with transseptal left heart catheterization. Am Heart J 1963; 65; 327–33.
10. Singleton RT, Scherlis L. Transseptal catheterization of the heart: observations in 56 patients. Am Heart J 1960; 60: 879–85.
11. Croft CH, Lipscomb K. Modified technique of transseptal left heart catheterization. J Am Coll Cardiol 1985; 5: 904–10.
12. Sherman W, Lee P, Hartley A. Transatrial septal catheterization using a new radiofrequency probe. Cathet Cardiovasc Interven 2005; 66: 14–17.
13. Kronzon I, Glassman E, Cohen M et al. Use of two dimensional echocardiography during transseptal catheterization. J Am Coll Cardiol 1984; 4: 425–8.
14. Ballal RS, Mahan EF III, Nanda NC et al. Utility of transesophageal echocardiography in interatrial septal puncture during percutaneous mitral balloon commissurotomy. Am J Cardiol 1990; 66: 230–2.
15. Sylvestry FE, Rodriquez LL, Herrmann H et al. Echocardiographic guidance and assessment of percutaneous repair of mitral regurgitation with the Evalve MitraClip. Am Soc Echocardiogr 2007; 20: 1131–40.
16. Hung JS, Fu M, Yeh KH et al. Usefullness of intracardiac echocardiography in complex transseptal catheterization during percutaneous transvenous mitral commissurotomy. Mayo Clin Proc 1996; 71:134–40.
17. Mitchel JF, Gillam LD, Sanzobrino BW et al. Intracardiac ultrasound imaging during transseptal catheterization. Chest 1995; 108: 104–8.
18. Herrmann H. ICE in interventional cardiology. In: Weigers S, Sylvestry F, eds. Intracardiac Echocardiography. London, UK: Taylor & Francis, 2005: 75–89.

37 Percutaneous mitral valve repair: percutaneous mitral annuloplasty via the coronary sinus

David G Reuter

BACKGROUND

Prevalence

Functional mitral regurgitation (FMR) is common among the 22 million people worldwide who suffer from heart failure.[1,2] Of patients with a dilated cardiomyopathy and New York Heart Class III–IV, approximately 90% have some degree of FMR.[3,4]

The efficiency of the ventricle is compromised by the development of FMR.[5] In patients with advanced heart failure, FMR increases the hemodynamic stress on the failing left ventricle (LV), resulting in progressive left ventricular dilation, progressive systolic dysfunction, higher left ventricular end diastolic pressure, and higher pulmonary capillary wedge pressure.[6]

The labile nature of FMR affects exercise tolerance. Studies have documented that, with exercise, FMR increases and there is a lower augmentation of the cardiac index.[6] Studies by Lebrun *et al.*[7] and Keren *et al.*[8] noted that the regurgitant volume of patients who underwent exercise testing almost doubled, while forward stroke volume substantially decreased. This increase in FMR by isometric exercise may be caused by elevated left ventricular afterload.[9] Functionally, Tada *et al.* demonstrated in 30 patients that even mild FMR had a detrimental effect on exercise.[10] The contribution of FMR to morbidity,[6,10,11] as well as mortality,[12–16] has been well characterized.

Anatomy and pathophysiology of functional mitral regurgitation

Redundant mechanisms exist to facilitate proper mitral valve closure. These anatomic and physiologic mechanisms include the following: (1) mitral annular dimensions that optimize the zone of coaptation; (2) elliptical shape of the mitral valve to minimize distance between anterior and posterior leaflets; (3) saddle-shaped geometry of the mitral annulus to facilitate mitral valve coaptation; (4) papillary muscle position to ensure proper chordal vectors to pull leaflets towards the apex of the heart; and (5) contraction of left ventricle and papillary muscles to augment the effect of the chordae tendinae. Each of these mechanisms, working in delicate concert, ensures the normal functioning of the mitral valve apparatus.

The compensatory changes that accompany the development of heart failure have a deleterious effect on the function of the mitral valve. The annular dilation, loss of elliptical geometry, and loss of saddle shape[17] all serve to reduce the zone of coaptation. Furthermore, the lateral displacement of the papillary muscles alters the vector that the chordae place on the mitral leaflets, thus tethering the leaflet and reducing leaflet motion.[18–20] Progression of this subvalvular pathology further increases the likelihood and severity of FMR.

Improved understanding of the anatomic and functional components of the mitral valve apparatus has affected therapeutic approaches designed to reduce FMR.

Surgical mitral annuloplasty

Despite the ventricular and annular contributions to FMR, surgical annular reduction alone has been shown to decrease FMR.[11,21] Because medical therapy continues to be the standard of care for patients with FMR,[22,23] the majority of surgical experience with ring annuloplasty stems from patients with FMR with concomitant coronary artery bypass graft surgery.[21,24,25] Although ring annuloplasty has been shown to increase the perioperative mortality,[26,27] it has also been shown to improve late survival.[21,28] The timing of intervention may be of import as well. Braun and colleagues have shown that the likelihood of reverse ventricular remodeling is highest when the left ventricular end diastolic diameter is less than 65 mm.[29]

To the extent that restoration of contractile function requires intervention prior to the onset of irreversible LV dysfunction,[30] therapeutic intervention earlier in the disease course may be ideal. Given the morbidity[18] and mortality associated with surgical repair, percutaneous interventions to treat FMR offer a potentially attractive alternative.

Relevant coronary sinus anatomy

The proximity of the coronary sinus (CS) and great cardiac vein (GCV) to the posterior leaflet of the mitral valve makes this venous structure amenable to percutaneous therapies. Several percutaneous mitral annuloplasty techniques are being developed which leverage this serendipitous anatomy.[31–33] The relevant anatomy that potentially affects the safety and efficacy of each therapeutic technique includes the following: (1) superior position of the CS relative to the mitral valve annulus; (2) relationship of the CS/GCV to the commissures of the mitral valve; (3) dilated and dynamic nature of the CS; and (4) relationship of the CS/GCV to coronary arterial anatomy.

The superior position of the CS relative to the mitral valve annulus has been well characterized. Yamanouchi et al. evaluated 50 human cadaver hearts, and measured the distance between the mitral valve annulus and the coronary sinus at five different positions along the posterior leaflet between 36° and 188°.[34] The shortest distance measured 8.2 ± 2.9 mm and the largest distance measured 10.9 ± 3.3 mm. A similar anatomic study using a different methodology was recently reported by Maselli et al. Using multidetector computed tomographic images, the distance from the coronary sinus to the mitral valve annulus was found to range from 3.2 to 19.7 mm.[35] Percutaneous CS-based devices must be compatible with this variable anatomy.

Equally important to the position of the CS relative to the mitral valve annulus is the position of the mitral valve commissures to the CS/GCV. As a general rule, the posterior commissure is adjacent to the coronary sinus ostium, and the anterior commissure is adjacent to the junction between the GCV and the anterior interventricular vein (AIV).

The CS is a dynamic structure throughout the cardiac cycle. The CS wall is relatively thick and, instead of smooth muscle forming a tunica media, it consists of striated myocardium continuous with the atrium. The CS narrows during atrial contraction in persons with normal sinus rhythm. Mild CS dilation was noted in patients with poorly contracting ventricles in both ischemic and non-ischemic cardiomyopathy patients.[36] In patients with advanced heart failure, the CS diameter is as much as twice the diameter of the CS in a normal subject.[37] The dilated CS is likely related to the chronically elevated right atrial pressures observed in heart failure patients. The altered mechanical properties of the CS must be taken into account by CS-based devices.

Two key valves are typically associated with the CS: the Thebesian valve and the Vieussens valve. The Thebesian valve is located at the junction between the right atrium and the coronary sinus ostium. This structure can range from a small crescent to a fenestrated valve.[38] The Vieussens valve is normally located at the junction between the CS and the GCV, near the insertion of the oblique vein of the left atrium (vein of Marshall). This valve can be either a monocuspid or a bicuspid valve. In an anatomic study of 37 human cadaver specimens, the Thebesian valve was present in 86% of cases, and the Vieussens valve was present in 57% of cases.[39]

The CS/GCV has a variable and intimate relationship with the coronary arterial anatomy. In a typical patient with a right dominant coronary arterial circulation, the left circumflex artery will cross over the CS/GCV soon after its bifurcation from the left main coronary artery (near the P1 scallop of the mitral valve). Pejkovic and Bogdanovic performed an anatomic study of 150 human cadaver hearts, and reported that the GCV is deep to the circumflex artery in 27% of cases, and is deep to the left anterior descending artery in 10% of cases.[40] Patients with a left dominant or codominant arterial circulation may have more than one obtuse marginal artery deep to the CS/GCV.

The terminal aspect of the right coronary artery may also lie in close proximity to the CS, although in most cases, these two vessels are sufficiently removed that device-related impingement is unlikely.

There are elements of the CS anatomy that may be advantageous to the function of mitral annuloplasty devices. For example, optimal leaflet coaptation is facilitated by the dynamic three-dimensional conformational changes of the mitral valve annulus.[41,42] Rigid annuloplasty rings prevent this dynamic motion. Since devices in the CS are able to modify the annular position, without directly restricting it, one is able to maintain the dynamic function of the annulus. A second example relates to restoration of the saddle-shaped nature of the annulus. Just as newer annuloplasty rings have been engineered with a three-dimensional shape to recreate the saddle-shaped nature of the mitral annulus, so too might CS devices apply not only an inward force, but also an upward force (based on its superior position) on the annulus so as to both reduce the septal lateral dimensions, and also partially restore the saddle shape of the annulus.

TECHNIQUES INVOLVED IN MANAGEMENT

Cardiac Dimensions technique

The Cardiac Dimensions procedure can be performed with either conscious sedation or general anesthesia.

Prior to accessing the CS, right and left coronary arteriograms are performed in order to characterize the arterial anatomy, and to determine the extent, if any, of coronary artery disease. In conjunction with the left arterial injection, the cine run may be extended in order to opacify the CS during the venous phase of the injection. An LAO caudal projection typically shows the plane of the CS well.

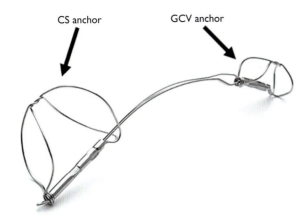

CS anchor   GCV anchor

Figure 37.1   CARILLON Mitral Contour System™.

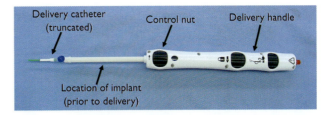

Delivery catheter (truncated)   Control nut   Delivery handle

Location of implant (prior to delivery)

Figure 37.2   CARILLON Delivery System. The rotational controls are used to deploy and lock the GCV and CS anchors, and decouple the device from the delivery system.

Deployment of the CARILLON™ Mitral Contour System™ requires cannulating the internal jugular vein, and positioning a 9 French delivery catheter at the distal end of the great cardiac vein, near the anterior commissure of the mitral valve. Implant selection depends upon the anatomic size of the CS/GCV in the anticipated locations of the distal and proximal anchor. Therefore, the next step in the procedure is to perform a venogram through the delivery catheter to characterize the CS/GCV diameters. Attention to detail at this point is important. Venograms performed in multiple projections (e.g., LAO caudal and RAO caudal) enable identification of the maximum vein diameter. In addition, a frame-by-frame review of the venous dimensions is important given the dynamic nature of the vein throughout the cardiac cycle. Once the venous dimensions are characterized, a marker catheter is inserted through the lumen of the delivery catheter, so as to determine the length of the vein from the CS ostium to the GCV/AIV junction.

The CARILLON device is a fixed-length, double-anchor device (Figure 37.1) that is designed to plicate tissue along the posterior mitral valve annulus to a variable degree, depending upon the amount of tension that is placed on the delivery system during device deployment. The goal of this adjustability is to optimize the effect of the device in a broad range of anatomic and pathologic conditions. Anticipating that approximately 4 cm of tension will be placed on the system, and knowing that the implant length is 6 cm, the target locations of the distal and proximal anchor are identified, characterized, and a device with appropriately sized anchors is selected.

The CARILLON implant, which is stored in the unlocked position, is advanced down the 9 French delivery catheter. The arched shape of the implant causes the anchors to consistently orient themselves toward the outside of the vein, and the ribbon element of the device to be directed toward the left atrial tissue, as it is advanced around the mitral valve. Utilizing the rotational controls of the delivery handle (Figure 37.2), the distal anchor of the implant is deployed in

the target location, typically near the anterior commissure of the mitral valve.

The anchors of the CARILLON implant consist of Nitinol wireforms that are shapeset into a helical configuration. Upon deployment of the distal anchor, the wireforms passively expand. In order to achieve the full height of the anchor, the delivery catheter is advanced forward to engage the distal anchor, and lock the wireforms into the appropriate location. This locking action increases the circumferential pressure that the wireforms exert on the venous endothelium because the anchor is designed to be oversized relative to the venous diameter by approximately a 1.5–2.0 ratio.

Once the distal anchor is deployed and locked into position, tension may be placed on the delivery system in order to pull the proximal anchor (which remains collapsed within the delivery catheter) closer to the CS ostium, near the posterior commissure of the mitral valve. By placing a graded amount of tension on the delivery system, a variable amount of tissue may be plicated. Since the impact of the device on the mitral regurgitation is monitored real-time with color Doppler, the user is able to adjust the amount of tissue plication needed in order to optimize the reduction in mitral regurgitation (Figure 37.3).

Given the intimate relationship of the coronary arteries to the CS and GCV, it is important to perform a coronary arteriogram immediately after plicating the peri-annular tissue. Several scenarios are possible. In many cases, no arteries are crossed with the device; therefore, there will be no impact on coronary flow. When arteries are crossed with the device, they will typically show no impact on flow, despite the annular reduction achieved during the deployment procedure. Occasionally, a reduction in coronary flow will be noted, but may be reversed (e.g., normal flow restored), with partial release of tension from the delivery system. In the final scenario, tensioning of the delivery system will create sufficient coronary artery compromise that recapture of the device is required.

Following the deployment of the distal anchor, and assessment of mitral regurgitation and coronary arterial flow, the proximal anchor of the device is released from the delivery catheter, and locked into position in a manner analogous to the locking of the distal anchor. With

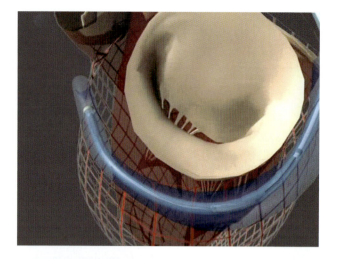

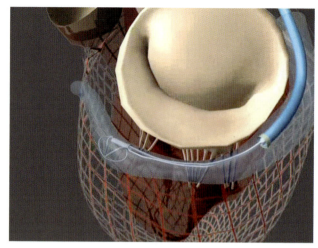

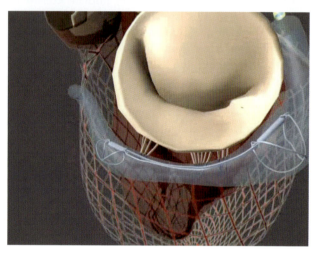

Figure 37.3 A 9 French delivery catheter is advanced to the distal aspect of the GCV, near the anterior commissure of the mitral valve. Once the distal anchor of the CARILLON Mitral Contour System is deployed, tension is placed on the system to plicate the peri-annular tissue. The proximal anchor is deployed near the posterior commissure of the mitral valve, and the device is released after safety and efficacy have been confirmed.

both anchors of the device deployed and anchored into position, echocardiographic assessment of the device can be performed. It is important to quantitate the reduction in mitral regurgitation using established methods (e.g., PISA and vena contracta). In addition to echocardiographic assessment of safety and efficacy, repeat coronary arteriography is worthwhile to confirm no deleterious impact on either right or left coronary arterial flow.

If reduction in mitral regurgitation is confirmed, and no safety issues are identified, the CARILLON Mitral Contour System is released from the delivery system. If there exists a clinical indication to recapture the implant, then advancement of the delivery catheter over the proximal and distal anchor wireforms will collapse the wires, and enable device recapture. The mechanism of device recapture allows for the deployment of a subsequent device in the CS/GCV, in the event that repositioning a second device would improve either safety or efficacy.

Edwards technique

MONARC system design

The Edwards MONARC system comprises a 12 French guide catheter, a 9 French delivery catheter (Figure 37.4), and a Nitinol shape memory implant (Figure 37.5). Using standard catheterization techniques, the Nitinol device is positioned in the CS, adjacent to the posterior portion of the mitral valve. The implant consists of four components: a self-expanding distal anchor, a self-expanding proximal anchor, a biodegradable element, and a spring bridge that connects the two anchoring segments. The anchors are designed such that they remain firmly in place acutely and encourage tissue in-growth, which provides a secure platform at both ends of the device. The biodegradable component is fabricated within the spring-like bridge and maintains the device in an elongated state at implant. After implant, the biodegradable element dissolves over 4–6 weeks, creating an active and sustained spring tension between the ostium of the CS and the distal GCV. As the device foreshortens, leaflet coaptation is improved, resulting in a reduction in mitral regurgitation.

The delayed release nature of this implant was designed to have minimal impact on adjacent cardiac structures and accommodate tissue movement. As the heart progresses through the remodeling process, the MONARC system compensates for changes in cardiac geometry with constant applied active tension to the mitral valve structure over time, allowing the heart to remodel and sustain this remodeling.

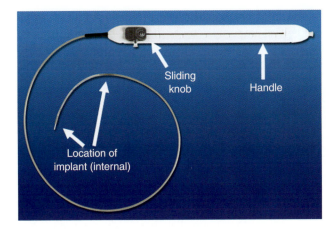

Figure 37.4   MONARC system delivery catheter.

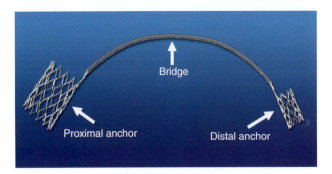

Figure 37.5   MONARC system implant.

Implant procedure and device sizing

The implant procedure starts with cannulation of the CS via a right internal jugular vein access and placement of a guide wire. The vein segment is then measured for diameter (distal and proximal) and length to determine the appropriate size device. Figure 37.6 illustrates the MONARC system implant in relation to the mitral valve and other pertinent cardiac structures.

Following device sizing and selection, the guiding catheter is inserted into the CS under fluoroscopic guidance. The delivery catheter is then passed through the guiding catheter and into the coronary venous system. Based on the previously identified landmarks, the distal anchor is deployed in the anterior interventricular vein by retraction of the outer restraining sheath with the thumb slider mechanism on the delivery catheter handle (Figure 37.4). After release of the distal anchor, slack is removed from the bridge element by withdrawing and tensioning the delivery catheter; this positions the proximal anchor just within the ostium of the CS, and retraction of the remaining outer sheath deploys the proximal anchor with the bridge lying along the inner radius of the sinus.

Viacor technique

Device description

The percutaneous transvenous mitral annuloplasty (PTMA) device (Viacor, Inc) is composed of two structural elements: a multilumen PTMA delivery catheter and PTMA rods. The PTMA delivery catheter is a 7 French, multilumen PTFE (Teflon) extrusion. It is designed to be advanced over the wire into the CS, GCV, and the proximal anterior interventricular vein. The distal tip of the device is made of a soft, nontraumatic molded silicone material. The PTMA delivery catheter includes three parallel lumens that travel the full length of the catheter. PTMA rods are solid Nitinol, custom ground to establish the desired stiffness properties. When placed within the PTMA delivery

catheter, PTMA rods produce a graded conformational change in the mitral annulus that reduces anterior-posterior diameter and increases leaflet coaptation. Rods are supplied in two hinge stiffnesses, six distal treatment lengths, and three tapers. The treatment part consists of two separated barrels (one proximal and one distal) supplied in different lengths for a total of 15 rod configurations. Up to three rods can be placed simultaneously within the PTMA delivery catheter, one in each lumen. By selectively increasing the number (1 to 3), stiffness, and length of stiffness of rods placed within the PTMA delivery catheter, the mitral annulus can be incrementally reshaped.[43]

Procedure

The procedure can be performed either in the operating room or the catheterization lab. Procedures are typically done under general anesthesia with transesophageal echocardiographic guidance. In the cath-lab, an 8 French sheath is introduced through the left subclavian vein, and the CS cannulated. After 2000 units of heparin are administered, venography is performed to verify CS and GCV anatomy. The PTMA delivery catheter is advanced over a soft tip 0.025 inch guide wire (Emerald guidewire, 150 cm/0.025 inch, Cordis Corp, Miami, FL) into the CS until the distal tip reaches the AIV. PTMA rods are inserted in the lumens of the PTMA delivery catheter under fluoroscopic guidance. PTMA rods are added or interchanged systematically, starting from modest pressure to more aggressive, to optimize the reduction in anterior-posterior annular dimensions and MR degree as assessed by transesophageal echocardiographic monitoring. After each PTMA rod adjustment, transesophageal echocardiography images are obtained. When maximal reduction of MR is achieved, the procedure is concluded.[43]

RECOMMENDED TECHNIQUES AND TOOLS TO ENSURE SUCCESS

Coronary sinus access

Devices intended for percutaneous mitral annuloplasty typically require either internal jugular venous access

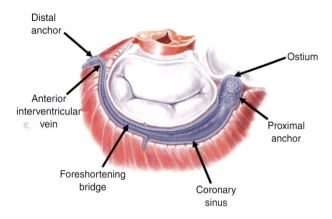

Figure 37.6 MONARC system implant illustration.

or subclavian vein access. Given the orientation of the CS ostium, this superior approach is ideal for CS access. In addition, because most procedures include a coronary arteriogram to characterize the arterial anatomy, the venous follow-through of this coronary injection provides a relevant road map of the CS. An LAO caudal projection is essentially perpendicular to the plane of the mitral valve annulus, and thus displays the CS/GCV clearly. An RAO caudal projection can also be used to cannulate the CS.

There are a variety of tools available to facilitate CS cannulation. The precise selection of tools depends in part on the size of the delivery catheter needed for each therapeutic procedure. The two general approaches include the use of either a deflectable catheter, or a guide wire and appropriately shaped diagnostic catheter. Each approach has its strengths and weaknesses.

Deflectable catheter approach

If one elects to cannulate the CS with a deflectable catheter, it is helpful to have the outside diameter (OD) of the deflectable catheter flush with the internal diameter (ID) of the delivery catheter. For example, if a 9 French delivery catheter is needed, the use of a 7 French deflectable catheter will minimize the risk of vein dissection as the delivery catheter is tracked along the deflectable catheter.

One advantage of the deflectable catheter is the spectrum of curves that can be imposed on the end of the catheter. Varying degrees of right atrial enlargement may require a larger or smaller radius of curvature in order to engage the CS ostium.[44] To facilitate engagement of the CS, it can be helpful to advance the deflectable catheter into the inferior vena cava. A curve is then placed on the end of the catheter, and the catheter is withdrawn into the right atrium while a gentle counterclockwise torque is placed on the handle. This maneuver will oftentimes help the tip of the catheter fall into the adjacent CS.

Once the deflectable catheter has engaged the CS, it can be slowly advanced toward the GCV/AIV junction.

Especially if a straight or stiff delivery catheter is to be used, it is important to keep the tip of the delivery catheter far back in the right atrium, so as to have minimal impact on the tip of the deflectable catheter. This will prevent excessive force from the rounded tip of the deflectable catheter being applied to the wall of the CS. At the junction of the CS and GCV, it is not uncommon to encounter increased resistance, likely due to the Vieussens valve. Increased force is not needed at this point. Rather, applying a slightly decreased radius of curvature (tighter curve) to the deflectable catheter, followed by gentle back and forth probing of the area while rotating the catheter, will frequently enable successful crossing of this region. Once the catheter tip has been advanced past the Vieussens valve, it will typically not encounter additional resistance. Because there is often an acute bend at the GCV/AIV junction, it is important to know where this junction is, and not to advance the tip of the catheter beyond the junction. Occlusion of a small GCV is inconsequential, as there is extensive collateral venous return.

Once the deflectable catheter is in the proper position near the GCV/AIV junction, backwards traction can be placed on the deflectable catheter while simultaneously advancing the delivery catheter over the deflectable catheter to the desired position. As long as the OD of the deflectable is flush with the ID of the delivery catheter, there is very little chance of the delivery catheter being caught on either the valve of Vieussens or venous tributaries that drain into the CS/GCV.

Many percutaneous mitral annuloplasty procedures require a venogram to characterize the venous dimensions. It is important to perform a small test injection through the delivery catheter to ensure that it is not caught in a side branch, or to confirm that it is not wedged at the GCV/AIV junction. Oftentimes the best venograms will be obtained if the delivery catheter is approximately two-thirds of the way around the vein. If additional advancement of the delivery catheter is required following a venogram, it is important never to advance the delivery catheter on its own. Furthermore, because of the distensible nature of the vein, it can be hazardous to advance the deflectable catheter out the end of the delivery catheter. The safest technique involves placing the tip of the deflectable catheter just proximal to the tip of the delivery catheter, then retracting the 9 French catheter all the way back out into the right atrium. This will minimize the force that the delivery catheter places on the deflectable tip, and thus minimizes the risk of CS perforation. The deflectable catheter can then be advanced to the GCV/AIV junction, followed by advancing the delivery catheter to the appropriate location.

The advantage of the deflectable catheter approach is essentially two-fold. First, the spectrum of curves available at the tip facilitates CS cannulation for a range of different anatomies. Second, the stiff body of the deflectable catheter facilitates the tracking of a stiff delivery catheter, without losing position. The major disadvantage is cost.

Guidewire/diagnostic catheter approach

Cannulating the CS with a diagnostic catheter requires selecting the appropriate shape catheter. Improved catheter shapes resulting from the experience with cardiac resynchronization therapy has made catheter availability and selection easier. In most cases, either a multipurpose catheter or an Amplatz L1 or L2 catheter provides an adequate shape to enable CS access.

Consistent with standard catheter techniques, it is important not to advance the catheter deep into the CS without the use of a guide wire. Even the softer tip of a diagnostic catheter can traumatize the wall of the CS if used inappropriately.

Although there are a variety of guide wires that one can use in the CS, a few common principles apply. A 0.035 inch wire should provide sufficient support over which to track the diagnostic catheter. A flexible wire with a J-tip is important to minimize venous trauma. Lastly, many individuals prefer a hydrophilic wire because of the ease with which it can be advanced through the CS/GCV, partially down the AIV. Examples of acceptable wires include the standard, hydrophilic-coated Glidewire with a flexible J-tip (Terumo, Inc), or the Standard Cordis STORQ guide wire with a modified J-tip (Johnson and Johnson, Inc).

Should the guide wire fail to advance past the Vieussens valve, one may advance the diagnostic catheter to the CS/GCV junction, thus providing greater support to navigate the guide wire past this valve. Once again, gentle probing with the guide wire will typically enable crossing the valve. Seating the end of the guide wire in the AIV will facilitate tracking the diagnostic catheter over the wire without the wire losing position.

To minimize the risk of traumatizing the CS, one should avoid tracking catheters with a sharply angled tip along a guide wire to the distal aspect of the CS/GCV. If an atypical shaped catheter is required to access the CS (e.g., left coronary bypass catheter), then that catheter should be exchanged over an exchange-length wire that has modest stiffness in the body so as to enable the use of a benign tipped catheter (e.g., multipurpose) to be advanced to the GCV/AIV junction.

Similar to the sizing of a deflectable catheter, it is beneficial if the OD of the diagnostic catheter is the same as the ID of the delivery catheter. This prevents the delivery catheter from catching on venous valves or venous tributaries as it is advanced around the posterior aspect of the mitral valve.

Coronary artery management

Analogous to surgical annuloplasty, where care must be taken when throwing stitches so as not to inadvertently ligate a coronary artery in the atrioventricular groove, similar care must be taken with CS-based mitral annuloplasty devices to insure that coronary flow is not compromised during device deployment.

The anatomic proximity of both the right and left coronary arteries to the CS/GCV necessitates a careful characterization of the native coronary anatomy, close monitoring during device placement, and attention to patient stability throughout the course of the procedure. Successful device delivery will typically be driven by both proper patient selection and vigilant monitoring of coronary arterial flow during the implant procedure.

Because of the anticipated infrequent rate of coronary artery compromise, most patients should be eligible to undergo an implant procedure independent of their underlying coronary artery anatomy and pathology. Patients who have severe coronary artery disease, potentially with occlusion of both the left anterior descending and the right coronary artery, may be poor candidates for a percutaneous CS-based procedure if the only blood supply to the left ventricle is via the circumflex artery, especially if the circumflex is deep to the CS. Either previous coronary angiography or angiography at the time of the index procedure should be sufficient to screen for these potentially high-risk patients.

As noted by Carabello in his extensive work to characterize the natural history of mitral regurgitation, patients whose ventricular dilation and mitral regurgitation become too severe are likely to experience irreversible left ventricular dysfunction.[30] Conversely, as noted by Braun *et al.*, the likelihood of achieving reverse ventricular remodeling following surgical annuloplasty is increased when surgery is performed before the left ventricular end diastolic diameter (LVEDD) exceeds 65 mm.[29] The principle of early intervention is ideal for percutaneous therapies. From a patient selection and coronary artery management vantage point, this approach has several benefits. Specifically, patients with only modest LV dilation and modest annular dilation likely require less tissue plication, or less septal-lateral reduction, to achieve the desired effect. With only modest forces required to effect a repair, the likelihood of coronary artery compromise is reduced. To the extent that many of the percutaneous devices designed to treat FMR should not preclude future cardiac surgery, or cardiac resynchronization implantation, future therapeutic options would not be compromised.

Intraprocedure coronary artery management begins with a careful characterization of the native coronary anatomy, and the degree of pre-existing coronary artery disease. A right and left coronary arteriogram is typically sufficient to characterize the anatomy. To the extent that there exists modest flexibility in the precise placement of each of the CS-based mitral annuloplasty devices, care can be taken to insure that devices are placed with the intention of minimizing potential adverse events. Although the exact mechanism of action is different for the spectrum of CS-based devices being developed, each of these devices exerts forces on the surrounding tissues, either by the anchored ends of the device or the connecting elements. As such, performing intermittent coronary arteriograms during the implant procedure, as well as monitoring for hemodynamic and electrocardiographic changes, is worthwhile.

In the event that a more thorough assessment of coronary flow is desired, a pressure wire could be used to assess the impact of the device on surrounding coronaries. As needed, infusion of adenosine may be important to achieve maximal arteriolar vasodilatation so as to obtain an accurate and reliable fractional flow reserve value.

Occasionally, alteration of coronary flow will be caused not by mechanical compression, but transient arterial spasms due to the influence of the device. Intravenous nitroglycerin helps to diagnose and treat this condition.

POSSIBLE COMPLICATIONS AND THEIR MANAGEMENT

Coronary sinus perforation

If cannulation of the CS or GCV results in dissection of the vein, no intervention is needed.[45] Unlike coronary arterial dissections, coronary venous dissections are benign and self-limited. To err on the side of caution, one may consider aborting and rescheduling an implant procedure if a significant dissection is noted.

CS perforation is a more severe complication. The rate of this event is likely to parallel or possibly exceed the rate of CS perforation noted in the cardiac resynchronization therapy (CRT) literature. Medtronic's MIRACLE trial reported a 2% rate of CS perforation in 453 patients.[46] Guidant's COMPANION trial reported a 1.1% rate of CS perforation in 1520 patients who were assigned to one of three arms: drug, CRT device, or CRT plus ICD.[47] Most recently, a study by Beshai et al. evaluating the effect of CRT in patients with narrow QRS complexes reported a 0.6% rate of CS perforation in 172 patients.[48]

Management of CS perforation depends upon the severity of the event. If, for example, the CS was only perforated with a guide wire, there is a high likelihood that no intervention will be required. Careful cardiopulmonary monitoring is important at this time. An echocardiogram is needed to characterize the degree of hemopericardium, and the progression or stabilization of the process.

If a larger catheter perforates the CS, it is unlikely that observation alone will suffice in the management of the complication. In this circumstance, placement of a pericardial drain using standard subxyphoid or parasternal techniques is recommended to evacuate the pericardial fluid and thus prevent or alleviate any cardiac tamponade. The volume of pericardial fluid accumulation should be carefully recorded, as it may take several hours before the process stabilizes and no additional fluid accumulation is noted.

Reversal of heparin may be required, especially if monitoring of the pericardial effusion confirms that a non-conservative approach is required.

In rare circumstances, mediastinal and pericardial adhesions (e.g., from prior cardiac surgery) may complicate the standard technique of pericardiocentesis. If transcutaneous pericardial access is not possible due to these adhesions, one may prep the skin with the appropriate antibacterial agent, then perform a small paraxyphoid cutdown with blunt dissection to expose the pericardial sac. From this point, the standard Seldinger technique should be successful to facilitate pericardial access.

Third-degree heart block

The proximity of the atrioventricular node adjacent to the coronary sinus ostium makes catheter-induced conduction disturbances a potential complication during attempts to cannulate the CS. Although the development of third-degree heart block is an infrequent complication of CS access, it is imperative to have back-up pacing capabilities readily available as needed. Since jugular venous access already exists, removing the delivery catheter and inserting a pacing lead into the right ventricle is a simple maneuver. For those patients with a history of AV node dysfunction, or left bundle branch block, one may consider placing a pacing lead in the right ventricle prophylacticly prior to the annuloplasty procedure.

Atrial fibrillation

Mechanical stimulation of the right atrium during the annuloplasty procedure increases the risk of inducing atrial fibrillation. The dilated atria of patients with long-standing heart failure, and tricuspid regurgitation, increases the likelihood of inducing atrial fibrillation. The altered atrial contractility may negatively affect the patient's hemodynamics. If the atrial arrhythmia does not automatically revert to sinus rhythm, then either pharmacologic cardioversion or electrical cardioversion, may be necessary.

Mitral stenosis

Although the creation of mitral stenosis has been reported infrequently following surgical annuloplasty, it is unlikely in CS-based annuloplasty given the superior position of the vein to the mitral annulus.[49] In a canine model of pacing-induced cardiomyopathy, mitral stenosis was not observed following deployment and tensioning of a distal anchor near the anterior commissure.[31] As needed, echocardiography can be used to assess transmitral pressure gradients.

Contrast-induced nephropathy

The majority of patients who have advanced heart failure and FMR also have renal insufficiency. As such, adequate hydration prior to the procedure, and judicious use of contrast during the procedure, are important to minimize the risk of contrast-induced nephropathy. Although a ventriculogram could be used to assess the degree of MR before or after device placement, the large amount of contrast required makes this imaging modality suboptimal. Quantitative echocardiography is a more benign means to assess the degree of MR around the time of the procedure. In this way, contrast use is only required to characterize and assess coronary artery flow, and to opacify the CS/GCV to facilitate anatomic measurements. A modest protective effect may be conferred by acetylcysteine administration in the pre- and periprocedural period.

Coronary sinus thrombosis

In general, the CS-based devices that are being designed have a sufficiently low profile that chronic CS thrombosis and occlusion is unlikely. In fact, both the Cardiac Dimensions device and the Edwards device would be expected to become endothelialized in the first months after device implantation. In the unlikely event that distal GCV thrombosis led to vessel occlusion, the surgical experience suggests that the event would be inconsequential due to the extensive and redundant venous system of the heart.

Acute thrombus formation during CS access has been reported in the CRT literature. Given the static column of blood in the delivery catheter, thrombus formation is possible during percutaneous mitral annuloplasty. Therefore, heparin should be administered during the procedure to achieve an activated clotting time (ACT) level > 300 seconds.[50]

CONCLUSION

FMR complicates the care of patients with heart failure. The CS represents a viable anatomy from which to effect a percutaneous repair. Several innovative techniques have been developed. Proper tools and techniques employed during CS access and device delivery can minimize the likelihood of complications. Appropriate clinical trials will be necessary to establish the unique risks and benefits for each device.

REFERENCES

1. American Heart Association. 2002 Heart and Stroke Statistical Update. Dallas, Tex.: American Heart Association, 2001.
2. Codd MB, Sugrue DD, Gersh BJ, Melton LJ. Epidemiology of idiopathic dilated and hypertrophic cardiomyopathy; a population-based study in Olmsted County, Minnesota, 1975–1984. Circulation 1989; 80: 564–72.
3. Patel JB, Borgeson DD, Barnes ME et al. Mitral regurgitation in patients with advanced systolic heart failure. J Card Fail 2004; 10(4): 285–91.
4. Ennezat PV, Marechaux S, Asseman P et al. Functional mitral regurgitation and chronic heart failure. Minerva Cardioangiol 2006; 54(6): 725–33.
5. Trichon BH, Felker GM, Shaw LK et al. Mitral regurgitation is an independent risk factor for mortality in patients with heart failure and left ventricular systolic dysfunction. J Am Coll Cardiol 2002; 39(5)(Suppl A): 1205-155–194A.
6. Junker A, Thayssen P, Nielsen B, Andersen PE. The hemodynamic and prognostic significance of echo-Doppler-proven mitral regurgitation in patients with dilated cardiomyopathy. Cardiology 1993; 83: 14–20.
7. Lebrun F, Lancellotti P, Peirard LA. Quantitation of functional mitral regurgitation during bicycle exercise in patients with heart failure. J Am Coll Cardiol 2001; 38: 1685–92.
8. Keren G, Katz S, Strom J et al. Dynamic mitral regurgitation: an important determinant of hemodynamic response to load alterations and inotropic therapy in severe heart failure. Circulation 1989; 80(2): 306–13.
9. Lachmann J, Shirani J, Prestis KA et al. Mitral ring annuloplasty: an incomplete correction of functional mitral regurgitation associated with left ventricular remodeling. Curr Cardiol Rep 2001; 3: 241–6.
10. Tada H, Tamai J, Takaki H et al. Mild mitral regurgitation reduces exercise capacity in patients with idiopathic dilated cardiomyopathy. Int J Cardiol 1997; 58: 41–5.
11. Bach DS, Bolling SF. Improvement following correction of secondary mitral regurgitation in end-stage cardiomyopathy with mitral annuloplasty. Am J Cardiol 1996; 78: 966–9.
12. Blondheim DS, Jacobs LE, Kotler MN et al. Dilated cardiomyopathy with mitral regurgitation: decreased survival despite a low frequency of left ventricular thrombus. Am Heart J 1991; 122: 763.
13. Trichon BH, Felker GM, Shaw et al. Relation of frequency and severity of mitral regurgitation to survival among patients with left ventricular systolic dysfunction and heart failure. Am J Cardiol 2003; 91: 538–43.
14. Grigioni F, Enriquez-Sarano M, Zehr KJ et al. Ischemic mitral regurgitation: long term outcome and prognostic implications with quantitative Doppler assessment. Circulation 2001; 103: 1759–64.
15. Koelling TM, Aaronson KD, Cody RJ et al. Prognostic significance of mitral regurgitation and tricuspid regurgitation in patients with left ventricular systolic dysfunction. Am Heart J 2002; 144: 524–9.
16. Lam BK, Gillinov AM, Blackstone EH et al. Importance of moderate ischemic mitral regurgitation. Ann Thorac Surg 2005; 79: 462–70.
17. Kaplan SR, Bashein G, Sheehan F et al. Three-dimensional echocardiographic assessment of annular shape changes in the normal and regurgitant mitral valve. Am Heart J 2000; 139(3): 378–87.
18. Calafiore AM, DiMauro M, Gallina S et al. Mitral valve surgery for chronic ischemic mitral regurgitation. Ann Thorac Surg 2004; 77: 1989–97.
19. Carabello BA. Mitral valve regurgitation. Curr Probl Cardiol 1998; 23(4): 202–41.
20. Levine RA, Hung J, Otsuji Y et al. Mechanistic insights into functional mitral regurgitation. Curr Cardiol Rep 2002; 4: 125–9.
21. Chen FY, Adams DH, Aranki SF et al. Mitral valve repair in cardiomyopathy. Circulation 1998; 98: II-124–II-127.
22. Bonow RO, Carabello BA, Chatterjee K et al. ACC/AHA 2006 guidelines for the management of patients with valvular heart disease: executive summary: a report of the American College of Cardiology/American Heart Association Task Force

on Practice Guidelines (Writing Committee to Develop Guidelines for the Management of Patients With Valvular Heart Disease). Published online before print July 10, 2006. Circulation 2006: 114–450–527.

23. Hunt SA, Abraham WT, Chin MH et al. ACC/AHA 2005 guideline update for the diagnosis and management of chronic heart failure in the adult: summary article: a report of the American College of Cardiology/American Heart Association Task Force on Practice Guidelines (Writing Committee to Update the 2001 Guidelines for the Evaluation and Management of Heart Failure). J Am Coll Cardiol 2005; 46: 1116–43.

24. Gillinov MA, Wierup PN, Blackstone EH et al. Is repair preferable to replacement for ischemic mitral regurgitation. J Thorac Cardiovasc Surg 2001; 122(6): 1125–41.

25. Tulner SA, Steendijk P, Klautz RJ et al. Clinical efficacy of surgical heart failure therapy by ventricular restoration and restrictive mitral annuloplasty. J Card Fail 2007; 13: 178–83.

26. Tahta SA, Oury JH, Maxwell MJ et al. Outcome of mitral valve repair for functional ischemic mitral regurgitation. J Heart Valve Dis 2002; 11: 11–19.

27. Gangemi JJ, Tribble CG, Ross SD et al. Does the additive risk of mitral valve repair in patients with ischemic cardiomyopathy prohibit surgical intervention? Ann Surg 2000; 231(5): 710–14.

28. Harris KM, Sundt T, Aeppli D, Sharma R, Barzilai B. Can late survival of patients with moderate ischemic mitral regurgitation be impacted by intervention on the valve? Ann Thorac Surg 2002; 74: 1468–75.

29. Braun J, Bax JJ, Versteegh MIM et al. Preoperative left ventricular dimensions predict reverse remodeling following restrictive mitral annuloplasty in ischemic mitral regurgitation. Eur J Cardiothorac Surg 2005; 27: 847–53.

30. Carabello BA. The pathophysiology of mitral regurgitation. J Heart Valve Dis 2000; 9: 600–8.

31. Maniu CV, Patel JB, Reuter DG et al. Acute and chronic reduction of functional mitral regurgitation in experimental heart failure by percutaneous mitral annuloplasty. J Am Coll Cardiol 2004; 44: 1652–61.

32. Webb JG, Harnek J, Munt B et al. Percutaneous transvenous mitral annuloplasty: initial human experience with device implantation in the coronary sinus. Circulation 2006; 113: 851–5.

33. Daimon M, Gillinov AM, Liddicoat JR et al. Dynamic change in mitral annular area and motion during percutaneous mitral annuloplasty for ischemic mitral regurgitation: preliminary animal study with real-time 3-dimensional echocardiography. J Am Soc Echocardiogr 2007; 20(4): 381–8.

34. Yamanouchi Y, Egawa O, Hisatome I. Activation mapping from the coronary sinus may be limited by anatomic variations. PACE 1998; 21: 2522–6.

35. Maselli D, Guarracino F, Chiaramonti F et al. Percutaneous mitral annuloplasty: an anatomic study of human coronary sinus and its relation with mitral valve annulus and coronary arteries. Circulation 2006; 114: 377–80.

36. D'Cruz IA, Shala B, Johns C. Echocardiography of the coronary sinus in adults. Clin Cardiol 2000; 23: 149–54.

37. D'Cruz IA, Johns C, Shala MB et al. Dynamic cyclic changes in coronary sinus caliber in patients with and without congestive heart failure. Am J Cardiology 1999; 83: 275–7.

38. Silver MA, Rowley NE. The functional anatomy of the human coronary sinus. Am Heart J 1988; 115: 1080–4.

39. Ortale JR, Gabriel EA, Iost C, Marquez CQ. The anatomy of the coronary sinus and its tributaries. Surg Radiol Anat 2001; 23: 15–21.

40. Pejkovic B, Bogdanovic D. The great cardiac vein. Surg Radiol Anat 1992; 14: 23–8.

41. Aybek T, Risteski P, Miskovic A et al. Seven years experience with suture annuloplasty for mitral valve repair. J Thorac Cardiovasc Surg 2006; 131; 99–106.

42. Herregods MC, Tau A, Vandeplas A et al. Values for mitral valve annulus dimensions in normals and patients with mitral regurgitation. Echocardiography 1997; 14: 529–33.

43. Dubreuil O, Basmadjian A, Ducharme A et al. Percutaneous mitral valve annuloplasty for ischemic mitral regurgitation: first in man experience with a temporary implant. Cathet Cardiovasc Interven 2007; 69: 1053–61.

44. Hansky B, Vogt J, Gueldner H et al. Left heart pacing–experience with several types of coronary vein leads. J Interven Card Electrophys 2002; 6: 71–5.

45. Meisel E, Pfeiffer D, Engelmann L et al. Investigation of coronary venous anatomy by retrograde venography in patients with malignant ventricular tachycardia. Circulation 2001; 104: 442–7.

46. Abraham WT, Fisher WG, Smith AL et al. Cardiac resynchronization in chronic heart failure. N Engl J Med 2002; 346: 1845–53.

47. Bristow MR, Saxon LA, Boehmer J et al. Cardiac-resynchronization therapy with or without an implantable defibrillator in advanced chronic heart failure. N Engl J Med 2004; 350: 2140–50.

48. Beshai JF, Grimm RA, Nagueh SF et al. Cardiac-resynchronization therapy in heart failure with narrow QRS complexes. N Engl J Med 2007; Dec 13; 357(24): 2461–71.

49. Savage EB, Ferguson TB Jr, DeSesa VJ. Use of mitral valve repair: analysis of contemporary United States experience reported to the Society of Thoracic Surgeons National Cardiac Database. Ann Thorac Surg 2003; 75(3): 820–5.

50. Chew DP, Bhatt DL, Lincoff AM et al. Defining the optimal activated clotting time during percutaneous coronary intervention. Circulation 2001; 103: 961–6.

38 Percutaneous left ventricular chamber and mitral annular remodeling

Wes R Pedersen, Peter Block, and Ted Feldman

INTRODUCTION

Functional mitral regurgitation (FMR) is a ventricular disease characterized by mitral insufficiency in the absence of structural valve abnormalities. It occurs either in the presence of dilated (non-ischemic) cardiomyopathy or in association with regional (ischemic) left ventricular dysfunction. Medical therapy is of limited benefit and currently treatment falls predominantly in the realm of open heart surgery, including either annuloplasty repair or prosthetic valve replacement. These cardiac surgical techniques suffer significantly from their failure to address the primary underlying problem of ventricular distortion and by virtue of their highly invasive nature. The need for a less invasive and a more integrated approach directed at reshaping the remodeled left ventricle and mitral valve annulus is now recognized. Two novel and related technologies, the surgical Coapsys® and the percutaneous iCoapsys® devices are currently under investigation.

Although the methods for delivering each of these devices are different, the actual implants are remarkably similar. Both devices consist of anterior and posterior epicardial pads connected by a subvalvular (i.e. transventricular) chord that passes midway between the papillary muscles (Figure 38.1). Sizing instruments are used to reduce the chord length between the two pads, resulting in septal-lateral reduction of the left ventricular and annular dimensions, thereby compressing the regurgitant orifice and reducing MR. No adverse consequences on ventricular systolic or diastolic function have been demonstrated in patients treated thus far with the surgical Coapsys system.[1-4]

COAPSYS

The Coapsys (surgical) device is delivered using an open chest approach through a median sternotomy. It is implanted on a beating heart in the absence of cardiopulmonary bypass or atriotomy using direct visualization of external landmarks and epicardial two-dimensional (2D) echocardiography of relevant internal structures.[1]

The Coapsys device is currently undergoing clinical evaluation. The initial feasibility trial, TRACE (Treatment of FMR without Atriotomy or Cardiopulmonary Bypass)

has been completed. A total of 34 non-randomized patients who participated in TRACE underwent combined beating heart coronary artery bypass grafting (CABG) and Coapsys implantation for ischemic MR. One year follow-up has been reported in the initial 29 patients, documenting sustained reduction in MR from 3.0 ± 0.55 to 1.1 ± 0.99.[2] The ongoing pivotal Randomized Evaluation of a Surgical Treatment for Off-Pump Repair of the Mitral Valve (RESTOR-MV) Trial is currently randomizing patients who need CABG and have grade 2 or greater ischemic MR to either CABG and conventional mitral annuloplasty repair or CABG and Coapsys implantation. In the initial 19 patients randomized to the Coapsys group, intraoperative MR grade was reduced from 2.7 ± 0.8 to 0.4 ± 0.7 ($p < 0.0001$) and epicardial to epicardial diastolic LV dimension from 8.5 ± 1.2 to 6.4 ± 0.8 cm ($p < 0.0001$).[5]

For the completed TRACE feasibility evaluation, primary adverse events (PAE) were defined as death, stroke, myocardial infarction, Coapsys structural failure, reoperation for bleeding, life-threatening arrhythmia, heart valve repair/replacement. Survival and freedom from PAE at the end of the 1-year follow-up period were 97% and 91%, respectively. A total of 3 PAEs were recorded in 3 (9%) patients. The early PAEs ($\leq$30 days postoperatively) were (1) perioperative death due to aortic dissection caused by use of an intra-aortic balloon pump (not Coapsys-related) and (2) development of ventricular arrhythmia resulting in reoperation for graft revision. The lone late PAE (>30 days postoperatively) was a case of reported stroke (neurologic impairment >24 hours) with CT evidence, but subsequent clinical examination showed absence of neurologic sequelae with a post-event echo showing no evidence of thrombus formation on or near the subvalvular chord. Over the follow-up duration, there was no evidence of Coapsys device failure, no reoperations for valve surgery, and no myocardial infarctions. Results of the RESTOR-MV trial are not yet available as the trial remains in the active enrollment phase.

ICOAPSYS

In order to further reduce the invasiveness of the procedure and perioperative risks inherent to all open

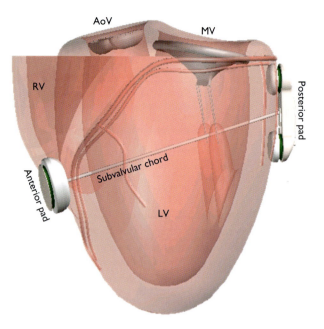

Figure 38.1 Schematic of an implanted iCoapsys® device. AoV, aortic valve; MV, mitral valve; RV, right ventricle; LV, left ventricle.

chest surgical approaches, a transcatheter implantation system, the iCoapsys, has been developed. The iCoapsys utilizes catheter-based technology for percutaneous, transpericardial delivery of a device designed to duplicate all the important elements of the surgical Coapsys implant. Safe delivery and accurate device positioning have been preliminarily demonstrated in acute animal models without MR.[6] Based on this early animal experience using the transcatheter system and preliminary findings thus far acquired from the ongoing Coapsys clinical trials, the VIVID (Valvular and Ventricular Improvement via iCoapsys Delivery) feasibility study has been developed and is now FDA approved. This phase I experience will include 15 to 30 patients with symptomatic ischemic or non-ischemic functional MR.

Preliminary evaluation of the iCoapsys transcatheter system was carried out by nine interventional cardiologists using an adult sheep model without MR. All devices were successfully delivered via a pericardial access system, and there were no episodes of prolonged hemodynamic or arrhythmic compromise. Post-mortem evaluation demonstrated no cases of coronary, mitral, or tricuspid valve, left ventricular or right ventricular outflow tract impingement. There was no cardiac trauma and no excessive bleeding seen in any animals.[6]

The iCoapsys device, similar to the Coapsys, consists of an anterior and posterior pad tethered by a transventricular chord. A series of specifically designed pericardial access, epicardial position finding, and implant delivery catheters are used for device implantation under coronary angiographic, epicardial, and transesophageal echo guidance.

The procedure is divided into four stages:

1. pericardial access
2. site identification
3. device implantation
4. sizing and therapeutic evaluation.

A brief description of procedural methods, potential complications, as well as preventative and treatment strategies will be discussed under each stage. Complications of this percutaneous procedure are only speculative, based on the lack of any clinical experience in man prior to this publication.

Pericardial access

Catheters and operative procedure

A specifically designed pericardial access system has been developed for implantation of the iCoapsys device (Figure 38.2). The pericardial access needle is equipped with a distal lancet tip and an adjacent penetration depth control (stop) to limit overadvancement into the myocardium. The pericardial space is percutaneously accessed from the subxiphoid approach with the assistance of fluoroscopic and coronary angiographic guidance. The anterior pericardial space is entered 4–5 cm medial to the mid left anterior descending artery (LAD). Pericardial entry is felt as a distinct 'pop' and confirmed with contrast injection delivered from an infusion port on the proximal end of the needle. Guide wire exchanges are then carried out, following which the pericardium and overlying soft tissue is predilated with a 20 to 24 mm peripheral balloon. The 52 French access sheath is then positioned and temporarily secured at the subxiphoid, percutaneous entry site.

Potential complications and avoidance/treatment strategies

Epicardial *coronary laceration*, resulting in pericardial bleeding with tamponade, should be minimized by pericardial needle delivery under coronary angiographic guidance. In the remote likelihood of this event, should hemostasis not occur with protamine reversal, intracoronary perfusion balloon inflations and, if necessary, covered stent deployment should be considered in combination with pericardial drainage. If significant bleeding persists, the procedure should ultimately be converted to an open chest operation.

Myocardial perforation secondary to overadvancement of the pericardial needle should be minimized with the depth control feature just proximal to the lancet needle tip. In addition, cautious advancement of the access needle along with contrast injection confirming entry into the pericardial space, is important in the prevention of this complication, as demonstrated by Schweikert

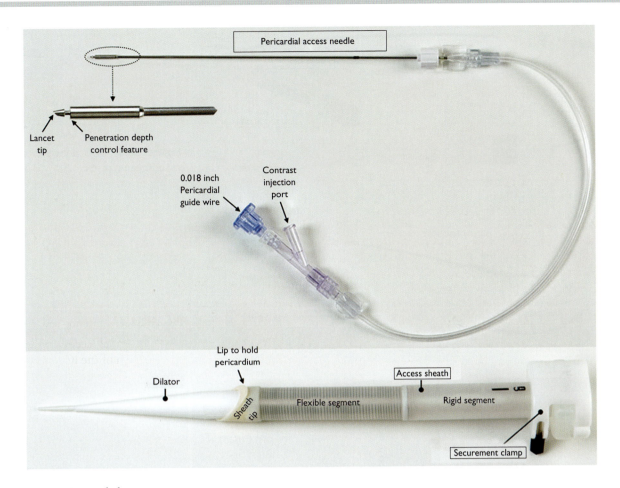

Figure 38.2   Pericardial access system.

et al.[7] in 48 patients who underwent epicardial ablation. Inadvertent myocardial perforation with the low profile needle should self-seal on withdrawal, in which case the procedure can be continued after a brief period of observation. If necessary, a pericardial drain can be left in place and the procedure aborted or converted to an open chest operation.

Trauma to adjacent structures, such as the liver, spleen, stomach, diaphragm, and phrenic nerve is unlikely using the characteristic external landmarks from the subxiphoid approach and pericardial needle delivery in a shallow trajectory toward the left shoulder. Pneumothorax may rarely occur as a result of entry into the pleural space and/or perforation of the underlying lung.

Site identification

Catheters and operative procedure

Three vacuum stabilized catheters are specifically designed for this stage to identify the anterior and posterior pad implantation sites. These catheters are delivered through the pericardial access sheath under fluoroscopic and coronary angiographic guidance. A co-axial,

intracardiac echo (ICE) delivery catheter (Figure 38.3) is initially positioned on the anterior cardiac surface of the heart 1 to 2 cm medial to the mid LAD and over the right ventricular outflow tract base. It is positioned during simultaneous left coronary angiography and right ventriculography. Additional 'fine' adjustments are made to display echocardiographic images of the left ventricle in cross-section (short axis) extending from the mid papillary muscles apically to the mitral annulus at the base. The posterior sighting catheter (Figure 38.4) is then delivered to the posterior left ventricle (LV) wall segment. Coronary angiography is used to guide distal vacuum cup placement 2 to 3 cm apical to the distal atrioventricular (AV) groove segment and free of major posterolateral branches. Further 'fine' adjustments of the posterior catheter are made using epicardial ICE guidance to establish precise placement mid way between the papillary muscles (Figure 38.5A and B), following which it is vacuum stabilized. Fluoroscopy is then performed in multiple angulated views to establish a 'sighting view', whereby precise superimposition of the anterior ICE imaging transducer over the posterior vacuum cup is achieved without further manipulation of the respective catheters. The ICE catheter is then removed from the anterior cardiac surface and the anterior sighting

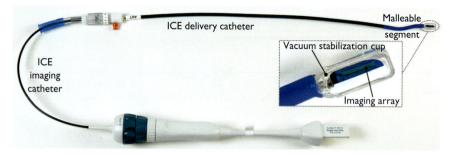

Figure 38.3 ICE delivery catheter with imaging probe.

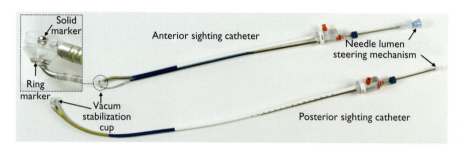

Figure 38.4 Anterior and posterior sighting catheters.

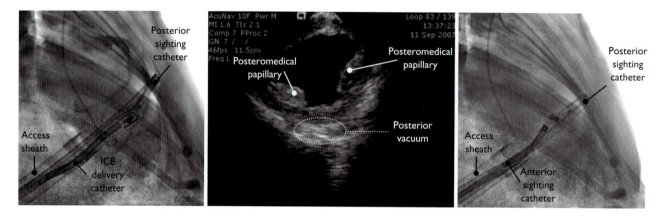

Figure 38.5 Positioned anterior and posterior catheters in the 'sighting view.' (A) Catheters positioned using coronary angiography. (B) Cross-sectional epicardial echo image. (C) Fluoroscopic image of sighting catheters.

catheter (Figure 38.4) is positioned in its place under fluoroscopic and coronary angiographic guidance while in the 'sighting view' (Figure 38.5C). Vacuum is then applied for temporary catheter fixation.

Potential complications and avoidance/treatment strategies

Although not seen in the preclinical (i.e. animal) experience, epicardial coronary trauma resulting from intrapericardial catheter manipulation may potentially occur. Pericardial bleeding with tamponade or coronary flow impingement with myocardial ischemia or infarction may result. Vacuum application for temporary distal catheter fixation over a coronary branch vessel should be avoided with coronary angiographic guidance. In this unlikely circumstance, risk of intracoronary thrombosis should be minimized with the recommended procedural heparin anticoagulation and

early recognition of coronary angiographic occlusion or constriction. Mechanical stimulation with epicardial catheter manipulation may provoke ventricular tachyarrhythmia, although this should be non-sustained with appropriate catheter adjustment. Although our animal experience demonstrated no sustained arrhythmia provocation, these were non-cardiomyopathic models and therefore possibly less prone to sustained tachyarrhythmias than patients with abnormal LV function might be.

Device implantation

Catheters and operative procedure

With the anterior and posterior sighting cups positioned appropriately on the epicardial surface, the needle lumen steering mechanism at the proximal end of each catheter

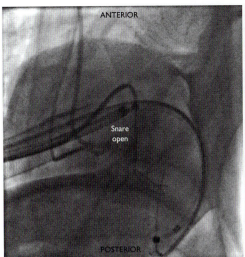
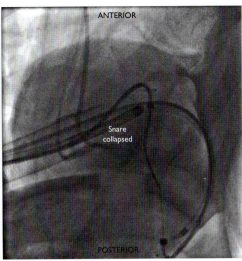

Figure 38.6 Fluoroscopic images of intraventricular snare and posterior needle.

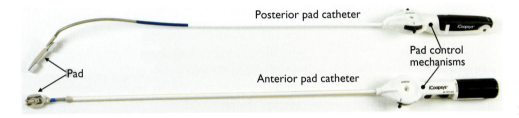

Figure 38.7 Epicardial pad delivery catheters.

is adjusted to precisely aim the anterior and posterior cups at each other. This is accomplished by centering the outer ring marker around its inner solid marker within the distal catheter cups while in the 'sighting view.'

The anterior needle assembly is inserted through the catheter's needle lumen under fluoroscopy, 3 to 4 cm into the LV chamber. After removing the needle stylet, a snare assembly is advanced into the LV through the needle lumen. The posterior needle assembly is then advanced through the posterior catheter's needle lumen into the LV chamber (Figure 38.6). The anterior snare is then used to grasp the posterior needle assembly which is pulled through the anterior wall and exteriorized on withdrawal of the anterior sighting catheter. The posterior sighting catheter is then withdrawn, exteriorizing the posterior limb of the now transventricular needle tube. The actual implanted subvalvular chord is then inserted into the posterior limb of the needle tube and pulled through the LV, leaving an anterior and posterior limb exteriorized. After attaching the posterior pad mounted on its delivery catheter to the exteriorized posterior limb (Figure 38.7), the pad is positioned on the posterior ventricular surface with coronary angiographic guidance. The anterior limb is then threaded through the anterior pad mounted on its delivery catheter. The anterior pad is then tracked over the transventricular chord and positioned on the anterior cardiac surface, again using coronary angiographic guidance to insure pad placement parallel and medial to the mid LAD.

Potential complications and avoidance/treatment strategies

If the anterior and posterior needle assemblies are not delivered with precision toward each opposing sighting catheter, the transventricular chord which is ultimately deployed may traverse the anterior and posterior ventricular walls tangentially. This, in turn, could potentially result in ventricular compromise due to a developing laceration which could be a possible source for myocardial bleeding. In this case, subacute or possibly more delayed tamponade may result. The sighting markers on these respective catheters are specifically designed to minimize tangential myocardial delivery, and this was not seen in the acute animal series.[6] Management of this complication would require percutaneous pericardial drainage and, ultimately, conversion to an open chest procedure if persistent bleeding is documented.

Delivery of the needles and snare is carried out under fluoroscopic guidance to avoid significant deflection within the LV. If either the anterior or posterior needle delivery system is delivered into the LV and permitted to encircle a subvalvular chord or papillary muscle, mitral valve leaflet excursion would be restricted and likely result in unresolved MR on transesophageal echocardiography (TEE) evaluation in the final sizing stage. After the posterior needle assembly is snared and pulled back across the anterior wall, TEE imaging should permit early visualization of abnormal leaflet excursion, easily remedied by way of needle and snare redelivery. Identification, even at the later sizing stage, would still permit full reversibility and an attempt at redeployment.

The epicardial implant pads differ in both size and shape and may, without appropriate caution using angiographic guidance, be positioned over an adjacent coronary branch. If not detected during device implantation, this would likely restrict coronary blood flow, resulting in either myocardial ischemia or infarction. The pad delivery catheters are equipped with steering levers at the proximal ends to permit precise longitudinal pad orientation on the epicardial surface to further insure avoidance of this potential complication. If reorientation or alternative pad sizes are not sufficient remedies to avoid coronary impingement, the procedure at this stage is fully reversible and can either be aborted or the system redelivered. Pad positioning was precise in all animals with no evidence of coronary artery impingement on subsequent direct post-mortem examination.[6]

Sizing and therapeutic evaluation

Catheters and operative procedure

Device sizing is carried out under TEE guidance to achieve significant MR reduction. This is accomplished by advancing the sizing instrument over the anterior limb of the subvalvular chord until it comes to rest on the surface of the anterior pad. This instrument is used to measure the epicardial to epicardial distance between pads prior to shortening, following which this distance is shortened to achieve a maximal MR reduction. After removing the sizing instrument, a staple deployment catheter is used to fix the chord to the anterior pad. Up to this point, the procedure is fully reversible. The anterior limb of the chord is then trimmed and the access sheath removed, completing the implant procedure.

Potential complications and avoidance/treatment strategies

The transventricular chord transverses not only the submitral position of the LV, but extends across a very short distance of the proximal right ventricular outflow tract (RVOT). Significant RVOT impingement may result in provocation of an outflow gradient and possible right heart failure. In turn, left ventricular outflow tract (LVOT) or left ventricle intracavitary obstruction may result in left heart failure. Excessive shortening of the epicardial to epicardial pad distance may also result in impaired ventricular filling and a reduction in cardiac output. This can be easily remedied prior to removing the sizing instrument. These potential complications should be easily avoidable while sizing under TEE guidance and hemodynamic monitoring, and has not been seen in the Coapsys surgical experience.[1,5]

Intraventricular conduction abnormalities may potentially arise as an early or possibly late event, more likely in the presence of chronic conduction system disease. This, in turn, may result in bradyarrhythmias which up to this point have not been demonstrated in either the Coapsys clinical[1,5] or iCoapsys animal experiences.[6] Bradyarrthymias, particularly if manifested late, would probably be best managed with chronic pacing, especially in the presence of significant reduction in MR and clinical benefit. If detected during the implantation, the option for aborting the procedure would exist.

OTHER POTENTIAL COMPLICATIONS

1. As with any foreign body implant, the possibility of *device-related infection* exists, the risk of which would predominantly occur at the time of implantation. To minimize this risk, strict sterile technique is necessary and should replicate other permanent implant procedures, such as permanent pacemaker implantation. Further, prophylactic antibiotics are recommended perioperatively to include *Staphylococcus* coverage. Refractory device-related infections would require open chest surgery for device explantation.

2. *Peripheral thromboembolism* including stroke remains a potential risk secondary to thrombus attachment to the left ventricular chord. If associated with the small segment of the cord transversing the RVOT, it may conceivably result in pulmonary emboli. However, the chord is made of a non-thrombogenic and braided material. In addition, prophylactic antithrombotic medical therapy, including some combination of antiplatelet therapy with or without warfarin, is recommended. Systemic vascular embolic events would require TEE evaluation and, if appropriate, at minimum a more aggressive antiplatelet regimen with or without the addition of warfarin. Recurrent episodes localized to the device would warrant surgical explantation. Strong consideration for 'early' device explantation would have to be given in the event that a large intraventricular thrombus is identified, especially if unresolved following a prolonged course of systemic anticoagulation. This complication has not been observed in the surgical Coapsys experience.[1]

3. Intravascular contrast administration is necessary by virtue of the requirement for selective coronary angiography to guide epicardial device positioning and to insure that coronary circulation is not compromised. The possible risk of contrast-induced renal failure in patients with renal insufficiency who are not already on chronic hemodialysis must be factored in accordingly in evaluating candidates for iCoapsys implantation. Appropriate steps should be taken to reduce the likelihood of renal failure in

those with mild to moderate baseline insufficiency, including sparing use of an isosmolar contrast agent in combination with pretreatment strategies, including aggressive hydration. Appropriate prophylaxis in patients with a history of significant contrast allergy should be initiated.

SUMMARY

With up to 4 years of patient follow-up in more than 120 surgical (Coapsys) implants thus far, there has been a remarkable dearth of device-related complications. The epicardial pads and transventricular chord are well tolerated and the chord has not led to any thromboembolic complications, mitral valve trauma, or impairment. The ability to precisely deliver the percutaneous (iCoapsys) implants in 12 acute animal studies without significant complications has now led to the initiation of the first-in-man study. The mechanics and potential complications of the novel pericardial access and delivery system will require some experience to define.

REFERENCES

1. Mishra YK, Mittal S, Jaguri P, Trehan N. Coapsys mitral annuloplasty for chronic functional ischemic mitral regurgitation: 1-year results. Ann Thorac Surg 2006; 81: 42–6.
2. Mittal S, Mishra YK, Jaguri P, Trehan N. Coapsys mitral valve repair improves 1 year outcomes in patients with ischemic mitral regurgitation undergoing off-pump CABG. J Am Coll Cardiol 2005; 45: 365A.
3. Mittal S, Mishra YK, Trehan N. The Coapsys, annuloplasty device reverses left ventricular remodeling along with reduction of mitral regurgitation. Circulation 2005; 112: II-591.
4. Grossi E, Woo YJ, Gangahar DM et al. Comparison of Coapsys annuloplasty and internal reduction mitral annuloplasty of the randomized treatment of functional mitral regurgitation: impact on the left ventricle. J Thorac Cardiovasc Surg 2006; 131: 1095–8.
5. Grossi EA, Saunders PC, Woo YJ et al. Intraoperative effects of the Coapsys annuloplasty system in a randomized evaluation (RESTOR-MV) of functional ischemic mitral regurgitation. Ann Thorac Surg 2005; 80: 1706–11.
6. Pedersen WR, Block P, Leon M et al. iCoapsys mitral valve repair system: percutaneous implantation in an animal model. CCI 2008 (in press).
7. Schweikert RA, Saliba WI, Tomassoni G et al. Percutaneous pericardial instrumentation for endo-epicardial mapping of previously failed ablations. Circulation 2003; 108: 1329–35.

39 Preventing and managing complications of percutaneous mitral leaflet repair using the Evalve Mitraclip

Ted Feldman

MITRAL REPAIR COMPLICATIONS

The Evalve mitral valve repair procedure is a novel approach for leaflet repair for mitral regurgitation (MR).[1-11] The potential for complications in this procedure remains largely unexplored territory, since this is a first in class and first-in-man effort, and no other parallel experience exists. The procedure is performed via transseptal catheterization. A guide catheter is placed in the left atrium above the mitral valve and used to steer the Evalve Mitraclip into position to grasp the mitral leaflets and create a double orifice, with resultant better approximation of the mitral leaflets and diminution of the degree of MR.

Most of the elements of the procedure are standard catheterization approaches. The details and flow of the procedure are important for an understanding of the potential complications.

The procedure is performed under general anesthesia using continuous transesophageal echocardiographic (TEE) guidance. After general anesthesia and placement of the echo probe, catheterization is performed via multiple femoral access. Left femoral venous and arterial sheaths are placed for right heart catheterization and arterial pressure measurements. A right femoral venous puncture is used for transseptal access and ultimately placement of the EVALVE guide catheter and clip.

After baseline hemodynamic and angiographic measurements are obtained, transseptal puncture is performed. The point of puncture is important to the ultimate deliverability of the clip. A puncture that is superior and posterior in the arc of the fossa ovalis optimizes the delivery trajectory for the clip (Figure 39.1). The demands to place the transseptal puncture have clearly led to some procedure complications.

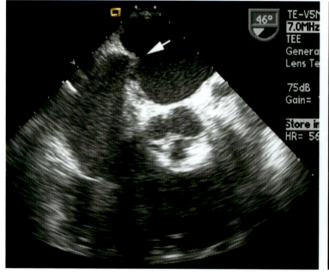 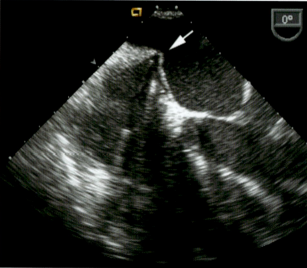

Figure 39.1 (Left) A short-axis transesophageal echo image obtained during transseptal puncture for an Evalve procedure. Tenting of the atrial septum is shown by the arrow, the arrow is in the left atrium, and the transseptal needle in the right atrium. This view shows that the puncture is posterior along the antero-posterior axis of the atrial septum. (Right) A long-axis view. The arrow, again in the left atrium, shows indentation of the septum from the needle. The shadow of the needle can be seen coming up from the inferior vena cava which is in the lower portion of the image. In this view, the tenting can be seen at the superior end of the septum. Thus, the puncture is posterior and superior, which allows an optimal trajectory for the clip delivery system toward the mitral valve.

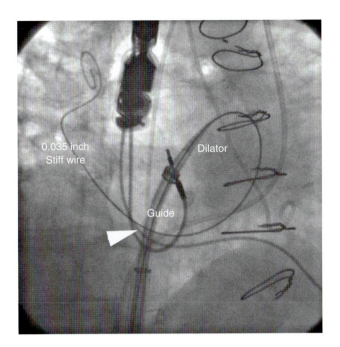

Figure 39.2 This fluoroscopic image shows the guide catheter and dilator being passed over a stiff guide wire into the left atrium. The transesophageal echo probe is seen coming from the top of the figure. The arrowhead shows the point at which the guide catheter crosses the atrial septum, marked here by the course of the stiff guide wire along the floor of the left atrium. The tip of the dilator has a metal wire coiled and embedded inside the dilator. This is highly echo reflective and allows some guidance from echocardiographic imaging as well as fluoroscopic imaging for positioning of the dilator within the left atrium.

After transseptal puncture has been accomplished, a stiff guide wire is placed in the left atrium or left upper lobe pulmonary vein and the guide catheter is passed across the atrial septum. The guide catheter has a tapered dilator, the tip of which is marked with wire coils for better visualizing using echocardiography (Figure 39.2). The guide catheter is 24 French at the skin insertion and 22 French at the point of the atrial septum. It is thus important to advance the guide very slowly so that the atrial septum may be dilated without tearing. The guide catheter is then positioned 1–2 cm beyond the left side of the atrial septum and the wire and dilator are removed. At this point the clip delivery system is inserted, flushed, and de-aired.

Multiple steering maneuvers are made to guide the clip delivery system and clip to the center of the mitral orifice (Figure 39.3). The clip arms are opened and a short axis view is used to insure that the clip arms are perpendicular to the line of mitral leaflet coaptation. At this point, the clip arms in an open position are advanced into the left ventricle, their position once again checked, and then the clip is pulled back with the arms opened so that the mitral leaflets will fall into the clip arms. A barbed gripper is lowered to sandwich the leaflets between the gripper and the clip arms and the clip arms are partially closed. At this point it is possible to evaluate the impact of the device on the degree of MR. If MR is diminished sufficiently, the clip is closed completely and then detached. Mitral regurgitation can be re-assessed and the clip delivery system removed. A second clip may be placed in a similar fashion if needed (Figures 39.4 and 39.5). It is critical that an evaluation of mitral area is made before a second clip is placed, so that if the mitral valve area is diminished by a first clip, a second clip will not be used to avoid causing or creating mitral stenosis (Figure 39.6).

EVALVE PROCEDURE COMPLICATIONS

An examination of the complications encountered during the treatment of the first 100 registry patients in the initial EVALVE phase 1 experience reveals the considerations for management and prevention of complications.[1,7] There have been no deaths related to placement of a clip. Importantly, the extensive manipulations of the EVALVE device in the mitral orifice have not led to hemodynamic stability during the procedure. Mechanical ventilation for more than 48 hours has occurred in a single patient, bleeding requiring transfusions of 2 or more units of blood in 4.7% of patients, and transseptal complications in 2.8% of patients. Possibly the most important occurrence related to this procedure is partial clip detachment, which has occurred in 9% of patients, either during clip placement, prior to hospital discharge, or within the first 30 days in the vast majority of patients.

FEMORAL ACCESS

The potential for complications of course begins with femoral access. Venous access for the large sheath requires no special considerations at the time of needle puncture. It has been my practice to use preclosure with suture closure devices at the time of initial sheath placement to minimize the need for prolonged compression of the large venous puncture at the conclusion of the procedure.[12–14] An important potential complication resulting from removal of these large sheaths would be prolonged compression with resultant deep vein thrombosis. Additionally, the puncture is large enough that oozing, even without frank bleeding, is a common problem in the periprocedure period. Accordingly, in my practice, suture closure using two 6 French Proglide devices deployed at right angles, or with a single 10 French ProStar device has resulted in my own practice and immediately hemostasis without need for any compression at all of the venous puncture. I believe this is an advantage for this procedure and similar procedures utilizing large bore venous

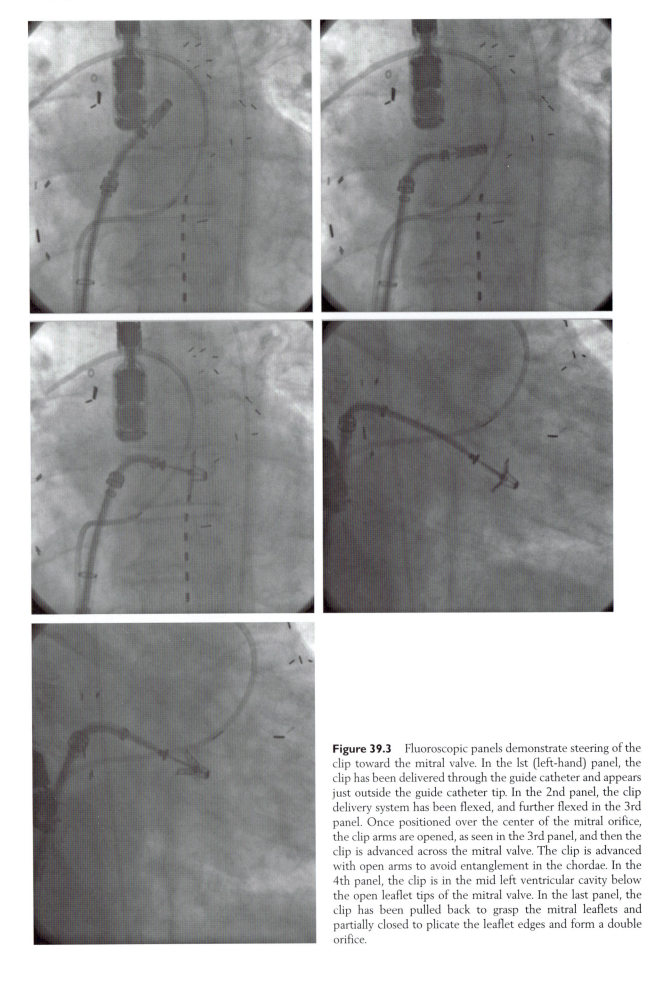

Figure 39.3 Fluoroscopic panels demonstrate steering of the clip toward the mitral valve. In the 1st (left-hand) panel, the clip has been delivered through the guide catheter and appears just outside the guide catheter tip. In the 2nd panel, the clip delivery system has been flexed, and further flexed in the 3rd panel. Once positioned over the center of the mitral orifice, the clip arms are opened, as seen in the 3rd panel, and then the clip is advanced across the mitral valve. The clip is advanced with open arms to avoid entanglement in the chordae. In the 4th panel, the clip is in the mid left ventricular cavity below the open leaflet tips of the mitral valve. In the last panel, the clip has been pulled back to grasp the mitral leaflets and partially closed to plicate the leaflet edges and form a double orifice.

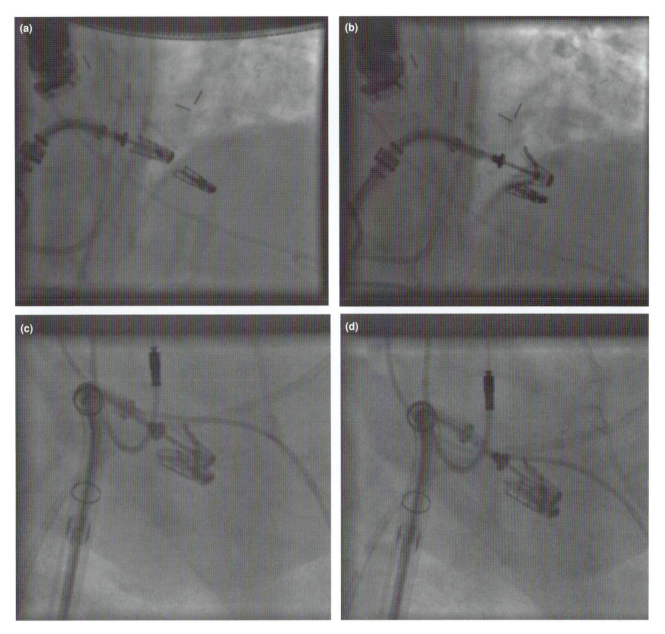

Figure 39.4   The sequence of images shows placement of a 2nd clip. In contrast to maneuvering the 1st clip, the 2nd clip is delivered across the mitral orifice with the clip arms closed to avoid dislodging the 1st clip. (A) The 2nd clip can be seen positioned on the left atrial side of the 1st clip, which has already been released. (B) The clip has been pulled back to grasp the mitral leaflets. (C and D) The clip is seen to be closed to minimize the degree of mitral regurgitation. When assessment of the mitral regurgitation has been completed, the clip is released.

access. The technique of suture closure in the venous circulation has been described and is effectively the same as for arterial puncture. The fundamental difference is that the lower pressure venous system does not result in brisk back bleeding from the Perclose device marker port. Thus, the Perclose device is inserted into the venous circulation and a few seconds must be taken to wait for back bleeding. Asking the patient to cough or take a deep breath will often result in back bleeding through the venous port. After this has been

observed, the remainder of the preclose deployment procedure is routine. After the sutures have been pulled back out of the skin, they are left dangling outside the puncture as the device is rewired for exchange for a large sheath or the guide catheter. It is my practice to leave the free sutures under betadine-soaked gauze since the sutures will be on the skin, outside of the body, for some time during the procedure and this may help minimize the potential for a suture closure device-related infection.

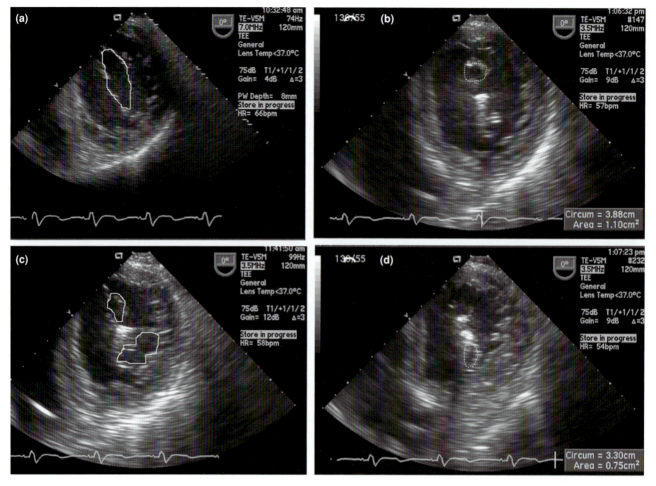

Figure 39.5 (A) A short-axis transgastric echocardiographic view of the mitral orifice prior to placement of a clip. The orifice has been outlined in a white line. (B) A single clip has been placed, and the double orifice areas assessed by planimetry. (C) After placement of two clips, the superior orifice (medial) is outlined. (D) The lower, or lateral, orifice is outlined separately. The combined area of the two orifices after double clip placement is 1.85 cm^2 which represents a degree of mitral stenosis unlikely to cause symptoms or impairment of mitral inflow.

TRANSSEPTAL PUNCTURE

The transseptal puncture is clearly one of the most important sources of potential complications.[15,16] The puncture is performed using standard transseptal 8 French equipment. Transesophageal echo (TEE) guidance is important to ensure that the puncture is in the superior and posterior aspect of the fossa ovalis (Figure 39.1). Attempts to make the puncture too far superiorly or too far posteriorly have resulted in transseptal-related cardiac perforations. The compromise between trying to optimize the location of the puncture and performing a safe puncture is challenging. Because the fossa represents an arc, the further posterior one goes in the limbus, the less superior the puncture will become. The optimal point of puncture is along the arc of the limbus where the superior and posterior locations are both maximized. In some cases the tissue of the fossa is highly distensible and the atrial septum is displaced towards the lateral wall of the left atrium, which may result in perforation of the lateral or superior left atrium as the transseptal needle is advanced. Patience during the procedure, willingness to replace the transseptal equipment over a wire into the superior vena cava and make another pass at the atrial septum, and judgment regarding the compromise of posterior and superior extremes are necessary for the optimal safety of the transseptal puncture.

GUIDE CATHETER

Passage of the guide catheter through the skin and across the atrial septum requires special care due to the large caliber and stiffness of the guide catheter (Figure 39.2). The guide system is compatible with a 0.035 inch guide wire. I ordinarily place an extra-stiff exchange-length guide wire into the left upper lobe pulmonary vein using either the Mullins sheath or a multipurpose catheter. The Mullins sheath is then withdrawn, and the guide catheter and dilator inserted through the skin. After the catheter has been passed across the septum, and the dilator removed, special care must be taken not to allow air to enter the guide catheter.

After the wire is placed a 14 French Inoue rigid dilator may be used to predilate the septum, prior to passing the tapered dilator and guide catheter.

A side stop cock port is built into the guide catheter and this is aspirated gently as the dilator is withdrawn with the guide wire. Thus, air that entrains into the hemostatic valve on the guide catheter as the dilator is being withdrawn can be removed. The hub end of the guide catheter is transparent so it is easy to directly visualize any air in the system at that point. Even with a back-bleed gasket, the 24 French end of the guide catheter will typically not be hemostatic, thus air management is a critical part of the procedure. During aspiration from the catheter to remove air, in some cases a substantial amount of blood will be aspirated. It is important to return this to the circulation via one of the other sheaths. Once the guide catheter is introduced into the left atrium and the position of the tip is verified by TEE to be 1–2 cm inside of the left atrial cavity, the clip delivery system can be introduced into the guide catheter. The clip delivery system is flushed continuously with pressure saline as it is introduced into the guide catheter. Aspiration of the guide in the same manner as during withdrawal of the dilator is necessary to be sure the system does not collect air as the clip delivery system is introduced. This attention to air management is a critical part of the procedure. To date, no instances of air emboli have been observed clinically.

STEERING THE CLIP INTO POSITION

After the clip system is introduced through the guide catheter into the left atrium, the next critical point in avoiding complications is to be sure that neither the guide nor the clip are extended into contact with the roof of the left atrium or the walls of the appendage (Figure 39.3). Careful echocardiographic guidance in multiple planes is key to steadily advancing and flexing the clip to reach a point above the mitral orifice without running the risk of chamber perforation.[17–19] This step is sometimes tedious or time consuming, but, due to the obvious need for both echocardiographic and fluoroscopic monitoring, has not been a source of complications in these procedures.

Once the clip is correctly positioned above the valve, and is seen to be centered over the Doppler origin of the regurgitant jet and that opened clip arms are perpendicular to the line of mitral leaflet coaptation,

the clip is advanced across the leaflets. This is typically performed with the clip opened to about 120°. The open clip helps to avoid the potential for chordal entanglement. Once the position of the clip in the left ventricle is verified by echocardiography, the clip is pulled back to grasp mitral leaflets. After the grippers are lowered and the clip is closed an assessment of the insertion of the leaflets into the clip is the next critical step. It is tempting to immediately focus on MR reduction, but it is critical to be sure the leaflets are well inserted into the clip as a next step. The potential for partial clip attachment is obviously minimized by careful echocardiographic interrogation to be sure that the leaflets are well inserted into the clip arms. This step requires multiple TEE imaging angles and careful observation through a few cardiac cycles. The appearance of some separation between the grippers and the clip arms is a sign of tissue insertion. Careful echo imaging will find a plane in which the leaflets can be visualized entering the clip. In the event that the regurgitant jet is not diminished, or the leaflet insertion appears to be inadequate, the clip can be opened, the grippers raised, and the system advanced into the left ventricle to disengage the mitral leaflets. Chordal entanglement at this point may be a problem. Ordinarily, simply waiting and occasionally moving the clip forward and backward very small amounts will usually result in freeing up of the entangled valve structures. In the event that the clip needs to be withdrawn into the left atrium, the arms are completely everted so that the clip may be safely pulled back into the left atrium. At this point a decision regarding abandoning the procedure and removing the clip entirely, or trying for another grasp, is usually made. It is typical for multiple grasps to be necessary to determine the optimal point of clip attachment for the best degree of reduction of MR.

SECOND CLIP

In almost one-third of cases a second clip must be placed to adequately reduce the severity of MR (Figures 39.4 and 39.5). The number of considerations is critical to avoiding complications at this step of the procedure. The potential to cause mitral stenosis exists with a second clip (Figure 39.6).[20,21] Baseline hemodynamic measurements include careful verification of the absence of a transmitral valve pressure gradient. Although simultaneous wedge pressure with left ventricular diastolic pressures is commonly used for this assessment, false gradients are common. Thus, verification that wedge and left atrial pressures are matched is critical during the baseline measurements. Ideally, after a first clip is placed the left atrial pressure is remeasured through the guide catheter with a simultaneous left ventricular catheter to assess the potential pressure

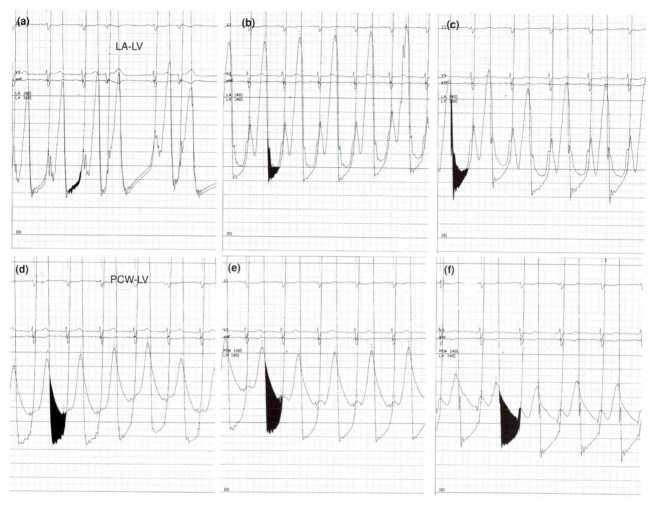

Figure 39.6   The upper sequence of panels (A–C) shows a comparison of left atrial (LA) and left ventricular (LV) pressures. The lower sequence of panels (D–F) shows a comparison of pulmonary capillary wedge (PCW) and left ventricular (LV) pressures, all from the same patient. (A) At baseline, before placement of a clip, there is virtually no pressure gradient between the left atrium and left ventricle. The large 'V'-wave of mitral regurgitation is clearly seen. (B) A small gradient is seen after placement of a single clip. (C) A small but slightly larger gradient is seen after placement of two clips. The height of the 'V'-wave can be seen to be greatly diminished in (C). The comparisons between pulmonary wedge and left ventricular pressure demonstrate one of the major pitfalls of relying on wedge rather than direct left atrial pressure. At baseline, there is the appearance of a sizeable gradient at rest when comparing the wedge, seen in panel D, with the left ventricular pressure. This is clearly a false gradient, as demonstrated by the absence of a gradient in the direct measurement of left atrial compared to left ventricular pressure in (A). Thus, if wedge pressure is to be used to assess gradients after clip placement, it must be carefully matched to directly measured left atrial pressure at baseline to verify that the wedge is an accurate measure. (E and F) After 1 and 2 clips, respectively, the wedge pressure is seen not to change appreciably.

gradient. An illustration of a clinical nature of this measurement comes from a recent case in our laboratory. A patient with apparent degenerative MR and severe prolapse had a first clip placed. This resulted in a significant but not completely adequate reduction in MR. At that point, a 3–4 mm pressure gradient was observed and a valve area by the Gorlin formula was 2 cm². It was clear that addition of a second clip would result in a valve area likely below 1.5 cm². Accordingly the first clip was removed and the procedure was abandoned. At operation the patient was found to have typical mitral valve prolapse but, in addition, also

changes in valve morphology consistent with rheumatic disease. Thus, the likely outcome of a second clip would have been mitral stenosis with hemodynamic compromise.

Another special consideration with placement of a second clip is taking particular care not to dislodge the first clip. Thus, positioning of the second clip is greatly facilitated by using the first clip as a landmark, but at the same time additional care must be taken before advancing the clip adjacent to the existing first clip to be sure the two are not directly in contact.

IMPACT ON POTENTIAL FOR FUTURE REPAIR

Does placement of one or two Evalve clips on the mitral leaflets diminish the potential for future surgical valve repair using standard methods? In the experience using this device to date, among patients in whom either a clip was placed on the leaflets and then removed acutely during the procedure, or among those in whom a clip was placed and left in place, who had severe mitral regurgitation subsequently, surgical repair using standard leaflet repair approaches has been possible.[22,23] Clips have been removed from the leaflets as late as a year and a half after having been attached, with successful leaflet resection, and a good outcome from surgical repair.[23] It is clear that at some point a tissue bridge will form around the clip, and, in some cases, this would eliminate the potential for a future leaflet resection. Of course, an initial surgical leaflet repair diminishes the chances for a future surgical repair in the same way that a clip repair ultimately will as well. It is important that in the early experience with this device, surgical options have been preserved for patients in whom the clip is not successful. The repair rate in this early Evalve experience has been over 65% overall, and over 80% in patients in whom repair was the intended surgical procedure.

OPERATOR VOLUMES

Operator volumes have been used as a surrogate for competence for other percutaneous procedures. Particularly, for coronary stent implantation, high volumes of procedures are required for certification in interventional training programs. The paradigm for operator volumes for percutaneous valve procedures will necessarily be different.[24] The pool of patients to undergo these procedures on heart valves is much smaller, and the procedures themselves more complex than for coronary artery disease. Thus, these are comparatively high-complexity and low-volume situations in which the expectation that operators may have a large experience in some training setting is not realistic. Surgical valve repair may be a better comparator, but even there, maintenance of high volumes has been difficult. The vast majority of surgical operators in the United States perform less than 35 surgical mitral valve repairs annually.[25] The lowest mortality and highest rates for successful repair exist only in the small minority of operators in whom the surgical volumes exceed 140 cases per year. In a recent Society for Thoracic Surgery (STS) database report, the number of hospitals in the United States with volumes >140 repair cases annually represents only 27 of 575 centers reporting cardiac surgery in the database.[25] Thus, as is the case for coronary intervention, a large number of lower volume operators is part of the landscape in valve surgery. The way that this will translate into volume as a surrogate for low complication rates and good outcomes in percutaneous valve therapy has yet to be determined.

REFERENCES

1. Feldman T, Wasserman HS, Herrmann HC et al. Percutaneous mitral valve repair using the edge-to-edge technique: 6 month results of the EVEREST Phase I Clinical Trial. J Am Coll Cardiol 2005; 46: 2134–40.
2. Feldman T, Leon MB. Prospects for percutaneous valve therapies. Circulation 2007; 11: 2866–77.
3. Feldman T. Percutaneous valve repair and replacement: challenges encountered, challenges met, challenges ahead. Circulation 2006; 113(6): 771–3.
4. Feldman T. Percutaneous mitral annuloplasty: not always a cinch. Cathet Cardiovasc Interven 2007; 69: 1062–3.
5. St. Goar FG, James FI, Komtebedde J et al. Endovascular edge-to-edge mitral valve repair: short-term results in a porcine model. Circulation 2003; 108: 1990–3.
6. Feldman T, Herrmann HC, St. Goar F. Percutaneous treatment of valvular heart disease: catheter based aortic valve replacement and mitral valve repair therapies. Am J Geriatric Cardiol 2006; 15: 291–301.
7. Herrmann HC, Feldman T. Percutaneous mitral valve edge-to-edge repair with the Evalve Mitraclip system: rationale and Phase I results. EuroInterven Suppl 2006; A: A36–9.
8. Leung R, Feldman T. Percutaneous mitral valve repair. Card Interven Today 2007; 27–31 March.
9. St. Goar FG, Fann JI, Feldman TE, Block PC, Herrmann HC. Percutaneous mitral valve repair with the edge-to-edge technique. In Herrman HC ed,. Contemporary Cardiology: Interventional Cardiology – Percutaneous Noncoronary Intervention. Totowa, NJ: Humana Press, 2005: 87–95.
10. Feldman T, Alfieri O, St. Goar F. Percutaneous leaflet repair for mitral regurgitation using the Evalve edge-to-edge clip technique. In Hijazi Z, Bonhoeffoer P, Feldman T, Ruiz C, eds, Transcatheter Valve Repair. Martin Dunitz & Parthenon Publishing/ Taylor & Francis Medical Books. London: 2006: 275–84.
11. Foster E, Wasserman HS, Gray W et al. Quantitative assessment of MR severity with serial echocardiography in a multi-center clinical trial of percutaneous mitral valve repair. Am J Cardiol 2007; 100: 1577–83.
12. Mylonas I, Sakata Y, Salinger MH, Sanborn T, Feldman T. The use of percutaneous suture-mediated closure for the management of 14 french femoral venous access. J Invas Cardiol 2006; 18: 299–302.
13. Feldman T. Percutaneous suture closure for management of large French size arterial and venous puncture. J Interven Cardiol 2000; 13: 237–42.
14. Sanborn TA, Feldman T. Status of femoral closure devices. Am Heart Hosp J 2003; 1: 212–15.
15. Feldman T, Fisher WG. Transseptal puncture. In Colombo A, Stankovic G, Problem Oriented Approaches in Interventional Cardiology, eds,. Taylor & Francis, Boca Raton, FL, 2007.
16. Sakata Y, Feldman T. Transcatheter creation of atrial septal perforation using radio frequency transseptal system: novel approach as an alternative to transseptal needle puncture. Cathet Cardiovasc Interven 2005; 64: 327–32.
17. Zamorano J, Perez de Isla L, Sugeng L et al. Non-invasive assessment of mitral valve area during percutaneous balloon mitral valvuloplasty: role of real time 3D echocardiography. Eur Heart J 2004; 25: 2086–91.

18. Silvestry S, Rodriguez L, Herrmann H et al. Echocardiographic guidance and assessment of percutaneous repair for mitral regurgitation with the Evalve MitraClip: Lessons Learned from EVEREST I. J Am Soc Echo 2007; 100: 1577–83.

19. Feldman T. Intra-procedure guidance for percutaneous mitral valve interventions: TTE, TEE, ICE or Xray? Cathet Cardiovasc Interven 2004; 63: 395–6.

20. Fusman B, Faxon D, Feldman T. Hemodynamic rounds: transvalvular pressure gradient measurement. Cathet Cardiovasc Interven 2001; 53: 553–61.

21. Herrmann HC, Rohatgia S, Wasserman HS et al. Effects of percutaneous edge to edge repair for mitral regurgitation on mitral valve hemodynamics. Cathet Cardiovasc Diagn 2006; 68: 821–6.

22. Fann JI, St Goar FG, Komtebedde J et al. Beating heart catheter-based edge-to-edge mitral valve procedure in a porcine model; efficacy and healing response. Circulation 2004; 110: 988–93:

23. role of real time 3D echocardiography. Eur Heart Journal 2004; 25: 2086–91.

23. Dang NC, Aboodi MS, Sakaguchi T et al. Surgical revision after percutaneous mitral valve repair with a clip: initial multi-center experience. Ann Thorac Surg 2005; 80(6): 2338–42.

24. Vassiliades TA Jr, Block PC, Cohn LH et al. An Interdisciplinary Position Statement-The Society of Thoracic Surgeons (STS), The American Association for Thoracic Surgery (AATS), The American College of Cardiology (ACC), and The Society of ardiovascular Angiography and Intervention (SCAI). Cathet Cardiovasc Diagn 65: 73–9, Annals of Thoracic Surgery 79: 1812–18, J Am Coll Cardiol 49: 1554–60. J Cardiovasc Thor Surg 2005; 129: 970–6.

25. Gammie JS, O'Brien SM, Griffith BP, Ferguson TB, Peterson ED. Influence of hospital procedural volume on care process and mortality for patients undergoing elective surgery for mitral regurgitation. Circulation 2007; 115: 881–7.

40 Complications of pericardiocentesis

Roy P Venzon and Ziyad M Hijazi

Percutaneous pericardiocentesis involves the removal of fluid from the pericardial sac and is a potentially life-saving procedure. Its use was first described in 1840, when it was performed by Franz Schuh on a patient with pericardial effusion secondary to malignancy.[1] Pericardiocentesis is primarily indicated for the treatment of cardiac tamponade. In addition, it may also be used to determine the cause of a pericardial effusion, to administer chemotherapeutic agents or antibiotics to patients with pericardial disease, or to remove massive pericardial effusions that compromise lung capacity.[2]

Pericardiocentesis was originally performed as a blind procedure and was fraught with morbidity and mortality. However, refinement in technique, improvement in needle and catheter design, and the introduction of several imaging modalities have all contributed to make pericardiocentesis a safe and effective procedure.

EQUIPMENT NEEDED

In emergent situations, the pericardium may be tapped in any medical setting. However, it is best to perform pericardiocentesis in a controlled environment where monitoring and resuscitation equipment are on hand. Pericardiocentesis kits are widely available, and should contain the necessary items needed to perform the procedure.

Needles

Puncture needles should be at least 5 cm long. A short bevel is preferred in order to minimize the risk of lacerating the myocardium or a coronary vessel. An 18-gauge thin-walled needle is ideal. However, in emergent settings where pericardiocentesis kits are not readily available, other needles, such as spinal or lumbar puncture needles, may also be used.

Catheters and wires

If the intention is to place an indwelling catheter to allow for extended drainage of pericardial fluid, the appropriate catheter should be available. A pigtailed or straight catheter with side holes is commonly preferred and is advanced into the pericardial space over a short guide wire with a floppy tip.

Monitoring equipment

Pressure monitoring equipment is needed to keep track of the patient's blood pressure, as well as right-sided cardiac pressures and pericardial pressures. Electrocardiographic (ECG) equipment is necessary to watch for any arrhythmias that may arise, and to monitor ST segment changes if an electrode is going to be attached to the puncture needle.

For these reasons, it is preferred that pericardiocentesis be performed in the cardiac catheterization laboratory, or similar setting.

Imaging equipment

Fluoroscopy,[3] two-dimensional echocardiography,[4–6] and computed tomography[7–9] have all been used to visualize the puncture needle and monitor its progress. These adjunctive imaging modalities have greatly improved the safety and success of pericardiocentesis and should be employed when performing the procedure.

TECHNIQUE

Patient preparation

The patient is propped up slightly to allow for the pericardial fluid to gravitate inferiorly. The chosen entry point is sterilized, and then infiltrated with local anesthesia. The entry point is typically the subxyphoid area, although parasternal or apical approaches may also be used.

Needle puncture

Once local anesthesia has been administered, the puncture needle is then advanced slowly, alternately aspirating and injecting more local anesthesia as needed. With the subxyphoid approach, the needle is directed towards the posterior of the left shoulder. As the needle is advanced, its progress should be monitored by fluoroscopy, echocardiography, or computed tomography. Once the pericardial space is reached, a 'give' or 'pop' is usually felt, and pericardial fluid can be aspirated through the needle.

Attaching an ECG lead to the needle may be used to monitor for ST segment changes. The development of ST segment elevation suggests that the needle has reached cardiac tissue and should be withdrawn. However, it is no longer recommended that ECG monitoring be the sole adjunct as it is not an adequate safeguard against potential complications.[10]

Confirmation of needle placement

In order to confirm that the needle is in the pericardial space, contrast may be injected and observed under fluoroscopy. Contrast injected into the pericardial space will slowly gravitate to dependent areas, whereas contrast injected into a cardiac chamber will be rapidly cleared away. Alternatively, agitated saline may also be injected and observed under echocardiography.

Drainage of the effusion

Once the position of the needle is confirmed, a soft-tipped guide wire is advanced into the pericardial space. The needle is then removed and the needle track dilated with a dilator. Afterwards, a pigtailed or straight catheter is advanced over the guide wire. The pericardial effusion is then drained. The catheter may be left in place to allow for further drainage of the effusion, and removed once the output has decreased to less than 50 ml per 24 hours.

COMPLICATIONS

Pericardiocentesis has evolved into a safe and effective procedure, in part due to the use of adjunctive imaging. Major complications, defined as complications needing treatment, have been reported to occur in 4% of fluoroscopy-guided[3] and 1.2% of echocardiography-guided pericardiocentesis.[5] Despite the relatively low incidence of morbidity, it remains imperative that one is cognizant of the possible complications of pericardiocentesis to be able to minimize the risk that these will occur, or to be able to manage them if they do happen.

Needle perforation and laceration

The majority of complications that occur during pericardiocentesis are caused by the puncture needle. Cardiac perforation occurs when the needle punctures the myocardium and enters a cardiac chamber. The right ventricle, because of its anterior location, is the most often punctured chamber (Figure 40.1). Using a needle with a short bevel is recommended to minimize the risk of needle contact with the heart. Monitoring the needle as it is being advanced with fluoroscopy or echocardiography is likewise important in avoiding cardiac perforation. A dilator or catheter should never be inserted if the needle or wire position in the pericardial space has not been confirmed. Cardiac perforation with a needle often seals itself off, is well tolerated, and rarely requires additional treatment. However, dilating a tract through a cardiac wall may lead to catastrophic results. If a needle puncture does occur, the needle should be withdrawn slowly until it is in the pericardial space. An indwelling catheter may be left in place to allow for subsequent drainage if the effusion reaccumulates.

Laceration of a cardiac wall or coronary vessel is a more serious complication of pericardiocentesis. In contrast to cardiac perforation, lacerations will often lead to rapid bleeding and the development of hemopericardium and severe cardiac tamponade. Immediate drainage should be done, and emergent surgical repair of the laceration is often necessary.

Bleeding

Bleeding, as a complication of pericardiocentesis, often occurs at the point of entry and its underlying tract, or from inadvertent puncture of a blood vessel. The subxyphoid approach is the most commonly used approach, and bypasses nearby vessels. However, if a parasternal approach is employed, care should be taken to avoid the internal mammary artery and intercostal blood vessels. The use of ultrasound to localize the internal mammary artery has been suggested when using this approach.[11]

Before proceeding with pericardiocentesis, it is important to determine if any bleeding diathesis is present. If the procedure is not emergently needed, any bleeding diathesis should first be corrected. In the case of patients who are on warfarin and have an elevated INR, vitamin K or fresh frozen plasma may be administered. For patients who are thrombocytopenic, platelet transfusion may be given.

Arrhythmias

The most common arrhythmia associated with pericardiocentesis is sinus bradycardia due to a vasovagal response. If bradycardia becomes symptomatic or is associated with hypotension, atropine and other supportive measures should be used.

Although rare, atrial fibrillation and ventricular arrhythmias immediately following pericardiocentesis have also been reported.[3,5] It is imperative that the cardiac catheterization laboratory has the appropriate

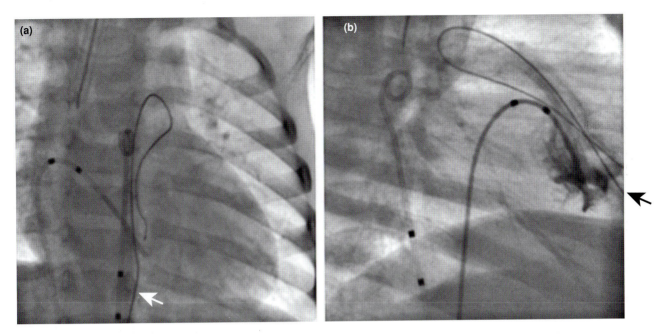

Figure 40.1   (A) Cine frame in the frontal projection in a 9-month-old infant with severe bilateral branch pulmonary artery stenosis and supravalvar aortic and pulmonic stenosis (non-Williams) who, when undergoing cardiac catheterization, suddenly became hypotensive and bradycardiac. At that time cardiac tamponade was suspected and the operators immediately punctured the subxyphoid area with a 21 gauge needle. A 0.021 inch guide wire was advanced under fluoroscopy to the area of the right ventricle outflow tract. At that time the operator realized that the wire was not inside the pericardial cavity. (B) Lateral projection during injection of contrast using a catheter positioned in the right ventricle. This demonstrated that the wire was indeed inside the heart and not the pericardial cavity. The wire was pulled out and the baby was observed by serial echocardiography over 24 hours with minimal increase in the amount of pericardial fluid.

medications and defibrillation equipment to manage these arrhythmias if they do arise.

Pulmonary edema

The development of pulmonary edema following pericardiocentesis is a rare complication of the procedure.[12–15] There have also been reports of right ventricular and biventricular failure following pericardiocentesis.[16,17] The exact mechanism of this phenomenon is not entirely clear. However, it has been postulated that the rapid drainage of pericardial effusion leads to a sudden increase in venous return that overwhelms the left ventricle and causes pulmonary edema. One suggestion has been to drain a maximum of 1000 ml of pericardial fluid at a time, particularly in patients with left ventricular dysfunction, to prevent pulmonary edema from happening. If it does occur, ventilatory and inotropic support may be needed and it is always prudent to ascertain the availability of these therapies prior to starting the procedure.

Infection

Infection complicating pericardiocentesis happens in less than 1% of cases in both fluoroscopy-guided and echocardiography-guided series.[3,5] Infection may occur along the needle tract, or in the form of pericarditis or peritonitis. It is important to maintain aseptic technique during the performance of pericardiocentesis. If a catheter is left in place for extended drainage, a closed system between the catheter, stop-cock, and aspiration syringe should be maintained. One recommendation is to keep the drainage catheter for only 48 hours, before removing it, to minimize the risk of infection.

Others

Other reported complications arising from pericardiocentesis include perforation of the stomach or colon, hemoperitoneum, pneumothorax, pneumopericardium, hypoxia, and intrapericardial thrombus formation.[2,17–20]

CONCLUSION

Pericardiocentesis is a potentially life-saving procedure. As with any other invasive intervention, complications can occur. The use of proper technique and adjunctive fluoroscopic and echocardiographic imaging minimizes the risk of these complications, and makes pericardiocentesis safe and effective.

REFERENCES

1. Kilpatrick Z, Chapman C. On pericardiocentesis. Am J Cardiol 1965; 16: 622.

2. Spodick DH. The technique of pericardiocentesis. J Crit Illness 1995; 10: 807–12.

3. Duvernoy O, Borowiec J, Helmius G, Erikson U. Complications of percutaneous pericardiocentesis under fluoroscopic guidance. Acta Radiol 1992; 33: 309–13.

4. Tsang TS, Freeman WK, Sinak LJ, Seward JB. Echocardiographically guided pericardiocentesis: evolution and state-of-the-art technique. Mayo Clin Proc 1998; 73: 647–752.

5. Tsang TS, Enriquez-Sarano M, Freeman WK et al. Consecutive 1127 therapeutic echocardiographically guided pericardiocentesis: clinical profile, practice patterns, and outcomes spanning 21 years. Mayo Clin Proc 2002; 77: 429–36.

6. Lindenberger M, Kjellberg M, Karlsson E, Wranne B. Pericardiocentesis guided by 2-D echocardiography: the method of choice for treatment of pericardial effusion. J Int Med 2003; 253: 411–17.

7. Duvernoy O, Magnusson A. CT-guided pericardiocentesis. Acta Radiol 1992; 33: 309–13.

8. Klein SV, Afridi H, Agarwal D, Coughlin BF. CT directed diagnostic and therapeutic pericardiocentesis: 8-year experience at a single institution. Emerg Radiol 2005; 11: 353–63.

9. Bruning R, Muehstaedt M, Becker C et al. Computed tomography–fluoroscopy guided drainage of pericardial effusions: experience in 11 cases. Invest Radiol 2002; 37: 328–32.

10. Maisch B, Seferovic PM, Ristic AD et al. Guidelines on the diagnosis and management of pericardial diseases. Eur Heart J 2004; 25: 587–610.

11. Kronzon I, Glassman LR, Tunick PA. Avoiding the left internal mammary artery during anterior pericardiocentesis. Echocardiography 2003; 20: 533–4.

12. Vandyke WH, Cure J, Chakko CS, Gheorghiade M. Pulmonary edema after pericardiocentesis for cardiac tamponade. N Engl J Med 1983; 309: 595–6.

13. Downey RJ, Bessler M, Weissman C. Acute pulmonary edema following pericardiocentesis for chronic cardiac tamponade secondary to trauma. Crit Care Med 1991; 19: 1323–5.

14. Chamoun A, Cenz R, Mager A et al. Acute left ventricular failure after large volume pericardiocentesis. Clin Cardiol 2003; 26: 588–90.

15. Armstrong WF, Feigenbaum H, Dillon JC. Acute right ventricular dilation and echocardiographic volume overload following pericardiocentesis for relief of cardiac tamponade. Am Heart J 1984; 107: 1266–70.

16. Ligero C, Leta R, Bayes-Genis A. Transient biventricular dysfunction following pericardiocentesis. Eur J Heart Fail 2006; 1: 102–4.

17. Bender F. Hemoperitoneum after pericardiocentesis in a CAPD patient. Perit Dial Int 1996; 3: 330.

18. Mullens W, Dupont M, Raedt H. Pneumopericardium after pericardiocentesis. Int J Cardiol 2007; 118: e57.

19. Muir AR, Lowry KG, Dalzell GW. Profound hypoxia complicating pericardiocentesis. Int J Cardiol 2007; 115; 406–7.

20. Calabrese P, Iliceto S, Rizzon P. Pericardiocentesis-induced intrapericardial thrombus: visualization of thrombus formation and spontaneous internal lysis by two-dimensional echocardiography. J Clin Ultrasound 1985; 13: 49–51.

41 Complications of endomyocardial biopsy in children

Daphne T Hsu

Endomyocardial biopsy has been used to establish a diagnosis in patients with myocardial dysfunction for over 40 years. The first procedures were performed to detect the presence of inflammation or specific pathologic findings associated with systemic diseases.[1–4] With the advent of heart transplantation, endomyocardial biopsy became an essential tool in the diagnosis of allograft rejection. Specialized catheters and techniques were developed to allow the procedures to be performed efficiently at minimal risk.[5–12] Endomyocardial biopsy procedures in infants and children offered additional challenges, and techniques were modified to accommodate smaller heart sizes and vessels.[13–18]

INDICATIONS

The indications for endomyocardial biopsy in adults and children have evolved over the years. In a recently published scientific statement sponsored by the American Heart Association, American College of Cardiology, and the European Society of Cardiology, the incremental diagnostic, prognostic, and therapeutic value of endomyocardial biopsy was estimated and compared with procedural risks in 14 clinical scenarios.[19] The clinical scenarios most relevant to the pediatric age range and designated as class I and class IIa recommendations are summarized in Table 41.1. In addition to these scenarios, endomyocardial biopsy was classified as reasonable in the presence of heart failure and left ventricular dilation with new ventricular arrhythmias or heart block if cardiac sarcoidosis or idiopathic granulomatous myocarditis was suspected, or in patients with eosinophilia and a suspicion of hypersensitivity cardiomyopathy. The use of endomyocardial biopsy to evaluate the patient with a dilated left ventricle and unexplained chronic heart failure, heart failure with unexplained hypertrophic cardiomyopathy, suspected arrhythmogenic cardiomyopathy, and unexplained ventricular arrhythmias is controversial and, in most cases, these scenarios are not considered indications for endomyocardial biopsy in children.

In children with cardiomyopathy entered in the NIH/NHLBI-sponsored Pediatric Cardiomyopathy Registry, an endomyocardial biopsy was associated with an increased ability to establish an etiology, particularly a

Table 41.1 Indications for endomyocardial biopsy: pediatric patients.[19]

Class I (endomyocardial biopsy should be performed)
- Unexplained, new-onset heart failure < 2 weeks' duration associated with normal-sized or dilated left ventricle and hemodynamic compromise
- New onset heart failure of 2 weeks' to 3 months' duration associated with a dilated left ventricle and new ventricular arrhythmias, second- or third-degree heart block or failure to respond to usual care within 1–2 weeks

Class IIa (endomyocardial biopsy is reasonable)
- Unexplained heart failure associated with suspected anthracycline cardiomyopathy
- Heart failure associated with unexplained restrictive cardiomyopathy
- Suspected cardiac tumor, with the exception of typical myxomas
- Unexplained cardiomyopathy in children

diagnosis of myocarditis.[20] Histologic evidence of lymphocytic, giant cell, or hypersensitivity myocarditis can provide important information and improve outcomes by allowing diagnosis-directed therapy to be instituted in a timely fashion. The finding of active lymphocytic myocarditis in a patient with ventricular dysfunction raises the possibility of recovery with supportive measures and may lead to an effort to avoid the use of transplantation in the acute phases of the disease. In patients with giant cell myocarditis and severe heart failure, earlier consideration of a ventricular assist device or transplantation may occur, because giant cell myocarditis is associated with worse outcome than patients with other causes of ventricular dysfunction.[21]

Endomyocardial biopsy remains the gold standard for the diagnosis and treatment of acute cellular rejection in the heart transplant recipient.[22] Although many techniques for the non-invasive assessment of graft function have been proposed, the sensitivity and/or specificity of these modalities have not been sufficient to obviate the need for surveillance endomyocardial biopsy.[23–28] The grading system used to classify allograft rejection was recently revised and is summarized

Table 41.2 International Society for Heart and Lung Transplant Cardiac Biopsy grading system.[22]

Grade	Histology
0	No rejection
Grade 1 R, mild	Interstitial and/or perivascular infiltrate with up to one focus of myocyte damage
Grade 2 R, moderate	Two or more foci of infiltrate with associated myocyte damage
Grade 3 R, severe	Diffuse infiltrate with multifocal myocyte damage ± edema ± hemorrhage ± vasculitis

in Table 41.2. The frequency of biopsy surveillance varies according to the age of the transplant recipient, the type of immunosuppressive therapy, and the protocol followed at the transplant institution. With the advent of newer immunosuppressive agents, the incidence of rejection appears to be decreasing, lessening the use of surveillance endomyocardial biopsy. However, asymptomatic late rejection still occurs, supporting the limited use of surveillance biopsy even late after transplantation.[28–30] In the transplant recipient who presents with new onset heart failure and ventricular dysfunction, endomyocardial biopsy is a key diagnostic tool, as it can distinguish among possible etiologies such as acute cellular rejection, humoral rejection, or graft atherosclerosis. The findings of the endomyocardial biopsy in this clinical situation often directly impact therapeutic decisions.

In addition to the detection of cellular rejection, there is increasing understanding of the impact of antibody-mediated (humoral) rejection on long-term graft survival.[25] The revised classification of allograft rejection includes a discussion of the endomyocardial biopsy findings of humoral rejection. The presence of antibody deposition and/or complement binding to the capillary endothelium are important criteria used in the definition of humoral rejection in recipients with ventricular dysfunction.[22]

TECHNIQUES OF ENDOMYOCARDIAL BIOPSY IN CHILDREN

Transvenous right ventricular biopsy is the standard approach to obtaining endomyocardial samples. As many cardiomyopathic processes primarily affect the left ventricle, there is a rationale for sampling the left ventricular endocardium. However, the incidence of ventricular arrhythmias and the potential for systemic embolic events has led to the virtual abandonment of this approach. The most common sites used for the endomyocardial biopsy are the right internal jugular vein and the femoral veins.[10, 31, 32] Modifications of the Caves–Schulton technique via the right internal jugular vein have included the development of disposable

bioptomes and ascertaining proper placement of the bioptome in the right ventricle under echocardiographic guidance to minimize fluoroscopic exposure.[33–40] In small children, the use of the femoral venous approach is usually preferred, given the higher degree of difficulty accessing the internal jugular veins, although the internal jugular vein has been used in infants when other sites are unavailable.[13,36,41–43] The use of ultrasound guidance to image the jugular vein can decrease the incidence of carotid artery puncture and other complications and decrease the time spent to access the vessel.[44]

TISSUE ANALYSIS

Endomyocardial biopsy samples should be obtained from multiple sites in the right ventricular septum. To avoid damage to the tissue, the specimens should be handled carefully and transferred to the fixative using a sterile needle not forceps. The fixative should be at room temperature to prevent the formation of contraction band artifacts.[19] In heart transplant recipients, a minimum of four samples are required, as rejection is a focal process.[22] In patients with unexplained heart failure, between four and five samples should be obtained for light microscopy and additional samples for electron microscopy, viral genome analysis, or molecular studies should be collected as indicated.[19]

Light microscopy is used to evaluate for the presence of suspected myocarditis based on the presence of lymphocytic infiltrate and myocyte necrosis and grading is performed using the Dallas criteria.[45] Light microscopy is also used to diagnosis other specific diseases, such as giant cell myocarditis, hypersensitivity myocarditis, amyloidosis, or iron overload. Electron microscopy can be diagnostic of glycogen storage diseases, lysosomal storage diseases, and other infiltrative disorders.

The presence of viral pathogens in the myocardium can be detected using polymerase chain reaction (PCR) techniques for viral genome analysis. Quantitative and qualitative PCR analysis of endomyocardial biopsy samples has provided evidence of viral infection in patients with heart failure and ventricular dysfunction in the absence of histologic evidence of myocarditis.[46–48] The diagnostic and prognostic implications of the detection of viral genome have not been well enough defined for this method to supplant the clinical and histologic diagnosis of myocarditis. Studies are ongoing and, if a molecular-based definition of myocarditis leads to institution of directed therapies, the use of the endomyocardial biopsy in unexplained heart failure may be expanded.[49,50] In heart transplant recipients, the detection of viral genome has been associated with acute rejection and graft loss.[51,52] This finding is undergoing continued study to determine the prognostic value of viral genome analysis in the management of the heart transplant recipient.

COMPLICATIONS OF ENDOMYOCARDIAL BIOPSY

In adult and pediatric series, the overall complication rate of endomyocardial biopsy has been reported to be between 1 and 10%.[12,53–57] The general catheterization-related complications from the use of sedation or repeated vascular access can occur, as well as specific complications related to the biopsy procedure.

COMPLICATIONS OF VASCULAR ACCESS

Complications from the internal jugular venous approach include hematoma formation with the potential for airway obstruction and respiratory distress. Vocal cord paresis, diaphragmatic paresis, or Horner's syndrome can also occur as a result of direct nerve injury or compression from a hematoma. Arteriovenous fistulae formation between the carotid artery and the internal jugular vein has been reported. In the event that the pleural or mediastinal space is entered, pneumothorax, hemothorax, and pneumomediastinum can also occur. In small children and infants, the use of general anesthesia and mechanical ventilation is necessary to safely gain access to the internal jugular vein, increasing the potential for anesthesia-related complications during the procedure.

The femoral venous approach is more commonly used in young children and infants. This requires the use of a long sheath to guide the bioptome into the right ventricle. As with any central venous access, hematoma formation (superficial or retroperitoneal), formation of an arteriovenous fistula, or vessel occlusion can occur. In addition to these common complications, there are reports of pulmonary embolus following deep vein thrombosis.[58]

PROCEDURAL COMPLICATIONS

Cardiac perforation and tamponade

The most serious procedural complication associated with endomyocardial biopsy procedures is cardiac perforation and tamponade. The incidence of cardiac perforation is reported to be in the range of 0.3–0.9%. In one of the largest pediatric series, 9 perforations occurred in 1000 procedures. Multivariate analysis demonstrated that the risk of perforation was higher in children being evaluated for possible myocarditis and those requiring inotropic support. Death resulting from perforation and tamponade has been reported rarely following endomyocardial biopsy.

Arrhythmias

Arrhythmias are a common occurrence during the endomyocardial biopsy procedure, and premature ventricular contractions are often elicited to confirm contact of the bioptome with the ventricular endocardium prior to sampling. The overall incidence of arrhythmias is reported to be 0.3–0.5%.[54,55] Atrial and ventricular tachyarrhythmias have been reported, including atrial fibrillation, ventricular tachycardia, and supraventricular tachycardia. Bradycardia, asystole, and heart block are also known to occur. Arrhythmias are often self-limited, but in some instances will require medical therapy, cardioversion, or temporary pacemaker placement. New right bundle branch block has also been reported to occur.[37]

Coronary artery fistula formation

Coronary artery fistula formation to the right ventricle can occur following endomyocardial biopsy. Reported incidence ranges between 3 and 5%.[59,60] The majority of biopsy-induced coronary-cameral fistulae are asymptomatic and detected by routine coronary angiography in heart transplant patients. Myocardial infarction has been reported secondary to a coronary steal phenomenon or thrombotic occlusion of the left anterior descending coronary artery distal to the entry point of the fistula into the right ventricle.[61] Coil occlusion or surgical closure has been performed in patients with hemodynamically significant left to right shunts.[62,63]

Tricuspid regurgitation

Damage to the tricuspid valve apparatus and tricuspid insufficiency have been described following transvenous endomyocardial biopsy. Incidences in small series range between 6 and 20%.[64,65] The mechanism is felt to be damage to the tricuspid valve cordae causing a flail leaflet during endomyocardial sampling.[66] It has been suggested that use of a long sheath positioned across the tricuspid valve and/or echocardiographic guidance may decrease the incidence of tricuspid valve incompetence.[32] In some cases, tricuspid valve replacement has been necessary due to the presence of right heart failure.[67]

Other complications

Anecdotal reports of complications have been reported, such as an allergic reaction to the reusable bioptome or pacemaker wire dislodgement.[56] In a small prospective series of adult transplant recipients undergoing routine surveillance biopsy, blood cultures were obtained pre- and postprocedure. Occult bacteremia with coagulase-negative staphylococcus was documented in 14/20 samples obtained postbiopsy.[68] In the same report, the authors reviewed the records of 249 recipients and found a 2.5% incidence of right-sided endocarditis that was felt to involve the tricuspid valve.

CONCLUSIONS

Endomyocardial biopsy is most commonly performed in children to evaluate for the presence of acute allograft rejection in the postheart transplant recipient. The nontransplant indications for endomyocardial biopsy in children include suspected lymphocytic, giant cell, and/or hypersensitivity myocarditis. The ability of quantitative and qualitative PCR analysis to detect viral genome in the myocardium may expand the indications for biopsy in heart transplant recipients and in patients with left ventricular dysfunction and dilatation. The complication rate following endomyocardial biopsy in children is low. Cardiac tamponade following perforation and significant tricuspid valve regurgitation carry the highest morbidity and mortality of the complications reported. Although reported series are small, it appears that younger age and non-transplant diagnoses are associated with a higher complication rate.

REFERENCES

1. Sakakibara S, Konno S. Endomyocardial biopsy. Jpn Heart J 1962; 3: 537–43.
2. Goldberger E. Endomyocardial Biopsy. Am J Cardiol 1964; 14: 723.
3. Wennemark JR, Sommers HM, Zitnik RS. Endomyocardial biopsy. Experimental study with a catheter technique. Am Heart J 1966; 72: 675–80.
4. Somers K, Hutt MS, Patel AK et al. Endomyocardial biopsy in diagnosis of cardiomyopathies. Br Heart J 1971; 33: 822–32.
5. Ali N, Ferrans VJ, Roberts WC et al. Clinical evaluation of transvenous catheter technique for endomyocardial biopsy. Chest 1973; 63: 399–402.
6. Billingham ME, Caves PK, Dong E Jr et al. The diagnosis of canine orthotopic cardiac allograft rejection by transvenous endomyocardial biopsy. Transplant Proc 1973; 5: 741–3.
7. Caves PK, Stinson EB, Billingham M et al. Percutaneous transvenous endomyocardial biopsy in human heart recipients. Experience with a new technique. Ann Thorac Surg 1973; 16: 325–36.
8. Caves PK, Stinson EB, Graham AF et al. Percutaneous transvenous endomyocardial biopsy. JAMA 1973; 225: 288–91.
9. Hirota Y, Khaja F, Abelmann WH. Effectiveness and hazard of endomyocardial biopsy in dogs: comparison of two methods. Am Heart J 1976; 92: 767–72.
10. Mason JW. Techniques for right and left ventricular endomyocardial biopsy. Am J Cardiol 1978; 41: 887–92.
11. Rose AG, Uys CJ, Losman JG et al. Evaluation of endomyocardial biopsy in the diagnosis of cardiac rejection. A study using bioptome samples of formalin-fixed tissue. Transplantation 1978; 26: 10–13.
12. Cooper DK, Fraser RC, Rose AG et al. Technique, complications, and clinical value of endomyocardial biopsy in patients with heterotopic heart transplants. Thorax 1982; 37: 727–31.
13. Schmaltz AA, Apitz J, Hort W. Endomyocardial biopsy in infants and children: technique; indications and results. Eur J Pediatr 1982; 138: 211–15.
14. Pegelow CH, Popper RW, de Wit SA et al. Endomyocardial biopsy to monitor anthracycline therapy in children. J Clin Oncol 1984; 2: 443–6.
15. Saji T, Matsuo N, Hashiguchi R et al. Endomyocardial biopsy findings in pediatric patients with post myocarditic state. Jpn Circ J 1986; 50: 1201–8.
16. Bhargava H, Donner RM, Sanchez G et al. Endomyocardial biopsy after heart transplantation in children. J Heart Transplant 1987; 6: 298–302.
17. Lurie PR. Revision of pediatric endomyocardial biopsy technique. Am J Cardiol 1987; 60: 368–70.
18. Mortensen SA, Baandrup U. Endomyocardial biopsy with a modified bioptome introducer sheath: focus on diagnostic yield and prevention of complications. Cathet Cardiovasc Diagn 1987; 13: 194–203.
19. Cooper LT, Baughman KL, Feldman AM et al. The role of endomyocardial biopsy in the management of cardiovascular disease: a scientific statement from the American Heart Association, the American College of Cardiology, and the European Society of Cardiology. Endorsed by the Heart Failure Society of America and the Heart Failure Association of the European Society of Cardiology. J Am Coll Cardiol 2007; 50: 1914–31.
20. Cox GF, Sleeper LA, Lowe AM et al. Factors associated with establishing a causal diagnosis for children with cardiomyopathy. Pediatrics 2006; 118: 1519–31.
21. Narula N, Narula J, Dec GW. Endomyocardial biopsy for non-transplant-related disorders. Am J Clin Pathol 2005; 123(Suppl): S106–18.
22. Stewart S, Winters GL, Fishbein MC et al. Revision of the 1990 working formulation for the standardization of nomenclature in the diagnosis of heart rejection. J Heart Lung Transplant 2005; 24: 1710–20.
23. Hsu DT. Can non-invasive methodology predict rejection and either dictate or obviate the need for an endomyocardial biopsy in pediatric heart transplant recipients? Pediatr Transplant 2005; 9: 697–9.
24. Law YM. Pathophysiology and diagnosis of allograft rejection in pediatric heart transplantation. Curr Opin Cardiol 2007; 22: 66–71.
25. Casarez TW, Perens G, Williams RJ et al. Humoral rejection in pediatric orthotopic heart transplantation. J Heart Lung Transplant 2007; 26: 114–19.
26. Leonard GT Jr, Fricker FJ, Pruett D et al. Increased myocardial performance index correlates with biopsy-proven rejection in pediatric heart transplant recipients. J Heart Lung Transplant 2006; 25: 61–6.
27. Kirklin JK. Is biopsy-proven cellular rejection an important clinical consideration in heart transplantation? Curr Opin Cardiol 2005; 20: 127–31.
28. Rosenthal DN, Chin C, Nishimura K et al. Identifying cardiac transplant rejection in children: diagnostic utility of echocardiography, right heart catheterization and endomyocardial biopsy data. J Heart Lung Transplant 2004; 23: 323–9.
29. Chin C, Akhtar MJ, Rosenthal DN et al. Safety and utility of the routine surveillance biopsy in pediatric patients 2 years after heart transplantation. J Pediatr 2000; 136: 238–42.
30. Levi DS, DeConde AS, Fishbein MC et al. The yield of surveillance endomyocardial biopsies as a screen for cellular rejection in pediatric heart transplant patients. Pediatr Transplant 2004; 8: 22–8.
31. Goy JJ, Gilliard D, Kaufmann U et al. Endomyocardial biopsy in cardiac transplant recipients using the femoral venous approach. Am J Cardiol 1990; 65: 822–3.
32. Anderson JL, Marshall HW. The femoral venous approach to endomyocardial biopsy: comparison with internal jugular and transarterial approaches. Am J Cardiol 1984; 53: 833–7.

33. Scheurer M, Bandisode V, Ruff P et al. Early experience with real-time three-dimensional echocardiographic guidance of right ventricular biopsy in children. Echocardiography 2006; 23: 45–9.

34. Balzer D, Moorhead S, Saffitz JE et al. Pediatric endomyocardial biopsy performed solely with echocardiographic guidance. J Am Soc Echocardiogr 1993; 6: 510–15.

35. Kawauchi M, Gundry SR, Boucek MM et al. Real-time monitoring of the endomyocardial biopsy site with pediatric transesophageal echocardiography. J Heart Lung Transplant 1992; 11: 306–10.

36. Appleton RS, Miller LW, Nouri S et al. Endomyocardial biopsies in pediatric patients with no irradiation. Use of internal jugular venous approach and echocardiographic guidance. Transplantation 1991; 51: 309–11.

37. Han J, Park Y, Lee H et al. Complications of 2-D echocardiography guided transfemoral right ventricular endomyocardial biopsy. J Korean Med Sci 2006; 21: 989–94.

38. Pytlewski G, Georgeson S, Burke J et al. Endomyocardial biopsy under transesophageal echocardiographic guidance can be safely performed in the critically ill cardiac transplant recipient. Am J Cardiol 1994; 73: 1019–20.

39. Nelson OL, Robbins CT. Comparison of echocardiography-guided and fluoroscopy-guided endomyocardial biopsy techniques. Vet Radiol Ultrasound 2005; 46: 131–4.

40. French JW, Popp RL, Pitlick PT. Cardiac localization of transvascular bioptome using 2-dimensional echocardiography. Am J Cardiol 1983; 51: 219–23.

41. Shaddy RE, Bullock EA. Efficacy of 100 consecutive right ventricular endomyocardial biopsies in pediatric patients using the right internal jugular venous approach. Pediatr Cardiol 1993; 14: 5–8.

42. Pass RH, Trivedi KR, Hsu DT. A new technique for endomyocardial biopsy in infants and small children. Cathet Cardiovasc Interven 2000; 50: 441–4.

43. Guccione P, Gagliardi MG, Bevilacqua M et al. Cardiac catheterization through the internal jugular vein in pediatric patients. An alternative to the usual femoral vein access. Chest 1992; 101: 1512–14.

44. Etheridge SP, Berry JM, Krabill KA et al. Echocardiographic-guided internal jugular venous cannulation in children with heart disease. Arch Pediatr Adolesc Med 1995; 149: 77–80.

45. Aretz HT. Myocarditis: the Dallas criteria. Hum Pathol 1987; 18: 619–24.

46. Kuhl U, Pauschinger M, Noutsias M et al. High prevalence of viral genomes and multiple viral infections in the myocardium of adults with 'idiopathic' left ventricular dysfunction. Circulation 2005; 111: 887–93.

47. Bowles NE, Richardson PJ, Olsen EG et al. Detection of Coxsackie-B-virus-specific RNA sequences in myocardial biopsy samples from patients with myocarditis and dilated cardiomyopathy. Lancet 1986; 1: 1120–3.

48. Jin O, Sole MJ, Butany JW et al. Detection of enterovirus RNA in myocardial biopsies from patients with myocarditis and cardiomyopathy using gene amplification by polymerase chain reaction. Circulation 1990; 82: 8–16.

49. Bowles NE, Bowles KR, Towbin JA. Viral genomic detection and outcome in myocarditis. Heart Fail Clin 2005; 1: 407–17.

50. Baughman KL. Diagnosis of myocarditis: death of Dallas criteria. Circulation 2006; 113: 593–5.

51. Shirali GS, Ni J, Chinnock RE et al. Association of viral genome with graft loss in children after cardiac transplantation. N Engl J Med 2001; 344: 1498–503.

52. Schowengerdt KO, Ni J, Denfield SW et al. Diagnosis, surveillance, and epidemiologic evaluation of viral infections in pediatric cardiac transplant recipients with the use of the polymerase chain reaction. J Heart Lung Transplant 1996; 15: 111–23.

53. Yoshizato T, Edwards WD, Alboliras ET et al. Safety and utility of endomyocardial biopsy in infants, children and adolescents: a review of 66 procedures in 53 patients. J Am Coll Cardiol 1990; 15: 436–42.

54. Cowley CG, Lozier JS, Orsmond GS et al. Safety of endomyocardial biopsy in children. Cardiol Young 2003; 13: 404–7.

55. Pophal SG, Sigfusson G, Booth KL et al. Complications of endomyocardial biopsy in children. J Am Coll Cardiol 1999; 34: 2105–10.

56. Baraldi-Junkins C, Levin HR, Kasper EK et al. Complications of endomyocardial biopsy in heart transplant patients. J Heart Lung Transplant 1993; 12: 63–7.

57. Deckers JW, Hare JM, Baughman KL. Complications of transvenous right ventricular endomyocardial biopsy in adult patients with cardiomyopathy: a seven-year survey of 546 consecutive diagnostic procedures in a tertiary referral center. J Am Coll Cardiol 1992; 19: 43–7.

58. Vorlat A, Conraads V, Vrintz C. Deep vein thrombosis after transfemoral endomyocardial biopsy in cardiac transplant recipients. J Heart Lung Transplant 2003: 1063.

59. Henzlova MJ, Nath H, Bucy RP et al. Coronary artery to right ventricle fistula in heart transplant recipients: a complication of endomyocardial biopsy. J Am Coll Cardiol 1989; 14: 258–61.

60. Lazar JM, Uretsky BF. Coronary artery fistula after heart transplantation: a disappearing entity? Cathet Cardiovasc Diagn 1996; 37: 10–13.

61. Drobinski G, Dorent R, Ghossoub JJ et al. Myocardial infarction after endomyocardial biopsy in a heart transplant patient. J Interven Cardiol 2002; 15: 403–5.

62. Eccleshall SC, Pitt M, Townend JN. Transcatheter embolisation of an enlarging acquired coronary arteriovenous fistula in a heart transplant recipient. Heart 1997; 78: 203–5.

63. Uchida N, Baudet E, Roques X et al. Surgical experience of coronary artery–right ventricular fistula in a heart transplant patient. Eur J Cardiothorac Surg 1995; 9: 106–8.

64. Wiklund L, Caidahl K, Kjellstrom C et al. Tricuspid valve insufficiency as a complication of endomyocardial biopsy. Transpl Int 1992; 5(Suppl 1): S255–8.

65. Lo CY, Chang HH, Hsu CP et al. Endomyocardial biopsy-related tricuspid regurgitation after orthotopic heart transplantation: single-center experience. J Chin Med Assoc 2007; 70: 185–92.

66. Tucker PA 2nd, Jin BS, Gaos CM et al. Flail tricuspid leaflet after multiple biopsies following orthotopic heart transplantation: echocardiographic and hemodynamic correlation. J Heart Lung Transplant 1994; 13: 466–72.

67. Alharethi R, Bader F, Kfoury AG et al. Tricuspid valve replacement after cardiac transplantation. J Heart Lung Transplant 2006; 25: 48–52.

68. Aziz T, Krysiak P, El-Gamel A et al. Bacteremia and endocarditis following endomyocardial biopsy. Transplant Proc 1996; 30: 2112–13.

42 Preventing complications of diagnostic cardiac catheterization: some cognitive and philosophical issues, and a couple of critical techniques

Ted Feldman

The usual chapter on complications of catheterization procedures would follow an outline listing the most frequent and most serious complications, with some discussion of how to deal with them. Most of the discussions focus on either the prognostic factors involved in predicting complications, risk scoring systems, the management of specific complications, or sometimes frightening illustrations of the worst outcomes in a variety of settings. The probability of each complication is delineated and referenced. It is sometimes confusing to read discussions of risk predictors for percutaneous coronary interventional procedures because risk scoring systems are derived from population statistics, and applying a probability score to an individual patient is intangible, usually not accurate, and highly unsatisfying. In fact, for an individual patient, the probability of a complication is either 0 or 100%. This 'boiler plate' book chapter on complications is available in many places, from many sources, and from excellent writers. I will take advantage of this chapter as an opportunity to approach the subject differently. Table 42.1 shows a classification for complications, based on the broad categories under which most complications fall. This discussion will not follow such an outline, but rather will relate some of the strategies involved in complication management that are more intangible, and are not part of the usual discourse of such a discussion. The performance of catheterization procedures certainly requires a substantial amount of didactic and technical training, and a great deal of practice to develop the skills necessary for the technical aspects of procedure performance. In training programs and at meetings we dwell on these technical details, including equipment choice, balloon compliance curves, pharmacodynamics, and the sizing of balloons and stents. Despite the technical demands of coronary interventional procedures, catheterization is at least more than 50% cognitive, and in my opinion is closer to 75 or 80% cognitive and/or philosophical. I will discuss some of the cognitive aspects of the prevention and management of complications during diagnostic cardiac catheterization, and touch on some

Table 42.1 Classification of complications.

Intraprocedure
Mechanical
Embolic
Thrombotic
Stupidity-related
Bad luck

Ischemic
Death
MI
Re-revascularization

Hemorrhagic
Access site
Anticoagulation

of the technical and procedural points I think are particularly important.

COGNITIVE AND PHILOSOPHICAL

Talk to your patients before, during, and after catheterization

Establishing a relationship prior to catheterization is a critical part of a positive outcome. Failed or less than successful procedures can have a positive outcome if patients' expectations are satisfied. Even if only for a couple of minutes, discussion with the patient and family members to define expectations about the procedure is critical. It is a great disservice to paint too optimistic a picture and suggest that neither complications nor a poor outcome are possibilities, and it is just as problematic to 'hang crepe' and suggest only the bleakest of outcomes. A balanced assessment of the potential risks and probable outcomes is key. For example, a patient who is admitted with high-risk unstable angina, including a troponin elevation and abnormal electrocardiographic ST segment changes, going into a diagnostic catheterization procedure faces a chance of about 5% to need coronary artery bypass graft surgery, 50–70% for an ad hoc coronary intervention, and a 10–20% chance of having a situation managed without a revascularization therapy. Painting a picture consistent with this expectation prior to the procedure goes a long way in the event that a left main stenosis is detected and surgery has to be discussed. Similarly, emphasizing that severe complications may ensue, even from a diagnostic catheterization, such as the rare events of stroke or renal failure, is necessary. The fact of these potential occurrences can be counterbalanced with a statement to the effect that they are like accidents while driving a car; they are infrequent enough to make the use of a car a highly positive decision-making balance, even though accidents can be lethal or debilitating.

The importance of talking to patients during a procedure is as important. In a recent procedure I stented a bifurcation lesion with two stents, the side branch stent being oversized enough for me to be concerned about an outlet dissection. The patient, an 82-year-old woman, began complaining of left shoulder and arm pain. I took multiple views of the stented segments, looked at six lead ECGs, and gave repeated doses of intracoronary nitroglycerine. The pain persisted at a 7/10 level, clearly too much to declare procedural success and close the femoral arterial access site. Finally, I started taking some history, and had the staff move the left arm, reproducing the pain, and making it clear that it was musculoskeletal rather than ischemic. Fifty extra cc of contrast was not as helpful as a brief conversation with the patient to clarify the nature of the pain.

Plan the case

A diagnostic catheterization even at its simplest requires some strategy. The main objective in terms of data gathering should be clearly in mind at the outset. For an obvious example, a patient with suspected coronary disease should have coronary angiography prior to left ventriculography. The left ventriculogram may be necessary to assess wall motion in conjunction with coronary disease, but defining the coronary anatomy is the first priority and should be accomplished before any unforeseen circumstances derail the procedure. Similarly, a patient in whom the assessment of cardiomyopathy is the main objective might best undergo a right heart catheterization, before any angiography, to help with an assessment of how much contrast load might be tolerated based on pulmonary artery and pulmonary wedge pressures. More complex anatomic or functional problems require greater planning. The patient with adult congenital heart disease may require some thought prior to embarking on the

catheterization procedure. For complex interventions, planning alternative strategies if the initial plan does not work is critical. Make a plan, stick to a plan, and modify the plan as needed. It is usually not a good idea to deviate too far afield from a planned procedure sequence. At the same time, it is, of course, not possible to remain rigid as circumstances change.

For example, in a patient with chest pain referred for coronary angiography, a routine procedure may become highly complicated if the coronaries cannot be located with the first few attempts, and after a catheter exchange or two. In this setting, aortic dissection must be suspected with a catheter pathway through a false lumen. Adjustments must be made to change the plan of assessment toward aortography and surgical consultation.

Similarly, during an apparently routine right heart catheterization, an unusual path of the right heart catheter may suggest a shunt, with the catheter crossing an atrial septal defect and appearing in the upper lung field in the left lung, extending far beyond the heart border, or even more bizarrely sometimes entering the coronary sinus and then a persistent left superior vena cava. At this point, angiography, oximetry, and plans for transesophageal echocardiography may supersede what appeared to be a simple right and left heart catheterization for a patient with heart failure.

Call a failure a failure

When complications occur, or it is not possible to achieve a satisfactory procedure outcome, it is critical to call it what it is. For the best management of a patient, recognizing what information may not have been gathered or what problems may have been created by a catheterization procedure are critical. Any hesitancy or lack of surety or clarity about calling a complication what it is to the patient and your colleagues will lead to a worse outcome than recognizing the situation in a matter-of-fact manner, and dealing with it efficiently and expeditiously.

In my own practice, when I create a significant femoral artery complication during the course of a procedure, I will immediately notify the patient that a complication has occurred and, before even leaving the procedure room for the control room, will instruct the staff to track down the vascular surgeon on call. Similarly, a coronary intervention that is in the downward spiral of extending dissection and vessel occlusion cannot be managed without at least notifying a surgical colleague so that, in the worse case, no extra delays are experienced in providing for backup.

During diagnostic catheterization vascular complications are certainly the most common, and the ability to recognize them and either treat or assess them with the help of colleagues and other disciplines will lead to best possible outcomes, good collegial working relationships, and the respect of your colleagues. In some cases it is lack of success rather than a complication that is the issue. Being straight with a patient and colleagues that a procedure failed, even in the absence of complications, is the best course. Complications will occur if you perform enough procedures, and managing them in any way other than the most direct and above board diminishes the chance of a successful or optimal outcome. Fortunately, the vast majority of the problems we create can be solved without lasting harm to our patients and this is best done in a clear and straightforward manner.

Ask for help

When faced with a challenging diagnostic problem, therapeutic dilemma, or procedure complication, there are vast resources available from our colleagues in cardiology, vascular and cardiovascular surgery, and radiology. Being able to ask for help when needed is the hallmark of an insightful practitioner. Most situations allow for time to ask questions and contact your colleagues. Beyond the day-to-day interaction with colleagues and the availability of on-site curb side consultations, the world has grown very small with the electronic era. I frequently use e-mail to send a digital cine loop or echocardiographic file to my colleagues around the country and around the world to gather expert opinions. The number of phone calls for help I have received from colleagues in the midst of procedures having a technical challenge or facing a difficult decision has been very gratifying. Many of our colleagues around the country and around the world are always willing to help with challenges during procedures. When a diagnostic dilemma presents itself during a catheterization, simply stopping and reviewing and discussing the case is a great option, rather than moving forward with a poorly conceived therapeutic plan. Waiting for or creating a difficult situation in the cath lab can sometimes be averted by discussing cases prior to or after catheterization so that a good procedure plan can be developed.

No other option is not an indication to do a procedure

An 85-year-old patient presents with rest angina, enzyme elevation, and ECG ST depression. You are called to perform a catheterization. You find that the patient has a serum Cr 3.4 mg/dl, Hb 8.1 g/dl with no clear etiology for the anemia, and dementia. You suggest conservative management. Two days later you are called again because the angina persists and the patient continues to leak troponin. The referring physician and family all want to be aggressive. Is the absence of other options an indication for catheterization? A diagnostic study with limited contrast has significant risk of precipitating contrast mediate nephropathy, and an intervention carries the additional substantial risk of bleeding in an already anemic, elderly patient. In this kind of setting a diagnostic study is easy to justify, with the hope that a simple target lesion might be identified, and that a bare metal stent could provide relief to a suffering patient without too great a commitment to anticoagulation. So you perform a catheterization. The right coronary is occluded, and the left main has a tight bifurcation lesion, with diffuse disease of the distal vasculature. Your cardiac surgery colleagues decline to operate due to the anemia, dementia, and generally poor condition of the patient. This is the situation where no other option is not an indication to go forward and do a procedure. The decision not to act requires more judgment and poses a greater challenge than forging ahead. In the long run, you will be respected for having good judgment and not subjecting patients to procedures that ultimately carry high risk with marginal or no benefits.

TECHNICAL

The most fundamental part of all procedures is femoral access. Bleeding complications are the most frequent and often the most serious. The seeds of intra- and postprocedure bleeding are sown with vascular puncture. Careful attention to arterial access can reduce the frequency of low or high punctures, and I will describe some simple methods that should be routinely practiced. Another technical and procedural skill I believe is not well taught is pericardiocentesis. The need is infrequent, and the situation that requires it unforgiving. Having given it any thought before the need arises may bail you and the patient out of a difficult and life-threatening situation. I will detail the simplest way to respond to this dire emergency.

Optimal femoral artery access

We are preoccupied with the coronary and cardiac complications of catheterization and intervention, but it is femoral arterial complications that occur more frequently, and are remembered by our patients. The incidence of vascular complications has been reduced by refinements in techniques and anticoagulation regimes to 2–3%, but they still remain frequent adverse events.[1] Before we think about complications we need to focus on optimal femoral arterial access. A good understanding of some key features of the local anatomy is essential for both optimal access and ideal management of the puncture site. Careful attention to access is key to both reduce sheath insertion trauma and ultimately to uncomplicated sheath removal.

It is important to puncture at the level of the common femoral artery. This allows compression of the vessel against the femoral head at the time of sheath removal. Punctures which are below the common femoral arterial bifurcation (thus in one of the branches, either the profunda femoris or the superficial femoral artery) are over soft tissue and are difficult to compress. Branch punctures have been shown to be associated with increased risk of pseudoaneurysms and arteriovenous fistula formation. When the puncture site is above the inguinal ligament (in the external iliac artery) the retroperitoneal space has been entered, which also represents an incompressible location. These high punctures are associated with the risk of retroperitoneal bleeding.[2,3]

Fluoroscopic landmarks are the best way to identify the location of the common femoral artery. About 75–80% of common femoral bifurcations are at or below the inferior border of the femoral head and 95% are at or below the mid femoral head.[4] The deep circumflex iliac artery is commonly used as a surrogate marker of the upper border of the common femoral artery since the inguinal ligament cannot be seen with fluoroscopy (Figure 42.1). This landmark is usually above the superior border of the femoral head. The deep circumflex iliac artery is the last arterial branch of the external iliac artery before the external iliac courses under the inguinal ligament and becomes the common femoral artery. The deep circumflex iliac artery arises from the lateral aspect of the external iliac artery nearly opposite the origin of the inferior epigastric artery. Puncture above the most inferior border of the course of the deep circumflex iliac artery, and thus above the inguinal ligament, is associated with increased risk of retroperitoneal hemorrhage.[2]

The technique of arterial access has changed very little since it was initially introduced. It can be improved by using fluoroscopy of bony landmarks to identify the likely course of the common femoral artery, followed by confirmation with femoral angiography after sheath insertion.[5] Entry into the common femoral artery at the mid femoral head or slightly above is ideal. The femoral skin crease, which is commonly used as a landmark for puncture, is distal to the common femoral bifurcation in 72% of cases and is a poor landmark. Younger patients tend have a mid femoral head location close to or above the femoral crease, and older patients usually have the femoral head significantly above the femoral crease, because with age the crease tends to sag. Obese patients may have two or sometimes even three femoral creases (Figure 42.1).

The optimal technique of puncture requires a few fluoroscopic steps. Before local anesthesia is given, a clamp or needle can be laid at the point where the pulse is most easily felt, just above the femoral crease. Fluoroscopy can be used to locate the position of the needle relative to the femoral crease and the center of the femoral head (Figure 42.1). Local anesthesia is given accordingly. After the local is given, the needle is advanced to a point just above the arterial wall, using palpation as a guide. The location of the needle is again visualized. This is a final chance to adjust the puncture to maximize the chance to enter the common femoral artery in the ideal landing zone. These few steps are worthwhile, despite taking an extra minute, and justify the extra time at the beginning of the procedure.

Once the sheath has been inserted, a sheath angiogram should be taken to verify the sheath insertion location. Usually an ipsilateral angulation of the image intensifier will show both the entry point of the sheath and the femoral arterial bifurcation. This shows whether or not there is atherosclerosis, calcification, or angulation, and the location of the puncture site. I prefer to do the sheath angiogram at the beginning of the procedure. Thus, decisions about closure and anticoagulation can be made before the procedure is actually undertaken. If the sheath has been inserted into the branch vessels below the bifurcation, this will often have an impact on ultimate sheath size, for example in the setting of bifurcation or chronic total occlusion intervention, and may impact the choice of anticoagulation. When the puncture is above the most inferior border of the deep circumflex iliac artery, it is likely that the retroperitoneal space has been entered with the sheath. In this instance, an option is to defer intervention until a later time. Full anticoagulation with the sheath in this location greatly increases the risk of retroperitoneal bleeding, which is one of the worst and more difficult local complications to manage.

Pericardiocentesis

Pericardiocentesis is required for management of acute pericardial effusions and cardiac tamponade complicating a variety of interventional procedures. This is a life-saving technique and few operators have adequate experience with the procedure. Unexplained hypotension during catheterization procedures may be caused by right ventricular perforation during pacing catheter placement, or by a right heart multipurpose or even balloon catheter, or coronary perforation. Pericardial tamponade also complicates about 1% of transseptal puncture procedures. Pericardiocentesis is an essential skill that should be acquired during the cardiac catheterization training experience. Because of the infrequent nature of the event many operators are not exposed to pericardiocentesis during training, and few have the volume of elective procedures to maintain skills after training, in the course of practice.

In a true emergency pericardiocentesis can be performed with tools available for every routine diagnostic catheterization. Finding and opening a drainage kit is not needed. In the emergency setting all that is needed is a standard 3.5 inch long 18 gauge thin-walled needle, a 0.035 or 0.038 inch wire, and a pigtail catheter.

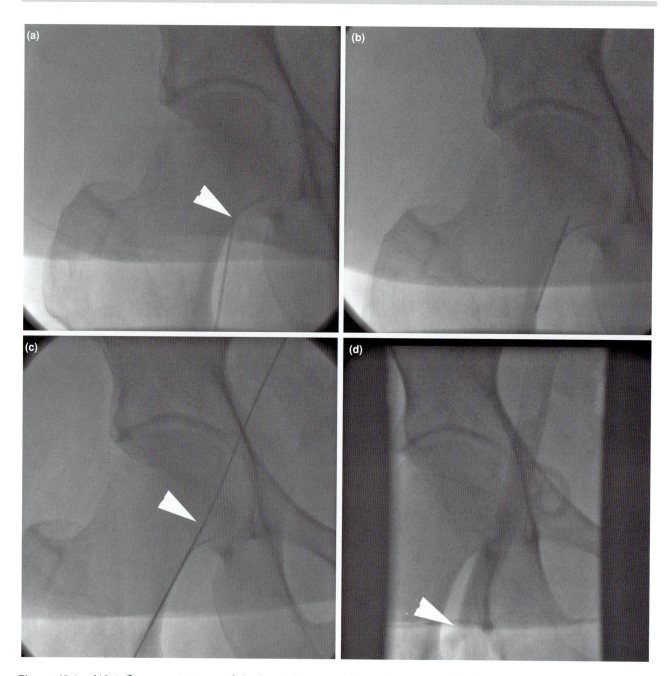

Figure 42.1 (A) A fluoroscopic image of the femoral head and femoral crease in a 230 kg patient. The arrowhead denotes the tip of a thin-walled 18-gauge needle that has been pushed against the femoral crease. (B) The needle, under fluoroscopic visualization, has been pushed up underneath the crease to the level of the inferior border of the femoral head. Local anesthesia is given at and below this location. (C) The needle has been passed into the femoral artery and a wire introduced. The arrowhead shows the point of entry of the needle into the femoral artery, with the 0.035 inch guide wire extending beyond the tip of the needle. At this point the needle and wire can be withdrawn and a better puncture location attempted after a few minutes of manual compression. (D) An angiogram has been taken through the femoral artery sheath with shallow right anterior oblique angulation. The arrowhead denotes the bifurcation of the femoral artery. The sheath is seen to insert into the vessel at the level of the inferior border of the femoral head. The deep circumflex iliac artery arises near the top of the femoral head and is commonly used as a surrogate marker of the inguinal ligament and retroperitoneal space. The angiogram was taken with 50% strength contrast. Note that collimators have been brought in to minimize radiation exposure to both patient and physician, and to yield a better image quality.

A sheath (5–7 French) can even be used without a pigtail, though I believe a pigtail is safer. Longer needles are usually not necessary.

Elective pericardiocentesis is often preceded by echocardiographic confirmation of the pericardial fluid, however tamponade is often acute. Echocardiography is not required and may be detrimental by delaying needed intervention. We always have an echo machine parked in our laboratory, but in the true emergency the boot-up time required by the machine is too long.

The preferred approach is the subxiphoid route but other sites are acceptable, depending on the location and volume of the effusion.[6–8] The advantage of the subxiphoid approach is the decreased likelihood of coronary and internal thoracic artery lacerations. In addition, the more lateral to the sternum the puncture, the greater the risk of pneumothorax. In the acute setting the sub-xiphoid approach is most easily identified and is most familiar to most operators. Other puncture locations are best assessed with transthoracic echo, to demonstrate proximity of the effusion to the skin, without intervening lung. Ideally, the patient is raised to a 30 to 45° head-up angle using a pillow or wedge. This permits pooling of pericardial fluid on the inferior surface of the heart closest to the xiphoid access approach. Local anesthesia is instilled through the thin-walled needle as it is advanced initially perpendicular to the skin and then at a sharp low angle. The route of approach is analogous to subclavian puncture where it is important to 'walk the needle' under the clavicle. In the case of pericardiocentesis the needle must be angled to clear below the level of the inferior rib edge above the xiphoid process. If the puncture is made too high up near the recess at the xiphoid angle, it is difficult to get under the rib. One finger breadth inferior and lateral to the edge of the xiphoid allows enough room for passage of the needle beneath the rib.

Aspiration of the needle during passage through the skin may block the needle with subcutaneous adipose tissue. Flush can be used liberally with either saline or lidocaine to clear any tissue that may have accumulated in the needle before passing through the pericardium. The pericardium is a rigid fibrous membrane so there is often a palpable 'pop' when the membrane is punctured. Acute pericardial effusions during catheterization procedures are bloody, do not generally clot in the syringe, and have a lower hematocrit than intravascular blood.

Immediate confirmation that the needle tip has entered the pericardial space can be obtained by observing the pressure wave form. Inadvertent right ventricular pressure can be recognized immediately. In case of tamponade, pericardial pressure will resemble right atrial pressure. Hemodynamic monitoring is preferred over echo- or ECG-guided pericardiocentesis for its ease of application in the catheterization laboratory. It is also critical to closely monitor arterial pressure by invasive or non-invasive techniques throughout the procedure. When echocardiographic imaging is used, the observance of echo contrast in the pericardial space is more useful than attempts to identify the tip of the needle. The plane of echo imaging will typically transect the body of the needle and give a false clue regarding the location of the tip of the needle.

Once the needle is in the pericardial space, as confirmed by fluid withdrawal, a soft guide wire is inserted under fluoroscopic guidance. It is typical for this wire to loop in the pericardial space. Should the wire go far beyond the heart border, it is possible that the pleural space or pulmonary artery, via the right

ventricle, has been entered. Injections of contrast through the needle may be necessary to identify that the position of the needle is in the pericardial space. Once the wire has been placed, a pigtail catheter or sheath can be passed into the pericardial space. Pigtail catheters are typically difficult to keep patent and when used in an emergency setting can be exchanged for a larger bore pericardial drainage catheter when the acute situation has stabilized. If there is a question regarding the exact position of the needle or catheter, X-ray contrast or echo contrast may be used to verify catheter position. Contrast medium pools in the dependent portion of the pericardial space, but will wash out of the vascular space rapidly if a cardiac chamber has been inadvertently entered.

Pericardial drainage catheters can be sutured in place and the volume of output monitored. Considerations for conservative or surgical management are made after the drain is in place. Right ventricular and most coronary guide wire perforations can be managed conservatively, but reversal of heparin may cause PCI vessel closure. Elective surgery or bypass may be a preferred option under these circumstances. Tamponade is particularly problematic to manage in patients who have received intravenous platelet inhibitors. The administration of platelets and fresh frozen plasma, and the time necessary for small molecule GPZB3A antiplatelet agents to be metabolized is critical.

The drainage catheter should be left in place overnight, or until there is less than 100 cc per 12–24 hours. In my opinion, it is a mistake to have successful drainage and rescue of the patient during the procedure and then pull the drain in the cath lab or immediately on the floor or in the unit. The potential for the effusion to recur, and the consequences, are too great to allow that risk.

Do not treat non-ischemic symptoms

Many patients present with clear history and ambiguous non-invasive testing, or ambiguous history and clear non-invasive testing. A third group presents with atypical or ambiguous symptoms, and borderline objective evidence for myocardial ischemia. This last group of patients frequently find themselves in the pathway for diagnostic catheterization, and then almost inevitable occlustenotic intervention if something is found anatomically during coronary angiography. While the diagnostic angiogram is often critically important for risk stratification, in the absence of significant ischemia on objective testing, or in the absence of symptoms you truly believe to be anginal, proceeding from the step of diagnostic to therapeutic catheterization, is fraught with unintended consequences. There is no mandate to proceed from diagnostic catheterization to percutaneous intervention in this setting, and our guidelines have long suggested that only those patients with significant ischemia on objective testing, or those with severe angina, benefit with either a mortality or symptom reduction.[9]

This is as true in other areas besides coronary artery disease. Recently, I saw a patient who had transient monocular blindness, interpreted in this young man as transient ischemic attacks. He was found to have a patent foramen ovale. The diagnostic evaluation was certainly warranted. The history of visual disturbance was, in retrospect, soft. Following device closure he had no relief of his symptoms, and then a new host of complaints related to the procedural venous access, and perceived ill effects of adjunctive antiplatelet therapy. This paradigm is found in many situations. More commonly is the setting in which catheterization is performed for atypical chest pain and a borderline stress test result. A focal stenosis is found, and a stent implanted. The cascade of unintended consequences may include repeated admissions for atypical chest pain with multiple catheterizations demonstrating patent stents, or in situations where there is moderate diffuse disease, a rollercoaster of additional stenting for borderline lesions in a patient who, at the outset, probably did not have angina anyway. The potential for complications to result from procedures that were not clearly indicated in the beginning is a syndrome many of us have encountered at one time or another.

Prevention of X-ray contrast nephropathy

Use less contrast. A great deal has been written about various fluids to use for hydration to prevent X-ray contrast nephropathy.[10–13] The use of acetylcysteine has been analyzed and meta-analyzed repeatedly, and while there may be benefits, especially in patients with elevated serum creatinine, the relative degree of renal 'protection' from pretreatment with acetylcysteine appears to be modest at best.

Most of the studies examining methods for minimizing the incidence of x-ray contrast nephropathy report the contrast volumes used. Radiology studies involving computed tomography typically employ between 75 and 125 ml of contrast, diagnostic catheterization studies utilize 100 to 150 ml, and interventional reports describe contrast volumes ranging between 150 and 300 ml, even in patients with elevated creatinine or diminished creatinine clearance at baseline.

Minimizing the use of contrast injections is not adequately discussed. In my experience, incidence of contrast nephropathy when volumes less than 50 ml are used is negligible. A well-planned single-vessel intervention can often be carried out with these very low volumes, and a diagnostic catheterization study can often be successfully completed with less than 50 ml as well. For interventional procedures, the use of baseline angiograms from prior studies obviates the need for repeat set-up pictures. For diagnostic studies, the use of biplane angiography, or careful selection of angulation with a single-plane system, will often diminish the need for multiple pictures. While two

views of each major arterial system and the large bifurcations are clearly necessary, this can often be achieved with two or three left system pictures and a rotating gantry right coronary injection. Left ventriculography should not be performed in these patients, and pre-procedure echocardiography will often answer many questions that simplify the study. An increasing number of coronary laboratories have digital subtraction angiography, and this can be used for femoral artery access angiography to plan for device closure, with no more than a couple of ml of dilute contrast. Whatever pretreatment is utilized in the guise of volume infusions, bicarbonate administration, or acetylcysteine, there is no substitute for a carefully planned study with a minimum amount of contrast injection.

REFERENCES

1. Dauerman HL, Applegate RJ, Cohen DJ. Vascular closure devices: the second decade. J Am Coll Cardiol 2007; 50: 1617–26.
2. Sherev DA, Shaw RE, Brent BN. Angiographic predictors of femoral access site complications: implication for planned percutaneous coronary intervention. Cathet Cardiovasc Interven 2005; 65: 196–202.
3. Ellis SG, Bhatt D, Kapadia S et al. Correlates and outcomes of retroperitoneal hemorrhage complicating percutaneous coronary intervention. Cathet Cardiovasc Interven 2006; 67: 541–5.
4. Schnyder G, Sawhney N, Whisenant B, Tsimikas S, Turi ZG. Common femoral artery anatomy is influenced by demographics and comorbidity: implications for cardiac and peripheral invasive studies. Cathet Cardiovasc Interven 2001; 53: 289–95.
5. Turi ZG. Optimizing vascular access: routine femoral angiography keeps the vascular complication away. Cathet Cardiovasc Interven 2005; 65: 203–4.
6. Ellis H. The clinical anatomy of pericardiocentesis. Br J Hosp Med 2007; 68(6): M98–9.
7. Strike PC. How to carry out pericardial aspiration. Br J Hosp Med 2005; 66(10): M48–9.
8. Aqel R, Mehta D, Zoghbi GJ. Percutaneous balloon pericardiotomy for the treatment of infected pericardial effusion with tamponade. J Invas Cardiol 2006; 18(7): E194–7.
9. Smith SC Jr, Feldman TE, Hirshfeld JW Jr et al. ACC/AHA/ACAI 2005 guideline update for percutaneous coronary intervention: a report of the American College of Cardiology/American Heart Association Task Force on Practice Guidelines ACC/AHA/SCAI Writing Committee to Update the 2001 Guidelines for Percutaneous Coronary Intervention). Circulation 2006; 113: 156–75. ACC website. Available at: http://www.acc.org/clinical/guidelines/percutaneous/update/ index.pdf.
10. Lee PT, Chou KJ, Liu CP et al. Renal protection for coronary angiography in advanced renal failure patients by prophylactic hemodialysis. A randomized controlled trial. J Am Coll Cardiol 2007; 50(11): 1015–20.
11. Briguori C, Airoldi F, D'Andrea D et al. Renal Insufficiency Following Contrast Media Administration Trial (REMEDIAL): a randomized comparison of 3 preventive strategies. Circulation 2007; 115(10): 1211–17.
12. Pannu N, Wiebe N, Tonelli M. Alberta Kidney Disease Network. Prophylaxis strategies for contrast-induced nephropathy. JAMA 2006; 295(23): 2765–79.
13. Pannu N. Tonelli M. Strategies to reduce the risk of contrast nephropathy: an evidence-based approach. Curr Opin Nephrol Hypertens 2006; 15(3): 285–90.

Index

page references followed by f indicate an illustrative figure; t indicates a table